Introduction to
Human Nutrition

Introduction to Human Nutrition

Edited on behalf of The Nutrition Society by

Michael J Gibney, Hester H Vorster and Frans J Kok

Blackwell
Science

© The Nutrition Society 2002

Blackwell Science Ltd, a Blackwell Publishing Company
Editorial Offices:
Osney Mead, Oxford OX2 0EL, UK
  Tel: + 44 (0)1865 206206
Blackwell Science, Inc., 350 Main Street,
Malden, MA 02148-5018, USA
  Tel: + 1 781 388 8250
Iowa State Press, a Blackwell Publishing Company,
2121 State Avenue, Ames, Iowa 50014-8300, USA
  Tel: + 1 515 292 0140
Blackwell Publishing Asia Pty Ltd, 550 Swanston Street,
Carlton South, Victoria 3053, Australia
  Tel: + 61 (0)3 9347 0300
Blackwell Wissenschafts Verlag,
Kurfürstendamm 57, 10707 Berlin, Germany
  Tel: + 49 (0)30 32 79 060

First published 2002 by Blackwell Science Ltd

Library of Congress
Cataloging-in-Publication Data is available

ISBN 0-632-05624-X

A catalogue record for this title is available from the
British Library

Set in Minion and produced by Gray Publishing,
Tunbridge Wells, Kent
Printed and bound in Great Britain by Ashford Colour
Press, Gosport

For further information on Blackwell Science,
visit our website:
www.blackwell-science.com

The Human Nutrition Textbook Series

The International Scientific Committee

Editor-in-Chief
Professor Michael J Gibney
Trinity College, Dublin, Ireland

Assistant Editor
Julie Dowsett
Trinity College, Dublin, Ireland

Professor Lenore Arab
University of North Carolina, USA

Professor Yvon Carpentier
Université Libre de Bruxelles, Belgium

Professor Marinos Elia
University of Southampton, UK

Professor Frans J Kok
Wageningen University, Netherlands

Professor Olle Ljunqvist
Ersta Hospital & Huddinge University Hospital, Sweden

Professor Ian McDonald
University of Nottingham, UK

Professor Barrie Margetts
University of Southampton, UK

Professor Kerin O'Dea
Menzies School of Health Research, Darwin, Australia

Dr Helen Roche
Trinity College Dublin, Ireland

Professor Hester H Vorster
Potchefstroom, South Africa

Textbook Editors

Introduction to Human Nutrition
Editor-in-Chief
Professor Michael J Gibney
Trinity College, Dublin, Ireland

Professor Hester H Vorster
Potchefstroom, South Africa

Professor Frans J Kok
Wageningen University, Netherlands

Nutrition and Metabolism
Editor-in-Chief
Professor Michael J Gibney
Trinity College, Dublin, Ireland

Professor Ian McDonald
University of Nottingham, UK

Dr Helen Roche,
*Trinity College Dublin,
Ireland*

Public Health Nutrition
Editor-in-Chief
Professor Michael J Gibney
Trinity College, Dublin, Ireland

Professor Lenore Arab
University of North Carolina, USA

Professor Barrie Margetts
University of Southampton, UK

Clinical Nutrition
Editor-in-Chief
Professor Michael J Gibney
Trinity College, Dublin, Ireland

Professor Marinos Elia
University of Southampton, UK

Professor Olle Ljunqvist
Ersta Hospital & Huddinge University Hospital, Sweden

The Human Nutrition Textbook series comprises:

Introduction to Human Nutrition

Introduction to Human Nutrition: a global perspective
  on food and nutrition
Body composition
Energy metabolism
Nutrition and metabolism of proteins and amino acids
Digestion and metabolism of carbohydrates
Nutrition and metabolism of lipids
Dietary reference standards
The vitamins
Minerals and trace elements
Measuring food intake
Food composition
Food policy and regulatory issues
Nutrition research methodology
Food safety: a public health issue of
  growing importance
Food and nutrition: the global challenge

Nutrition and Metabolism

Core concepts of nutrition
Molecular nutrition
The regulation of food intake
Integration of metabolism 1: Energy
Integration of metabolism 2: Carbohydrates and lipids
Integration of metabolism 3: Protein and amino acids
Phytochemicals
Pregnancy and lactation
Growth and ageing
Gastrointestinal tract
Cardiovascular system
The skeletal system
The immune and inflammatory systems
The sensory systems
Physical activity
Overnutrition
Undernutrition
The brain

Public Health Nutrition

An overview of public health nutrition
Nutrition epidemiology
Food choice
Assessment of nutritional status at individual and
  population level
Assessment of physical activity
Overnutrition
Undernutrition
Eating disorders, dieting and food fads
PHN strategies for nutrition: intervention at the level
  of individuals
PHN strategies for nutrition: intervention at the
  ecological level
Food and nutrition guidelines
Fetal programming
Cardiovascular disease
Cancer
Osteoporosis
Diabetes
Vitamin A deficiency
Iodine deficiency
Iron deficiency
Maternal and child health
Breast feeding
Adverse outcomes in pregnancy

Clinical Nutrition

General principles of clinical nutrition
Metabolic and nutritional assessment
Overnutrition
Undernutrition
Metabolic disorders
Eating disorders
Adverse reactions to foods
Nutritional support
Ethical and legal issues
Gastrointestinal tract
The liver
The pancreas
The kidney
Blood and bone marrow
The lung
Immune and inflammatory systems
Heart and blood vessels
The skeleton
Traumatic diseases
Infectious diseases
Malignant diseases
Pediatric nutrition
Cystic fibrosis
Clinical cases
Water and electrolytes

Contents

Series Foreword   xii

Preface   xiii

Contributors   xv

1. Introduction to Human Nutrition: A Global Perspective on Food and Nutrition   1
HH Vorster and J Hautvast

  1.1   Orientation to human nutrition   1
  1.2   An integrated approach   2
  1.3   A conceptional framework for the study of nutrition   2
  1.4   Relationship between nutrition and health   3
  1.5   Nutrients: the basics   4
  1.6   Global malnutrition   5
  1.7   Relationship between nutrition science and practice   6
  1.8   Nutrition milestones: the development of nutrition as a science   7
  1.9   Future challenges for nutrition research and practice   9
  1.10   Perspectives on the future   10
       Further reading   11

2. Body Composition   12
P Deurenberg and R Roubenoff

  2.1   Introduction   12
  2.2   Five levels of body composition   13
  2.3   Relationships between different levels of body composition   14
  2.4   Body composition techniques   15
  2.5   Direct methods   15
  2.6   Indirect methods   16
  2.7   Doubly indirect methods   22
  2.8   Perspectives on the future   28
       Further reading   29

3. Energy Metabolism   30
MI Goran and A Astrup

  3.1   Introduction   30
  3.2   Energy intake   32
  3.3   Energy expenditure   34
  3.4   Factors that influence energy expenditure   36
  3.5   Energy requirements   39
  3.6   Energy balance in various conditions   40
  3.7   Obesity   42
  3.8   Perspectives on the future   45
       Further reading   45

4. Nutrition and Metabolism of Proteins and Amino Acids   46
VR Young and PJ Reeds

  4.1   Introduction   46
  4.2   A historical perspective   48

4.3	Structure and chemistry of amino acids	49
4.4	Classification of amino acids	50
4.5	Biology of protein and amino acid requirements	54
4.6	Estimation of protein and amino acid requirements	59
4.7	Meeting protein and amino acid needs	63
4.8	Factors other than diet affecting protein and amino acid requirements	66
4.9	Perspectives on the future	67
	Further reading	67

5.   Digestion and Metabolism of Carbohydrates   **69**
J Mathers and T Wolever

5.1	Introduction: carbohydrates in foods	69
5.2	Digestive fate of dietary carbohydrates	70
5.3	Glycemic carbohydrates	72
5.4	Non-glycemic carbohydrates	74
5.5	Carbohydrates and dental caries	79
5.6	Perspectives on the future	80
	Further reading	80

6.   Nutrition and Metabolism of Lipids   **81**
SC Cunnane and BA Griffin

6.1	Introduction: the history of lipids in human nutrition	81
6.2	Terminology of dietary fats	82
6.3	Lipid components of the diet	86
6.4	Digestion, absorption and transport of dietary fat	87
6.5	Circulating lipids: lipoprotein structures and metabolism	93
6.6	Body lipid pools	98
6.7	Long-chain fatty acid metabolism	100
6.8	Nutritional regulation of long-chain fatty acid profiles and metabolism	106
6.9	Nutritional and metabolic effects of dietary fatty acids	107
6.10	Cholesterol synthesis and regulation	109
6.11	Effect of diet on serum lipids and lipoproteins	109
6.12	Perspectives on the future	114
	Further reading	115

7.   Dietary Reference Standards   **116**
KM Younger

7.1	Introduction	116
7.2	Terminology and conceptual approaches to setting nutrient recommendations	116
7.3	Interpretation and uses of dietary recommendations	119
7.4	The use of reference values to assess the adequacy of the nutrient intakes of population groups	120
7.5	Methods used to determine requirements and set dietary recommendations	121
7.6	Methods used to determine requirements	122
7.7	Perspectives on the future	124
	Further reading	124

8. **The Vitamins**   125
    DA Bender

    8.1   Introduction   125
    8.2   Vitamin A   127
    8.3   Vitamin D   134
    8.4   Vitamin E   138
    8.5   Vitamin K   141
    8.6   Vitamin B_1 (thiamin)   143
    8.7   Vitamin B_2 (riboflavin)   146
    8.8   Niacin   149
    8.9   Vitamin B_6 153
    8.10 Vitamin B_{12} 157
    8.11 Folic acid   160
    8.12 Biotin   166
    8.13 Pantothenic acid   167
    8.14 Vitamin C (ascorbic acid)   169
    8.15 Perspectives on the future   174
          Further reading   176

9. **Minerals and Trace Elements**   177
    JJ Strain and KD Cashman

    9.1   Introduction   177
    9.2   Calcium   178
    9.3   Magnesium   183
    9.4   Phosphorus   186
    9.5   Sodium and chloride   189
    9.6   Potassium   192
    9.7   Iron   194
    9.8   Zinc   197
    9.9   Copper   200
    9.10 Selenium   205
    9.11 Iodine   208
    9.12 Manganese   212
    9.13 Molybdenum   214
    9.14 Fluoride   215
    9.15 Chromium   217
    9.16 Other elements   219
    9.17 Perspectives on the future   219
          Further reading   224

10. **Measuring Food Intake**   225
    IHE Rutishauser and AE Black

    10.1 Introduction   225
    10.2 Indirect measurements of food intake   227
    10.3 Household food surveys   228
    10.4 Direct measures of food intake   229
    10.5 Basic concepts   230
    10.6 Options for measuring intake on specified days   232

10.7   Options for measuring intake over the longer term   234
10.8   Sources of error in dietary studies   235
10.9   Day-to-day variation in intake   239
10.10   Choosing a dietary method   240
10.11   Biological measures to validate energy and nutrient intake   243
10.12   Characteristics of low energy reporters   245
10.13   Evaluation of food intake data   245
10.14   Assessment of dietary adequacy   246
10.15   Perspectives on the future   248
        Further reading   248

11.   **Food Composition**   249
        CE West and HC Schönfeldt

11.1   Introduction   249
11.2   Foods   250
11.3   Nutrients, nonnutrients and energy   254
11.4   Information required on sources of data in tables   257
11.5   Overcoming the inadequacies of food composition tables   257
11.6   Description of food composition tables and how to retrieve data   260
11.7   Converting foods to nutrients   260
11.8   Perspectives on the future   261
        Further reading   261

12.   **Food Policy and Regulatory Issues**   263
        BO Schneeman and JR Lupien

12.1   Introduction   263
12.2   Food and nutrition monitoring   264
12.3   Food policy and food production   265
12.4   Regulatory aspects of food safety   266
12.5   Nutritional aspects of food policy   270
12.6   Research on food, nutrition and health   272
12.7   International work on food policy   273
12.8   Perspectives on the future   273
        Further reading   274

13.   **Nutrition Research Methodology**   275
        JA Martínez and MA Martínez González

13.1   Introduction   275
13.2   Statistical analysis and experimental design   275
13.3   *In vitro* studies   280
13.4   Animal models in nutrition research   281
13.5   Human studies   283
13.6   Epidemiological designs   285
13.7   Perspectives on the future   291
        Further reading   291

14.   **Food Safety: A Public Health Issue of Growing Importance**   292
        A Reilly, C Tlustos, W Anderson, L O'Connor, B Foley and P Wall

14.1   Introduction   292
14.2   Factors contributing to food safety concerns   293

14.3 Food-borne bacteria   296
14.4 Food-borne viruses   301
14.5 Food-borne parasites   303
14.6 Transmissible spongiform encephalopathies and food   307
14.7 Chemicals affecting food safety   308
14.8 Food safety control programs   316
14.9 Perspectives on the future   317
     Further reading   317

15. **Food and Nutrition: The Global Challenge**   **318**
     P Shetty

15.1 Introduction   318
15.2 Malnutrition through the life cycle   319
15.3 Hidden hunger: the global problem of micronutrient deficiency   325
15.4 Food, nutrition and the emerging burden of obesity and chronic diseases 328
15.5 Food and nutrition and the promotion of public health   330
15.6 Perspectives on the future   331
     Further reading   333

Index   **335**

Series Foreword

The early decades of the twentieth century were a period of intense research on constituents of food essential for normal growth and development, and saw the discovery of most of the vitamins, minerals, amino acids and essential fatty acids. In 1941, a group of leading physiologists, biochemists and medical scientists recognized that the emerging discipline of nutrition needed its own learned society and the Nutrition Society was established. Our mission was, and remains, "*to advance the scientific study of nutrition and its application to the maintenance of human and animal health*". The Nutrition Society is the largest learned society for nutrition in Europe and we have over 2000 members worldwide. You can find out more about the Society and how to become a member by visiting our website at www.nutsoc.org.uk

The ongoing revolution in biology initiated by large-scale genome mapping and facilitated by the development of reliable, simple-to-use molecular biological tools makes this a very exciting time to be working in nutrition. We now have the opportunity to obtain a much better understanding of how specific genes interact with nutritional intake and other lifestyle factors to influence gene expression in individual cells and tissues and, ultimately, affect our health. Knowledge of the polymorphisms in key genes carried by a patient will allow the prescription of more effective, and safe, dietary treatments. At the population level, molecular epidemiology is opening up much more incisive approaches to understanding the role of particular dietary patterns in disease causation. This excitement is reflected in the several scientific meetings that the Nutrition Society, often in collaboration with sister learned societies in Europe, organizes each year. We provide travel grants and other assistance to encourage students and young researchers to attend and participate in these meetings.

Throughout its history a primary objective of the Society has been to encourage nutrition research and to disseminate the results of such research. Our first journal, *The Proceedings of the Nutrition Society*, recorded, as it still does, the scientific presentations made to the Society. Shortly afterwards, *The British Journal of Nutrition* was established to provide a medium for the publication of primary research on all aspects of human and animal nutrition by scientists from around the world. Recognizing the needs of students and their teachers for authoritative reviews on topical issues in nutrition, the Society began publishing *Nutrition Research Reviews* in 1988. More recently, we launched *Public Health Nutrition,* the first international journal dedicated to this important and growing area. All of these journals are available in electronic, as well as in the conventional paper form and we are exploring new opportunities to exploit the web to make the outcomes of nutritional research more quickly and more readily accessible.

To protect the public and to enhance the career prospects of nutritionists, the Nutrition Society is committed to ensuring that those who practice as nutritionists are properly trained and qualified. This is recognized by placing the names of suitably qualified individuals on our professional registers and by the award of the qualifications Registered Public Health Nutritionist (RPHNutr) and Registered Nutritionist (RNutr). Graduates with appropriate degrees but who do not yet have sufficient postgraduate experience can join our Associate Nutritionist registers. We undertake accreditation of university degree programs in public health nutrition and are developing accreditation processes for other nutrition degree programs.

Just as in research, having the best possible tools is an enormous advantage in teaching and learning. This is the reasoning behind the initiative to launch this series of human nutrition textbooks designed for use worldwide. The Society is deeply indebted to its former President, Professor Mike Gibney, for his foresight, and to him and his team of editors for their innovative approaches and hard work in bringing this major publishing exercise to successful fruition. Read, learn and enjoy.

John Mathers
President of the Nutrition Society

Preface

Nutrition has as its core the physiology and biochemistry of human metabolism and surrounding that core are studies on the factors influencing the nature of the food supply, on factors influencing food choice, on public health nutrition programs to prevent diet-related diseases and on the role of diet in the clinical management of disease. As an academic subject, nutrition has grown enormously in recent years and with it the need for specialist textbooks on the subject. The decision of The Nutrition Society to produce a series of four textbooks in nutrition was in response to this need. The introductory textbook is designed for students of nutrition and also for the many students who take nutrition as part of their coursework but who major in other subjects such as pharmacy, food science or nursing. The second textbook provides a detailed coverage of nutrition in metabolism and will be the next essential step for all students of nutrition. Thereafter, some may opt to pursue clinical nutrition, public health nutrition or elements of both, and the third and fourth books in the series cover these topics. From an editorial viewpoint, a major decision involved overlap between texts and given that several of the texts could be stand-alone textbooks, we opted not to eradicate overlap but rather to harmonize coverage. Thus, in the introductory text,

the student is introduced to calcium and vitamin D nutrition. In the nutrition and metabolism text, the physiology and biochemistry of bone metabolism are covered. Osteoporosis as a public health disorder is covered in the *Public Health Nutrition* textbook, while skeletal metabolism in the clinical setting is covered in the textbook on *Clinical Nutrition*. In these circumstances, overlap is inevitable but we hope that we have managed it to the maximum benefit of students.

This may not be the first time that a learned society has produced its own textbook, but it is probably the most ambitious yet undertaken. In total, nearly 130 authors from more than 20 countries have been involved in the writing of 80 chapters. Each chapter has been reviewed by the editors at the outline stage and following first and second drafts. Authors of related chapters have worked together to manage inevitable overlap. On behalf of the members of the Nutrition Society, I thank the Society for their investment in this project, all of the long-suffering authors, my fellow editors and, in particular, Julie Dowsett, who has worked so cheerfully and so hard as assistant editor to the series.

Michael J Gibney
Editor-in-Chief

www.nutritiontexts.com

A unique feature of the Nutrition Society Textbook Series is that each chapter has its own website, accessible at www.nutritiontexts.com. In the course of time, each will have downloadable teaching aids, suggestions for projects, updates on the content of each chapter and sample multiple choice questions. With input from teachers and students we will have a vibrant, informative and social website.

Contributors

Wayne Anderson
Food Safety Authority of Ireland,
Dublin, Ireland

Professor Arne Astrup
Director of the Research Department
of Human Nutrition,
The Royal Veterinary and Agricultural University,
Frederiksberg, Denmark

Dr David A Bender
Sub-Dean (Teaching),
Royal Free and University College Medical School,
Department of Biochemistry and Molecular Biology,
University College London, UK

Dr Alison Black
Formerly with Medical Research Council
Resource Centre for Human Nutrition Research,
Cambridge, UK

Professor Kevin Cashman
Department of Nutritional Sciences,
University College Cork,
Ireland

Dr Stephen Cunnane
Department of Nutritional Sciences,
Faculty of Medicine,
University of Toronto,
Canada

Professor Paul Deurenberg
Associate Professor in Nutrition,
Department of Human Nutrition,
Wageningen University,
The Netherlands
Visiting Professor,
University Tor Vergata, Rome, Italy
Nutrition Consultant, Singapore

Barbara Foley
Food Safety Authority of Ireland,
Dublin, Ireland

Professor Michael J Gibney
Department of Clinical Medicine,
Trinity College, Dublin,
Ireland

Professor Michael Goran
Professor of Preventive Medicine
and Associate Director,
Institute for Prevention Research,
University of Southern California,
Los Angeles, USA

Dr Bruce Griffin
Reader in Nutritional Metabolism,
Centre for Nutrition and Food Safety,
University of Surrey, Guildford, UK

Professor Joseph Hautvast
Director of the Wageningen Centre for
Food Sciences,
The Netherlands

Professor Frans J Kok
Chair and Head of Division,
Human Nutrition and Epidemiology,
Wageningen University,
The Netherlands

Dr John Lupien
Ex-Director of the Food and Nutrition Division,
Food and Agriculture Organization
(FAO) of the United Nations,
Rome, Italy

Professor Alfredo Martínez
Department of Physiology and Nutrition,
University of Navarra,
Spain

Dr Miguel A Martínez González
Department of Epidemiology and Public Health,
University of Navarra,
Spain

Professor John Mathers
Human Nutrition Research Centre,
Department of Biological and
Nutritional Sciences,
University of Newcastle, UK

Lisa O'Connor
Food Safety Authority of Ireland,
Dublin, Ireland

Professor Peter Reeds
Professor of Nutritional Sciences,
Department of Animal Sciences,
University of Urbana Champaign,
Illinois, USA

Dr Alan Reilly
Food Safety Authority of Ireland,
Dublin, Ireland

Professor Ronenn Roubenoff
Associate Professor of Medicine and Nutrition,
Chief of Nutrition, Exercise Physiology and
Sarcopenia (NEPS) Lab,
Jean Mayer USDA Human Nutrition
Research Centre on Aging,
Tufts University,
Boston, USA

Dr Ingrid Rutishauser
Honorary Fellow,
School of Health Sciences,
Deakin University, Geelong Campus,
Australia
Adjunct Associate Professor,
Nutrition Program,
University of Queensland,
Brisbane, Australia

Professor Barbara Schneeman
Professor of Nutrition,
Department of Nutrition,
University of California,
Davis, USA

Professor Hettie Schönfeldt
Director: Centre of Nutrition,
University of Pretoria,
South Africa

Dr Prakash Shetty
Food and Nutrition Division,
Food and Agriculture Organization (FAO) of the
United Nations,
Rome, Italy

Professor JJ (Sean) Strain
Professor of Nutrition,
Northern Ireland Centre for Diet and Health,
University of Ulster,
Coleraine, Northern Ireland

Christina Tlustos
Technical Executive,
Food Safety Authority of Ireland,
Dublin, Ireland

Professor Hester H Vorster
Director of Focus Area 9.1: Health Research,
Faculty of Health Sciences,
Lipid Clinic PU for CHE,
Potchefstroom, South Africa

Dr Pat Wall
Chief Executive,
Food Safety Authority of Ireland,
Dublin, Ireland

Dr Clive West
Division of Human Nutrition
and Epidemiology,
Wageningen Agricultural University,
The Netherlands

Professor Tom Wolever
Department of Nutrition,
University of Toronto,
Canada

Professor Vernon Young
Laboratory of Human Nutrition,
Massachusetts Institute of Technology,
Cambridge, USA

Dr Kate Younger
Lecturer in Human Nutrition,
Department of Biological Sciences,
Dublin Institute of Technology,
Ireland

1
Introduction to Human Nutrition: A Global Perspective on Food and Nutrition

Hester H Vorster and Jo Hautvast

Key messages

- Human nutrition is a complex, multifaceted scientific domain indicating how substances in foods provide essential nourishment for the maintenance of life.
- To understand, study, research and practice nutrition, a holistic integrated approach from molecular to societal level is needed.
- Optimal, balanced nutrition is a major determinant of health. It can be used to promote health and well-being, to prevent ill-health and to treat disease.
- The study of the structure, chemical and physical characteristics, and physiological and biochemical effects of the more than 50 nutrients found in foods underpins the understanding of nutrition.
- The hundreds of millions of food- and nutrition-insecure people globally, the coexistence of undernutrition and overnutrition, and inappropriate nutritional behaviors are challenges that face the nutritionist of today.
- Nutrition practice has a firm and well-developed research and knowledge base. There are, however, many areas where more information is needed to solve global, regional, communal and individual nutrition problems.
- The development of ethical norms, standards and values in nutrition research and practice is needed.

1.1 Orientation to human nutrition

The major purpose of this series of four textbooks on nutrition is to guide the nutrition student through the exciting journey of discovery of nutrition as a science. As apprentices in nutrition science and practice students will learn how to collect, systemize and classify knowledge by reading, experimentation, observation and reasoning. The road for this journey was mapped out millennia ago. The knowledge that nutrition – what we choose to eat and drink – influences our health, well-being and quality of life is as old as human history. For millions of years the quest for food has helped to shape human development, the organization of society and history itself. It has influenced wars, population growth, urban expansion, economic and political theory, religion, science, medicine and technological development.

It was only in the second half of the eighteenth century that nutrition started to experience its first renaissance with the observation by scientists that intakes of certain foods, later called nutrients, and eventually other substances not yet classified as nutrients, influence the function of the body, protect against disease, restore health and determine people's response to changes in the environment. During this period, nutrition was studied from a medical model or paradigm by defining the chemical structures and characteristics of nutrients found in foods, their physiological functions, biochemical reactions and human requirements to prevent, first, deficiency diseases and later also chronic noncommunicable diseases.

Since the late 1980s nutrition has experienced a second renaissance with the growing perception that the knowledge gained did not equip mankind to solve the global problems of food insecurity and malnutrition. The emphasis shifted from the medical or pathological paradigm to a more psychosocial, behavioral one in which nutrition is defined as a basic human right, not only essential for human development, but also as an outcome of development.

In this first, introductory text, the focus is on principles and essentials of human nutrition, with the main purpose of helping the nutrition student to develop a holistic and integrated understanding of this complex, multifaceted scientific domain.

1.2 An integrated approach

Human nutrition describes the processes whereby cellular organelles, cells, tissues, organs, systems and the body as a whole obtain and use necessary substances obtained from foods (nutrients) to maintain structural and functional integrity. For an understanding of how humans obtain and utilize foods and nutrients from a molecular to a societal level, and of the factors determining and influencing these processes, the study and practice of human nutrition involve a spectrum of other basic and applied scientific disciplines. These include molecular biology, genetics, biochemistry, chemistry, physics, food science, microbiology, physiology, pathology, immunology, psychology, sociology, political science, anthropology, communications and economics. The multidisciplinary nature of the science of nutrition, lying in both the natural (biological) and social scientific fields, demands that students of nutrition should have a basic understanding of many branches of science, and should be able to integrate different concepts from these different disciplines. It implies that students should choose their accompanying subjects (electives) carefully and that they should read widely in these different areas.

1.3 A conceptional framework for the study of nutrition

In the journey of discovery into nutrition science it will often be necessary to put new knowledge, or new applications of old knowledge, into the perspective of the holistic picture. For this, a conceptual framework of the multidisciplinary nature of nutrition science and practice may be of value. Such a conceptual framework, illustrating the complex interactions between internal or constitutional factors and external environmental factors which determine nutritional status and health, is given in Figure 1.1.

On a genetic level it is now accepted that nutrients dictate phenotypic expression of an individual's genotype by influencing the processes of transcription,

translation or post-translational reactions. In other words, nutrients can directly influence genetic (DNA) expression, determining the type of RNA formed (transcription) and also the proteins synthesized (translation). For example, glucose, a carbohydrate macronutrient, increases transcription for the synthesis of glucokinase, the micronutrient iron increases translation for the synthesis of ferritin, while vitamin K increases post-translational carboxylation of glutamic acid residues for the synthesis of prothrombin. Nutrients, therefore, influence the synthesis of structural and functional proteins, by influencing gene expression within cells.

Nutrients also act as substrates and cofactors in all of the metabolic reactions in cells necessary for the growth and maintenance of structure and function. Cells take up nutrients (through complex mechanisms across cell membranes) from their immediate environment, also known as the body's internal environment. The composition of this environment is carefully regulated to ensure optimal function and survival of cells, a process known as homeostasis.

Nutrients and oxygen are provided to the internal environment by the circulating blood, which also removes metabolic end-products and harmful substances from this environment for excretion through the skin, the kidneys and the large bowel.

The concerted function of different organs and systems of the body ensures that nutrients and oxygen are extracted or taken up from the external environment and transferred to the blood for transport and delivery to the internal environment and cells. The digestive system, for example, is responsible for the ingestion of food and beverages, the breakdown (digestion and fermentation) of these for extraction of nutrients, and the absorption of the nutrients into the circulation, while the respiratory system extracts oxygen from the air. These functions are co-ordinated and regulated by the endocrine and central nervous systems in response to the chemical and physical composition of the blood and internal environment, and to cellular needs.

The health or disease state of the different organs and systems will determine the nutrient requirements of the body as a whole.

The central nervous system is also the site or "headquarters" of the higher, mental functions related to conscious or cognitive spiritual, religious and cultural behaviors, which will determine, in response to the internal and external environments, what and how

Levels of human function (Factors)	Accompanying scientific disciplines of study
Constitutional	
• Cell nucleus DNA ⇌ RNA (Genetic level)	• Molecular biology, foods
• Cells: metabolism • Internal environment • Circulation • All organ systems, *also* • Central nervous system	• Biochemistry, foods • Biochemistry, physiology, foods • Physiology, pathology, foods, pharmacology, etc. • Psychology, pathology, foods, pharmacology, etc.
Nutritional status Health/Ill-health	
External environment	
• Food security/insecurity; • Household characteristics; care; • Social circumstances; • Economic circumstances; • Housing, sanitation, politics; • Agriculture, health services (resources; ideologies)	• Foods, agriculture, food systems, sociology, anthropology, economics, politics, policy, etc.

Figure 1.1 Conceptual framework for a holistic, integrated understanding of human nutrition.

much will be eaten. What and how much is eaten will further depend on what is available, influenced by a host of factors determining food security. All of these factors, on an individual, household, community, national or international level, shape the external environment.

During the first renaissance of nutrition, emphasis was placed on the study of nutrients and their functions. A medical, natural science or biological model underpinned the study of the relationships between nutrition and health or ill-health. During the second renaissance, these aspects are not neglected, but expanded to include the study of all other external environmental factors that determine what and how much food and nutrients are available on a global level. These studies are underpinned by social, behavioral, economic, agricultural and political sciences. The study of human nutrition therefore seeks to understand the complexities of both social and biological factors on how individuals and populations maintain optimal function and health, how the quality, quantity and balance of the food supply are influenced, what happens to food after it is eaten and the way that diet affects health and wellbeing. This integrated approach has led to a better understanding of the causes and consequences of malnutrition, and of the relationship between nutrition and health.

1.4 Relationship between nutrition and health

Figure 1.2 shows that individuals can be broadly categorized into having optimal nutritional status, or being undernourished, overnourished or malnourished. The major causes and consequences of these nutritional states are indicated. It is important to realize that many other lifestyle and environmental factors, in addition

Nutritional situation	Health consequences, outcomes
Optimum nutrition Food secure individuals with adequate, balanced and prudent diets	→ Health, well being, normal development, high quality of life
Undernutrition: Hunger Food insecure individuals living in poverty, ignorance, political unstable environments, disrupted societies, war	→ • Decreased physical and mental development; • Compromised immune systems; • Increased infectious diseases; • Vicious circle of undernutrition, underdevelopment, poverty
Overnutrition Overconsumption of food, especially macronutrients, plus: • low physical activity • smoking, stress, etc.	→ Obesity, metabolic syndrome, cardiovascular disease, type 2 diabetes mellitus, certain cancers: chronic noncommunicable diseases (NCDs), often characterized by overnutrition of macronutrients and micronutrient undernutrition
Malnutrition Nutrition transition: individuals and communities previously food insecure → confronted with abundance of palatable foods → some undernourished, other too much macronutrients and too little micronutrients	→ Double burden of infectious plus NCDs, often characterized by overnutrition of macronutrients and micronutrient undernutrition

Figure 1.2 Relationship between nutrition and health.

to nutrition, influence health and well-being, but nutrition is a major, modifiable and powerful factor in promoting health, preventing and treating disease and improving quality of life.

1.5 Nutrients: the basics

People eat food, not nutrients; however, it is the combination and amounts of nutrients in consumed foods that determine health. To read one must know the letters of the alphabet; to do sums one must be able to count, add, subtract, multiply and divide. To understand nutrition, one must know about nutrients. The study of nutrients, the ABC and numeric calculations of nutrition, will form a major part of the student's nutrition journey, and should include:

- the chemical and physical structure and characteristics of the nutrient
- the food sources of the nutrient, including food composition, the way in which foods are grown, harvested, stored, processed and prepared, and effects

of these on nutrient composition and nutritional value
- the digestion, absorption, circulatory transport and cellular uptake of the nutrient, as well as regulation of all these processes
- the metabolism of the nutrient, its functions, storage and excretion
- physiological needs (demands or requirements) for the nutrient in health and disease, and during special circumstances (pregnancy, lactation, sport events), as well as individual variability
- interactions with other nutrients, nonnutrients (phytochemicals), antinutrients and drugs
- the consequences of underconsumption and overconsumption of nutrients
- the therapeutic uses of the nutrient
- factors influencing food and nutrition security and food safety.

There are more than 50 known nutrients (including amino acids and fatty acids) and many more chemicals in food thought to influence human function and health

Box 1.1 Classes of nutrients for human nutrition

Class/category	Subclass/category	Nutrient examples
Carbohydrates (macronutrients)	Monosaccharides and disaccharides	Glucose, fructose, galactose, sucrose, maltose, lactose
Proteins (macronutrients)	Plant and animal source proteins	Amino acids ($n = 20$): aliphatic, aromatic, sulfur-containing, acidic, basic
Fats and oils (lipids) (macronutrients)	Saturated fatty acids Monounsaturated fatty acids Polyunsaturated fatty acids (n-3, n-6, n-9)	Palmitic and stearic acid Oleic (*cis*) and elaidic (*trans*) fatty acids Linoleic, α-linoleic, arachidonic, eicosapentanoic, docosahexanoic acid
Minerals (micronutrients)	Minerals and electrolytes Trace elements	Calcium, sodium, phosphate, potassium, iron, zinc, selenium, copper, manganese, molybdenum, fluoride, chromium
Vitamins (micronutrients)	Fat soluble	Retinol (A), calciferols (D), tocopherols (E), vitamin K, ascorbic acid (C), thiamine (B_1), riboflavin (B_2), niacin (B_3), pyridoxine (B_6), folate, cobalimine (B_{12})
Water	Water	Water

(see Box 1.1). Nutrients do not exist in isolation, except for water and others in some pharmaceutical preparations. In foods, in the gut during digestion, fermentation and absorption, in the blood during transport, and in cells during metabolism, nutrients interact with each other. Therefore, a particular nutrient should not be studied in isolation, but integrated with other nutrients and seen in the context of total body function. The study of nutrition also includes how to determine nutrient requirements to make recommendations for intakes and how nutritional status is monitored by measuring intakes, anthropometry, body composition, biochemical markers reflecting nutritional status and the clinical signs of malnutrition.

This knowledge of nutrients and their functions will enable the nutritionist to advise individuals what and how much to eat. However, this knowledge is not sufficient to understand and address the global problem of malnutrition facing mankind today. This perception has resulted in the cultivation of social science disciplines to support knowledge from the biological sciences to address global malnutrition.

1.6 Global malnutrition

It is a major tragedy that millions of people currently live with hunger and fear starvation. This is despite the

Box 1.2

Food insecurity: when people live with hunger and fear starvation.

Food security: access for all, at all times, to a sustainable, affordable supply of nutritionally adequate and safe food for normal physical and mental development and healthy, productive lives.

fact that food security or "access for all at all times, to a sustainable supply of nutritionally adequate and safe food for normal physical and mental development and healthy, productive lives" is a basic human right embedded in the constitution of most developing countries. It is also despite the fact that sufficient food is produced on a global level (see Box 1.2). Food insecurity is an obstacle to human rights, quality of life and human dignity. It was estimated that during the last decade of the twentieth century, 826 million people were undernourished: 792 million in developing countries and 34 million in developed countries. In developing countries, more than 199 million children under the age of 5 years suffer from acute or chronic protein and energy deficiencies. An estimated 3.5–5 billion people are iron deficient, 2.2 billion iodine deficient and 140–250 million vitamin A deficient. This has led to several global initiatives and commitments, spearheaded by a number of United Nations organizations, to reduce global undernutrition, food insecurity, hunger, starvation and micronutrient deficiencies. Some of these initiatives are:

- the 1990 United Nations Children's Fund (UNICEF)-supported World Summit for Children, with a call to reduce severe and moderate malnutrition among children under 5 years of age by half the 1990 rate by the year 2000, including goals for the elimination of micronutrient malnutrition;
- the 1992 World Health Organization/Food and Agriculture Organization (WHO/FAO) International Conference on Nutrition that reinforced earlier goals and extended them to the elimination of death from famine;
- the 1996 FAO-supported World Food Summit during which 186 heads of state and governments pledged their political will and commitment to a plan of action to reduce the number of undernourished people to half their 1996 number by 2015;
- the establishment in 1997 of the Food Insecurity and Vulnerability Information and Mapping System (FIVIMS) and their Intern-Agency Working Group (IAWG), which consists of 26 international organizations and agencies with a shared commitment to reduce food insecurity and vulnerability and its multidimensional causes rooted in poverty. Information about these initiatives can be accessed at: http://www.fao.org/

A 2001 report from the FAO indicated that in 1997–1999 there were 815 million undernourished people in the world, of whom 777 million were in developing countries, 27 million in transitional countries and 11 million in the industrialized countries. The annual decrease in undernourished people from the 1990–1992 period was 6 million. To reach the World Food Summit goal of halving the number of undernourished in developing countries by 2015, it is estimated that the annual decrease required is 22 million.

Clearly, this is a huge challenge for food and nutrition scientists and practitioners. It would need a holistic approach and understanding of the complex, interacting factors that contribute to malnutrition on different levels. These include immediate, intermediate, underlying and basic causes:

- individual level or immediate causes: food and nutrient intake, physical activity, health status, social structures, care, taboos, growth, personal choice;
- household level or intermediate causes: family size and composition, gender equity, rules of distribution of food within the household, income, availability of food, access to food;
- national level or underlying causes: health, education, sanitation, agriculture and food security, war, political instability, urbanization, population growth, distribution and conflicts, war, natural disasters, decreased resources;
- international level or basic causes: social, economic and political structures, trade agreements, population size, population growth distribution, environmental degradation.

To address these causes of undernutrition food-insecure and hungry communities and individuals must be empowered to be their own agents of food security and livelihood development. Complicating the task of fighting food insecurity and hunger are natural disasters such as droughts, floods, cyclones and extreme temperatures, ongoing wars and regional conflicts, as well as the devastating impact of the human immunodeficiency virus (HIV) and the acquired immunodeficiency syndrome (AIDS), especially in sub-Saharan Africa.

In many developing countries, indigenous people have changed their diets and physical activity patterns to those followed in industrialized countries. Supplementary feeding programs in these countries have often been associated with increasing trends towards obesity, insulin resistance and the emergence of chronic diseases of lifestyle in some segments of these populations, while other segments are still undernourished.

The coexistence of undernutrition and overnutrition, leading to a double burden of infectious and chronic, noncommunicable diseases, and the multifactorial causes of malnutrition, call for innovative approaches to tackle both undernutrition and overnutrition in integrated nutrition and health-promoting programs, focusing on optimal nutrition for all.

1.7 Relationship between nutrition science and practice

The journey through the scientific domain of nutrition will, at a specialized stage, fork into different roads. These roads will lead to the different scopes or branches of nutrition science that are covered in the second, third and fourth texts of this series. These different branches of nutrition science could lead to the training of nutrition specialists for specific practice areas.

The main aim of nutrition professionals is to apply nutrition principles to promote health and well-being, to prevent disease and/or to restore health (treat disease) in individuals, families, communities and the population. To help individuals or groups of people to eat a balanced diet, in which food supply meets nutrient needs, involves application of nutrition principles from a very broad field to almost every facet of human life. It is therefore not surprising that these different branches or specialities of nutrition have evolved and are developing. They include clinical nutrition, community nutrition, public health and public nutrition. It can be expected that there will be overlap in the practice areas of these specialities.

- The clinical nutritionist will counsel individuals from a biomedical–disease-behavioral paradigm to promote health, prevent disease or treat disease. The clinical nutritionist will mostly work within the health service (hospitals, clinics, private practice).
- The community nutritionist, with additional skills from the psychosocial behavioral sciences, should be aware of the dynamics within particular communities responsible for nutritional problems. These would include household food security, socioeconomic background, education levels, child-care practices, sanitation, water, energy sources, healthcare services and other quality-of-life indicators. The community nutritionist will design, implement and monitor appropriate, community-participatory programs to address these problems.
- The public health or public nutritionist covers the health and care practice areas but will also be concerned with food security (agricultural) and environmental issues on a public level. The public health or public nutritionist will, for example, be responsible for nutrition surveillance, and the design, implementation and monitoring of dietary guidelines that address relevant public health problems. A background knowledge in economics, agriculture, political science and policy design is essential for the formulation and application of nutrition policy in a country.

Many developing countries will not have the capacity or the financial resources to train and employ professionals for different specialities. However, future specialized training and employment of different professionals could result in a capacity to address nutritional problems more effectively.

1.8 Nutrition milestones: the development of nutrition as a science

Ancient beliefs

Throughout human existence people have attributed special powers to certain foods and developed beliefs and taboos regarding foods. These were often based on climatic, economic, political or religious circumstances and principles, but also on observations regarding the relationship between the consumption of certain foods and health.

Recorded examples are ancient Chinese and Indian philosophers who advised on the use of warming and cooling foods and spices for certain conditions and for "uplifting the soul", the Mosaic laws documented in the Old Testament which distinguished between clean and unclean foods, the fasting and halal practices of Islam, and the Benedictine monks from Salerno who preached the use of hot and moist versus cold and dry foods for various purposes. Hippocrates, the father of modern medicine, who lived from 460 to about 377 BC, and later Moses Maimonides, who lived in the twelfth century, urged people to practice abstemiousness and a prudent lifestyle. They, and others, advised that for a long and healthy life, one should avoid too much fat in the diet, eat more fruit, get ample sleep and be physically active – advice that is still incorporated in the modern, science-based dietary guidelines of the twenty-first century!

Cultural beliefs

The perception that food represents more than its constituent parts is still true. Eating together is an accepted form of social interaction. It is a way in which cultural habits and customs, social status, kingship, love, respect, sharing and hospitality are expressed. Scientists and nutrition professionals realize that when formulating dietary guidelines for traditional living people, cultural beliefs and taboos should be taken into account and incorporated. There are numerous examples of traditional food habits and diets, often based on what was available. Today, with the world becoming a global village, cultures have learned from each other and dietary patterns associated with good health, such as the Mediterranean diet, are becoming popular among many cultures.

The first renaissance: development of an evidence base

The knowledge of the specific health effects of particular diets, foods and nutrients is now firmly based on the results of rigid scientific experimentation. Nutrition developed gradually as a science, but advanced with rapid strides during the twentieth century. There are numerous meticulously recorded examples of how initial (often ancient and primitive) observations about diet and health relationships led to the discovery, elucidation of function, isolation and synthesis of the different nutrients. Perhaps the most often quoted example is James Lind's description in 1772 of how citrus fruit could cure and prevent scurvy in seamen on long voyages. The anti-scurvy factor (ascorbic acid or vitamin C) was only isolated in 1921, characterized in 1932 and chemically synthesized in 1933. Other examples of nutritional milestones are the induction of beriberi in domestic fowl by Eijkman in 1897, the observation of Takaki in 1906 that beriberi in Japanese sailors could be prevented by supplementing their polished rice diets with wheat bread, and eventually the isolation of the responsible factor, thiamine or vitamin B_1, by Funk in 1911. Others are the Nobel Prize-winning discovery by Minot and Murphy in 1926 that pernicious anemia is a nutritional dis-order due to a lack of vitamin B_{12} in the diet, the description of kwashiorkor as a protein-deficiency state by Cecily Williams in 1935, and the discovery of resistant starch and importance of colonic fermentation for humans by nutritionists of the Dunn Clinical Nutrition Centre in the 1980s.

The history of modern nutrition as practiced today is an exciting one to read, and students are encouraged to spend some time on it. It is often characterized by heartbreaking courage and surprising insights. An example of the former is the carefully documented clinical, metabolic and pathological consequences of hunger and starvation by a group of Jewish doctors in 1940 in the Warsaw ghetto: doctors who themselves were dying of hunger. An example of the latter is the studies by Price, an American dentist, who tried to identify the dietary factors responsible for good dental and overall health in people living traditional lifestyles. He unwittingly used a fortigenic paradigm in his research, examining the strengths and factors that keep people healthy, long before the term was defined or its value recognized.

At present, thousands of nutrition scientists examine many aspects of nutrition in laboratories and field studies all over the world and publish in more than 100 international scientific nutrition journals. This means that nutrition science generates new knowledge based on well-established research methodologies. The many types of experiments, varying from molecular experimentation in the laboratory, through placebo-controlled, double-blinded clinical interventions, to observational epidemiological surveys, and experiments based on a health (fortigenic) or a disease (pathogenic) paradigm, will be addressed in this volume (Chapter 13). The peer-review process of published results has helped in the development of guidelines to judge how possible, probable, convincing and applicable results from these studies are. New knowledge of nutrients, foods and diet relationships with health and disease is, therefore, generated through a process in which many scientists examine different pieces of the puzzle all over the world in controlled scientific experiments. Therefore, nutrition practice today has a firm research base that enables nutritional professionals to practice evidence-based nutrition.

The second renaissance: solving global malnutrition

There is little doubt that improved nutrition has contributed to the improved health and survival times experienced by modern humans. However, global figures on the prevalence of both undernutrition and overnutrition show that millions of people do not have enough to eat, while the millions who eat too much suffer from the consequences of obesity. It is tempting to equate this situation to the gap between the poor and the rich or between developing and developed countries, but the situation is much more complex. Obesity, a consequence of overnutrition, is now a public health problem not only in rich, developed, food-secure countries, but also in developing, food-insecure countries, especially among women. Undernutrition, the major impediment to national development, is the biggest single contributor to childhood death rates, and to impaired physical growth and mental development of children in both developing and developed countries. Moreover, a combination of undernutrition and overnutrition in the same communities, in single households and even in the same individual is often reported. Examples are obese mothers with undernourished children and obese women with certain micronutrient deficiencies. The perception that these global problems of malnutrition will only be solved in innovative, multidisciplinary and multisectoral ways has led to the second, very recent renaissance in nutrition research and practice.

1.9 Future challenges for nutrition research and practice

Basic, molecular nutrition

The tremendous development in recent years of molecular biology and the availability of sophisticated new techniques are opening up a field in which nutrient–gene interactions and dietary manipulation of genetic expression will receive increasing attention. The effects of more than 12 000 different substances in plant foods, not yet classified as nutrients, will also be examined. These substances are produced by plants for hormonal, attractant and chemoprotective purposes, and there is evidence that many of them offer protection against a wide range of human conditions. It is possible that new functions of known nutrients, and even new nutrients, may be discovered, described and applied in the future.

Clinical and community nutrition

Today, the focus has moved from simple experiments with clear-cut answers, to studies where sophisticated statistics have to be used to dissect out the role of specific nutrients, foods and diets in multifactorial diseases. Nutrition epidemiology is now established as the discipline in which these questions can be addressed. A number of pressing problems will have to be researched and the results applied, for example:

- the biological and sociological causes of childhood obesity, which is emerging as a global public health problem;
- the nutrient requirements of the elderly: in the year 2000, more than 800 million of the Earth's inhabitants were older than 60 years. To ensure a high-quality life in the growing elderly population, much more needs to be known about their nutrient requirements;
- the relationships between nutrition and immune function and how improved nutrition can help to defend against invading micro-organisms; in the light of the increasing HIV/AIDS pandemic, more information in this area is urgently needed;
- dietary recommendations: despite sufficient, convincing evidence about the effects of nutrients and foods on health, nutritionists have generally not been very successful in motivating the public to change

their diets to more healthy ones. We need to know more about why people make certain food choices in order to design culturally sensitive and practical dietary guidelines that will impact positively on dietary choices. The food-based dietary guidelines that are now being developed in many countries are a first step in this direction.

Public health nutrition

The single most important challenge facing mankind in the future is probably to provide adequate safe food and clean water for all in an environmentally safe way that will not compromise the ability of future generations to meet their needs. In addition to the hundreds of millions not eating enough food to meet their needs for a healthy, active life, an additional 80 million people have to be fed each year. The challenge to feed mankind in the future calls for improved agriculture in drought-stricken areas such as sub-Saharan Africa, the application of biotechnology in a responsible way, interdisciplinary and intersectorial co-operation of all involved, and a better distribution of the food supply so that affordable food is accessible by all. The need for sustained economic growth in poor countries is evident.

Nutritionists have an important part to play in ensuring food security for all, a basic human right, in the future. One of their main functions would be to educate and inform populations not to rely too heavily on animal products in their diet, the production of which places a much heavier burden on the environment than plant foods. A major challenge would be to convince political leaders and governments that addressing undernutrition (the major obstacle in national development) in sustainable programs should be the top priority in developing and poor communities. Another challenge is to develop models based on the dynamics within communities and, using a human rights approach, to alleviate undernutrition without creating a problem of overnutrition. There are examples where such models, incorporated into community development programs, have been very successful (e.g. in Thailand).

Functional foods: a new development

Functional foods are new or novel foods, developed to have specific health benefits, in addition to their usual functions. Examples are spreads with added phytosterols, to lower serum low-density lipoprotein cholesterol and the risk of coronary heart disease, and

Microbial contamination Bacteria and mould (fungi) producing toxins and aflatoxins. Toxins cause îfood poisoningî and aflatoxins are carcinogenic.	
Natural toxins Such as cyanide in cassava, solanine in potatoes; can be produced by abnormal circumstances, could be enzyme inhibitors or antivitamins.	Agricultural residues Pesticides such as DDT or hormones used to promote growth such as bovine somatotrophin.
Environmental contamination Heavy metals and minerals; criminal adulteration, industrial pollution; substances from packaging materials; changes during cooking and processing of foods.	Intentional additives artificial sweetners; preservatives; phytochemicals; modified carbohydrates (for functional foods).

Figure 1.3 Potential hazardous substances in food.

the development of starchy products with resistant starch and lower glycemic indices, to help control blood glucose levels. The development and testing of functional foods is an exciting new area. These foods may help to improve or restore nutritional status in many people. However, much more should be known about suitable biomarkers to test their efficacy, variability in human response to specific food products, safety, consumer understanding, and how their health messages must be formulated, labeled and communicated.

Food safety

The continued provision of safe food, free from micro-organisms, toxins and other hazardous substances that cause disease, remains a huge challenge. Recent experiences with animals suffering from bovine spongiform encephalopathy (BSE or mad cow disease) or from foot-and-mouth disease, have shown how quickly a national problem can become an international one because of global marketing of products. The list of possible hazardous substances in foods emphasizes the need for continuous monitoring of the food supply by health officials (see Figure 1.3).

1.10 Perspectives on the future

Nutrition research and practice, although it has been around for many years, is in its infancy as a basic and applied scientific discipline. The present and future nutrition student will take part in this very exciting

Box 1.3 Future challenges that require exceptional leadership

- Basic molecular nutrition
  - Nutrient–gene interactions
  - Role of phytochemicals in health
  - New nutrients? New functions?
- Community and public health nutrition
  - Childhood obesity
  - Requirements of the elderly
  - Dietary recommendations
  - Nutrition of HIV/AIDS patients
- Public nutrition
  - To feed mankind
  - Food security
- Functional foods
  - To ensure that novel foods are effective and safe
- Food safety
  - Continuous monitoring
- Partnerships with other disciplines
- Leadership

second renaissance of nutrition and see its maturation. However, to influence effectively the nutrition and health of individuals and populations, the nutritionist will have to forge links and partnerships with other health professionals and policy makers, and will have to develop lateral thinking processes. The magnitude and complexity of nutritional problems facing mankind today demand concerted multidisciplinary and multisectorial efforts from all involved to solve them. Therefore, the principal message to take on a nutrition science journey is that teamwork is essential: one cannot travel this road on one's own; partners from different disciplines are needed. Another essential need is the continuous development of leadership in nutrition. Leaders on every level of research and practice are necessary to respond to the existing challenges of global malnutrition and to face future challenges.

The modern advances in molecular biology and biotechnology on the one hand, and the persistence of global malnutrition on the other, increasingly demand a re-evaluation of ethical norms, standards and values for nutrition science and practice. Direction from responsible leaders is needed (see Box 1.3).

The student in nutrition, at the beginning of this journey of discovery of nutrition as a science, must make use of the many opportunities to develop leadership qualities. May this be a happy, fruitful and life-long journey with many lessons that can be applied in the research and practice of nutrition to make a difference in the life of all.

Further reading

Websites

http://www.ahsl.arizona.edu/journals/ejrnls/subjresult.cfm?name=
    Nutrition
http://arborcom.com/frame/medicus.htm
http://nutrition.cabweb.org
http://www/wku.edu.nhrtm/nut-jrnl.htm
http://www/fao.org/es/ESN/NUTRI.HTM
http://www.wri.org/
http://wally.rit.edu/pubs/guides/nutritionj.html
http://www.sciencekomm.at/journals/food.html

2
Body Composition

Paul Deurenberg and Ronenn Roubenoff

Key messages

- Body composition data are used to evaluate nutritional status, growth and development, water homeostasis and specific disease states.
- Human body composition is studied at atomic, molecular, cellular, tissue and whole body levels. The levels are interrelated.
- A "normal-weight" human body consists of approximately 98% oxygen, carbon, hydrogen, nitrogen and calcium; of 60–70% water, 10–35% fat (depending on gender), 10–15% protein and 3–5% minerals.
- The variation in body composition between individuals is large, mainly because of variations in fat mass.
- Variations in fat-free mass are smaller.
- Several direct, indirect and doubly indirect techniques are available to measure body composition, each with its own distinct advantages and disadvantages.
- The choice of method will be influenced by the availability of instrumentation, invasiveness and radiation danger to subjects, price, accuracy required and application objectives.
- Interpretation and application of data from body composition measurements should be done with care and should take into account the limitations of the method used, age, gender and ethnic group.

2.1 Introduction

Mankind has long been fascinated with the composition of the human body. Centuries ago, the Greeks dissected human cadavers to obtain an insight into the structure and build of the human body, and drawings from the Middle Ages of gross muscle structures grace the walls of many famous art galleries. They are prized not only for their artistic merit, but also for what they reveal of the work of the dissectionists of that era. With progress in the development of analytical chemical methods in the twentieth century, these studies of body composition were applied to body tissues, fetuses and cadavers of newborns. Scientists such as Mitchell, Widdowson and Forbes performed the most important work of chemical analyses in adult cadavers during the 1940s and 1950s. Today, neutron activation analysis allows the chemical composition of the human body to be studied *in vivo*. These early chemical analyses of the body gave insights into the changes occurring during growth and development. They also form the basis for a number of methods now widely used to assess body composition *in vivo*.

Today it is known that many diseases and disorders are related to abnormal body composition or to changes in body composition. The most common of these conditions is obesity, in which the amount of body fat is excessively high, leading to abnormalities in lipid and carbohydrate metabolism, high blood pressure and adult-onset diabetes. At the other end of the nutritional spectrum, energy and protein malnutrition results in a decrease in the amount of fat and protein stores in the body, and many diseases are related to abnormalities in total body water or to the distribution of body water across the intracellular and extracellular spaces.

Because of the high variability between subjects in chemical body composition, mainly due to the high variation in body fat stores, the concept of fat-free mass (FFM) was introduced at the end of the nineteenth century. If body composition data are expressed as a proportion of the FFM, data become much more consistent between individuals. For example, the fraction of water in the FFM (0.73 ± 0.02) is very consistent across individuals, whereas the between-subject variation is two to three times higher if expressed per kilogram of body weight. This high variability in body components led to the definition of a "reference man", an imaginary person with a given body composition.

In this chapter a (global) description of the composition of the healthy human body is given and discussed at the following levels:

- atomic
- molecular
- cellular
- tissue
- whole body.

Of the many methods available to measure body composition, a few are highlighted and a short description of each is given. For more detailed information the books by Forbes (1987) and Roche *et al.* (1996) on human body composition are recommended for further reading.

2.2 Five levels of body composition

Human body composition can be studied at the atomic, molecular, cellular, tissue and whole body level. These five levels are related to each other. For example, information at the atomic level can be used, subject to certain assumptions, to provide information at the whole body level.

Atomic level

Many chemical elements (atoms) are found in the human body, but the six elements oxygen, carbon, hydrogen, nitrogen, calcium and phosphorus are the most abundant and together account for more than 98% of body weight (Table 2.1). Indeed, the 11 most common elements account for 99.5% of the atomic body composition. This information was initially based on chemical analysis of carcasses, but today the information can also be obtained by *in vivo* neutron activation analysis (IVNAA). The classical chemical cadaver analysis, as carried out mainly in the 1940s, still forms the basis for many *in vivo* techniques that are used to assess body composition.

Table 2.1 Body composition at the atomic level of a 70 kg reference man

Atomic element	Amount (kg)	Amount (% body weight)
Oxygen	43	61
Carbon	16	23
Hydrogen	7	10
Nitrogen	1.8	2.6
Calcium	1.0	1.4
Phosphorus	0.6	0.8
Total	69.4	98.8

Box 2.1

The water content in the body varies with age. In a fetus the water content slowly decreases from more than 90% after conception to about 80% before delivery at about 7 months of age. A newborn has about 70% body water, which is about 82% of the fat-free mass. This value slowly decreases further to 72% of the fat-free mass until the body is chemically mature at age 15–18 years. In general, males have more body water (related to body weight) than females, as their body fat content is lower.

Molecular level

The chemical elements in the human body are bound in molecules and, in very global terms, the main compartments are water, lipids, proteins, minerals and carbohydrates. The total amount of water in the body is high and, depending on the body fat content, can be as high as 60–70% of total body weight. Total body water can be divided into intracellular water and extracellular water, and the ratio of the two is an important health parameter that is disturbed in many diseases (Box 2.1).

Lipids appear in the human body in different forms. Essential structural lipids such as the phospholipids (cell membranes) and sphingomyelin (nervous system) form only a minor part of the total lipids in the body. The nonessential lipids, mostly triglycerides or triacylglycerol (fat), are the most abundant. They are the energy store of the adult human body, insulate against cold, protect vital organs such as the kidneys against mechanical damage and, to a certain extent, enhance the body's appearance. In a "normal-weight" healthy adult, the amount of body fat varies between 10 and 25% in males and between 15 and 35% in females. In obesity body fat can be as high as 60–70% of body weight.

Table 2.2 Body composition at the molecular level of a 70 kg reference man

Component	Amount (kg)	Amount (% body weight)
Water		
Extracellular	18	26
Intracellular	24	34
Lipid		
Essential	1.5	2.1
Non-essential	12	17
Protein	10.1	14.4
Mineral	3.7	5.3
Carbohydrate	0.5	0.6
Total	69.8	99.4

Table 2.3 Body composition at the tissue level of a 70 kg reference man

Tissue/organ	Amount (kg)	Amount (% body weight)
Muscle	28	40
Adipose tissue	15	21.4
Blood	5.5	7.9
Bone	5	7.1
Skin	2.6	3.7
Liver	1.8	2.6
Total	57.9	82.7

Body protein varies between 10 and 15%. It is higher in males than in females, as males generally have more muscles. There is no protein storage in the body and, generally speaking, loss of protein coincides with a loss of functionality given the high protein content and high protein turnover rates in vital organs.

The amount of minerals in the body varies between 3 and 5%, again dependent on body fat. Calcium and phosphorus are the two main minerals. They are found mainly in bones. Carbohydrates are found in the body as glucose (blood sugar) and glycogen, a polysaccharide in muscle and liver cells that serves as a short-term energy store. The amount of carbohydrates in the body rarely exceeds 500 g. Table 2.2 gives the body composition of the reference man at a molecular level.

Cellular level

At the cellular level, body composition can be described in terms of body cell mass, extracellular fluids and extracellular solids. The body cell mass includes the cells with all their contents, such as water, proteins and minerals. Extracellular fluid contains about 95% water, which is plasma in the intravascular space and interstitial fluid in the extravascular space. Extracellular solids are mainly proteins (e.g. collagen) and minerals (bone minerals and soluble minerals in the extracellular fluid). Body composition at the cellular level is not easy to measure, owing to its complex nature. As will be discussed later, the ^{40}K method can be used to assess body cell mass and some dilution techniques, for example bromide dilution, can be used to assess extracellular water.

Tissue level

Cells with equal functions form tissues, including muscular, connective, epithelial and nervous tissue. Bones are connective tissue and consist mainly of hydroxyapatite, $[Ca_3(PO_4)_2]_3Ca(OH)_2$, bedded in a protein matrix. A rather simple body composition model at the tissue level would be:

$$Body\ weight = adipose\ tissue + skeletal\ muscle + bone + organs + rest$$

Several of these components can now be measured with, for example, computed tomography (CT) or magnetic resonance imaging (MRI) for adipose tissue, creatinine excretion or N-methyl-histidine excretion in 24 h urine for skeletal muscle, dual-energy X-ray absorptiometry (DXA) for bones and MRI or ultrasound for organs. Body composition at the tissue level is given in Table 2.3.

Whole body level

Body composition measurements at the whole body level use simple body parameters to give an insight into body composition. Formulae, based on statistical relationships that have been established in earlier studies between body parameters (e.g. skinfold thickness) and information on body composition (e.g. body fat by density), also enable the assessment of body composition. Another example is the assessment of body water based on weight, height, age and gender.

2.3 Relationships between different levels of body composition

The five levels of body composition are interrelated. This means that information at one level can be translated to another level. This is important as it forms the

Box 2.2

Adipose tissue is made of adipocytes, cells that store triglycerides in the form of small fat droplets. Adipose tissue contains about 80% triglycerides and some 1–2% protein (enzymes), and the remaining part is water plus electrolytes. During weight loss adipose tissue decreases: the actual fat loss will be about 80% of the actual weight loss.

Table 2.4 Methods used to determine body composition

Direct	Indirect	Doubly indirect
Carcass analyses	Densitometry	Weight/height indices
IVNAA	Deuterium oxide dilution	Skinfolds/ultrasound
	^{40}K counting	Circumferences/diameters
	More-compartment models	Impedance
	DXA	Infrared interactance
	CT/MRI scans	Creatinine excretion

IVNAA: *in vivo* neutron activation analysis; DXA: dual-energy X-ray absorptiometry; CT: computed tomography; MRI: magnetic resonance imaging.

basis of many techniques used to determine body composition. In the context of this chapter, only a few examples are given. After determining the amount of calcium in the body by, for example, IVNAA (atomic level), the amount of bone can be calculated assuming that a certain amount of total body calcium is in the skeletal tissue. Determination of total body potassium (by ^{40}K or IVNAA) enables the assessment of the body cell mass, as most of the body potassium is known to be intracellular. Skinfold thickness measurements (total body level) enable the assessment of body fat (molecular level). Formulae used for these calculations are component based, property based or sometimes a combination. Component-based formulae are based on fixed relationships between components. An example is the calculation of total body water from measured hydrogen: the chemical formula of water determines the factor. Property-based formulae are based on established statistical relationships between variables. An example is the prediction of body fat per cent (body composition parameter) from skinfolds (property) (Box 2.2). Property-based formulae tend to be population specific.

Most body composition techniques that are in use today are based on assumptions, often derived from carcass analyses or experimentally derived from observational studies. Violation of these assumptions leads to biased results and some methods are more prone to bias than others. In the following short description of different methodologies, the most important assumptions are highlighted.

2.4 Body composition techniques

Body composition techniques can be described in terms of direct, indirect and doubly indirect methods.

- In direct methods the body component of interest is determined directly without or with only minor assumptions. Examples are chemical carcass analyses and IVNAA for the atomic components.
- In indirect techniques, the body component of interest is determined indirectly. Examples are the determination of body protein from body nitrogen, assuming a constant conversion factor of 6.25 from nitrogen to protein, and the determination of body cell mass using ^{40}K. In both examples assumptions are used. These assumptions may not be valid in the given situation or for the subject(s) under study and hence could lead to biased results.
- Doubly indirect methods rely on a statistical relationship between easy measurable body parameter(s) and the body component of interest. Examples are the assessment of skeletal muscle mass by creatinine excretion and the assessment of body fat from skinfold thickness. Table 2.4 gives an overview of the most common methods.

2.5 Direct methods

Carcass analysis

The (chemical) analysis of carcasses is a time-consuming exercise and requires very precise approaches to the task. The carcass has to be carefully dissected into the different tissues that are then exactly weighed, after which the chemical analyses have to be performed. To avoid errors it is important that no unaccounted water losses occur during the analytical work. As early as the nineteenth century, it was recognized that the variation in chemical body composition was reduced when results were expressed as fraction of the fat-free body. The data on the chemical composition of only a few human cadavers form the basis for the assumptions that are normally used in indirect methods. These chemical analyses were performed in five males and one female. It was concluded that, on the basis of FFM, the mean amounts of water, protein and minerals in the body are 72.6%, 20.5% and 6.9%, respectively. The variability in these figures is about 13% for protein and minerals and 4% for water. Although one can question the quality of these data as a basis for other methods (low number, high variation in age, variation in gender, some carcasses were not analyzed immediately after death), they form the basis for many indirect and doubly indirect body composition methods. Chemical carcass analysis also revealed that the amount of potassium in the FFM is fairly constant. This fact is used as the basis for the calculation of the amount of FFM or for body cell mass from total body potassium, determined by ^{40}K scanning.

In the 1980s, cadaver studies were performed again in the Brussels study. Unfortunately, only information at a tissue level and not at atomic or molecular level was collected. However, the need for cadaver studies has greatly diminished given that the same information can now be obtained *in vivo* by IVNAA.

In vivo *neutron activation analysis*

IVNAA is a relatively new body composition technique that allows the determination of specific chemical elements in the body. The body is bombarded with fast neutrons of known energy level. The neutrons can be captured by chemical elements (as part of molecules) in the body, resulting in a transition state of higher energy for that element, energy that is finally emitted as gamma rays. For example, capture of neutrons by nitrogen results in the formation of the isotope ^{15}N, which will emit the excess energy as gamma rays:

$$^{14}N + {}^1n \rightarrow {}^{15}N^* + \text{Gamma rays}$$

where ^{14}N = nitrogen with atomic mass 14, ^{15}N = nitrogen with atomic mass 15, and ^1n = neutron.

With IVNAA, many elements in the body can be determined, including calcium, phosphorus, nitrogen, oxygen, potassium and chlorine.

The information obtained at the atomic level can be converted to more useful information. For example, from total body nitrogen total body protein can be calculated as 6.25 times total nitrogen, assuming that body protein consists of 16% nitrogen. The advantage of the method is that the chemical body composition can be determined *in vivo* and can be compared with other, indirect techniques. For fundamental studies and for validation of existing techniques in special groups of subjects, for example in different ethnic groups, elderly subjects, obese subjects or in the diseased state, the methodology can be of great importance. The disadvantage of IVNAA is not only the price. The subject is irradiated, with the radiation dose used depending on the number and kind of elements to be determined. It is relatively low for nitrogen (0.26 mSv) but high for calcium (2.5 mSv).

2.6 Indirect methods

Densitometry

The densitometric method assumes that the body consists of two components, a fat mass, in which all "chemical" fat is located, and the FFM, which consists of (fat-free) bones, muscles, water and organs. Chemically, the FFM consists of water, minerals, protein and a small amount of carbohydrate, the latter often being neglected. The density of the fat mass is 0.900 kg/l and, from carcass analysis data, the density of the FFM can be calculated as 1.100 kg/l, depending on the relative amount of minerals, protein and water in the FFM (Box 2.3).

The density of the total body depends on the ratio of fat mass to FFM. Once the density of the body has

---

Box 2.3

The density of the fat-free mass (FFM) can be calculated if its composition is known.

In the calculation example below it is assumed that the FFM consists of 73.5% water, 19.6% protein and 6.9% minerals with densities (at 37°C) of 0.993, 1.340 and 3.038 kg/l, respectively. In addition, it is assumed that the volumes of the separate compartments can be added up to the total volume of the FFM (in fact, the compartments do not "mix"). Thus, the volume of the FFM equals the sum of the other compartments:

$$\text{FFM}_{volume} = \text{Water}_{volume} + \text{Mineral}_{volume} + \text{Protein}_{volume}$$

As volume is weight/density, the equation can be written as:

$$100/\text{Density}_{FFM} = 73.5/0.993 + 6.9/3.038 + 19.6/1.340$$

From this, the density of the FFM can be calculated as 1.0999 kg/l.

It is obvious that differences in composition of the FFM will result in a different density.

Box 2.4

Siri's formula can be derived assuming that the body consists of fat mass and fat-free mass (FFM). If body weight is assumed to be 100% and body fat is x%, then FFM is $100 - x$%. It is assumed that the volumes of these two compartments can be added up to total body volume. Then:

$$Body_{volume} = FM_{volume} + FFM_{volume}$$

As volume is weight/density, the equation can be written as:

$$100/body\ density = x/0.9 + 100 - x/1.1$$

From this, body fat percentage can be calculated as:

$$BF\% = 495/density - 450$$

The general formula to calculate body fat percentage from density is:

$$BF\% = \frac{1}{D_b} \times \left(\frac{D_{FFM} \times D_{FM}}{D_{FFM} - D_{FM}} \right) - \left(\frac{D_{FM}}{D_{FFM} - D_{FM}} \right)$$

In general, a lower density of the FFM than 1.1 kg/l will result in an overestimation of body fat per cent if Siri's formula is used. It is likely that the density of the FFM is lower in elderly people, owing to bone mineral loss (osteoporosis).

Figure 2.6 shows that densitometry (using Siri's equation) overestimates body fat compared with a four-compartment model.

Figure 2.1 Underwater weighing. The subject is submerged completely and breathes via a respirometer (1) for simultaneous residual lung volume measurement. Weight (2) under water is recorded and density is calculated as $D_{body} = W_{air}/(W_{air} - W_{uw})$. Corrections are made for water temperature and lung volume: $BF\% = 495/D_{body} - 450$.

been determined, the percentage of fat in the body (BF%) can be calculated by Siri's formula (Box 2.4):

$$BF\% = [495/body\ density] - 450$$

Body density can be determined by several techniques, the oldest and perhaps most accurate being underwater weighing. Behnke first used the technique, showing that excess body weight in football players was due not to excess fat but to enlarged muscle mass.

In underwater weighing, the weight of the subject is first measured in air and then while totally immersed in water. The difference between weight in air and weight under water is the upwards force, which equals the weight of the displaced water (Archimedes' law), from which, after correction for the water temperature (density), the displaced water volume (and thus the body volume) can be calculated. Corrections must be made for residual lung volume and air in the gut. Figure 2.1 shows an underwater weighing. The technique gives very reproducible results within about 1% point of body fat percentage. The absolute error in determined body fat is assumed to be maximal 3% point of body fat percentage. This error is mainly due to violation of the assumption that the density of the FFM equals 1.100 kg/l in the subject under study. It can be argued

that in certain subjects or groups of subjects this assumption may be violated, as for example in young children and in pregnant women. Use of Siri's formula will then lead to biased conclusions. Some laboratories have attempted to use water displacement instead of underwater weighing, but the technique failed, mainly because of the difficulty in accurately reading the water level in the tank.

An air-displacement method has been commercially available since 1995. This method measures body volume after placing the subject in a small, air-tight chamber and increasing the pressure by adding a known amount of air into the chamber. Boyle Gay-Lussac's law enables the calculation of body volume. Corrections are made for temperature and humidity changes, and lung volume is assessed simultaneously. Research to date has generally shown good agreement between underwater weighing and air displacement. Air displacement is better accepted by the volunteers, but some experience difficulties because of the breathing pattern to be followed or because of claustrophobia.

Dilution techniques

Carcass analyses revealed that the amount of water in the FFM is relatively constant at about 73%. Total body water (TBW) can be determined by dilution techniques. Dilution techniques are generally based on the equation:

$$C_1 \times V_1 = C_2 \times V_2 = \text{Constant}$$

where C = tracer (deuterium oxide, tritium or ^{18}O water) concentration and V = volume.

When a subject is given a known amount of a tracer ($C_1 \times V_1$) which is known to be diluted in a given body compartment, the volume of that body compartment can be calculated from the dose given and the concentration of the tracer in that compartment after equilibrium has been reached. Suitable tracers for the determination of TBW are deuterium oxide, tritium oxide and ^{18}O-labeled water. Other tracers can also be used, such as alcohol and urea, but they are less suitable because they are partly metabolized (alcohol) or because they are actively excreted from the body (urea) during the dilution period. After giving a subject the tracer and allowing around 3 h for equal distribution throughout the body, determination of the concentration of deuterium in blood, saliva or urine allows the calculation of TBW (Box 2.5).

Alternatively, other tracers can be used, such as tritium oxide and ^{18}O-labeled water, and the tracer can be given intravenously, which is advantageous when the subject has gastrointestinal disorders. The reproducibility of the method is 1–3%, depending on the tracer used and the analytical method chosen. From TBW, the FFM, and hence fat mass, can be calculated, assuming that 73% of the FFM is water:

$$BF\% = 100 \times (\text{Weight} - \text{TBW}/0.73)/\text{Weight}$$

The precision for estimations of body fat is about 3–4% of body weight. As with the densitometric method, this error is due to violations of the assumption used (i.e. that the relative amount of water in the FFM is constant and equals 73% of the FFM). In subjects with a larger than 73% water content in the FFM (pregnant women, morbid obese subjects and patients with edema), the factor 0.73 will result in an overestimation of the FFM.

A three-compartment model of the body that contains fat mass, water and dry FFM has a lower bias than a two-compartment model. An overestimation of body fat by densitometry, for example because of a relatively high amount of water in the FFM, will be counteracted

Box 2.6

For the computation of body composition from DXA, especially body fat and lean tissue, several assumptions are made, one of which is a constant hydration of the fat-free mass (FFM). The figure shows that the bias in calculated body fat per cent depends on the hydration of the FFM.
   Reference is a four-compartment model.

by an underestimation of the dilution method (see also Box 2.6).

The use of tracers that do not cross the cell membrane enables the determination of extracellular water (ECW). Commonly used tracers in this respect are bromide salts or sodium-24. Intracellular water (ICW) cannot be determined directly and is calculated as the difference between TBW and ECW.

Total body potassium

Chemical carcass analysis has revealed that the amount of potassium in the fat-free body is relatively constant, although the amount of potassium in different tissues varies widely. The determination of total body potassium (TBK) is relatively easy, owing to the natural occurrence of three potassium isotopes (^{39}K, ^{40}K and ^{41}K), in constant relative amounts, of which ^{40}K is radioactive (gamma emission). Counting the emission of the gamma rays from the body reveals the amount of radioactive potassium, from which total body potassium and hence FFM can be calculated. The chamber in which the subject is scanned has to be carefully shielded to avoid any background radiation (cosmic radiation). The scanning of the body for potassium lasts for 20–30 min and the reproducibility is 2–3%.

Several authors have shown that the amount of potassium in the FFM is different between males and females, is lower in obese subjects and is probably also age dependent. Thus, TBK is much more useful as a measure of body cell mass (BCM) than as a measure of FFM. However, this discrepancy can be used to calculate the "quality" of FFM, defined as the ratio of cellular to extracellular components of FFM, or operationally as BCM/FFM. Thus, when TBK is used to assess BCM, and another method such as hydrodensitometry or DXA is used to assess FFM independently, it can be shown that the quality of FFM declines with age, along with the quantity (see Figure 2.2). When potassium values are used to calculate intracellular water, BCM or FFM, assuming constant amounts of potassium in these body components, the same errors can occur as with densitometry and dilution techniques.

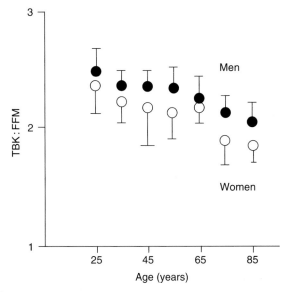

Figure 2.2 Difference in potassium content (TBK) of the fat-free mass (FFM) between men and women and the relationship with age.

Although the technique is easy to apply in patients, the high cost of the scanning instrumentation limits its use other than in research settings.

Dual-energy X-ray absorptiometry

During DXA (also known as DEXA), the body or part of the body is scanned with X-rays of two distinct levels of energy. The attenuation of the tissues for the two different levels of radiation depends on its chemical composition and is detected by photocells. The instrument's software generates a two-dimensional picture of the body or the body compartment under study. The software can calculate several body components: bone mineral content and bone mineral density, lean mass and adipose tissue fat mass. These calculations are possible for each of the body compartments, e.g. for legs, trunk, spine, femur and arms. However, the method cannot distinguish between subcutaneous adipose tissue and discrete adipose tissue sites such as perirenal adipose tissue. The reproducibility of DXA is very high, varying from about 0.5% for bone mineral density to about 2% for total body composition. The reproducibility for regional body composition is less. The method is quick and easy to perform and places very few demands on the subject. The radiation dose (0.02 mSv) is only a fraction of the radiation dose of a normal chest X-ray, and hardly higher than the normal background. Apart from repeated scanning, the radiation dose should not be a limiting factor in terms of volunteers being exposed to hazardous levels of radiation. A disadvantage of the method is that the attenuation of the X-rays depends on the thickness of the tissue. Therefore, correction for the body size has to be made. Compared with traditional methods, DXA scanning is easy and widely available which, in turn, leads to prediction equations for body composition based on DXA. However, as with other methods, DXA relies on certain assumptions (Box 2.6) and there are many publications showing that the error in body composition measurements using DXA can be considerable (see also Figure 2.3). Moreover, identical machines, even using the same software versions, can give different results in scanning the same person.

Multicompartment models

Two-compartment models, consisting of fat mass and FFM, lack validity in many situations where the composition of the body is "abnormal". Examples already mentioned are pregnancy, morbid obesity and the elderly. A combination of techniques often results in more valid estimates, as is the case when, for example, body density and body water are combined.

In this particular case the body is divided into three compartments:

$$\text{Body weight} = \text{Fat mass} + \text{Body water} + \text{Dry fat-free mass}$$

In this three-compartment model the variation of the water content in the FFM is accounted for. There are fewer assumptions in this model, leading to more valid results. Modern techniques as DXA enable the valid and precise measurement of bone mineral, from which total body mineral can be estimated. When the mineral content of the body is combined with body density and body water, a four-compartment model of the body is generated:

$$\text{Body weight} = \text{Fat mass} + \text{Water} + \text{Minerals} + \text{Protein}$$

In this model most of the variation in the amounts of the chemical components is accounted for, resulting in a very reliable body composition measure (Box 2.7). Four-compartment models can also be obtained using other techniques. For example, the measurement of calcium, phosphorus and nitrogen with IVNAA in combination with TBW provides information for a model

Figure 2.3 DXA scan using a HOLOGIC whole-body dual-energy X-ray absorptiometer (QDR-4500). Subcutaneous body fat, bone and muscle are distinguished by different colors.

Box 2.7

The first bar represents a two-compartment model of body composition, in which the body is divided into fat mass and fat-free mass (FFM). In the second bar the FFM is divided into water and a "dry" FFM, consisting of protein and mineral. The third bar shows a four-compartment model in which the body is divided into water, protein, mineral and fat. The four-compartment model shown has only minor assumptions and provides body composition data that are very accurate.

consisting of fat, minerals, protein and water. In the literature, models based on six compartments are also described. However, they do not provide much additional information and the increased technical error negates the methodological advantage.

More-compartment models enable the best possible estimate of body composition for populations as well as for individuals. Although some studies comparing body composition from four-compartment models show that mean values generally agree with simpler approaches, there are also studies showing directional bias of two-compartment body composition models. For this reason, more-compartment models should ideally be used as a reference (gold standard). However, only a limited number of laboratories can perform all of the necessary measurements for the calculation of maximum compartment models. Moreover, the data are expensive to collect, and measurements are time consuming and not very practical in clinical situations.

Imaging techniques

CT scanning enables the visualization of tissues in cross-sectional slices of the body. The thickness of those slices can vary, but is normally about 1 cm. During CT scanning a source of X-rays rotates perpendicularly around the body or a body segment, while photodetectors, opposite to the source, register the attenuation of the X-rays after they have passed through the body in the various directions. The information received by the photodetectors is used to generate images. Software enables the calculation of the amounts of tissues with different attenuation, for example adipose tissue against nonadipose tissue. The CT technique was introduced for body composition assessments in the 1980s and is now widely used, predominantly for measurements of body fat distribution. Figure 2.4 shows a scan of the abdomen at the level of the umbilicus, made by MRI, a technique that gives comparable information. The precision of the calculation of a tissue area or tissue volume from the same scan(s) is very accurate, with an error of about 1%. Partial volume effects (pixels that contain tissue with different attenuation) may influence the accuracy and reproducibility of the method.

A single CT scan provides only relative data, for example in a scan of the abdomen the relative amount of visceral adipose tissue to subcutaneous adipose tissue. Multiple CT scanning allows the calculation of tissue volumes. From adipose tissue volumes (tissue level) and an assumed density and composition of the adipose

Figure 2.4 Magnetic resonance imaging scan at the L4 level in an obese subject. The white areas in the image are adipose tissue. Subcutaneous adipose tissue and intra-abdominal adipose tissue are separated by the abdominal muscles.

tissue, the amount of fat mass (molecular level) can be calculated. Multiplying tissue volumes with specific densities of these tissues (determined *in vitro*) allows a recalculation of the body weight, a necessary but not sufficient exercise for validation of a whole body technique. Research in this area has shown that the CT technique allows the determination of total body composition, with an error of estimate for fat mass of 3–3.5 kg (compared with densitometry).

CT scanning is expensive and, because of the relatively high level of radiation, the method is limited to subjects for whom scanning is indicated on clinical grounds. An alternative method for CT scanning is MRI, which has the advantage that no radiation is involved.

During MRI, the signals emitted when the body is placed in a strong magnetic field are collected and, as with CT scanning, the data are used to generate a visual cross-sectional slice of the body in a certain region. The determination of adipose tissue versus nonadipose tissue is based on the shorter relaxation time of adipose tissue compared with other tissues that contain more protons or differ in resonance frequency. MRI has the advantage over CT scanning that the subject is not exposed to radiation. However, the time necessary to make an MRI image is relatively long (minutes versus seconds using CT), which has implications for the quality of the image. Any movement of the subject, even the movements of the intestinal tract when making images in the abdominal region, will decrease the quality of the image.

As with CT scanning, images can be combined to obtain information on total body composition. Information about organ size can be obtained with a high accuracy. For example, MRI was used to study the contribution of various organs to the resting metabolic rate of the total body.

Both CT scanning and MRI are expensive and therefore their use will remain limited to a few laboratories and for very specific situations.

2.7 Doubly indirect methods

Anthropometry

Weight/height indices

A weight/height index aims to correct body weight for height. As a measure of body composition, for example body fat, a weight/height index should have a high correlation with body fat, but also a low correlation with body height, otherwise in short people body fat would be systematically overestimated or underestimated.

In the literature, a number of weight/height indices have been proposed. Examples are the Quetelet index or body mass index (BMI:weight/height^2), the Broca index [weight/(height $-$ 100)] and the Benn index (weight/height^p, in which the exponent p is population specific). The Quetelet index or BMI is the most widely used index today. Its correlation with body fat is high (depending on the age group $r = 0.6$–0.8) and the correlation with body height is generally low. The World Health Organization (WHO) promotes the BMI as a crude indicator for weight judgement. In Table 2.5 the cut-off points for underweight, normal weight, overweight and obesity according to the WHO are given. These cut-off values are based on the relation of BMI with mortality and with risk factors for disease as found in Caucasian populations. The WHO is presently considering adaptation of these cut-off points for other populations.

The cut-off values for BMI as in Table 2.5 cannot be used in children. In younger children, weight compared to height is relatively low, and so is the BMI. During growth, the increase in weight is larger than the increase in height and, consequently, the BMI increases with age during the pubertal phase of life.

Table 2.5 Classification of weight in adults according to body mass index. Reproduced with permission of the World Health Organization.

Classification	Body mass index (kg/m^2)	Risk of comorbidities
Underweight	<18.5	Low
Normal range	18.5–24.9	Average
Overweight	>25.0	
Preobese	25.0–29.9	Increased
Obese class I	30.0–34.9	Moderate
Obese class II	35.0–39.9	Severe
Obese class III	>40	Very severe

Box 2.8

Recent studies have shown that the relationship between body mass index (BMI) and body fat per cent differs among ethnic groups. For example, compared with Caucasian populations some Asian populations have 3–5% more body fat for the same BMI, age and gender. These differences can be explained by differences in body build or frame size, subjects with a smaller frame having more body fat at the same BMI.

These differences can have important consequences for the definition of obesity (based on BMI cut-off values) and the prevalence of obesity in a population. In Indonesia, obesity has recently been redefined as BMI $\geq$ 27 kg/m^2. At this BMI, Indonesians have a comparable body fat with Caucasians with a BMI of 30 kg/m^2. The lowering of the cut-off point for obesity from 30 to 27 kg/m^2 increased the prevalence of obesity from less than 5% to over 10%.

There are age-related BMI cut-off values for obesity for children.

The BMI can also be used as a predictor for the percentage of body fat. Several studies have been published in which a good relationship between the BMI and the amount of body fat (either as fat mass or as body fat percentage) was demonstrated. The relationship between BMI and body fat percentage is age and gender dependent and is different among certain ethnic groups (Box 2.8). When using such age- and gender-specific prediction equations, body fat percentage can be predicted with an error of 3–5%. This error is comparable with the prediction error of other doubly indirect methods, for example skinfold thickness or total body bioelectrical impedance measurements. The disadvantage of these prediction formulae is that they cannot be used in certain subjects or groups of subjects such as pregnant women or body-builders. However, other predictive methods also have their limitations in these subjects.

Box 2.9

From Table 2.6 it can be seen that for the same amount of sub-cutaneous fat (identical skinfold thickness) women have more body fat than men. This is due to the higher internal (organ) fat content in women. It can also be seen (in both females and males) that at equal skinfold thickness older people have more body fat: with age the amount of internal fat increases.

TBW can also be predicted from weight and height and numerous prediction formulae have been published. The standard error of estimate of these equations is, however, considerable.

Skinfold thickness measurements

Body fat is located both internally and subcutaneously. If one assumes a constant relationship between subcutaneous fat and total body fat, then total body fat can be estimated by measuring the amount of the subcutaneous adipose tissue. The amount of subcutaneous tissue can be estimated by measuring the thickness of the subcutaneous fat layer at different sites of the body using a skinfold caliper, infrared interactance or ultrasound measurements. In a given age group, the relation between subcutaneous fat and total fat is indeed relatively constant. However, the relationship is different between males and females, females having relatively more internal fat (Box 2.9). Thus, it is possible by using age- and gender-specific prediction equations to assess the total amount of body fat by measuring skinfolds at different sites of the body.

Skinfolds can be measured all over the body. The most often measured skinfolds for the assessment of total body fat are skinfolds on the upper arm biceps (see Figure 2.5) and triceps, under the scapula (subscapular) and above the iliac crest (suprailiac). The sum of more skinfolds is normally used to reduce the error in measurement and to correct for possible differences in subcutaneous body fat distribution between subjects within the same age and gender group. Various prediction formulae for body fat from skinfold thickness have been published. For children, in whom the relationship between skinfold thickness and body fat depends on biological age, separate formulae must be used.

Measuring skinfolds adequately requires a trained and experienced observer, otherwise excessively large errors in the assessment of the body fat can occur.

Figure 2.5 Measurement of the biceps skinfold.

A disadvantage of the method is that the subject has to be partly undressed. This hampers the use of the method in epidemiological studies. In bed-ridden or seriously ill patients the measurement of the trunk skinfold thicknesses can be difficult. This can be overcome by measuring only the skinfold thickness at the upper arm, for example the triceps. However, the error can be large because the triceps does not necessarily represent the total amount of subcutaneous fat. With advancing age, the triceps skinfold becomes less representative of total body fat.

In elderly subjects, the correlation between skinfold thickness and total body fat as measured by densitometry is generally lower than in young and middle-aged adults. This is due to an increased amount of internal fat in the elderly. Obese subjects are difficult to measure and the error is large even when measured by trained observers. This is also the case in subjects with edema, in whom the thickness of the subcutaneous adipose tissue is easily overestimated. In patients with human immunodeficiency virus (HIV) lipodystrophy, peripheral subcutaneous fat may be almost

Table 2.6 Body fat per cent from the sum of four skinfolds (biceps, triceps, subscapular, suprailiac) in males and females of different ages[a]

Skinfolds (mm)	Age (Males)					Age (Females)				
	17–29	30–39	40–49	⩾50	60–87	17–29	30–39	40–49	⩾50	60–87
20	8	12	12	13	24	14	17	20	22	34
30	13	16	18	19	27	20	22	25	27	37
40	16	19	21	23	29	23	26	28	30	39
50	19	22	25	27	31	27	28	31	33	41
60	21	24	27	29	32	29	31	33	36	42
70	23	25	29	32	33	31	33	35	38	43
80	25	27	31	34	34	33	34	37	40	44
90	26	28	33	36	35	35	36	38	41	45
100	28	29	34	37	36	36	37	40	43	46
110	29	30	36	39	37	38	39	41	44	47
120	30	31	37	40	37	39	40	42	45	48
130	31	32	38	42	38	40	41	43	46	48
140	32	33	39	43	38	41	42	44	47	49
150	33	34	40	44	39	42	43	45	48	49

[a]Based on data from Durnin and Womersley (1974) for the age groups 17 to ⩾50 and on Visser *et al.* (1994) for the elderly. Reproduced with permission.

absent, while abdominal fat is increased. In this situation, skinfolds can be very misleading as indicators of total body fat, and should be used only to assess regional fat.

The calculation of the body fat percentage once the skinfolds have been measured is very simple. For a given skinfold thickness, the amount of body fat can be read from a table (see Table 2.6).

The prediction error in body fat percentage is 3–5% points compared with densitometry, depending on age, gender and level of body fatness. Given the possible error in densitometry (3% points), this means that in extreme cases body fat from skinfolds can be as much as 10–15% points off.

Other anthropometric variables

Measurements of widths of skeletal diameters provide an indication of the amount of skeletal mass. There are formulae that allow the calculation of the skeletal mass from body height, wrist diameter and knee diameter. The current reference data for ideal weight in the USA use the elbow diameter to classify people into three types of body build.

In elderly subjects, the measurement of stature can be difficult owing to kyphosis and/or shrinkage of the spinal vertebrae. Knee height can then be used to predict the maximal stature during lifetime. Arm span is also used for that purpose. However, one has to real-ize that the current prediction formulae are developed in younger populations, in which the relationship between stature and surrogate measurements may be different. In addition, the prediction error (3–5 cm) is relatively high. Knee height can also be used by itself (without predicting total stature), when comparing stature-adjusted body composition between young and old people.

Circumferences of the extremities or the trunk are used to obtain information on body composition. From the mid-arm circumference, in combination with the triceps skinfold thickness, information on muscle mass and fat mass of the upper arm can be obtained. Circumferences of the trunk at waist, hip and upper thigh level are used as indicators of body fat distribution. The WHO suggests an upper limit waist-to-hip circumference ratio above 0.85 for females and 1.00 for males for abdominal fat distribution. Diameters can also be used to gain insights into body fat distribution. A high sagittal diameter compared to transverse diameter of the abdomen is indicative of an enlarged amount of visceral fat. However, it has to be kept in mind that the relationship between these anthropometric parameters of body fat distribution and the intra-abdominal fat determined by CT or MRI scan is generally low. Changes in internal fat detected by MRI are only weakly associated with changes in these anthropometric parameters of fat distribution.

Infrared interactance

The principle of infrared interactance is based on differences in absorbance and reflection of infrared light in different tissues. When the absorbance of near-infrared light (700–1100 nm) is measured at well-defined sites of the body, information on the thickness of the subcutaneous adipose tissue layer can be obtained. In the prediction formulae used, many other parameters are included, such as weight, height, age and gender, and it has been argued that the prediction of body fat depends more on these parameters than on the measured infrared interaction.

Ultrasound measurements

Ultrasound measurements can also be used to study several aspects of body composition. With ultrasound measurements, the thickness of the subcutaneous fat layer can be determined and total body fat can be calculated. A good reflection signal depends heavily on the absence of connective tissue between adipose tissue and muscle. The main difficulty in ultrasound measurements is the exact application of the ultrasound transducer perpendicular to the tissue without any pressure. In the literature, several studies report a good correlation between skinfold thicknesses measured by calipers and measured by ultrasound. The correlation of skinfolds with total body fat was higher compared with ultrasound, suggesting that skinfold thickness measurements have a better predictive value.

Internal abdominal body fat can also be assessed with ultrasound. Studies have shown that ultrasound measurements provide a better method than anthropometry to assess internal abdominal fat depots.

Bioelectrical impedance

In bioelectrical impedance, a small alternating current is applied to the body. It is assumed that the body consists of different components, of which water and dissolved electrolytes are able to conduct the current. Hence, body impedance is a measure of body water. The electrical resistance or impedance of an electrolyte solution depends on several factors, of which the most important are the amount of electrolytes (pure water does not conduct the current), the kind of electrolytes and the temperature of the solution. If currents of low frequency (<5 kHz) are used, body impedance is a measure of ECW, as a low-frequency current cannot penetrate the cell membrane, which acts, with its layers of protein, lipids and proteins, as an electrical capacitor. With increasing frequencies the capacitor features of the cell membrane diminish and gradually ICW also participates in the conductance of the current, resulting in lower impedance values at higher frequencies. Hence, at higher frequencies, TBW is measured. TBW and ECW can be predicted from impedance at high and low frequency, respectively, using empirically derived prediction formulae. Other parameters are often taken into consideration, such as body weight, age and gender.

Most prediction equations are based on statistical relationships between empirically measured impedance index values (height^2/impedance) and body water values obtained by dilution techniques such as deuterium oxide dilution (for TBW) and bromide dilution (for ECW). As body water in healthy subjects is an assumed fixed part (73%) of the FFM, bioelectrical impedance measurements can also be used for the prediction of the FFM and hence body fat percentage. For those prediction equations, the impedance index was related to measures of FFM, normally obtained by densitometry or by DXA.

Body impedance depends on the frequency of the current used and on body water distribution between the extracellular and intracellular space and between the different geometrical body compartments (legs, trunk and arms). This calls for extreme caution in the interpretation of calculated body composition values in situations where body water distribution can be disturbed, as is the case, for example, in dialysis patients and in ascites. In general, prediction formulae based on impedance values are strongly population specific, and age and gender are important contributors. Differences between populations and individual errors are partly caused by differences in body build (e.g. relatively long legs), which is not surprising, as the legs contribute most to total body impedance relative to other parts of the body (Box 2.10).

Currently available impedance analyzers vary in their electrical features and in their principles. Many companies have developed impedance analyzers for personal use, anticipating considerable interest among the public in determining their body fat percentage. There are instruments that measure impedance from foot to foot while standing on a weighing scale and provide not only body weight but also body fat percentage. Other instruments measure impedance from hand to hand and allow the reading of body fat percentage, using a built-in software program in which weight, height, age and gender have to be entered. Combinations of foot-to-foot and hand-to-hand impedance analyzers are also marketed.

As for all other impedance analyzers, the incorporated formulae are population specific and have a prediction error of 4–5%. This means that apart from a systematic error (prediction formula is not valid), the value can be as much as 10% points off in extreme cases. This kind of error is comparable with the possible error in skinfold thickness measurements and hence impedance is no better than skinfold thickness measurements. The advantage is that there is no need to undress and measurements are less prone to observer bias.

Total body electrical conductivity

Total body electrical conductivity (TOBEC) was developed in the 1970s. The principle of the method is that conductive material (body water and dissolved electrolytes) that is placed in an electromagnetic field will cause an inductive current, which is related to the amount of conductive material. In practice, the subject lies on a stretcher, which enters the inner space of an electric wire coil, through which a high-frequency current (2.5–5 MHz) passes. The measurement is very quick (it takes only seconds), painless and without any risk to the subject. The reproducibility of a measurement is within 2% and the error in the predicted FFM was found to be about 3 kg in a group of adult subjects, which is comparable with, for example, skinfold thickness measurements or impedance measurements. The TOBEC method is especially suitable for measurements in infants and young children, in whom bioelectrical impedance measurements are difficult or impossible to perform, owing to movement. The main disadvantage of the method is the high price.

Creatinine excretion and N-*methyl-histidine* excretion

In the muscle cell, creatine phosphate, necessary for the energy metabolism of the cell, degenerates to creatinine at a constant daily rate of about 2%. It is assumed that 1 g of excreted creatinine is equivalent to 18–22 kg of muscle mass. As the cell cannot recycle creatinine, the kidneys excrete it. Since metabolized creatine phosphate is not the only source of urinary creatinine (e.g. creatinine in ingested meat is also excreted immediately), the validity of the method is dubious. A day-to-day coefficient of variation in the excretion of creatinine of almost 20% is reported, when the subject is free living and the urine is sampled over constant periods of 24 h. The high variation is due to the ingestion of creatinine with nonvegetarian meals, differences in physical activity levels and variation in creatinine excretion within the phase of the menstrual cycle. After careful standardization, which includes a controlled diet, the day-to-day variability in excretion can be decreased to about 5%. To obtain a reliable assessment of the creatinine excretion, sampling of urine over multiple 24 h periods is necessary.

The excretion of 3-methylhistidine has also been proposed as a measure for muscle mass. FFM determined by densitometry correlates well with excreted 3-methylhistidine. The chemical determination of 3-methylhistidine is, however, more complicated than that of creatinine. A unique feature of 3-methylhistidine is that it gives a measure of muscle protein breakdown. Given the greater expense of measuring 3-methylhistidine and the limited benefit for muscle mass estimates, it is probably best to use it primarily for turnover studies.

The main disadvantages of creatinine and 3-methylhistidine excretion as measures for body composition are the large variability in excretion, the necessity to follow a controlled (meat-free) diet for several days before and during the urine collections and the difficulties associated with collecting 24 h urine samples.

Use and misuse of body composition data

Information on the body composition of groups of subjects or individuals is important, as body composition is an indicator of nutritional status and also provides information about acute water homeostasis. Depending on what information is needed, several methods are available. However, all have their advantages and

Table 2.7 Buyer's guide to different methods used to determine body composition

Method	Accuracy	Expenses	Radiation	Time	Convenience for subject
Carcass analysis	+++	−−			
Neutron activation	+++	−−	−−	++	++
Densitometry	++	+		++	+/−
Dilution method	++	+/−	(−)	+	+
^{40}K method	++	−		++	++
DXA	+++	+/−	−	++	++
More-compartment models	+++	−	−	−	+
CT scanning	++	−	−−	++	++
MRI scanning	++	−		++	+
Anthropometry	+	+++		++	+
Infrared interactance	+	++		++	++
Bioelectrical impedance	+	+		+++	+++
TOBEC	+	−		++	++
Creatinine/N-methylhistidine excretion	+	+		−	−

DXA: dual-energy X-ray absorptiometry; CT: computed tomography; MRI: magnetic resonance imaging; TOBEC: total body electrical conductivity.

+++: excellent; ++: very good; +: good; +/−: reasonable; −: bad; −−: very bad.

limitations. The price of the method (both the instrument and the required personnel), the eventual stress and danger (e.g. radiation) for the subject and the time necessary to obtain the information determine the choice of the method, as well as the required accuracy. The use in epidemiological studies is different to that in clinical situations or in physiological research. Table 2.7 provides a "buyer's guide" to the several methods discussed in this chapter. It is difficult to generalize as to which method should be used in a given study. Apart from the factors mentioned in Table 2.7, availability plays an important role. Some situations are discussed below.

For the description of body fatness of a large general population group, the calculation of the body fat percentage from the BMI may be as good as or even better than the more expensive information obtained from bioelectrical impedance or the laborious measurement of skinfold thicknesses. Whichever method is to be used for the prediction of body fat percentage in the population, it is important to remember that the formulae used should have been validated in the population under study. The fact that a formula is cross-validated by the authors who published the formula does not mean that the formula is valid in another population. The use of the Durnin and Womersley equations for estimating body fat from the sum of four skinfolds may be correct if the population is adult but younger than about 60 years. In older subjects, the amount of body fat is likely to be underestimated with these formulae. Therefore, their use and thoughtless interpretation in the elderly would lead to completely wrong conclusions about body composition in the elderly and changes in body composition with age. For the same reason, the BMI as an indicator of body fatness is only suitable when corrections for age and gender are made; for example, a BMI of $25 \, \text{kg/m}^2$ at the age of 20 years reflects a much lower percentage of body fat than at the age of 70 years. Body fat in females is always higher than body fat in males with the same BMI and age. Recent studies have shown that the relationship between BMI and body fat percentage also differs among ethnic groups. Prediction equations based on impedance are dependent on body build, among other factors, and there are no universally valid prediction equations based on impedance. Choice of method to assess body composition in a population would also take into consideration within- and between-observer variability. Thus, impedance may be better than skinfold thickness measurements in a study of 1000 people, where variability between technicians is important. One may argue that for population studies, a slight overestimation or underestimation of body fat is not important. However, if for example, obesity is defined as a certain amount of body fat that is achieved at a certain distinct level of BMI, even minor differences in body fat percentage or in BMI will result in large differences in the prevalence of obesity.

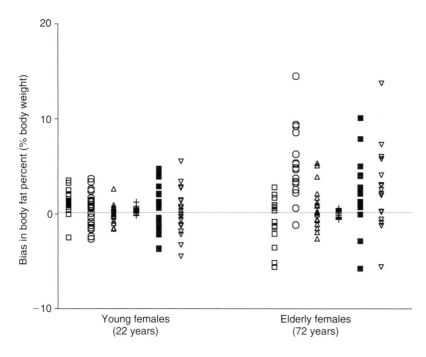

Figure 2.6 Individual differences in measured body fat percentage compared with a chemical four-compartment model in 20 young and 20 elderly females using various techniques. *y*-axis: BF% from four-compartment model minus: □, densitometry (Siri); ○, deuterium dilution; △, DXA; +, three-compartment model (Siri); ■, skinfold thickness; ▽, bioelectrical impedance.

In physiological studies where, for example, energy metabolism has to be corrected for body composition, a systematic bias in body composition results may lead to completely wrong conclusions. When a body composition formula or method systematically overestimates the FFM in obese subjects, a "normal" resting metabolic rate in obese subjects would be underestimated after "correction" for differences in body composition (expressed as kJ/kg FFM). This may lead to the conclusion that obese subjects have lower metabolic rates, which might have caused their excess adipose tissue stores. This argument does not even imply whether the FFM can be treated as one entity in different populations instead of different components such as the heart, liver or muscles. These considerations are important for comparative studies between groups (e.g. obese versus nonobese, elderly versus young or middle-aged), but also for longitudinal studies (e.g. weight-loss studies).

The use of bioelectrical impedance to predict changes in FFM, TBW or body fat during weight loss is questionable. The difference in body water distribution (anatomically as well as intracellular/extracellular) before and after weight loss may be considerable, leading to a different and systematic bias of the prediction equation. In such a study it may be better to report changes in impedance values instead of changes in predicted body composition. Another example is the very low change in impedance after water removal in patients with ascites. Despite the fact that a considerable amount of water is removed from the body, the change in total body impedance is low as the trunk hardly contributes to total body impedance.

All methods have their limitations, doubly indirect more than indirect methods. Figure 2.6 shows the individual errors in body fat percentage from densitometry, DXA, deuterium dilution, a chemical three-compartment model, skinfold thicknesses and bioelectrical impedance in young and elderly females compared with body fat percentage obtained from a four-compartment model. It is obvious that errors can be considerable, both at a group level and especially at an individual level in the elderly. Many of these errors can be explained by the violation of assumptions. This clearly shows that information on body composition must be used with an awareness of the limitations of the techniques.

2.8 Perspectives on the future

Given the importance of body composition to evaluate nutritional status and to gain information on certain disease processes, it can be expected that more easy-to-use methods and instrumentation will be developed and become available in the future. Application and interpretation of data from these methods should be used with an awareness of possible limitations, as mentioned above. There is a growing perception that because of differences in body build, frame size and possibly also other variables, there are differences in the relationship between BMI and body fat percentage among ethnic groups. It seems that some Aboriginal and Asian people have a higher fat percentage and therefore greater risk for several chronic diseases at a given BMI than Caucasian populations. Conversely, Africans often have higher bone density than Caucasians. Much more research is needed to define the optimal BMI values that will correlate with optimal health and the lowest risk of disease for different populations.

Further reading

Durnin JVGA, Womersley J. Body fat assessed from total body density and its estimation from skinfold thickness: measurements on 481 men and women aged from 17 to 72 years. Br J Nutr 1974; 32: 77–97.

Forbes GB. Human Body Composition. New York: Springer, 1987.

Lukaski HC, Bolonchuk WW, Hall CB, Siders WA. Validity of tetrapolar bioelectrical impedance method to assess human body composition. J Appl Physiol 1986; 60: 1327–1332.

Roche AF, Heymsfield SB, Lohman TG. Human Body Composition. Champaign, IL: Human Kinetics, 1996.

Segal KR, Van Loan M, Fitzgerald PI, Hodgdon JA, Van Itallie TB. Lean body mass estimation by bio-electrical impedance analysis: a four site cross-validation study. Am J Clin Nutr 1988; 47: 7–14.

Siri WE. Body composition from fluid spaces and density: analysis of methods. In: Techniques for Measuring Body Composition (J Brozek, A Henschel, eds), pp. 223–244. Washington, DC: National Academy of Sciences, 1961.

Snijder WS, Cook MJ, Nasset ES et al. Report of the Task Group on Reference Man. Oxford: Pergamon Press, 1984.

Visser M, Heuvel van den E, Deurenberg P. Prediction equations for the estimation of body composition in the elderly using anthropometric data. Br J Nutr 1994; 71: 823–833.

Wang Z-M, Pierson RN, Heymsfield SB. The five-level model: a new approach to organise body composition research. Am J Clin Nutr 1992; 56: 19–28.

World Health Organization. Obesity – preventing and managing the global epidemic. Geneva: WHO, 1998.

3
Energy Metabolism

Michael I Goran and Arne Astrup

Key messages

- Energy balance in the body is the balance between how much energy is consumed and how much is expended. Positive balance is when intake exceeds expenditure and is associated with increases in body energy stores (weight gain). During negative balance, as in periods of starvation, body energy stores are depleted.
- Energy intake is the consumption of macronutrients in foods. Carbohydrate provides 16.8 kJ/g, protein also 16.8 kJ/g, fat 37.8 kJ/g and alcohol 29.4 kJ/g.
- Total energy expenditure comprises approximately two-thirds of the energy expended by the body to maintain basic physiological functions plus the thermic effect of a meal and energy expended during physical movement. The basic physiological functions include heart beat, muscle function and respiration (resting or basal metabolic rate). The thermic effect of a meal is about 10% of the caloric value of the meal, needed to digest, metabolize and store ingested macronutrients. The energy expended during physical activity is energy expended when skeletal muscles are used for any type of physical movement. In infants and children, the cost of growth is added.
- Energy requirement is the amount of food energy needed to balance energy expenditure in order to maintain body size, body composition and level of physical activity, consistent with long-term good health. This includes the energy needs for optimal growth and development in children, and the needs of pregnancy and lactation (deposition of tissue and secretion of milk).
- Body mass index (BMI) classifies weight relative to height squared and is the most accepted and widely used crude index of obesity. A BMI of $18–24.9\,kg/m^2$ is regarded as normal for adults, between 25 and $29.9\,kg/m^2$ as overweight and $>30\,kg/m^2$ as obese.
- Energy expenditure can be measured by direct methods (calorimetry) or indirect methods, in which oxygen consumption and carbon dioxide production are used to calculate energy expenditure. However, the modern gold standard is measurement by doubly labeled water, which is a noninvasive method used to measure total energy expenditure over periods of 7–14 days while subjects are living in their usual environments.
- Hunger is the physiological need to eat and results in actions to attempt to obtain food for consumption. Appetite is a psychological desire to eat and is related to the pleasant sensations that are often associated with food. Thus, hunger is more of an intrinsic instinct, whereas appetite is often a learned response.

3.1 Introduction

Definition and conceptualization of energy balance

The average adult human consumes close to one million calories (4000 MJ) per year. Despite this huge energy intake, most healthy individuals are able to strike a remarkable balance between how much energy is consumed and how much energy is expended, thus resulting in a state of energy balance in the body. This accurate balance between energy intake and energy expenditure is an example of homeostatic regulation and results in maintenance of body weight and body energy stores. This regulation of energy balance is achieved over the long term despite large fluctuations in both energy intake and energy expenditure within and between days. The accuracy and precision by which the body maintains energy balance is highlighted by the fact that even a small error in the system can have detrimental consequences over time. If energy intake chronically exceeds energy expenditure by as little as 105 kJ/day, then over time, a person will become substantially obese. The achievement of energy balance is driven by the first law of thermodynamics, which states that energy can be neither destroyed nor created. This principle necessitates that when energy intake equals energy expenditure, body energy stores must remain constant. This chapter explains how the body is able to achieve this state of energy balance through regulation of energy intake and energy expenditure. In addition, the various ways that body energy stores can be measured and some examples of conditions in which energy balance may be disrupted are summarized. Particular emphasis is placed on obesity, which is the end-result of a positive energy balance and is now considered one of the major nutritional disorders.

Components of energy balance

Energy intake
Energy intake is defined as the caloric or energy content of food as provided by the major sources of dietary energy: carbohydrate (16.8 kJ/g), protein (16.8 kJ/g), fat (37.8 kJ/g) and alcohol (29.4 kJ/g).

Energy storage
The energy that is consumed in the form of food or drinks can either be stored in the body in the form of fat (the major energy store), glycogen (short-term energy/carbohydrate reserves) or protein (rarely used by the body for energy except in severe cases of starvation and other wasting conditions, as discussed later in the chapter), or be used by the body to fuel energy-requiring events.

Energy expenditure
The energy that is consumed in the form of food is required by the body for metabolic, cellular and mechanical work such as breathing, heart beat and muscular work, all of which require energy and result in heat production. The body requires energy for a variety of functions. The largest use of energy is needed to fuel the basal metabolic rate (BMR), which is the energy expended by the body to maintain basic physiological functions (e.g. heart beat, muscle contraction and function, respiration). BMR is the minimum level of energy expended by the body to sustain life in the awake state. It can be measured after a 12 h fast while the subject is resting physically and mentally, and maintained in a thermoneutral, quiet environment. The BMR is slightly elevated above the metabolic rate during sleep, because energy expenditure increases above basal levels owing to the energy cost of arousal. Because of the difficulty in achieving basal metabolic rate under most measure-

ment situations, resting metabolic rate (RMR) is frequently measured using the same measurement conditions stated for BMR. Thus, the major difference between BMR and RMR is the slightly higher energy expended during RMR (~3%) due to less subject arousal and nonfasting conditions. Because of this small difference, the terms basal and resting metabolic rate are often used interchangeably. RMR occurs in a continual process throughout the 24 h of a day and remains relatively constant within individuals over time. In the average adult human, RMR is approximately 4.2 kJ/min. Thus, basal or resting metabolic rate is the largest component of energy expenditure and makes up about two-thirds of total energy expenditure.

In addition to RMR, there is an increase in energy expenditure in response to food intake. This increase in metabolic rate after food consumption is often referred to as the thermic effect of a meal (or meal-induced thermogenesis) and is mainly the energy that is expended to digest, metabolize, convert and store ingested macronutrients, named obligatory thermogenesis. The measured thermic effect of a meal is usually higher than the theoretical cost owing to a facultative component caused by an activation of the sympathoadrenal system, which increases energy expenditure through peripheral β-adrenoceptors. The energy cost associated with meal ingestion is primarily influenced by the composition of the food that is consumed, and also is relatively stable within individuals over time. The thermic effect of a meal usually constitutes approximately 10% of the caloric content of the meal that is consumed. The third source of energy expenditure in the body is the increase in metabolic rate that occurs during physical activity, which includes exercise as well as all forms of physical activity. Thus, physical activity energy expenditure (or the thermic effect of exercise) is the term frequently used to describe the increase in metabolic rate that is caused by use of skeletal muscles for any type of physical movement. Physical activity energy expenditure is the most variable component of daily energy expenditure and can vary greatly within and between individuals owing to the volitional and variable nature of physical activity patterns.

In addition to the three major components of energy expenditure, there may be a requirement for energy for three other minor needs.

- The energy cost of growth occurs in growing individuals, but is negligible except within the first few months of life.

- Adaptive thermogenesis is heat production during exposure to reduced temperatures, but rarely occurs in humans except during the initial months of life and during fever and other pathological conditions.
- Thermogenesis is increased by a number of agents in the environment, including in foods and beverages. Nicotine in tobacco is the most important one, and heavy smokers may have a 10% higher energy expenditure than nonsmokers of similar body size and composition, and physical activity. Caffeine and derivatives in coffee, tea and chocolate, capsaicin in hot chillies and other substances in foods and drinks may possess minor thermogenic effects that affect energy expenditure.

Energy balance

Energy balance occurs when the energy content of food is matched by the total amount of energy that is expended by the body. An example of energy balance would be the scenario cited at the onset of this chapter where, over a year, the average adult consumes and expends one million calories, resulting in no net change in the energy content of the body. When energy intake exceeds energy expenditure, a state of positive energy balance occurs. Thus, positive energy balance occurs when excessive overfeeding relative to energy needs occurs, and the body increases its overall energy stores. Examples of positive energy balance include periods around major festivals when overeating and inactivity generally prevail, and during pregnancy and lactation when the body purposefully increases its stores of energy. When energy intake is lower than energy expenditure, a state of negative energy balance occurs, for example during periods of starvation. It is important to note that energy balance can occur regardless of the levels of energy intake and expenditure; thus, energy balance can occur in very inactive individuals as well as in highly active individuals provided that adequate energy sources are available. It is also important to think of energy balance in terms of the major sources of energy, i.e. carbohydrate, protein and fat. For example, carbohydrate balance occurs when the body balances the amount of carbohydrate ingested with that expended for energy.

3.2 Energy intake

Sources of dietary energy

As mentioned above, the sources of energy in the food we eat include the major macronutrients: protein,

carbohydrate and fat, as well as alcohol. Carbohydrate and protein provide 16.8 kJ of energy for each gram; alcohol provides 29.4 kJ/g, while fat is the most energy dense, providing 37.8 kJ/g. Note that 4.2 kJ is defined as the amount of heat that is required to raise the temperature of 1 litre of water by 1°C. The energy content of food can be measured by bomb calorimetry, which involves combusting a known weight of food inside a sealed chamber and measuring the amount of heat that is released during this process. Thus, 1 g of pure fat would release 37.8 kJ during its complete combustion, while 1 g of pure carbohydrate would release 16.8 kJ. Thus, if the gram quantities of any type of food are known, the energy content can easily be calculated. For example, if a protein-rich nutrition snack contains 21 g of carbohydrate, 6 g of fat and 14 g of protein, then the total energy content is $(21 \times 16.9) + (6 \times 37.8) + (14 \times 16.8) = 814.8$ kJ. The macronutrient composition of food is typically assessed in the percentage contribution of each macronutrient to the total number of calories. In this example, the carbohydrate content is 21 g, which is 352.8 kJ, or 43% of the total energy in the bar, the fat content is 6 g, or 226.8 kJ, equivalent to 28% of the energy, and the protein contributes 14 g, 226.8 kJ and 29% of the energy.

Regulation of food intake

Appetite, hunger and satiety

The quality and quantity of food that is consumed are closely regulated by the body. Food intake is regulated by a number of factors involving complex interactions among various hormones, neuroendocrine factors, the central nervous system and organ systems (e.g. brain and liver), and environmental and external factors.

Appetite is usually defined as a psychological desire to eat and is related to the pleasant sensations that are often associated with specific foods. Scientifically, appetite is used as a general term of overall sensations related to food intake.

Hunger is usually defined as the subjective feeling that determines when food consumption is initiated and can be described as a nagging, irritating feeling that signifies food deprivation to a degree that the next eating episode should take place.

Satiety is considered as the state of inhibition over eating that leads to the termination of a meal, and related to the time interval until the next eating episode. Thus, hunger and satiety are more intrinsic instincts, whereas appetite is often a learned response.

The internal factors that regulate the overall feeling of hunger and satiety include the central nervous system (primarily the hypothalamus and the vagus nerve), the major digestive organs such as the stomach and liver, and various hormones. In addition, environmental factors (e.g. meal pattern and composition, food availability, smell and sight of foods, climate), emotional factors (e.g. stress) and some diseased states (e.g. anorexia, trauma, infection) may influence the feelings of both hunger and appetite. The factors that influence appetite include factors external to the individual (e.g. climate, weather), specific appetite cravings, specific learned dislikes or avoidance (e.g. alcohol), intrinsic properties of food (e.g. taste, palatability, texture), cultural practices or preferences, specific effects of some drugs and diseases, and metabolic factors such as hormones and neurotransmitters. Some of these factors are described in further detail below.

Factors influencing food intake

Digestive factors
Several factors in the digestive system exert a short-term influence over food intake. The presence of food and drink in the stomach and intestine and the resultant pressure that they exert may regulate food intake. This effect is known as gastrointestinal distension. In addition, the stomach produces a hormone called cholecystokinin (CCK) in response to food intake, which may, in turn, regulate food intake. Furthermore, when subjects have fat or carbohydrate infused directly into the small intestine, they report feelings of satiety. This suggests that factors in the intestine regulate food intake. Indeed, receptors in the intestine have been identified that recognize the presence of specific macronutrients; these receptors are linked to the brain and therefore can communicate directly with the central nervous system, resulting in regulation of energy balance. In addition, other gastrointestinal hormones, such as glucagon-like peptide-1 and -2 (GLPs), CCK and glucose-dependent insulinotropic polypeptide (GIP), are likely to play a role in the mediation of gut events and brain perception of hunger and satiety.

Central nervous system factors
The main contributory factor regulating food intake in the central nervous system is the hypothalamus. The hypothalamus is linked to specific parts of the brain that are known to modify feeding behavior, specifically the paraventicular nuclei and the nigrostriatal tract. These

areas of the brain respond to various neurotransmitters as well as sympathetic nervous system activity. In general, food intake will decrease as sympathetic nervous system activity increases, and vice versa.

Circulating factors
After consumption of a meal food is broken down into its basic components (i.e. carbohydrate is broken down to glucose, protein to amino acids, and fats or triglycerides to glycerol and fatty acids) and the circulating levels of some of these breakdown products increase in the blood. Consequently, glucose, amino acids, glycerol and fatty acids are further metabolized, primarily in the liver, or used for immediate energy (e.g. in muscle or brain). There is evidence to suggest that this resultant metabolism, especially in the liver, may in turn regulate food intake. After meal consumption, the circulating levels of nutrients fall (within minutes for glucose, several hours for triglycerides) and the feelings of hunger return. The link from nutrient metabolism to central control of food intake occurs through signals from the liver to the brain via the vagus nerve. Thus, circulating factors provide a link between the digestive system and the central nervous system which provides another system for regulating food intake.

Neurological and hormonal factors
Numerous hormones, neuroendocrine factors and drugs are known to influence eating behavior through their direct or indirect effects on neurotransmitters in the brain. These factors may have specific or general effects on food intake. Examples of hormonal influences include insulin, cortisol, glucagon and the gastrointestinal hormones (e.g. secretin, CCK, GIP, GLP-1). Insulin is of particular importance because it can modify initiation as well as completion of food intake. Examples of neurotransmitters (or neuroendocrine factors) include histamine (decreases food intake), neuropeptide Y (linked to carbohydrate craving), serotonin (linked to food intake in general) and galanin (linked to dietary fat intake). Another important and recently discovered hormone that may regulate food intake is leptin. Leptin is a hormone that is produced by fat cells and communicates with the central nervous system through leptin receptors in the hypothalamus. Reduced production of leptin, or lack of sensitivity of the hypothalamus to leptin, may regulate food intake and play a key role in the etiology of rare forms of obesity in humans.

External factors

Various nonphysiological or external factors are also known to modify food intake, and these effects may be mediated through the intrinsic factors described above. Psychological factors such as depression may lead to either increased or decreased food intake, or changes in the consumption of specific types of foods. Environmental factors are also important, the most obvious being food availability. Even when food is available, some of the specific properties of food make them more or less appealing, thereby modifying food intake. Important physical characteristics of food include taste, texture, color, temperature and presentation. Other cultural influences in the environment, such as time of day, social factors, peer influence and cultural preferences, can also play a role in influencing food intake.

3.3 Energy expenditure

Concept of energy expenditure

The process of energy expenditure and the oxidation or combustion of food for energy in the body is analogous to a wood-stove that burns wood to release heat in a controlled fashion. In this analogy, large chunks of wood are fed to the stove and the wood is gradually combusted in the presence of oxygen to release carbon dioxide, water vapor and heat. Similarly, in the body, the food consumed is oxidized or combusted in the presence of oxygen to release carbon dioxide, water and heat. When ingested food is used for energy, however, the release and transfer of energy occur through a series of tightly regulated metabolic pathways in which the potential energy from food is released slowly and gradually over time. This process ensures that the body is provided with a gradual and constant energy store, rather than relying on a sudden release of energy from an immediate combustion of ingested food. As a simple example of how the body uses food for energy, consider the combustion of a simple glucose molecule:

$$C_6H_{12}O_6 + 6O_2 \rightarrow 6H_2O + 6CO_2 + Heat$$

Similar chemical reactions can be described for the combustion of other sources of energy, such as fat and other types of carbohydrates. These types of reaction occur continuously in the body and constitute energy expenditure. As discussed previously, the three major sources of energy expenditure in the body are to fuel RMR, the thermic effect of meals and physical activity.

As discussed in more detail below, energy expenditure can be measured by assessment of total heat production in the body (direct calorimetry) or by assessment of oxygen consumption and carbon dioxide production (indirect calorimetry).

Historical aspects of energy expenditure

The burning or combustion of food in the body was originally described in the classic experiments of Lavoisier, who worked in France in the late eighteenth century. Lavoisier discovered that a candle would only burn in the presence of oxygen. In addition, he was the first to describe how living organisms produced heat in a similar way, as they required oxygen for life and combusted food as they released heat. His experiments were the first to document the heat production of living organisms. Working before the invention of electricity, he built the first calorimeter in which a small animal was placed in a sealed chamber. Lavoisier packed ice into a sealed pocket around the chamber (he could only perform these studies in the winter when ice was collected from the ground), and then placed the chamber and ice layer inside an insulated chamber. Lavoisier then collected and measured the volume of melting water. Since the ice layer was insulated from the outside world, the only way that the ice could melt was by the increase in heat produced by the living animal. Lavoisier therefore measured the volume of melted ice water, and by so doing, was able to calculate accurately the amount of heat that had to be produced by the animal to melt the measured amount of ice.

Measurement of energy expenditure

Lavoisier's device was the first calorimeter that was used to measure heat production. This approach is termed direct calorimetry because heat production is measured directly. Direct calorimeters have been designed for measuring heat production in humans, but this approach is technically demanding, especially in human studies, and is now infrequently used. Indirect calorimetry measures energy production via respiratory gas analysis. This approach is based on oxygen consumption and carbon dioxide production that occurs during the combustion (or oxidation) of protein, carbohydrate, fat and alcohol, as shown in the example of glucose combustion. Respiratory gas analysis can easily be achieved in humans either over short measurement periods at rest or during exercise using a face mask, mouthpiece or canopy system for gas collection, and over longer periods of 24 h (and longer) with subjects living in a metabolic chamber. BMR is typically measured by indirect calorimetry under fasted conditions while subjects lie quietly at rest in the early morning for 30–40 min. The thermic effect of a meal is typically measured by monitoring the changes in metabolic rate by indirect calorimetry for 3–6 h following consumption of a test meal of known caloric content. The energy expended in physical activity can be measured under laboratory conditions, also using indirect calorimetry during standard activities. In addition, free-living physical activity-related energy expenditure over extended periods of up to 2 weeks can be measured by the combination of doubly labeled water (DLW) to measure total energy expenditure (see below), and indirect calorimetry to measure resting energy expenditure and the thermic effect of a meal. Indirect calorimetry has an added advantage in that the ratio of carbon dioxide production to oxygen consumption (the respiratory quotient, or RQ) is indicative of the type of substrate (i.e. fat versus carbohydrate) being oxidized, for example carbohydrate oxidation has an RQ of 1.0 and fat oxidation has an RQ close to 0.7.

Energy expenditure can be assessed from indirect calorimetry in a simple, less accurate way by ignoring the contribution of protein oxidation or by collecting urine during the measurement to analyze the excreted nitrogen. The latter approach is preferable because it gives a more accurate estimate of energy expenditure and RQ.

Step 1

First, the contribution of protein oxidation to oxygen consumption ($\dot{V}_{O_2}$) and carbon dioxide production ($\dot{V}_{CO_2}$) is estimated based on the knowledge that the nitrogen content of protein is 1/6.25:

$$\dot{V}_{O_2(prot)} = n \times 6.25 \times 0.97$$
$$\dot{V}_{CO_2(prot)} = n \times 6.25 \times 0.77$$

where V = volume, 0.97 and 0.77 are litres of O_2 consumed and CO_2 produced by the biological oxidation of 1 g of protein, and prot = protein.

Step 2

Next, nonprotein $\dot{V}_{O_2}$ ($\dot{V}_{O_2(nonprot)}$) and nonprotein $\dot{V}_{CO_2}$ ($\dot{V}_{CO_2(nonprot)}$) are calculated:

$$\dot{V}_{O_2(nonprot)} = \dot{V}_{O_2} - \dot{V}_{O_2(prot)}$$
$$\dot{V}_{CO_2(nonprot)} = \dot{V}_{CO_2} - \dot{V}_{CO_2(prot)}$$

$$\dot{V}_{O_2(nonprot)} = C \times 0.828 + F \times 2.03$$
$$\dot{V}_{CO_2(nonprot)} = C \times 0.828 + F \times 1.43$$

where C and F are grams of oxidized carbohydrate and fat and can be found by solving the two equations with two unknowns. O_2 and CO_2 produced by the combustion of 1 g of carbohydrate equal 0.828 l, while the combustion of 1 g triglyceride consumes 2.03 l O_2 and produces 1.43 l CO_2. The protein oxidation (P) is $n \times 6.25$ g.

Step 3

The RQ is defined as:

$$\dot{V}_{CO_2}/\dot{V}_{O_2}$$

Nonprotein RQ ($RQ_{(nonprot)}$) is calculated by the equation:

$$RQ_{(nonprot)} = \dot{V}_{CO_2(nonprot)}/\dot{V}_{O_2(nonprot)}$$

Step 4

Next, energy expenditure can be calculated:

$$\text{Energy expenditure (kJ/min)} = [19.63 + 4.59 \, (RQ_{(nonprot)} - 0.707] \times \dot{V}_{O_2(nonprot)} + 18.78 \times \dot{V}_{O_2(nonprot)}$$

or:

$$\text{Energy expenditure (kJ/min)} = 17 \times P + 17.5 \times C + 38.9 \times F$$

where 17, 17.5 and 38.9 are the heat produced (kJ) by the combustion of 1 g of protein, glycogen and triglyceride.

The equations are produced by the insertion of the heat equivalent for carbohydrate and fat, and are valid even though there is a quantitative conversion of carbohydrate to lipid (*de novo* lipogenesis) or glyconeogenesis.

The caloric equivalent for O_2 is similar to the three main substrates: 21 kJ/l O_2 for carbohydrate, 19 kJ/l O_2 for fat and 17.8 kJ/l O_2 for protein (which only contributes modestly to energy expenditure). Energy expenditure can therefore be calculated with reasonable accuracy by the equation:

$$\text{Energy expenditure (kJ/min)} = 20 \, \text{kJ/l} \times \dot{V}_{O_2} \, \text{(l/min)}$$

With pure fat oxidation the RQ is 0.707, with pure carbohydrate oxidation it is 1.0 and with pure protein oxidation it is approximately 0.8.

Step 5

Oxidation of protein (P), carbohydrate (C) and fat (F) can be calculated by the following equations, where n is the unit g/min:

$$P \text{ (g/min)} = 6.25 \times n$$
$$C \text{ (g/min)} = 4.55 \times \dot{V}_{CO_2} - 3.21 \times \dot{V}_{O_2} - 2.87$$
$$F \text{ (g/min)} = 1.67 \times \dot{V}_{O_2} - 1.67 \times \dot{V}_{CO_2} - 1.92 \times n$$

3.4 Factors that influence energy expenditure

Resting metabolic rate

Each of the components of energy expenditure is determined by various factors. RMR is highly variable between individuals ($\pm 25\%$), but is very consistent within individuals ($<5\%$). Since RMR occurs predominantly in muscle and the major organs of the body, the main source of individual variability in resting metabolic rate is an individual's amount of organ and muscle mass. Thus, fat-free mass (FFM; the total mass of the body that is not fat, i.e. predominantly organs and muscle) explains 60–80% of the variation in resting metabolic rate between individuals. This concept can be explained using the wood-stove analogy; the larger the wood-stove (or FFM), the larger the amount of heat production (or the larger the resting metabolic rate). Since FFM is a heterogeneous mixture of all nonfat body components, the metabolic rate associated with each kilogram of FFM is dependent on the quality of the FFM, in terms of hydration and relative contribution of the different organs that make up the FFM. For example, skeletal muscle compromises approximately 43% of total mass in an adult, but only contributes 22–36% of the RMR, whereas the brain, which constitutes approximately only 2% of mass, contributes 20–24% of the RMR. In addition, the metabolic cost of each kilogram of FFM decreases with developmental progression, probably owing to developmental increases in the muscle mass to organ mass ratio within FFM. Thus, the relationship between RMR and FFM is not linear across all ages and is estimated to be 331.8 kJ/kg between the ages of 0 and 2.5 years, 151.2 kJ/kg in 4–7-year-old children, 88.2 kJ/kg during adolescence and 151.2 kJ/kg in adulthood.

RMR is also influenced by fat mass, even though fat mass is generally thought to be metabolically inert. Fat mass contributes in the order of 42.0–54.6 kJ/kg to RMR. In healthy adults, RMR declines with age, over and

above that expected given the age-related decline in FFM. RMR is also influenced by gender, in that males have a higher value than females by approximately 210 kJ/day. This difference is independent of the gender difference in FFM; in other words, if one studied a group of males and females of identical FFM and similar age, RMR would be higher in males than females by around 210.0 kJ/day. This gender difference is consistent across the lifespan, and the source of the difference is not well understood (see Table 3.1). More active people tend to have a higher RMR than inactive individuals. This difference may be explained in part by the residual effects of chronic exercise on metabolic rate. In other words, RMR appears to be elevated because of the long-lasting effects of the thermic effect of exercise. However, other factors are also involved, since the higher RMR in more active individuals persists long after the last bout of exercise has been completed. Collectively, FFM, fat mass, age, gender and physical activity explain 80–90% of the variance in RMR. In addition, a portion of the unique variance in RMR across individuals has been ascribed to genetic factors, although the specific source of this genetic variation has not yet been identified. Other factors that have been shown to influence metabolic rate include thyroid hormones (higher levels increase metabolic rate) and sympathetic nervous system activity.

Table 3.1 Variation in total energy expenditure (TEE) as a function of resting metabolic rate (RMR) among various populations

Study group	Average TEE/RMR (range)
5-year-old children in Arizona, USA	1.37 (1.15–1.70)
Obese women in the UK	1.39 (1.20–1.77)
Elderly women in Vermont, USA	1.42 (1.25–1.82)
5-year-old children in Vermont, USA	1.44 (1.11–1.77)
Elderly men in Vermont, USA	1.50 (1.30–2.11)
Obese Pima Indians	1.56 (1.03–1.99)
Adolescents in the UK	1.56
Dutch adults	1.64
Obese women in New York, USA	1.68
Young men in Boston, USA	1.70 (1.38–2.32)
Obese women in New York, USA	1.73
Elderly men in Boston, USA	1.74
Young men in the UK	1.88 (1.44–2.57)
Young men in Boston, USA	1.98 (1.57–2.60)
Mount Everest climbers	
Tour de France cyclists	
Burn patients	

Range of TEE/RMR is given in parentheses for studies in which the individual data were reported.

Table 3.2 Simple equations for estimating resting metabolic rate (RMR) from body weight according to gender and age

| Age (years) | RMR (kJ/day) | |
	Equation for males	Equation for females
0–3	$(60.9 \times$ wt$) - 54$	$(61.0 \times$ wt$) - 51$
3–10	$(22.7 \times$ wt$) + 495$	$(22.5 \times$ wt$) + 499$
10–18	$(17.5 \times$ wt$) + 651$	$(12.2 \times$ wt$) + 746$
18–30	$(15.3 \times$ wt$) + 679$	$(14.7 \times$ wt$) + 496$
30–60	$(11.6 \times$ wt$) + 879$	$(8.7 \times$ wt$) + 829$
>60	$(13.5 \times$ wt$) + 487$	$(10.5 \times$ wt$) + 596$

wt: body weight (kg).

Several prediction equations have been developed to estimate RMR from other simple measures. These equations are often useful for making estimates in clinical situations when measurement of RMR cannot be achieved, or for estimating energy needs for other individuals. The classic equations of Harris and Benedict are frequently used for this purpose. These equations were developed from limited measures performed in the early 1900s, and predict RMR from age, height and weight, and may be of limited accuracy. More recent equations have been developed in larger groups of subjects and can predict RMR from body weight (Table 3.2). These new equations have been shown to be more accurate.

Thermic effect of feeding

The thermic effect of meal ingestion is primarily influenced by the quantity and macronutrient quality of the ingested calories. The thermic effect of food has also been termed meal-induced thermogenesis, or the specific dynamic action of food. The increase in metabolic rate that occurs after meal ingestion occurs over an extended period of at least 5 h; the cumulative energy cost is equivalent to around 10% of the energy ingested. In other words, if one consumed a mixed meal of 2.1 MJ, the body would require 210.0 kJ to digest, process and metabolize the contents of the meal. The thermic effect of feeding is higher for protein and carbohydrate than for fat. This is because for fat, the process of energy storage is very efficient, whereas for carbohydrate and protein, additional energy is required for metabolic conversion to the appropriate storage form (i.e. excess glucose converted to glycogen for storage, and excess amino acids from protein converted to fat for storage). In addition to the obligatory energetic cost of processing

and storage of nutrients, a more variable facultative thermogenic component has been described. This component is mainly pertinent to carbohydrates, which through increased insulin secretion produce a diphasic activation of the sympathoadrenal system. The initial phase in an insulin-mediated increase in sympathetic activity, which produces a β-adrenoceptor mediated increase in energy expenditure. The second and later phase occurs when a counter-regulatory increase in plasma adrenaline is elicited by the falling blood glucose. This increase in adrenaline has a similar slight stimulatory effect on energy expenditure. As a result of the mediation by β-adrenoceptors the thermic effect of carbohydrate-rich meals can be slightly reduced by pharmacological β-adrenoceptor antagonists.

Energy expenditure related to physical activity

Physical activity energy expenditure encompasses all types of activity, including sports and leisure, work-related activities, general activities of daily living and fidgeting. The metabolic rate of physical activity is determined by the amount or duration of activity (i.e. time), the type of physical activity (e.g. walking, running, typing) and the intensity at which the particular activity is performed. The metabolic cost of physical activities is frequently expressed as metabolic equivalents (METs), which represent multiples of RMR. Thus, by definition, sitting quietly after a 12 h fast is equivalent to 1 MET. Table 3.3 provides MET equivalents for other typical physical activities. The cumulative total daily energy cost of physical activity is highly variable both within and between individuals. Therefore, physical activity provides the greatest source of plasticity or flexibility in the energy expenditure system, and is the component through which large changes in energy expenditure can be achieved.

Total energy expenditure: measurement by doubly labeled water

The integrated sum of all components of energy expenditure is termed total energy expenditure. Until recently, there was no good way to measure total energy expenditure in humans living under their habitual conditions. Total energy expenditure can be measured over 24 h or longer in a metabolic chamber, but this environment is artificial and is not representative of the normal daily pattern of physical activity. The DLW

Table 3.3 Examples of metabolic equivalence (MET) values for various physical activities

Activity	MET
Basketball	8.0
Chopping wood	6.0
Cleaning house	2.0–4.0
Cycling for pleasure	8.0
Gardening	5.0
Kayaking	5.0
Mowing lawn (power mower)	4.5
Painting house	4.0–5.0
Playing musical instrument	2.0–4.0
Running slowly (8–11 km/h)	8.0–10.0
Running quickly (14–16 km/h)	16.0–18.0
Soccer	7.0–10.0
Strength training	6.0
Stretching	4.0
Tennis	6.0–8.0
Skiing	7.0–14.0
Swimming laps	6.0–12.0
Walking	3.0–5.0
Water skiing	6.0

technique can be used to obtain an integrated measure of all components of daily energy expenditure over extended periods, typically 7–14 days, while subjects are living in their usual environment. The technique was first introduced in the 1950s as an isotopic technique for measuring the carbon dioxide production rate in small animals. Unfortunately, it was not possible to apply the technique to humans because the dose required was cost prohibitive given the relatively poor sensitivity of the required instrumentation at that time. It was not for another 20 years that the inventors of this technique described the feasibility of applying the technique to measure free-living energy expenditure in humans, and 10 years later this concept became a reality.

The DLW method requires a person to ingest small amounts of "heavy" water that is isotopically labeled with deuterium and oxygen-18 (^2H_2O and $H_2{}^{18}O$). These forms of water are naturally occurring, stable (nonradioactive) isotopes of water that differ from the most abundant form of water. In deuterium-labeled water, the hydrogen is replaced with deuterium, which is an identical form of water except that deuterium has an extra neutron in its nucleus compared with hydrogen, and is thus a heavier form of water; similarly, ^{18}O-labeled water contains oxygen with an additional two extra neutrons. Thus, these stable isotopes act as molecular tags so that water can be tracked in the body. After a loading

dose, deuterium-labeled water is washed out of the body as a function of body water turnover; ^{18}O is also lost as a function of water turnover, but is lost via carbon dioxide production as well. Therefore, using a number of assumptions, the rate of carbon dioxide production and energy expenditure can be assessed based on the different rates of loss of these isotopes from the body.

The major advantages of the DLW method are that the methodology is truly noninvasive and nonobtrusive (subjects are entirely unaware that energy expenditure is being measured), and measurement is performed under free-living conditions over extended periods (7–14 days). Moreover, when used in combination with indirect calorimetry for assessment of resting metabolic rate, physical activity-related energy expenditure can be assessed by the difference (i.e. total energy expenditure minus resting metabolic rate, minus the thermic effect of meals = physical activity energy expenditure). The additional power of assessing total energy expenditure with the DLW method is that this approach can provide a measure of total energy intake in subjects who are in energy balance. This is because, by definition, in a state of energy balance, total energy intake must be equivalent to total energy expenditure. This aspect of the technique has been used as a tool to validate energy intakes using other methods such as food records and dietary recall. For example, it has been known for some time that obese subjects report a lower than expected value for energy intake. At one time it was thought that this was due to low energy requirements in the obese due to low energy expenditure and reduced physical activity. However, using DLW, it has now been established that obese subjects systematically underreport their actual energy intake by 30–40% and actually have a normal energy expenditure, relative to their larger body size.

The major disadvantages of the technique are the periodic nonavailability and expense of the ^{18}O isotope (around US$550 for a 70 kg adult), the need for and reliance on expensive equipment for analysis of samples, and that the technique is not well suited to large-scale epidemiological studies. Furthermore, although the technique can be used to obtain estimates of physical activity energy expenditure, it does not provide any information on physical activity patterns (i.e. type, duration and intensity of physical activity periods during the day).

The DLW technique has been validated in humans in several laboratories around the world by comparison with indirect calorimetry in adults and infants.

These studies generally show the technique to be accurate to within 5–10%, relative to data derived by indirect calorimetry for subjects living in metabolic chambers. The theoretical precision of the DLW technique is 3–5%. However, the experimental variability is ±12% under free-living conditions, owing to fluctuations in physical activity levels, and ±8% under more controlled sedentary living conditions. The good accuracy and reasonable precision of the technique therefore allow the DLW method to be used as a "gold standard" measure of free-living energy expenditure in humans against which other methods can be compared.

3.5 Energy requirements

How much energy do we need to sustain life and maintain our body energy stores? Why do some people require more energy and others less? In other words, what are the energy requirements of different types of people? Based on our earlier definition of energy balance, the energy needs or energy requirements of the body to maintain energy balance must be equal to total daily energy expenditure. Total daily energy expenditure is the sum of the individual components of energy expenditure as discussed previously, and represents the total energy requirements of an individual that are required to maintain energy balance. Until recently, there was no accurate way to measure total energy expenditure or energy needs of humans. The DLW technique has provided a truly noninvasive means to measure accurately total daily energy expenditure, and thus energy needs, in free-living humans. Before DLW, energy requirements were usually assessed by measurement or prediction of RMR, the largest component of energy requirements. However, since the relationship between RMR and total energy expenditure is highly variable because of differences in physical activity, the estimation of energy needs from knowledge of RMR is not that accurate and requires a crude estimate of physical activity level. Nevertheless, reasonable estimates can be made to estimate daily energy budgets for individuals (Table 3.4).

Following the validation of DLW in humans, this technique has been applied to many different populations. Total energy expenditure is often compared across groups or individuals using the ratio of one's total energy expenditure to RMR, or physical activity level (PAL). Thus, for example, if the total energy expenditure was

Table 3.4 Typical daily energy budgets for a sedentary and a physically active individual of identical occupation, body weight and resting metabolic rate of 6.0 MJ/day (4.2 kJ/min)

Activity	Activity index	Minutes per day		MJ per day	
		Sedentary	Active	Sedentary	Active
Sleep	1.0	480	480	2.0	2.0
Daily needs	1.06	120	120	5.3	5.3
Occupational	1.5	480	480	3.0	3.0
Passive recreation	2.0	360	300	3.0	2.5
Exercise	12.0	0	60	0	3.0
Total		1440	1440	8.6	11.1
				PAL = 1.4	PAL = 1.8

Thus, the sedentary individual would need to perform 60 min of vigorous activity each day at an intensity of 12.0 to increase the physical activity level (PAL) from a sedentary 1.4 to an active and healthy 1.8.

12.6 MJ/day and the RMR was 6.3 MJ/day, the PAL factor would be 2.0. This value indicates that total energy expenditure is twice the RMR. The PAL factor has been assessed in a variety of types of individual. A low PAL indicates a sedentary lifestyle, whereas a high PAL represents a highly active lifestyle. The highest recorded sustained PAL in humans was recorded in cyclists participating in the Tour de France road race. These elite athletes could sustain a daily energy expenditure that was up to five times their RMR over extended periods. Smaller animals, such as migrating birds, have a much higher ceiling for achieving higher rates of total energy expenditure, which can reach up to 20 times their RMR.

Factors such as body weight, FFM and RMR account for 40–60% of the variation in total energy expenditure. Total energy expenditure is similar between lean and obese individuals after taking into account differences in FFM. Thus, fatness has negligible effects on total energy expenditure, other than the small effect on RMR, as discussed previously. The lack of effect of increased body fat on total energy expenditure is probably due to the opposing effects of:

- the additional energy cost of weight-bearing activities in subjects with greater body fat and the greater RMR associated with the increased fat mass, versus
- the decreased likelihood of physical activity that is associated with carrying additional fat mass.

With regard to age, some studies suggest that only a limited change in total energy expenditure (relative to RMR) occurs from childhood to adulthood, but that a decline occurs in the elderly. Recent data also suggest a gender-related difference in total energy expenditure, in addition to that previously described for RMR. In a meta-analysis that examined data from a variety of published studies, absolute total energy expenditure was significantly higher in males than in females by 3.1 MJ/day (10.2 ± 2.1 MJ/day in females, 13.3 ± 3.1 MJ/ day in males), and nonresting energy expenditure remained higher in men by 1.1 MJ/day.

Individuals who have sedentary occupations and do not participate frequently in leisure pursuits that require physical activity probably have a PAL factor in the region of 1.4. Those who have occupations requiring light activity and participate in light physical activities in leisure time probably have a PAL around 1.6 (this is a typical value for sedentary people living in an urban environment). Individuals who have physically active occupations and lifestyles probably have a PAL greater than 1.75. It has been suggested that the optimal PAL that protects against the development of obesity is around 1.8 or higher. Increasing one's physical activity index from 1.6 to 1.8 requires 30 min of daily vigorous activity, or 60 min of light activity (Table 3.4).

3.6 Energy balance in various conditions

Infancy and childhood

Changes in energy intake during infancy have been well characterized. During the first 12 months of life, energy intake falls from almost 525 kJ/kg per day in the first month of life to a nadir of 399 kJ/kg per day by the eighth month, then rises to 441 kJ/kg per day by the 12th month. However, total energy expenditure in the first year of life is relatively constant at around 252–294 kJ/kg per day. In infants, the large difference between total energy expenditure and energy intake is explained by a positive energy balance to account for growth. In the first 3 months of life it is estimated that the energy accretion due to growth is 701.4 kJ/day, or approximately 32% of energy intake, falling to 151.2 kJ/day, or 4% of energy intake, by 1 year of age. Individual growth rates and early infancy feeding behavior are at least two known factors that would cause variation in these figures.

There is now substantial evidence to suggest that existing recommendations may overestimate true energy needs, based on measurement of total energy expenditure in infants. In the first year of life, traditional values of energy requirements overestimate those derived from measurement of total energy expenditure and adjusted for growth by 11%. Between 1 and 3 years of age the discrepancy is more striking, where the traditional values for requirements are 20% higher than those derived from total energy expenditure and adjusted for growth. For example, in 3-year-old children total energy expenditure by DLW averages 5.1 MJ/day, while the currently recommended intake for these children is 6.2 MJ/day. Thus, newer estimates of the energy needs of infants are needed based on assessment of total energy expenditure data.

Several laboratories have reported measurements of total energy expenditure in young, healthy, free-living children around the world. Despite marked differences in geographical locations, the data are similar, although environmental factors such as season and sociocultural influences on physical activity can influence total energy expenditure and thus energy requirements. In the average 5-year-old child weighing 20 kg, total energy expenditure is approximately 5.5–5.9 MJ/day, which is significantly lower than the existing recommended daily allowance for energy in children of this age, by approximately 1.7–2.1 MJ/day. Thus, as with infants, newer estimates of energy needs in children are needed based on assessment of total energy expenditure data.

Aging

In the elderly, two different problems related to energy balance can be recognized. In one segment of the elderly population there is a decline in food intake that is associated with dynamic changes in body composition where there is a tendency to lose FFM, which leads to loss in functionality. In others there is a tendency to gain fat mass, which increases the risk for obesity, cardiovascular disease and noninsulin-dependent diabetes. These two opposing patterns suggest that the ability to self-regulate whole body energy balance may diminish with aging. Thus, prescription of individual energy requirements may serve as a useful tool to prevent the age-related deterioration of body composition. Other special considerations in the elderly relate to meeting energy needs in special populations, such as those suffering from Alzheimer's and Parkinson's disease, which frequently can lead to malnourished states and a diminishing of body weight. It was thought that these neurological conditions may lead to body weight loss because of an associated hypermetabolic condition in which metabolic rate may increase above normal, thus increasing energy needs. However, more recent studies have clearly shown that the wasting or loss of body weight often associated with these conditions is explained by a reduction in food intake, probably due to a loss in functionality.

Energy requirements in physically active groups

The DLW technique has been used to assess energy requirements in highly physically active groups of people. The most extreme case is a study that assessed the energy requirements of cyclists performing in the 3-week-long Tour de France bicycle race. The level of total energy expenditure recorded (PAL factor of 5.3, or approximately 35.7 MJ/day) was the highest recorded sustained level in humans. In another study involving young male soldiers training for jungle warfare, energy requirements were 19.9 MJ/day (PAL factor of 2.6). The total energy expenditure of four mountaineers climbing Mount Everest was 13.6 MJ/day (PAL 2.0–2.7), which was similar to energy expenditure during on-site preparation prior to climbing (14.7 MJ/day). Total energy expenditure in free-living collegiate swimmers was almost 16.8 MJ/day in men and 10.9 MJ/day in women. In elite female runners previously performed studies of energy intake suggested unusually low energy requirements. However, in a study in nine highly trained young women, free-living energy expenditure was 11.9 ± 1.3 MJ/day, compared with the reported energy intake of 9.2 ± 1.9 MJ/day. This study suggests that elite female runners underreport true levels of energy intake and confirms the absence of energy-saving metabolic adaptations in this population.

Regular participation in exercise is traditionally thought to elevate energy requirements through the additional direct cost of the activity, as well as through an increase in RMR. However, in some situations energy requirements are not necessarily altered by participation in regular physical activity. For example, in a study of an elderly group of healthy volunteers, there was no significant change in total energy expenditure in the last 2 weeks of an 8 week vigorous endurance training program. The failure to detect an increase in total energy expenditure occurred despite a 10% increase in RMR (6703.2 ± 898.8 to 7404.6 ± 714 kJ/day), as well as an additional 630 kJ/day associated with the exercise program. These increases in energy expenditure were counteracted by a significant reduction in the energy expenditure of physical activity during nonexercising time (2.4 ± 1.6 versus 1.4 ± 1.9 MJ/day). The lack of increase in total energy expenditure in this study is probably explained by a compensatory energy-conserving adaptation to this vigorous training program leading to a reduction in spontaneous physical activity and/or a reduction in voluntary physical activities, similar to that observed in several animal studies. Thus, it should not automatically be assumed that energy requirements are elevated by participation in activity programs, and the ultimate change in energy requirements may be dictated by the intensity of the training program and the net sum of change in the individual components of energy expenditure. An important area of research is to identify the optimal program of exercise intervention in terms of exercise mode, type, duration and intensity, that can have optimal effects on all components of energy balance.

Energy requirements in pregnancy and lactation

Pregnancy and lactation are two other examples in which energy metabolism is altered in order to achieve positive energy balance. The specific changes in energy requirements during pregnancy are unclear and the various factors affecting this change are complex. Traditional government guidelines suggest that energy requirements are raised by 1.3 MJ/day during pregnancy. This figure is based on theoretical calculations based on the energy accumulation associated with pregnancy. However, these figures do not include potential adaptations in either metabolic efficiency or PAL during pregnancy. In a study that performed measures in 12 women every 6 weeks during pregnancy the average increase in total energy expenditure was 1.1 MJ/day. The average energy cost of pregnancy (change in total energy expenditure plus change in energy storage) was 1.6 MJ/day. However, there was considerable variation among the 12 subjects for the increase in average total energy expenditure (264.6 kJ/day to 3.8 MJ/day) and the average energy cost of pregnancy (147 kJ/day to 5.2 MJ/day).

Metabolic adaptations during lactation have been examined in well-nourished women using the DLW technique. The energy cost of lactation was calculated to be 3.7 MJ/day. Just over half of this energy cost was achieved by an increase in energy intake, while the remainder was met by a decrease in physical activity energy expenditure (3.2 MJ + 873.6 kJ/day at 8 weeks of lactation compared with 3.9 + 1.1 MJ/day in the same women prior to pregnancy).

Energy requirements in disease and trauma

The DLW technique has been used in various studies to assess the energy requirements of hospitalized patients. Information on energy requirements during hospitalization for disease or trauma is important because:

- energy expenditure can be altered by the disease or injury
- physical activity is often impaired or reduced
- both underfeeding and overfeeding of critically ill patients can lead to metabolic complications. Therefore, correct assessment of energy requirements during recovery is an important part of therapy.

The metabolic response during recovery from a burn injury includes an increase in RMR, although this is not necessarily a function of the extent of the burn. The widely used formula to predict energy needs in burn patients are not based on measurement of energy expenditure and estimate that most patients require 2–2.5 times their estimated RMR. However, using the DLW technique, total energy expenditure was 6.7 + 2.9 MJ/day in 8-year-old children recovering from burn injury, which was only equivalent to 1.2 times the nonfasting RMR. The lower than expected values for total energy expenditure in children recovering from burns suggest that RMR is not as elevated in burn patients as previously speculated, and that RMR is not a function of burn size or time after the injury, probably owing to improvements in wound care which reduce heat loss. In addition, energy requirements in patients recovering from burn injury are reduced because of the sedentary nature of their hospitalization.

In a study of anorexia nervosa patients, total energy expenditure was not significantly different compared with controls (matched for age, gender and height). However, physical activity-related energy expenditure was 1.3 MJ/day higher in anorexia nervosa patients, which was compromised by a 1.3 MJ/day lower RMR. Thus, energy requirements in anorexia nervosa patients are normal, despite alterations in the individual components of total energy expenditure. In infants with cystic fibrosis, total energy expenditure was elevated by 25% relative to weight-matched controls, although the underlying mechanism for this effect is unknown.

Developmental disabilities appear to be associated with alterations in energy balance and nutritional status at opposite ends of the spectrum. For example, cerebral palsy is associated with reduced fat mass and FFM, whereas half of myelodysplasia patients are obese. It is unclear whether the abnormal body composition associated with these conditions is the end-result of inherent alterations in energy expenditure and/or food intake, or whether alterations in body composition are an inherent part of the etiology of the specific disability. In addition, it is unclear how early in life total energy expenditure may be altered and whether reduced energy expenditure is involved with the associated obese state. Nevertheless, prescription of appropriate energy requirements may be a useful tool in the improvement of nutritional status in developmental disabilities.

Total energy expenditure has been shown to be lower in adolescents with both cerebral palsy and myelodysplasia, partly owing to reduced RMR, but primarily to reduced physical activity. Based on measurements of total energy expenditure, energy requirements of adolescent cerebral palsy and myelodysplasia are not as high as previously speculated. In nonambulatory cerebral palsy patients, energy requirements are estimated to be 1.2 times RMR, and in the normal range of 1.6–2.1 times RMR in ambulatory cerebral palsy patients.

3.7 Obesity

Basic metabolic principles

Obesity is the most common form of a disruption in energy balance and now constitutes one of the major and most prevalent disorders of nutrition. Because of the strong relationship between obesity and health risks, obesity is now considered a disease.

Although the body continuously consumes a mixed diet of carbohydrate, protein and fat, and sometimes alcohol, the preferred store of energy is fat. There is a clearly defined hierarchy of energy stores that outlines a preferential storage of excess calories as fat. For alcohol, there is no storage capacity in the body. Thus, alcohol that is consumed is immediately oxidized for energy. For protein, there is a very limited storage capacity and, under most situations, protein metabolism is very well regulated. For carbohydrate there is only a very limited storage capacity, in the form of glycogen, which can be found in the liver and in muscle. Glycogen provides a very small and short-term energy store, which can easily be depleted after an overnight fast or after a bout of exercise. Most carbohydrate that is consumed is immediately used for energy. Contrary to popular belief, humans cannot convert excess carbohydrate intake to fat. Instead, when excess carbohydrates are consumed, the body adapts by preferentially increasing its use of carbohydrate as a fuel, thus, in effect, burning off any excessive carbohydrate consumption. Large excesses of carbohydrate may induce *de novo* lipogenesis, but normally this process is quantitatively minor. However, no such adaptive mechanism for fat exists. In other words, if excess fat is consumed, there is no mechanism by which the body can increase its use of fat as a fuel. Instead, when excess fat calories are consumed, the only option is to accumulate the excess fat as an energy store in the body. This process occurs at a very low metabolic cost and is therefore an extremely efficient process. To store excess carbohydrate as glycogen is much more metabolically expensive and therefore a less efficient option. There is another important reason why the body would prefer to store fat rather than glycogen. Glycogen can only be stored in a hydrated form that requires 3 g of water for each gram of glycogen, whereas fat does not require any such process. In other words, for each gram of glycogen that is stored, the body has to store an additional 3 g of water. Thus, for each 4 g of storage tissue, the body only stores 16.8 kJ, equivalent to just 4.2 kJ/g, compared with the benefit of fat which can be stored as 37.8 kJ/g.

Thus, a typical adult with 15 kg of fat carries 567.0 MJ of stored energy. If he or she did not eat and was inactive, they might require 8.4 MJ/day for survival, and their energy stores would be sufficient for almost 70 days. This length is about the limit of human survival without food. Given that glycogen stores require 4 g to store 4.2 kJ (3 g of water plus 1 g of glycogen = 16.8 kJ), we can calculate that to carry this much energy in the form of glycogen requires 135 kg of weight. It is no wonder therefore that the body's metabolism favors fat as the preferred energy store.

Definition of obesity

Obesity has traditionally been defined as an excess accumulation of body energy, in the form of fat or adipose tissue. Thus, obesity is a disease of positive energy balance, which arises as a result of dysregulation in the energy balance system. It is now becoming clear that the increased health risks of obesity may be conferred by the distribution of body fat. In addition, the influence of altered body fat and/or body fat distribution on health risk may vary across individuals. Thus, obesity

is best defined by indices of body fat accumulation, body fat pattern and alterations in health risk profile.

The body mass index (BMI) is now the most accepted and most widely used crude index of obesity. This index classifies weight relative to height squared. The BMI is therefore calculated as weight in kilograms divided by height squared in meters, and expressed in the units of kg/m^2. Obesity in adults is defined as a BMI above $30.0 \, kg/m^2$, while the normal range for BMI in adults is $18.5–24.9 \, kg/m^2$. A BMI in the range of $25–30 \, kg/m^2$ is considered overweight. In children, it is more difficult to classify obesity by BMI because height varies with age during growth; thus, age-adjusted BMI percentiles must be used.

One of the major disadvantages of using the BMI to classify obesity is that this index does not distinguish between excess muscle weight and excess fat weight. Thus, although BMI is strongly related to body fatness, at any given BMI in a population, there may be large differences in the range of body fatness. A classic example of misclassification that may arise from the use of the BMI is a heavy football player or body-builder with a large muscle mass, who may have a BMI above $30 \, kg/m^2$, but is not obese, rather has a high body weight for his height resulting from increased FFM.

Since the health risks of obesity are related to body fat distribution, and in particular due to excess abdominal fat, other anthropometric indices of body shape are useful in the definition of obesity. Traditionally, the waist-to-hip ratio has been used as a marker of upper versus lower body-fat distribution. More recent studies suggest that waist circumference alone provides the best index of central body-fat pattern and increased risk of obesity-related conditions. The recommended location for the measurement of waist circumference is at the midpoint between the lowest point of the rib cage and the iliac crest. The risk of obesity-related diseases is increased above a waist circumference of 94 cm in men and above 80 cm in women.

Etiology of obesity: excess intake or decreased physical activity

Stated simply, obesity is the end-result of positive energy balance, or an increased energy intake relative to expenditure. It is often stated, or assumed, that obesity is simply the result of overeating or lack of physical activity. However, the etiology of obesity is not as simple as this, and many complex and interrelated factors are likely to contribute to the development of obesity; it is extremely unlikely that any single factor causes obesity. Many cultural, behavioral and biological factors drive energy intake and energy expenditure, and contribute to the homeostatic regulation of body energy stores, as discussed earlier in the chapter. In addition, many of these factors are influenced by individual susceptibility, which may be driven by genetic, cultural and hormonal factors. Obesity may develop very gradually over time, such that the actual energy imbalance is negligible and undetectable.

Although there are genetic influences on the various components of body-weight regulation, and a major portion of individual differences in body weight can be explained by genetic differences, it seems unlikely that the increased global prevalence of obesity has been driven by a dramatic change in the gene pool. It is more likely and more reasonable that acute changes in behavior and environment have contributed to the rapid increase in obesity, and genetic factors may be important in the differing individual susceptibilities to these changes. The most striking behavioral changes that have occurred have been an increased reliance on high-fat and energy-dense fast foods, with larger portion sizes, coupled with an ever-increasing sedentary lifestyle. The more sedentary lifestyle is due to an increased reliance on technology and labor-saving devices which has reduced the need for physical activity for everyday activities. Examples of energy-saving devices are:

- increased use of automated transport rather than walking or cycling
- central heating and the use of automated equipment in the household, e.g. washing machines
- reduction in physical activity in the workplace due to computers, automated equipment and electronic mail, which all reduce the requirement for physical activity at work
- increased use of television and computers for entertainment and leisure activities
- use of elevators and escalators rather than using stairs
- increased fear of crime, which has reduced the likelihood of playing outdoors
- poor urban planning, which does not provide adequate cycle lanes or even pavements in some communities.

Thus, the increasing prevalence, numerous health risks and astounding economic costs of obesity clearly justify widespread efforts towards prevention.

The relationship between obesity and lifestyle factors reflects the principle of energy balance. Weight maintenance is the result of equivalent levels of energy intake and energy expenditure. Thus, a discrepancy between energy expenditure and energy intake depends on either food intake or energy expenditure, and it is becoming clear that physical activity provides the main source of plasticity in energy expenditure. In addition, lifestyle factors such as dietary and activity patterns are clearly susceptible to behavioral modification and are likely targets for obesity prevention programs. A second, yet related, reason that control of the obesity epidemic will depend on preventive action is that both the causes and health consequences of obesity begin early in life and track into adulthood. For example, both dietary and activity patterns responsible for the increasing prevalence of obesity are evident in childhood.

Role of physical activity and energy expenditure in the development of obesity

Although it is a popular belief that reduced levels of energy expenditure and physical activity lead to the development of obesity, this hypothesis remains controversial and has been difficult to prove. There are certainly good examples of an inverse relationship between physical activity and obesity (e.g. athletes are lean and nonobese individuals), as well as good examples of the positive relationship between obesity and physical inactivity (obese individuals tend to be less physically active). However, not all studies provide supporting evidence. For example, several studies suggest that increased television viewing (as a marker for inactivity) increases the risk of obesity, whereas others do not. Similar to the results for physical activity, some studies suggest that a low level of energy expenditure predicts the development of obesity, and others do not support this hypothesis.

Physical activity is hypothesized to protect people from the development of obesity through several channels. First, physical activity, by definition, results in an increase in energy expenditure due to the cost of the activity itself, and is also hypothesized to increase RMR. These increases in energy expenditure are likely to decrease the likelihood of positive energy balance. However, the entire picture of energy balance must be considered, particularly the possibility that increases in one or more components of energy expenditure can result in a compensatory reduction in other components (i.e.

resting energy expenditure and activity energy expenditure). Secondly, physical activity has beneficial effects on substrate metabolism, with an increased reliance on fat relative to carbohydrate for fuel utilization, and it has been hypothesized that highly active individuals can maintain energy balance on a high-fat diet.

Cross-sectional studies in children and adults have shown that energy expenditure, including physical activity energy expenditure, is similar in lean and obese subjects, especially after controlling for differences in body composition. Children of obese and lean parents have also been compared as a model of preobesity. Some studies show that children of obese parents had a reduced energy expenditure, including physical activity energy expenditure, whereas another study did not. A major limitation of the majority of studies that have examined the role of energy expenditure in the etiology of obesity is their cross-sectional design. Because growth of individual components of body composition is likely to be a continuous process, longitudinal studies are necessary to evaluate the rate of body fat change during the growing process. Again, some longitudinal studies support the idea that reduced energy expenditure is a risk factor for the development of obesity, whereas others do not. Finally, intervention studies have been conducted to determine whether the addition of physical activity can reduce obesity. These studies tend to support the positive role of physical activity in reducing body fat.

Several possibilities could account for such discrepant findings. First, the ambiguous findings in the literature may be explained by the possibility that differences in energy expenditure and physical activity and their impact on the development of obesity are different at the various stages of maturation. This hypothesis is supported by previous longitudinal studies in children, showing that a reduced energy expenditure is shown to be a risk factor for weight gain in the first 3 months of life, but not during the steady period of prepubertal growth. Secondly, there could be individual differences in the effect of altered energy expenditure on the regulation of energy balance. Thus, the effect of energy expenditure on the etiology of obesity could vary among different subgroups of the population (e.g. boys versus girls, different ethnic groups) and could also have a differential effect within individuals at different stages of development. It is conceivable that susceptible individuals fail to compensate for periodic fluctuations in energy expenditure. Third, explanations related to the methodology can also be offered because of the complexity of the nature of physical activity and its measurement. The success of controlled exercise interventions in improving body composition indicates an extremely promising area for the prevention of obesity. However, further studies are required to elucidate the specific effects of different types of exercise on the key features of body weight regulation.

3.8 Perspectives on the future

Much is known about how the body balances energy intake and expenditure. There are, however, areas that need further research. The technology to determine total energy expenditure with doubly labeled water has been standardized. Most of the data from using this method have been obtained in populations living in industrialized countries. More studies on infants, children, adolescents, adults, pregnant and lactating women, and the elderly living in developing countries are indicated. Doubly labeled water is an expensive method. There is a need to develop more cost-effective methods that can be used in field studies and to determine the energy cost of specific activities of people throughout the life cycle in developing countries. Obesity has recently been defined as a disease by the WHO. The growing problem of obesity worldwide, and in children and in people who were previously food insecure and malnourished, needs to be addressed with better information about the behavioral and cultural factors that influence energy balance. This demands a more holistic, integrated approach to the study of obesity in the future.

Further reading

Bjorntorp P, Brodoff BN, eds. Obesity. Philadelphia, PA: JB Lippincott, 1992.

Frayn KN. Metabolic Regulation: A Human Perspective. Portland, OR: Portland Press.

McArdle WD, Katch FI, Katch VL, eds. Exercise Physiology: Energy, Nutrition and Human Performance. Philadelphia, PA: Lea & Febiger, 1991.

Roche AF, Heymsfield SB, Lohman TG, eds. Human Body Composition. Champaign, IL: Human Kinetics, 1996.

World Health Organization. Obesity: Preventing and Managing the Global Epidemic. Report of a WHO Consultation on Obesity, Geneva, 3–5 June 1997.

4
Nutrition and Metabolism of Proteins and Amino Acids

Vernon R Young and Peter J Reeds

Key messages

- Protein is the most abundant nitrogen-containing compound in the diet and the body. Proteins are formed when L-α-amino acids polymerize via peptide bond formation.
- Amino acids have similar central structures with different side-chains determining the multiple metabolic and physiological roles of free amino acids.
- Indispensable (essential) amino acids cannot be synthesized by humans from materials ordinarily available to cells at a speed commensurate with the demands of human growth and maintenance.
- The requirements for indispensable amino acids can be defined as "the lowest level of intake that achieves nitrogen balance or that balances the irreversible oxidative loss of the amino acid, without requiring major changes in normal protein turnover and where there is energy balance with a modest level of physical activity". For infants, children, pregnant and lactating women, requirements would include protein deposited and secretion of milk proteins.
- "Conditionally" indispensable amino acids are those for which there are measurable limitations to the rate at which they can be synthesized because their synthesis requires another amino acid, and because only a number of tissues is able to synthesize them, and probably only in limited amounts. The metabolic demands for these amino acids may rise above the biosynthetic capacity of the organism.
- Protein and amino acid requirements are determined by the processes of protein synthesis, and maintenance

of cell and organ protein content, as well as the turnover rates of protein and amino acid metabolism, including synthesis, breakdown, interconversions, transformations, oxidation and synthesis of other nitrogen-containing compounds and urea. These processes are influenced by genetics, phase of life cycle, physical activity, dietary intake levels, how energy needs are met, route of delivery of nutrients, disease, hormones and immune system products.
- Protein and amino acid requirements can be determined by nitrogen excretion and balance, factorial estimations and/or tracer techniques.
- Existing recommendations on requirements differ by various authorities because of a lack of data when some were formulated, different interpretations of data and different criteria for judging adequate intakes.
- The United Nations plans to publish new recommendations for protein and amino acids during 2002/2003.
- Apparent protein digestibility, measured in the past as the difference between nitrogen intake and faecal nitrogen output, underestimates "true" digestibility because faecal nitrogen is derived, in part, from endogenous nitrogen sources.
- Tracer techniques have shown that "true" digestibility of most dietary proteins is high. The quality of food protein can be assessed as the protein digestibility-corrected amino acid score (PDCAAS).
- Animal protein foods generally have higher concentrations of indispensable amino acids than plant foods. Lysine is often the most limiting amino acid, followed by sulfur amino acids (methionine and cystine) and tryptophan and threonine.

4.1 Introduction

Protein is the most abundant nitrogen-containing compound in the diet and in the body. It is one of the five classes of complex biomolecules present in cells and tissues, the others being DNA, RNA, polysaccharides and lipids. The polymerization of L-α-amino acids through synthesis of peptide bonds contributes

Table 4.1 Some functions of amino acid and proteins

Function	Example
Amino acids	
Substrates for protein synthesis	Those for which there is a codon
Regulators of protein turnover	Leucine, arginine?
Regulators of enzyme activity (allosteric)	Arginine and NAG synthase
	Phenylalanine and PAH activation
Precursor of signal transducer	Arginine and nitric oxide
Methylation reactions	Methionine
Neurotransmitter	Tryptophan (serotonin), glutamine
Ion fluxes	Taurine, glutamate
Precursor of "physiological" molecules	Arginine (creatinine), Glu (NH$_2$)-purines
Transport of nitrogen	Alanine, Glu (NH$_2$)
Regulator of gene transcription	Amino acid depletion and asparagine synthase gene activation
Regulator of mRNA translation	Leucine: alters activity of initiation factor 4E-BP and
	P70 (6SK) via MTOR signaling pathway
Proteins	
Enzymic catalysis	Branched-chain ketoacid dehydrogenase
Transport	B$_{12}$ binding proteins, ceruloplasmin, apolipoproteins, albumin
Messengers/signals	Insulin, growth hormone
Movement	Kinesin, actin
Structure	Collagens, elastin
Storage/sequestration	Ferritin, metallothionein
Immunity	Antibodies, TNF, interleukins
Growth, differentiation, gene expression	Peptide growth factors, transcription factors

NAG: *N*-acetylglutamate; PAH: phenylalanine hydroxylase; Glu (NH$_2$): glutamine; TNF: tumor necrosis factor.

to the formation and structural framework of proteins. These may contain two or more polypeptide chains forming multimeric proteins, with the individual chains being termed subunits. Proteins are the workhorses in cells and organs and their building blocks are the amino acids, which are joined together according to a sequence directed by the base sequence of the DNA (the genome), and so they serve as the currency of protein nutrition and metabolism. There appear to be about 35 000 genes, whereas there may be hundreds of thousands of proteins that are responsible for giving a human its particular characteristics and uniqueness. Proteins and amino acids fulfil numerous functions, many of which are summarized in Table 4.1. Some amino acids, such as glutamine (Tables 4.2, 4.3), play multiple roles. It is not surprising, therefore, that inappropriate intakes of proteins and/or of specific amino acids can have important consequences for tissue and organ function, and the maintenance of health and the well-being of the individual.

This chapter begins with a short historical perspective and then moves in Sections 4.3 and 4.4 to discuss

Table 4.2 Multiple functions of an amino acid, using glutamine as an example

Substrate of protein synthesis (codons: CAA, CAG)
Anabolic/trophic substance for muscle, intestine (competence factor)
Controls acid–base balance (renal ammoniagenesis)
Substrate for hepatic ureagenesis
Substrate for hepatic/renal gluconeogenesis
Fuel for intestinal enteroctyes
Fuel and nucleic acid precursor and important for generation of cytotoxic products in immunocompetent cells
Ammonia scavenger
Substrate for citrulline and arginine synthesis
Nitrogen donor (nucleotides, amino sugars, coenzymes)
Nitrogen transport (one-third of circulating N) (muscle, lung)
Precursor of GABA (via glutamate)
Shuttle for glutamate (CNS)
Preferential substrate for GSH production?
Osmotic signaling mechanism in regulation of protein synthesis?
Stimulates glycogen synthesis
L-Arginine NO metabolism
Taste factor (umami)

GABA: γ-aminobutyric acid; CNS: central nervous system; GSH: reduced glutathione; NO: nitric oxide.

Table 4.3 Biochemical roles of amino acids not directly related to protein metabolism

Amino acid	Biochemical function
Integration of carbon and nitrogen metabolism	
Leucine, isoleucine, valine	Ubiquitous nitrogen donors and metabolic fuel
Glutamate	Ubiquitous nitrogen donor, extracellular transporter of four-carbon units
Glutamine	See Table 4.2
Alanine	Ubiquitous nitrogen donor, extracellular transporter of three-carbon units
Aspartate	Ubiquitous nitrogen donor, transfer form of nitrogen from cytoplasmic amino acids to urea
Single carbon metabolism	
Methionine	Donor and acceptor of methyl groups, hence important role in single carbon metabolism
Glycine	Donor of methylene groups
Serine	Donor of hydroxymethylene groups
Neurotransmitter synthesis	
Histidine	Precursor for histamine synthesis
Phenylalanine and tyrosine	Precursors for tyramine, dopamine, adrenaline and noradrenaline synthesis
Tryptophan	Precursor for serotonin synthesis
Glutamate	Precursor for γ-aminobutyric acid synthesis
Miscellaneous	
Arginine	Immediate precursor for urea
	Precursor for nitric oxide synthesis
Cysteine	Potential intracellular thiol buffer
	Precursor for taurine synthesis
Glycine	Nitrogen donor for heme synthesis

the classification, structure, chemistry and classification of amino acids. Section 4.5 is concerned with the biology of protein and amino acid requirements, with Sections 4.6 and 4.7 describing how the requirements are established and how they may be met, respectively. Finally, Section 4.8 examines how factors other than dietary protein can influence the requirements for proteins and amino acids.

4.2 A historical perspective

The early history of protein metabolism and nutrition is closely tied to the discovery of nitrogen and its distribution in nature. The reason for this is that proteins, on average, contain about 16% nitrogen by weight (to convert nitrogen to protein it is necessary to multiply by 6.25). Daniel Rutherford, in Edinburgh, can be regarded as the discoverer of nitrogen, which he called "phlogisticated air" in his Doctorate in Medicine thesis in 1792. The first amino acid to be discovered was cystine, which was extracted from a urinary calculus by

Wallaston in England in 1810. It was not until 1935 that threonine, the last of the so-called nutritionally indispensable (essential) amino acids for mammals, including man, was discovered by WC Rose at the University of Illinois. Finally, the term "protein" was invented by the Swedish chemist Jons Jakob Berzelius (1779–1848) and this was later accepted and promoted by the influential Dutch chemist Gerhardus Mulder in 1838.

The nutritional importance of nitrogenous components in the diet was first recognized in 1816 by Magendie. He described experiments in dogs that received only sugar and olive oil until they died within a few weeks. It was concluded that a nitrogen source was an essential component of the diet. Magendie's insightful views on nitrogen metabolism and nutrition were followed by studies carried out by the French scientific school, including Justus von Leibig, who investigated the chemical basis of protein metabolism and discovered that urea was an end-product of protein breakdown in the body. Later, Leibig founded a school of biochemical studies in Gissen and later in Munich, Germany, from which Carl Voit emerged as a distinguished scientist and laid the foundations of modern studies of body nitrogen balance. He, in turn, trained many famous scientific celebrities, including Max Rubner, from Germany, who studied the specific dynamic action of proteins and their effects on energy metabolism, and Wilbur Atwater and Graham Lusk, from the USA, who studied food composition, protein requirements and energy metabolism. Through their work, and that of others, theories of protein metabolism were proposed and challenged, leading to the more or less contemporary view which was established through the seminal work of Rudolf Schoenheimer, conducted at Columbia University, New York, in the mid-1930s and early 1940s. He applied the new tracer tool of stable isotope enriched compounds, especially amino acids, in the study of dynamic aspects of protein turnover and amino acid metabolism. Stable isotopes (such as ^{13}C, ^{18}O and ^{15}N) are naturally present in our environment, including the foods we eat, and they are safe to use in human metabolic studies. Using this approach, Schoenheimer established the fundamental biological principle of a continued tissue and organ protein loss and renewal, which forms the basis for the dietary need for protein or supply amino acids and a utilizable form of nitrogen.

4.3 Structure and chemistry of amino acids

With one exception, the amino acid proline, the amino acids that make up peptides and proteins have the same central structure (Figure 4.1; the A in this figure and

$$
\begin{array}{c}
H \\
| \\
-C-COOH \\
| \\
NH_2
\end{array}
$$

subsequent figures represent the $-C-COOH$ moiety).

The carboxylic acid and amino nitrogen groups are the components of the peptide bond that links the amino acids within the linear peptide structure, while the side-chains distinguish the physical and chemical properties of each chemical class of amino acid. In addition, some features of the amino acid-side chains are critical to the metabolic and physiological roles of free, as opposed to protein-bound, amino acids (Table 4.3, Figures 4.1, 4.2). These roles are reflections of either their specific chemical properties or specific metabolic interrelationships. Examples of the former are

Figure 4.1 Structures of some of the nutritionally important amino acids. All are components of proteins and they are coded by DNA. (a) Nutritionally indispensable (essential) includes also tryptophan and histidine; (b) nutritionally conditionally indispensable; (c) nutritionally dispensable.

Figure 4.2 Physiologically important amino acid metabolites.

Figure 4.3 Some amino acids that arise via a post-translational modification of a polypeptide-bound amino acid. These amino acids are not coded by DNA but are important determinants of the structural and functional characteristics of proteins.

the facility of methionine to donate a methyl group in one-carbon metabolism and the propensity for the amide group of glutamine to serve as a nitrogen source for pyrimidine synthesis. Examples of the latter are:

- the metabolic relationship between alanine and glutamic acid and their transamination partners, the keto acids pyruvate and α-ketoglutarate
- the similarity between the catabolic oxidation pathway of the branched-chain amino acids and the β-oxidation pathway of saturated fatty acids.

The former metabolic relationship allows alanine and glutamate (and glutamine) to provide a link between carbohydrate and protein metabolism; the latter enables the branched amino acids to function when required, as a "universal" fuel throughout the body.

Some of these amino acid and nitrogen compounds are derivatives of other amino acids:

- creatine is formed from glycine, arginine and methionine, and serves in intracellular energy transduction
- dopamine is formed from tyrosine and fulfils a neurotransmitter function

- ornithine can be formed from glutamate and serves as both an intermediate in the urea cycle and a precursor of the polyamines, spermine and spermidine, used in DNA packaging.

Finally, other amino acids (Figure 4.3) appear in proteins via a post-translational modification of a specific amino acid residue in the polypeptide chain that is being formed during protein synthesis. Some examples of this are:

- the formation of hydroxyproline, from proline, involved in the maturation of the different types of collagens in cells
- the methylation of a specific histidine in the muscle protein actin.

It could be that this modification gives this protein its ability to function effectively in the contractile activities of the skeletal muscles that help us to move about.

4.4 Classification of amino acids

"Indispensability" as a basis of classification

For most of the past 60 years amino acids have been divided into two general, nutritional categories: indispensable (essential) and dispensable (nonessential). This categorization provided a convenient and generally useful way of viewing amino acid nutrition at the time. The original definition of an indispensable amino acid was:

> One which cannot be synthesized by the animal organism out of materials *ordinarily available* to the cells *at a speed* commensurate with the demands for *normal growth*.

There are three important phrases in this definition: *ordinarily available*, *at a speed* and for *normal growth*.

The phrase "ordinarily available" is an important qualifier within this definition because a number of nutritionally essential amino acids, for example the branched-chain amino acids, phenylalanine and methionine, can be synthesized by transamination of their analogous α-keto acids. However, these keto acids are not normally part of the diet and so are not "ordinarily available to the cells". They may be used in special situations such as in nitrogen-accumulating diseases, including renal failure, where they may assist in maintaining a better status of body nitrogen metabolism.

The phrase "at a speed" is equally important, because there are circumstances in which the rate of synthesis of an amino acid may be constrained, such as by the availability of appropriate quantities of "nonessential" nitrogen. Further, the rate of synthesis becomes of particular importance when considering a group of amino acids, exemplified by arginine, cysteine, proline and probably glycine. These amino acids are frequently described as being conditionally indispensable. That is, their indispensability is dependent upon the physiological or pathophysiological condition of the individual.

Finally, the phrase "normal growth" is critical in two respects. First, it serves to emphasize that the definitions were originally constructed in the context of growth. For example, for the growing rat arginine is an indispensable amino acid but the adult rat does not require the presence of arginine in the diet and so it becomes a dispensable amino acid at that later stage of the life cycle. Of course, if the capacity to synthesize arginine is compromised by removing a significant part of the intestine which produces citrulline, a precursor of arginine, then the adult rat once again requires arginine as part of adequate diet. Secondly, by confining the definition to growth, this fails to consider the importance of amino acids to pathways of disposal other than protein deposition. This aspect of amino acid utilization will be considered below.

Table 4.4 Structural features that render amino acids indispensable components of the diet of mammals

Amino acid	Structural feature
Leucine, isoleucine, valine	Branched aliphatic side-chain
Lysine	Primary amine
Threonine	Secondary alcohol
Methionine	Secondary thiol
Tryptophan	Indole ring
Phenylalanine	Aromatic ring
Histidine	Imidazole ring

Chemical and metabolic characteristics as bases of classification

It is also possible to classify amino acids according to their chemical and metabolic characteristics rather than on the basis of their need for growth. Examination of the amino acids that are generally considered to be nutritionally indispensable for humans and most other mammals indicates that each has a specific structural feature, the synthesis of which cannot be accomplished owing to the absence of the necessary mammalian enzyme(s) (Table 4.4). Indeed, in obligatory carnivores, such as cats, the further loss of some critical enzyme(s) renders these animals particularly dependent on dietary sources of specific amino acids, such as arginine. The lack of arginine in a single meal when given to a cat can be fatal. However, even within this view, the important term is "*de novo* synthesis" because some amino acids can be synthesized from precursors that are structurally very similar. For example, methionine can be synthesized both by transamination of its keto acid analogue and by remethylation of homocysteine. According to this metabolic assessment of amino acids, threonine and lysine are the only amino acids that cannot be formed via transamination or via conversion from another carbon precursor. In this narrower metabolic view, they are truly indispensable amino acids. A contemporary nutritional classification of amino acids in human nutrition is given in Table 4.5.

Strictly speaking, a truly dispensable amino acid is one that can be synthesized *de novo* from a nonamino acid source of nitrogen (e.g. ammonium ion) and a carbon source (e.g. glucose). Accordingly, and from a knowledge of biochemical pathways, the only true metabolically indispensable amino acid is glutamic acid, and possibly also glycine. This is because they can be synthesized from glucose and ammonium ion, in the case of glutamate, and from carbon dioxide and ammonium ion, in the case of glycine. However, the *in vivo* condition may differ in both qualitative and quantitative terms from studies in test-tubes or in isolated cells in culture; amino acid metabolism *in vivo* is inherently more complex than is immediately evident from a simple consideration of biochemical pathways alone.

Table 4.5 Dietary amino acids of nutritional significance in humans

Indispensable	Conditionally indispensable	Dispensable
Valine	Glycine	Glutamic acid (?)
Isoleucine	Arginine	Alanine
Leucine	Glutamine	Serine
Lysine	Proline	Aspartic acid
Methionine	Cystine	Asparagine
Phenylalanine	Tyrosine	
Threonine	(Taurine)[a]	
Tryptophan	(Ornithine)[a]	
Histidine	(Citrulline)[a]	

[a] Nonproteinogenic amino acids, which have nutritional value in special cases.

Sources of nonspecific nitrogen for humans

In earlier texts it would have been stated that, given a sufficient intake of the indispensable amino acids, all that is then additionally needed to support body protein and nitrogen metabolism would be a source of "nonspecific" nitrogen (NSN) and that this could be in the form of a simple nitrogen-containing mixture, such as urea and diammonium citrate. However, this is no longer a sufficient description of what is actually required to sustain an adequate state of protein nurture in the human. This can be illustrated by considering the nitrogen cycle, on which all life ultimately depends (Figure 4.4). From this it can be seen that some organisms are capable of fixing atmospheric nitrogen into ammonia, and plants are able to use either the ammonia or soluble nitrates (that are reduced to ammonia) produced by nitrifying bacteria. However, vertebrates, including humans, must obtain dietary nitrogen in the form of amino acids or other organic compounds, possibly as urea and purine and pyrimidines. Glutamate and glutamine provide a critical entry of the ammonia from the nitrogen cycle into other amino acids. It is therefore important to

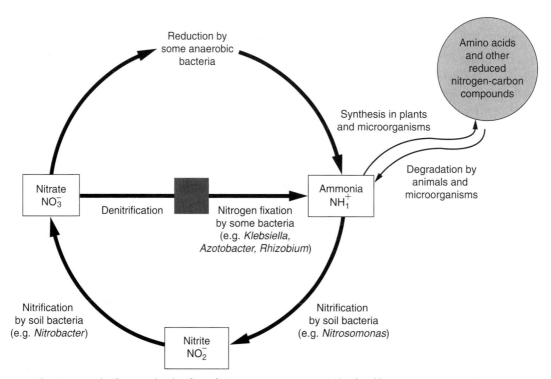

Figure 4.4 The nitrogen cycle. The most abundant form of nitrogen is present in air, which is four-fifths molecular nitrogen (N_2). The total amount of nitrogen that is fixed in the biosphere exceeds 10^{11} kg annually.

examine briefly the way in which the human body may obtain this NSN so as to maintain the nitrogen economy of the individual.

Ammonia can be introduced into amino acids: (1) by ubiquitous glutamate ammonia ligase (glutamine synthetase) that catalyzes the following reaction:

$$\text{Glutamate} + NH_4^+ + ATP$$
$$\rightarrow \text{Glutamine} + ADP + P_i + H^+ \quad (4.1)$$

and (2) via the glutamate dehydrogenase reaction:

$$\alpha\text{-Ketoglutarate} + NH_4^+ + NADPH$$
$$\rightleftharpoons \text{L-Glutamate} + NADP + H_2O \quad (4.2)$$

However, because K_m for NH_4^+ in this reaction is high (>1 mM), this reaction is thought to make only a modest contribution to net ammonia assimilation in the mammal.

In bacteria and plant chloroplasts, glutamate is produced by the action of glutamate synthase, according to the reaction:

$$\alpha\text{-Ketoglutarate} + \text{glutamine} + NADPH + H^+$$
$$\rightarrow 2 \text{ Glutamate} + NADP \quad (4.3)$$

The sum of the glutamate synthase (Eqn 4.3) and glutamine synthetase (Eqn 4.1) reactions is, therefore:

$$\alpha\text{-Ketoglutarate} + NH_4^+ + NADPH + ATP$$
$$\rightarrow \text{Glutamate} + NADP + ADP + P_i \quad (4.4)$$

Hence, the two reactions combined (Eqn 4.4) give a net synthesis of one molecule of glutamate. However, because glutamate synthetase is not present in animal tissues, a net incorporation of ammonia nitrogen via this nitrogen cycle arises primarily from glutamate rather than from glutamine. A net accumulation of glutamine would be achieved via the glutamine synthetase reaction that uses ammonia, which would be derived from various sources including glutamate, other amino acids or via hydrolysis of urea by the microflora on the intestinal lumen.

A net incorporation of ammonia into glycine might also be achieved via the glycine synthase (glycine cleavage) reaction, as follows:

$$CO_2 + NH_4^+H^+ + NAD + N_5, N_{10}\text{-Methylenetetrahydrofolate}$$
$$\rightleftharpoons \text{Glycine} + NAD^+ + \text{Tetrahydrofolate} \quad (4.5)$$

The glycine could then be incorporated into proteins and into such compounds as glutathione, creatine and the porphyrins, as well as being converted to serine. The nitrogen of serine would then either be available

for cysteine (and taurine) synthesis or be released as ammonia via the serine dehydratase reaction. However, the glycine cleavage reaction appears to be more important in glycine catabolism than for its synthesis. Therefore, the glycine–serine pathway of ammonia incorporation into the amino acid economy of the organism would appear to have only a limited effect on a net nitrogen input into the amino acid economy of the body. Serine can be formed from glucose via 3-phosphoglycerate, which comes from carbohydrate metabolism, and its nitrogen obtained from glutamic acid synthesis via transamination with 2-ketoglutarate.

This suggests, therefore, the possibility that glutamate is a key amino acid in making net amino nitrogen available to the mammalian organism; this glutamate would be derived ultimately from plant protein. In this sense, glutamate or its lower homologue, aspartic acid, which could supply the α-amino nitrogen for glutamate or its derivative, glutamine, would be required as a source of α-amino nitrogen. While additional research is necessary to determine whether glutamate, or one of these metabolically related amino acids, would be the most efficient source of α-amino nitrogen, these considerations potentially offer a new perspective on the NSN component of the total protein requirement. In 1965, a United Nations expert group stated:

> The proportion of nonessential amino acid nitrogen, and hence the E/T [total essential or indispensable amino acids to total nitrogen] ratio of the diet, has an obvious influence on essential amino acid requirements. … To make the best use of the available food supplies there is an obvious need to determine the minimum E/T ratios for different physiological states. … Finally, the question arises whether there is an optimal pattern of nonessential amino acids.

This statement can just as well be repeated today, but clearly recent studies are beginning to provide deeper metabolic insights into the nature of the NSN needs of the human body.

"Conditional" indispensability

A contemporary nutritional classification of amino acids in human nutrition is given in Table 4.5 and some points should be made here about the "conditionally" indispensable amino acids, a term that is used to indicate that there are measurable limitations to the rate at which they can be synthesized. There are several important determinants. First, their synthesis requires the provision of another amino acid, either as the carbon donor (e.g. citrulline in the case of arginine synthesis or serine in the case of glycine synthesis) or as a donor of an accessory group (e.g. the sulfur group of methionine for cysteine synthesis). The ability of the organism to synthesize a conditionally essential amino acid is, therefore, set by the availability of its amino acid precursor. Secondly, some of these amino acids are synthesized in only a limited number of tissues. The best example of this is the crucial dependence of the synthesis of proline and arginine on intestinal metabolism. Thirdly, most evidence suggests that even in the presence of abundant quantities of the appropriate precursors, the quantities of conditionally essential amino acids that can be synthesized may be quite limited. Thus, there are circumstances, for example in immaturity and during stress, under which the metabolic demands for the amino acids rise to values that are beyond the biosynthetic capacity of the organism. This appears to be the case with regard to the proline and arginine nutrition of severely burned individuals, and cysteine and perhaps glycine in the nutrition of prematurely delivered infants.

4.5 Biology of protein and amino acid requirements

Body protein mass

A major and fundamental quantitative function of the dietary α-amino acid nitrogen and of the indispensable amino acids is to furnish substrate required for the support of organ protein synthesis and the maintenance of cell and organ protein content. Therefore, in the first instance the body protein mass is a factor that will influence the total daily requirement for protein. Adult individuals of differing size but who are otherwise similar in age, body composition, gender and physiological state would be expected to require proportionately differing amounts of nitrogen and indispensable amino acids. Changes in the distribution and amount of body protein that occur during growth and development and later on during agng may be considered, therefore, as an initial approach for understanding the metabolic basis of the dietary protein and amino acid needs. (For more detailed considerations of body composition please refer to Chapter 2 of this volume.)

Direct measures of total body protein cannot yet be made in living subjects, although there are various indirect measures from which it is possible to obtain a picture of the body nitrogen (protein) content at various stages of life. From these approaches it is clear that that body nitrogen increases rapidly from birth during childhood and early maturity, reaching a maximum by about the third decade. Thereafter, body nitrogen decreases gradually during the later years, with the decline occurring more rapidly in men than in women. A major contributor to this age-related erosion of body nitrogen is the skeletal musculature. Strength training during later life can attenuate or partially reverse this decline in the amount of protein in skeletal muscles and improve overall function.

The protein requirement of adults is usually considered to be the continuing dietary intake that is just sufficient to achieve a "maintenance" of body nitrogen, often measured only over relatively short experimental periods. For infants and growing children and pregnant women an additional requirement is needed for protein deposition tissues. However, this concept is oversimplified since the chemical composition of the body is in a dynamic state and changes occur in the nitrogen content of individual tissues and organs in response to factors such as diet, hormonal balance, activity patterns and disease. Thus, proteins are being continually synthesized and degraded, an overall process that is referred to as turnover. The rate of turnover and the balance of synthesis and degradation of proteins, in addition to the mass of protein, are also important determinants of the requirements for nitrogen and amino acids, and these aspects will be discussed in the following section.

Turnover of proteins and amino acid metabolism

Protein synthesis, degradation and turnover

The principal metabolic systems responsible for the maintenance of body protein and amino acid homeostasis are shown in Figure 4.5. They are:

- protein synthesis
- protein breakdown or degradation
- amino acid interconversions, transformation and eventually oxidation, with elimination of carbon dioxide and urea production
- amino acid synthesis, in the case of the nutritionally dispensable or conditionally indispensable amino acids.

Dietary and nutritional factors determine, in part, the dynamic status of these systems; such factors include

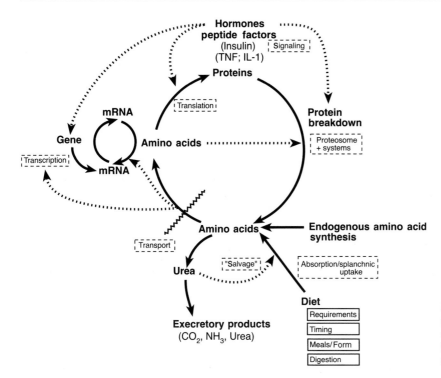

Figure 4.5 The major systems in amino acid uptake, utilization and catabolism, with an indication of the processes involved and some factors that can affect them.

the dietary intake levels relative to the host's protein and amino acid requirements, the form and route of delivery of nutrients, i.e. parenteral (venous) and enteral (oral) nutritional support, and timing of intake during the day, especially in relation to the intake of the major energy-yielding substrates, which are the carbohydrates and fats in foods. Other factors, including hormones and immune system products, also regulate these systems. This will be a topic for discussion in the following volume. Changes in the rates and efficiencies of one or more of these systems lead to an adjustment in whole body nitrogen (protein) balance and retention, with the net direction and the extent of the balance depending upon the sum of the interactions occurring among the prevailing factor(s).

In effect, there are two endogenous nitrogen cycles that determine the status of balance in body protein:

- the balance between intake and excretion
- the balance between protein synthesis and breakdown (Figure 4.6).

In the adult these two cycles operate so that they are effectively in balance (nitrogen intake = nitrogen excretion and protein synthesis = protein breakdown), but the intensity of the two cycles differs, the flow of

Figure 4.6 The two endogenous nitrogen cycles that determine the status of body protein (nitrogen) balance. (Adapted from Waterlow, 1999.)

nitrogen (and amino acids) being about three times greater for the protein synthesis/breakdown component than for nitrogen intake/excretion cycle.

Protein synthesis rates are high in the premature newborn, possibly about 11–14 g protein synthesized per kilogram of body weight per day, and these rates decline with growth and development so that in term babies and young adults these rates are about 7 g and 4–5 g protein/kg per day, respectively. Three points relevant to nutritional requirements may be drawn from these data. First, the higher rate of protein synthesis in the very young, compared with that in the adult, is related not only to the fact that a net deposition of protein occurs during growth, which may account for about 30% of the total amount of protein synthesized in the 6-month-old infant, but also to a high rate of protein turnover (synthesis and breakdown) associated with tissue remodeling and repair, as well as due to removal of abnormal proteins. In the adult the protein turnover is associated with cell and organ protein maintenance since there is no net tissue growth under most circumstances. Secondly, as will be seen later, at all ages in healthy subjects the rates of whole body protein synthesis and breakdown are considerably greater than usual intakes (the latter are about 1–1.5 g protein/kg per day in adults) or those levels of dietary protein thought to be just necessary to meet the body's needs for nitrogen and amino acids (about 0.8 g protein/kg per day). It follows, therefore, that there is an extensive reutilization within the body of the amino acids liberated during the course of protein breakdown. If this were not the case it might be predicted that we would be obligate carnivores and this, undoubtedly, would have changed the course of human evolution. Thirdly, although not evident from this discussion alone, there is a general as well as functional relationship between the basal energy metabolism or resting metabolic rate and the rate of whole body protein turnover. Protein synthesis and protein degradation are energy-requiring processes, as will be described elsewhere in these volumes, and from various studies, including interspecies components, it can be estimated that about 15–20 kJ (4–5 kcal) of basal energy expenditure is expended in association with the formation of each gram of new protein synthesis and turnover. In other words, protein and amino acid metabolism may be responsible for about 20% of total basal energy metabolism. Because basal metabolic rate accounts for a significant proportion of total daily energy expenditure, it should be clear from this discussion that there are significant, quantitative interrelationships between energy and protein metabolism and their nutritional requirements. For these reasons it would not be difficult to appreciate that both the level of dietary protein and the level of dietary energy can influence the balance between rates of protein synthesis and protein breakdown and so affect body nitrogen balance. Their effects are interdependent and their interactions can be complex. This can be illustrated by the changes in body nitrogen balance that occur for different protein and energy intakes (Figure 4.7); as seen here, the level of energy intake, whether above or below requirements, determines the degree of change in the nitrogen balance that

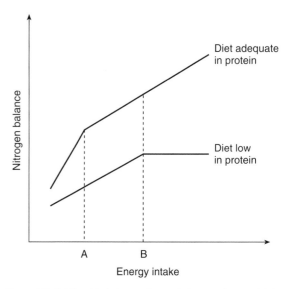

Figure 4.7 Relationship between nitrogen balance and energy intake with diets of different protein levels. Between energy intake A (low) and B (higher) the two lines are parallel. (Reproduced from Munro and Allison, 1964, Vol. 1, p. 381 with permission.)

occurs in response to a change in nitrogen intake. Conversely, the level of nitrogen intake determines the quantitative effect of energy intake on nitrogen balance. Therefore, optimum body protein nutrition is achieved when protein and energy intakes (from sources such as carbohydrates and lipids) are sufficient to meet or balance the needs for amino acids, nitrogen and the daily energy expenditure or, in the case of growth, the additional energy deposited in new tissues.

Amino acids as precursors of physiologically important nitrogen compounds

As already pointed out, amino acids are also used for the synthesis of important nitrogen-containing compounds that, in turn, play critical roles in cell, organ and system function. In carrying out these particular roles the amino acid-derived metabolites also turn over and they need to be replaced ultimately by the nitrogen and indispensable amino acids supplied by protein intake. Estimates on the quantitative utilization of these precursor and nonproteinogenic roles of amino acids in human subjects are limited but it is possible to give some examples.

- Arginine is the precursor of nitric oxide (NO); the total amount of NO synthesized (and degraded)

MITOCHONDRION

Figure 4.8 The urea cycle enzymes and their distribution in the liver. CPS: carbamoyl phosphate synthetase; OTC: ornithine transcarbamylase; Asy: argininosuccinic synthetase; AS: argininosuccinate; Arg: arginase.

per day represents less than 1% of whole body arginine flux and less than 1% of the daily arginine intake.

- In contrast, the rate of synthesis and degradation of creatinine is relatively high and accounts for 10% of the whole body flux of arginine and for 70% of the daily intake of arginine.
- Similarly, the synthesis and turnover of glutathione (a major intracellular thiol and important antioxidant, formed from glutamate, glycine and cysteine) accounts for a high rate of cysteine utilization such that it greatly exceeds the equivalent of the usually daily intake of cysteine. Since continued glutathione synthesis involves a reutilization of endogenous cysteine, a low intake of dietary methionine and cyst(e)ine would be expected to have an unfavorable influ-ence on glutathione status and synthesis. This has been shown experimentally to be the case, especially in trauma patients and those suffering from the acquired immunodeficiency syndrome (AIDS). Because glutathione is the most important intracellular antioxidant that protects cells against damage by reactive oxygen species, this would mean that particular attention should be paid to such amino acids in nutritional therapy in these groups of patients.

Urea cycle enzymes and urea production

Finally, with reference to the major processes depicted earlier in Figure 4.5, the urea cycle enzymes, which are distributed both within the mitochondrion and in the cytosol (Figure 4.8), are of importance. The production of urea may be viewed largely, but not entirely, as a pathway involved in the removal of amino nitrogen and contributing to an adjustment of nitrogen loss to nitrogen intake under various conditions. The five enzymes of urea biosynthesis associate as a tightly connected metabolic pathway, called a metabalon, for conversion of potentially toxic ammonia as well as removal of excess amino acids via their oxidation with transfer of the nitrogen to arginine and ultimately urea. This is especially important when the supply of protein or amino acids is high owing to variations in the exogenous intake or where there is a high rate of whole body protein breakdown in catabolic states, as occurs in severe trauma and following overwhelming infection.

Altered intakes of indispensable amino acids and of total nitrogen result in changes in rates of amino acid oxidation and the output of urea nitrogen in urine. There is a roughly parallel change in urea production and excretion throughout a relatively wide range of

Table 4.6 Essential amino acid composition of mixed body protein of immature mammals

| | Amino acid composition (mg/g protein) | | | | | | | |
	Lysine	Phenylalanine	Methionine	Histidine	Valine	Isoluecine	Leucine	Threonine
Rat	77	43	20	30	52	39	85	43
Human	72	41	20	26	47	35	75	41
Pig	75	42	20	28	52	38	72	37
Sheep	75	42	17	23	53	33	79	47
Calf	69	39	18	27	42	30	74	43

From Reeds (2000). Reproduced with permission of the publisher.

change in the level of dietary nitrogen intake above and below physiological requirement levels. Part of this urea enters the intestinal lumen, where there is some salvaging of urea nitrogen, via intestinal hydrolysis of urea to form ammonia. This ammonium nitrogen can be made available to the host for the net synthesis of dispensable or conditionally indispensable amino acids. However, the quantitative extent to which this pathway of nitrogen flow serves to maintain whole body N homeostasis and retention under normal conditions is a matter of uncertainty. The ammonia from urea could also enter the nitrogen moiety of the indispensable amino acids, but this would be essentially by an exchange mechanism and so would not contribute to a net gain of these amino acids in the body.

Summary of the metabolic basis for protein and amino acid requirements

It should be evident from this account of the underlying aspects of the needs for α-amino nitrogen and indispensable amino acids, that the "metabolic" requirement can usefully be divided: first, into those needs directly associated with protein deposition, a critical issue in infants, early childhood nutrition and during recovery from prior depletion due to disease or malnutrition; and secondly, into those needs associated with the maintenance of body protein balance, which accounts for almost all of the amino acid requirement in the healthy adult, except for that due to the turnover and loss of the various physiologically important nitrogen-containing products, some of which were mentioned above. Quantifying the minimum needs for nitrogen and for indispensable amino acids to support growth should be relatively easy, in principle, because these needs are simply the product of the rate of protein nitrogen deposition and the amino acid composition of the proteins that

are deposited. Here, it may be pointed out that the gross amino acid composition of whole body proteins shows essentially no difference among a variety of mammals, including humans (Table 4.6). Thus, at the major biochemical level the qualitative pattern of the needs of individual amino acids to support protein deposition would be expected to be generally similar.

In humans, in contrast to rapidly growing mammals such as the rat and pig, the obligatory amino acid needs for the purposes of net protein deposition are for most stages in life a relatively minor portion of the total amino acid requirement. Hence, most of the requirement for nitrogen and amino acids is associated with the maintenance of body protein stores (or body nitrogen equilibrium). A major portion of the maintenance nitrogen and amino acids needs is directly associated with protein metabolism and reflects two related factors.

- Amino acids released from tissue protein degradation are not recycled with 100% efficiency.
- Amino acid catabolism is a close function of the free amino acid concentration in tissues, and so the presence of the finite concentrations of free amino acids necessary to promote protein synthesis inevitably leads to some degree of amino acid catabolism and irreversible loss.

The other metabolic component of the requirement for nitrogen and amino acids, as mentioned above, is due to the turnover of functionally important products of amino acid metabolism, which are also necessary to maintain health. Although this may not necessarily be a major quantitative component of the daily requirement, it is qualitatively and functionally of considerable importance; health depends on the maintenance of this component of the protein need.

Table 4.7 Involvement of amino acids in physiological systems and metabolic function

System	Function	Product	Precursor
Intestine	Energy generation	ATP	Glu, Asp, Glu
	Proliferation	Nucleic acids	Glu, Gly, Asp
	Protection	Glutathione	Cys, Glu, Gly
		Nitric oxide	Arg
		Mucins	Thr, Cys, Ser, Pro
Skeletal muscle	Energy generation	Creatine	Gly, Arg, Met
	Peroxidative protection	Taurine (?)	Cys
Nervous system	Transmitter synthesis	Adrenergic	Phe
		Serotinergic	Try
		Glutaminergic	Glu
		Glycinergic	Gly
		Nitric oxide	Arg
	Peroxidative protection	Taurine (?)	Cys
Immune system	Lymphoctye proliferation	(?)	Glu, Arg, Asp
	Peroxidative protection	Glutathione	Cys, Glu, Gly
Cardiovascular	Blood pressure regulation	Nitric oxide	Arg
	Peroxidative protection (?)	Red cell glutathione	Cys, Glu, Gly

Finally, four physiological systems appear to be critical for health: the intestine, to maintain absorptive and protective function; the immune and repair system and other aspects of defense; the skeletal musculature system; and the central nervous system. Within each system it is possible to identify critical metabolic roles for some specific amino acids (Table 4.7). Also of note is that, with certain exceptions (the involvement of phenylalanine and tryptophan in the maintenance of the adrenergic and serotinergic neurotransmitter systems, and methionine as a methyl group donor for the synthesis of creatine, as well as the branched-chain amino acids as nitrogen precursors for cerebral glutamate synthesis), the necessary precursors shown here are the dispensable and conditionally indispensable amino acids.

4.6 Estimation of protein and amino acid requirements

Having considered the biology of protein and protein requirements, this section now considers how these factors may be used to estimate the requirement for protein and for amino acids. The first section discusses nitrogen balance and the definition of protein requirements, before discussing how these vary with age and for various physiological groups. Subsequent sections cover the estimation of the requirements for the indispensable amino acids.

Nitrogen balance and definition of requirement

The starting point for estimating total protein needs has been, in most studies, the measurement of the amount of dietary nitrogen needed for zero nitrogen balance, or equilibrium, in adults. In the growing infant and child and in women during pregnancy and lactation, or where repletion is necessary following trauma and infection, for example, there will be an additional requirement associated with the net deposition of protein in new tissue and that due to secretion of milk. Thus, a United Nations (UN) Expert Consultation in 1985 defined the dietary need for protein as follows.

> The protein requirement of an individual is defined as the lowest level of dietary protein intake that will balance the losses from the body in persons maintaining energy balance at modest levels of physical activity. In children and pregnant or lactating women, the protein requirement is taken to also include the needs associated with the deposition of tissues or the secretion of milk at rates consistent with good health.

Most estimates of human protein requirements have been obtained directly, or indirectly, from measurements of nitrogen excretion and balance (Nitrogen balance = Nitrogen intake − Nitrogen excretion via urine, feces, skin and other minor routes of nitrogen loss). It must be recognized that the nitrogen balance technique has serious technical and interpretative limitations and so it cannot serve as an entirely secure or sufficient basis for establishing the protein and amino acid needs for human subjects. Thus, there are:

- a number of inherent sources of error in nitrogen balance measurements that should be considered
- a number of experimental requirements that must be met if reliable nitrogen balance data are to be obtained.

These include

- the need to match closely energy intake with energy need, for the various reasons discussed earlier
- an appropriate stabilization period to the experimental diet and periods long enough to establish reliably the full response to a dietary change
- timing and completeness of urine collections
- absence of milk infections and of other sources of stress.

Reference to detailed reviews of the concepts behind and techniques involved in the nitrogen balance approach is given in the reading list at the end of this chapter.

Where direct nitrogen balance determinations of the protein requirement data are lacking, as is the case for a number of age groups, an interpolation of requirements between two age groups is usually made simply on the basis of body weight considerations. A factorial approach may also be applied; here, the so-called obligatory urine and faecal nitrogen losses are determined (after about 4–6 days of adaptation to a protein-free diet in adults), summated together with other obligatory losses, including those via sweat and the integument. For children, estimates of nitrogen deposition or retention are also included. In the case of very young infants the recommendations for meeting protein requirements are usually based on estimated protein intakes by fully breast-fed infants.

Protein requirements for various age and physiological groups

The protein requirements for young adult men and women have been based on both short- and long-term nitrogen balance studies. This also applies to healthy elderly people, whose protein requirements have been judged not to be different from those of younger adults. In order to make practical recommendations to cover the requirements for most individuals, it is necessary

Table 4.8 United Nations (1985 FAO/WHO/UNU) recommendations for a safe practical protein intake for selected age groups and physiological states. Reproduced with permission.

Group	Age (years)	Safe protein level (g/kg per day)
Infants	0.3–0.5	1.47
	0.75–1.0	1.15
Children	3–4	1.09
	9–10	0.99
Adolescent	13–14 (girls)	0.94
	13–14 (boys)	0.97
Young adults	≥19	0.75
Elderly		0.75
Women		
pregnant	2nd trimester	+6 g daily
	3rd trimester	+11 g daily
lactating	0–6 months	~ +16 g daily
	6–12 months	12 g daily

Values are for proteins such as those of quality equal to hen's eggs, cow's milk, meat or fish.

to adjust the average or mean requirement for a group by a factor that accounts for the variation in protein requirements among apparently similar individuals in that group. This factor is usually taken to be the coefficient of variation (CV) around the mean requirement and traditionally a value of $2 \times CV$ (SD/mean) is added to the mean physiological requirement, so that the needs of all but 2.5% of individuals within the population would be covered. This adjusted requirement value is taken to be the safe practical protein intake for the healthy adult (Table 4.8). Most individuals would require less than this intake to maintain an adequate protein nutritional status.

It is worth emphasizing two points: first, the current UN recommendations shown in Table 4.8 apply to healthy individuals of all ages. However, it is highly likely that the needs of sick or less healthy patients would differ from and usually exceed those of healthy subjects. In this case, the values given in this table can only be regarded as a basis from which to begin an evaluation of how disease and stress, including surgery, affect the needs for dietary protein. Unfortunately, the quantitative needs for protein (total nitrogen) in sick, hospitalized patients can only be very crudely approximated at this time.

Secondly, the values shown in Table 4.8 apply to high-quality food proteins, such as eggs, milk, meat and fish. The differing nutritional value of food proteins will be considered below.

Definition and determination of indispensable amino acid requirements

Definition

It is possible to modify slightly the earlier definition for the requirements for protein (nitrogen) for a specific, indispensable amino acid, which can be stated, therefore, as:

> the lowest level of intake of an indispensable amino acid that achieves nitrogen balance or that balances the irreversible oxidative loss of the amino acid, without requiring major changes in normal protein turnover and where there is energy balance with a modest level of physical activity. For infants, children and pregnant and lactating women, the requirements for the amino acid will include the additional amount of the amino acid needed for net protein deposition by the infant, child or fetus and conspectus and for the synthesis and secretion of milk proteins.

The foregoing is an operational definition of requirement, as in the case of protein. Ideally, a functional definition and determination of these requirements inherently would be preferable. However, the choice and nature of the functional index or (indices) (such as maximum resistance to disease or enhanced physical performance) and its quantitative definition remain a challenge for future nutrition and health-related research.

Determination

In general, the approaches and methods that have been most often used to determine specific indispensable amino acid requirements are similar to those used for estimation of total protein needs, that is, nitrogen excretion and balance and factorial estimation. Thus, amino acid requirements have been assessed by nitrogen balance in adults, and by determining the amounts needed for normal growth and nitrogen balance in infants, preschool children and school-aged children. For infants they have also been approached by assessment of the intakes provided by breast milk or those supplied from intakes of good quality proteins. In addition, factorial predictions of the amino acid requirements of infants and adults have been made. One such factorial approach for use in adults includes the following assumptions.

- The total obligatory nitrogen losses (those losses occurring after about 4–6 days of adjustment to a protein-free diet) are taken to be approximately 54 mg/kg nitrogen per day in an adult, or equivalent to 0.36 g protein/kg per day.
- The average amino acid composition of body proteins can be used to estimate the contribution made by each amino acid to this obligatory nitrogen output (equivalent, therefore, to the obligatory amino acid losses).
- At requirement intake levels, an absorbed amino acid is used to balance its obligatory oxidative loss with an assumed efficiency of about 70%.

This predictive or factorial approach is analogous to the factorial method for estimating the total nitrogen (protein) requirement of individuals at various ages (where various routes of nitrogen excretion and nitrogen gains are summated and an efficiency factor is used to estimate the intake needed to balance this summation).

Tracer techniques

With advances in the routine measurement of stable isotope enrichment in biological matrices and the expanded use of tracers enriched with these isotopes in human metabolic research, a series of tracer studies was begun at the Massachusetts Institute of Technology, USA, in the early 1980s to determine amino acid requirements in adults. Since that time several research groups have used different paradigms in tracer-based studies of human amino acid requirements. These can be distinguished according to the choice of tracer and protocol design applied:

- studies involving use of a labeled tracer of the dietary amino acid being tested and with its rate of oxidation (O) at various test intake levels [the direct amino acid oxidation (DAAO) technique, e.g. [^{13}C]lysine as a tracer to determine the lysine requirement]. This technique has been used to assess the requirements in adults for leucine, valine, lysine, threonine and phenylalanine;
- studies involving use of an "indicator" tracer to assess the status of indicator amino acid oxidation (IAAO) or indicator amino acid balance (IAAB) with varying levels of a test amino acid. Examples of the IAAO and IAAB approaches are where the rate of [^{13}C]phenylalanine oxidation (Figure 4.9) is measured or a [^{13}C]leucine balance determined at varying levels of lysine intake to estimate the lysine requirement;
- kinetic studies designed to assess the retention of protein during the postprandial phase of amino acid metabolism, using [^{13}C]leucine as a tracer: the

postprandial protein utilization (PPU) approach. This last and promising approach has not yet found an extensive use in studies of human amino acid requirements.

None of these methods is without its limitations, but at present the IAAO and IAAB approaches, involving tracer studies lasting for a continuous 24 h day, would appear to be the "reference method" for estimating amino acid requirements in adults.

Figure 4.9 Schematic outline of the concept of the indicator amino acid oxidation (IAAO) technique for estimation of indispensable amino acid requirements. Here the indicator is [^{13}C]phenylalanine and the dietary requirement being estimated for either leucine or lysine.

Indispensable amino acid requirement values

There is still debate and uncertainty about the precise requirements for amino acids in humans of all ages. Three major sets of proposed amino acid requirement values for healthy subjects should be noted in this text. First, there are the requirements proposed by the UN in 1985 for the various age groups, which are presented in Table 4.9. Secondly, another expert group in 1994 (IDECG) also has assessed the amino acid needs of infants by using a factorial method and these turned out to be much lower than those shown in Table 4.9 for infants. It should be noted, however, that the 1994 IDECG values approximate the average requirements, whereas the requirement intakes derived from estimates of breast milk intake (shown in Table 4.9) would be expected to be well above the requirement for virtually all infants and certainly well above the mean or average requirement. It is not surprising, therefore, that the UN and IDECG requirements disagreed. This also shows why recommendations by different national and international expert groups differ; they interpret the same data differently, use different data and also may choose to set different criteria for judging the adequacy of intake.

Further, as is characteristic of various estimates of human nutrient requirements in general, it must be appreciated that the values given in Table 4.9 are based on limited data; the values for the preschool children are derived from a single set of investigations carried out at the Institute for Central America and Panama,

Table 4.9 1985 FAO/WHO/UNU[a] estimates of amino acid requirements at different ages (mg/kg per day)

Amino acid	Infants (3–4 months)	Preschool children (2 years)	Schoolboys (10–12 years)	Adults
Histidine	28	?	?	(8–12)
Isoleucine	70	31	28	10
Leucine	161	73	44	14
Lysine	103	64	44	12
Methionine and cystine	58	28	22	13
Phenylalanine and tyrosine	125	69	22	14
Threonine	87	37	28	7
Tryptophan	17	12.5	3.3	3.5
Valine	93	38	25	10
Total	714	352	216	84
Total per g protein[b]	434	320	222	111

[a] FAO/WHO/UNU (1985). Reproduced with permission.
[b] Total mg/g crude protein.
Taken from Table 4, p. 65, and Table 38, p. 121, of the above reference and based on all amino acids minus hisitidine.

while those for the school-age children come from studies conducted by a single group of investigators in Japan. Those for adults are based importantly on the nitrogen balance studies in men carried out in the 1950s and 1960s. There are multiple reasons for questioning the precise reliability and nutritional significance of the adult values, and they include the facts that adult amino acid requirement values (Table 4.9) are greatly influenced by:

- the inappropriate experimental design used earlier for estimation of requirements
- the inadequacy of the nitrogen balance technique and the criterion of nitrogen balance that has been used to judge the nutritional adequacy of the levels of amino acid intake tested.

Therefore, some contemporary and newly proposed amino acid requirement estimates for adults are shown in Table 4.10. The more recent values are generally very different from the recommendations made in 1985. It is important to stay tuned in nutrition, as these texts will emphasize. At the time of writing this text, a new UN expert group is meeting to consider all of the new data that have been accumulated in the past 15 years. It is expected that new recommendations will be made in 2002 or 2003 and these will replace the figures in Table 4.10. The important point, however, is that all is not set in stone. Nutritional knowledge continues to

advance and with it the recommendations must change or at least be responsive to this new information.

4.7 Meeting protein and amino acid needs

Knowledge of the requirements for the specific indispensable amino acids and for total protein provides the basis for evaluating the relative capacity (or quality) of individual protein foods or mixtures of food protein sources to meet human amino acid requirements.

The two major determinants of the nutritional quality of food proteins are:

- the content of indispensable amino acids in the protein
- the extent to which the indispensable amino acids are available to host metabolism.

Digestibility and intestinal amino acid metabolism

Traditionally, the assessment of the availability of dietary proteins and amino acids under practical conditions has been based on "apparent digestibility", that is, the difference between nitrogen intake and faecal nitrogen output. However, for two reasons this method is unsatisfactory for the precise estimation of the digestibility of individual amino acids. First, faecal nitrogen consists largely of bacterial protein and because the composition of bacterial protein differs markedly from that of common dietary proteins, it gives very little information on the digestibility of different food-derived amino acids. Secondly, the bacterial nitrogen is not only derived from undigested protein. This is because proteins secreted into the intestinal lumen, as well as the urea nitrogen that has diffused from the blood, are important contributors to colonic nitrogen flow. Studies in both animals and humans using ^{15}N-labeled amino acids suggest that at least 50% of the faecal nitrogen is derived from the body rather than directly from undigested dietary protein.

Recently, ^{15}N-labeled dietary proteins have been given to adults and by measuring the flow of ^{15}N from the terminal ileum it is possible to calculate the "true" digestibility of the dietary source. There have also been a number of studies in pigs in which ^{15}N-amino acids have been infused intravenously for prolonged periods. This labels the host proteins so that the ^{15}N labeling of ileal proteins allows the calculation of the endogenous contribution of the lumenal protein pool.

Table 4.10 The earlier and two contemporary suggested patterns of amino acid requirements in healthy adults

Amino acid	United Nations[a] 1985	University of Surrey[b] 1999	MIT[c] 2000
Isoleucine	10[d](13)[e]	18(30)	23(35)
Leucine	14(19)	26(44)	23(65)
Lysine	12(16)	19(31)	30(50)
Methionine + cystine	13(17)	16(27)	13(25)
Phenylalanine + tyrosine	14(19)	20(33)	39(65)
Threonine	7(9)	16(26)	15(25)
Tryptophan	3.5(5)	4(6)	6(10)
Valine	10(13)	14(23)	20(35)

[a] FAO/WHO/UNU (1985).
[b] Millward (1999).
[c] Young and Borgonha (2000). With permission.
[d] Values expressed as mg/kg per day.
[e] Values expressed as mg amino acid/g protein required for effectively meeting total protein and amino acid needs.

By and large, the results of all these studies lead to the same conclusion; namely, that the true digestibility of most dietary proteins is very high and that at least 50% of the faecal nitrogen is derived from host metabolism rather than from the diet.

Most of the evidence favors the conclusion that there is an almost complete digestion of most dietary proteins in the small bowel. It is also quite clear that a considerable amount of amino acid metabolism occurs in the tissue of the splanchnic bed, in general, and in the intestinal mucosa, in particular, before the amino acids, liberated from food proteins during the digestive process, reach organs such as the liver, kidneys and skeletal muscles. Calculations based on recent isotopic studies suggest that intestinal amino acid utilization (both from the diet and via the blood supply to the intestine; the mesenteric arterial circulation) can account for as much as 50% of the body's utilization of amino acids. It is also important to note that the degree to which individual amino acids are utilized by the gut varies markedly (Table 4.11). Among the indispensable amino acids, threonine utilization is particularly high and virtually all of the dietary glutamate and aspartate are utilized within the mucosa. In addition, the magnitude of splanchnic amino acid metabolism varies with age, being apparently greater in infants and also perhaps in the elderly. This can affect the efficiency with which the amino acids derived from the protein ingested are used to support overall body nitrogen and amino acid homeostasis and balance.

Protein nutritional quality

Not all proteins have the same capacity to meet the physiological requirements for total nitrogen and the indispensable amino acids. The concentration and availability of the individual indispensable amino acids are major factors responsible for the differences in the nutritive values of food proteins. Thus, the content and balance of indispensable amino acids differ among plant and animal protein foods. For the present purpose a summary is given in Table 4.12, listing the four indispensable amino acids that are most likely to be limiting, or in shortest supply and especially in food proteins of plant origin. As can be seen, lysine is present in a much lower concentration in all the major plant food groups than in animal protein foods and is most frequently the most limiting amino acid.

The nutritional significance of these differences can be assessed in a number of ways. One useful approach is an amino acid scoring procedure that compares the content of amino acids in a protein with a reference human amino acid requirement pattern.

In 1991 a UN Expert Consultation reviewed the appropriate methods for measuring quality of food proteins for the nutrition of human populations. This consultation concluded that the most appropriate method available was the protein digestibility-corrected amino acid score (PDCAAS) method, and it was recommended for international use. This amino acid scoring procedure, including a correction for digestibility, uses the amino acid requirement pattern for the 2–5 year-old child (shown in Table 4.9). This is the reference amino acid requirement pattern for this purpose, expressing the amino acid requirement in relation to the total protein requirement.

The PDCAAS is estimated from the following equation:

$$\text{PDCAAS} = \frac{\text{Concentration of most limiting, digestibility-corrected amino acid in a test protein}}{\text{Concentration of that amino acid in the 1991 FAO/WHO amino acid scoring reference pattern (preschool child: see Table 4.9).}}$$

Table 4.11 Uptake of dietary amino acids by the visceral tissues

Amino acid	Utilization by the liver and gut (human) (% of intake)	Utilization by the gut (piglet) (% of intake)
Leucine	26	37
Lysine	32	45
Phenylalanine	39	53
Threonine	No data	65
Glutamine	53	50
Glutamate	88	95

Table 4.12 Amino acid content of different food protein sources

Food source	Amino acid (mg/g protein)			
	Lysine	Sulfur amino acids	Threonine	Tryptophan
Legumes	64 ± 10[a]	25 ± 3	38 ± 3	12 ± 4
Cereals	31 ± 10	37 ± 4	32 ± 4	12 ± 2
Nuts, seeds	45 ± 14	46 ± 17	36 ± 3	17 ± 3
Fruits	45 ± 12	27 ± 6	29 ± 7	11 ± 2
Animal foods	85 ± 9	38	44	12

From Young et al. (1998). With permission of Oxford University Press, Inc.
[a] Mean ± SD.

In addition to establishing the amino acid reference pattern for use in the PDCAAS method, the UN Consultation considered the procedures for measuring and estimating amino acids and digestibility. This approach offers considerable benefits over that of animal bioassays, which traditionally have been used to assess the quality of food protein in human diets. An important benefit is that PDCAAS approach uses human amino acid requirements as the basis of evaluation, which ensures that appropriate levels of indispensable amino acids will be provided in the diet. In addition, use of the proposed amino acid scoring procedure facilitates an evaluation of blending of

Table 4.13 Protein digestibility-corrected amino acid score (PDCAAS) of wheat, rice, maize, sorghum and millet

Protein source	PDCAAS
Wheat	40 (L)
Rice	56 (L)
Maize	43 (L)
Sorghum	33 (L)
Millet	53 (L)
Beef	>100 (S)

From Young *et al.* (1998). With permission of Oxford University Press, Inc.
(L): lysine first limiting amino acid; (S): sulfur amino acids (methionine + cystine).

foods to optimize nitrogen utilization and meet protein and amino acid needs. A listing of some calculated PDCAAS values for selected food protein sources is given in Table 4.13 and a worked example for a mixture of food proteins is presented in Table 4.14.

The development of an internationally derived procedure for evaluating protein quality using the amino acid scoring concept is a step that had long been required. This PDCAAS procedure can be modified as new knowledge about specific amino acid requirements emerges, as the determination of availability of dietary amino acids is improved, and as the factors affecting digestibility and availability are better understood. For the present, the PDCAAS procedure would appear to be very useful for evaluating the nutritional quality of human food protein sources.

Major sources of food proteins in the diet

The relative proportions in the diet of food proteins of animal and plant origin differ according to geographical region and other socioeconomic and cultural factors. Broadly, animal protein foods account for 60–70% of the total protein intake in the developed regions (Table 4.15). In contrast, plant proteins make up about 60–80% of the total protein intake in developing regions, with cereals being the dominant source in this case. Given the differences in amino acid

Table 4.14 Worked example of a PCDAAS for a mixture of wheat, chickpea and milk powder

	Analytical data							Quantities in mixture				
	Weight (g)	Protein (g/100 g)	Lys	SAA (mg/g protein)	Thr	Trp	Digestibility factor	Protein (g)	Lys (mg)	TSAA (mg)	Thr (mg)	Trp (mg)
	A	B	C	D	E	F	G	A × B/100 = P	PXC	PXD	PXE	PXF
Wheat	350	13	25	35	30	11	0.85	45.5	1138	1593	1365	501
Chickpea	150	22	70	25	42	13	0.80	33.0	2310	825	1386	429
Milk powder	50	34	80	30	37	12	0.95	17.0	1360	510	629	204
Totals								95.5	4808	2928	3380	1134
Amino acids mg/g protein [Total for each amino acid/Total protein]									50	31	35	12
Reference scoring pattern used			58	25	34	11						
Amino acids scoring for mixture amino acid/g protein divided by reference pattern									0.86	1.24	1.03	1.09
Weighted average protein digestibility sum of [protein × factor (PXG)] divided by protein total							0.85					
Score adjusted for digestibility (PDCAAS) (0.85 × 0.86)									0.73 (or 73%) with lysine limiting			

From Table 10 in FAO (1991).
SAA: Sulfur amino acids.

Table 4.15 Protein supplies per caput per day for selected regions

Region	Animal protein Total (g)	(%)	Plant protein Total (g)	(%)	Cereal protein Total (g)	(%)	Total protein (g)
World	26	36	46	64	33	46	72
Developing regions							
Africa	11	20	46	80	31	54	58
Asia	16	25	49	75	36	56	65
Latin America	32	45	39	55	25	36	70
Developed regions							
North America	72	64	41	36	25	22	113
Western Europe	62	60	41	40	25	24	103
Oceania	71	69	32	31	19	19	102

From Young *et al*. (1998). With permission of Oxford University Press, Inc.

Table 4.16 Calculated mean values per caput for the availability of specific indispensable amino acids in developed and developing regions

Region	Amino acid (mg/day) Lys	SAA	Try	Thr	Amino acid (mg/g protein) Lys	SAA	Try	Thr
Developing[a]	2947	2160	693	2204	49	36	11	37
Developed and transitional[b]	6149	3619	1177	3799	64	38	12	40

From Young *et al*. (1998). With permission of Oxford University Press, Inc.
[a]Data for 61 countries.
[b]Data for 29 countries.

content of food proteins mentioned above it is not surprising there are distinct differences in the intakes of the indispensable amino acids by different population groups worldwide. An example of such differences in given in Table 4.16. As already noted, the four amino acids of greatest importance and the ones most likely to be most limiting in intake, relative to requirements, are lysine, the sulfur amino acids (methionine and cystine), tryptophan and threonine.

4.8 Factors other than diet affecting protein and amino acid requirements

Not everyone of the same age, body-build and gender has the same nutrient requirements. These differences may be due, in part, to variations in genetic background. Various environmental, physiological, psychological and pathological influences affect the variability in physiological requirements for nutrients among individuals (Table 4.17). For example, as already discussed,

the growing infant or child requires higher nutrient intakes per unit of body weight than does the adult. Besides energy, for which the daily requirement declines with age because of reduced physical activity, it appears that the nutrient needs of healthy aged subjects do not differ significantly from those of young adults. Nevertheless, a characteristic of agng is an increased incidence of disease and morbidity, which is likely to be far more important than age per se in determining practical differences between the nutrient requirements of younger adults and elderly people.

Thus, superimposed infection, altered gastrointestinal function and metabolic changes that often accompany chronic disease states would all be expected to reduce the efficiency of dietary nitrogen and amino acid utilization. The metabolic response to acute infection in healthy young men has been characterized in experiments involving different types of intracellular infection, and involves an increased loss of body nitrogen,

Table 4.17 Agent, host and environment factors that affect protein and amino acid requirements and the nutritional status of the individual

Agent (dietary) factors
  Chemical form of nutrition (protein and amino acid source)
  Energy intake
  Food processing and preparation (may increase or
    decrease dietary needs)
  Effect of other dietary constituents
Host factors
  Age
  Gender
  Genetic make-up
  Pathological states
    Drugs
    Infection
    Physical trauma
    Chronic disease, cancer
Environmental factors
  Physical (unsuitable housing, inadequate heating)
  Biological (poor sanitary conditions)
  Socioeconomic (poverty, dietary habits and food choices,
    physical activity)

together with increased losses of several other nutrients including potassium, magnesium, phosphorus and vitamin C. This increased loss clearly implies increased needs for nitrogen, amino acids and other nutrients.

In addition to the catabolic response of body nitrogen metabolism to infection and trauma, there is a corresponding anabolic component that is of major importance during recovery from these stressful conditions. Anabolic responses occur not only during recovery but also in the early phase of illness, when anabolism is associated with increased production of immunocompetent cells such as phagocytes and other leukocytes, and the induction of several tissue enzymes and immunoglobulins.

During recovery from infection two characteristics of the anabolic period that follows are that the increased nitrogen retention seen during this period is greater than that measured during the preincubation phase, and its duration is much longer than the catabolic period. This may be due, in part, to the effect of protein depletion antedating an acute episode, which may be the case in poor communities. However, in spite of the potential for disease states to increase protein and amino acid needs there are too few studies that help to assess precisely their quantitative influence on nutrient utilization and dietary requirements.

4.9 Perspectives on the future

The purpose of this chapter was to provide a general overview of human protein and amino acid metabolism and a basis for an improved appreciation of the metabolic determinants of the requirements for protein (nitrogen) and for specific amino acids. With the recent beginning of the postgenome era, functional genomics, proteomics and metabolomics will take on an increasingly important basic and applied research focus in biology. Thus, it will be even more critical for students to understand the physiology of human protein metabolism at its various levels of biological complexity (cell, organ and whole body) and its nutritional corollaries.

There are certain areas of research in protein nutrition where more knowledge will equip nutritionists to make the best use of available food supplies. An example is the influence of the ratio of total essential or indispensable amino acids to total nitrogen and amino acid requirements for different physiological states. Another is the need for a functional definition of protein requirements (e.g. indices) for maximum resistance to disease and enhanced physical performance. These are some of the challenges facing nutritionists in the future. It is hoped that this chapter will serve as an appropriate catalyst for further learning in this area of human nutrition.

Further reading

Cohen PP. In: Nitrogen Metabolism in Man (JC Waterlow, JML Stephen, eds), p. 215. London: Applied Science, 1981.

FAO. Protein quality evaluation. FAO Food and Nutrition Paper 51, 66 pp. Rome: Food and Agriculture Organization of the United Nations, 1991.

FAO/WHO/UNU. Technical Report Series No. 724. Geneva: World Health Organization, 1985.

Garrow JS, Halliday D, eds. Substrate and Energy Metabolism in Man. London: John Libbey, 1985.

Lehninger AL, Nelson DL, Cox MM. Principles of Biochemistry, 2nd edn. New York: Worth, 1993.

Millward DJ. Proc Nutr Soc 1999; 58: 249–260.

HN Munro, ed. Mammalian Protein Metabolism, Vol. III. New York: Academic Press, 1969.

HN Munro, ed. Mammalian Protein Metabolism, Vol. IV. New York: Academic Press, 1970.

HN Munro, JB Allison, eds. Mammalian Protein Metabolism, Vols I and II. New York: Academic Press, 1964.

Reeds PJ. Dispensable and indispensable amino acids for humans. J Nutr 2000; 130: 1835S–1840S. American Society for Nutritional Sciences.

Waterlow JC. The mysteries of nitrogen balance. Nutr Res Rev 1999; 12: 25–54.

Waterlow JC, Garlick PJ, Millward DJ. Protein Turnover in Mammalian Tissues and in the Whole Body. Amsterdam: North-Holland, 1978.

Wolfe RR. Radioactive and Stable Isotope Tracers in Biomedicine: Principles and Practice of Kinetic Analysis. New York: Wiley-Liss, 1992.

Young VR, Borgonha S. Nitrogen and amino acid requirements: the Massachusetts Institute of Technology Amino Acid Requirement Pattern. J Nutr 2000; 130: 1841S–1849S. American Society for Nutritional Sciences.

Young VR, Scrimshaw NS, Pellett PL. In: Feeding a World Population of More than Eight Billion People, by Rank Prize Funds (JC Waterlow, DG Armstrong, L Fowder and R Riley, eds), pp. 206–212. New York: Oxford University Press, Inc, 1998.

Young VR, Yu Y-M, Fukagawa NK. Energy and Protein Turnover in Energy Metabolism: Tissue Determinants and Cellular Corollaries (JM Kinney, HN Tucker, eds), pp. 439–466. New York: Raven Press, 1992.

5
Digestion and Metabolism of Carbohydrates

John Mathers and Tom Wolever

Key messages

- Carbohydrates are the single most abundant and economic sources of food energy in the human diet, comprising 40–80% of total energy intake in different populations.
- Carbohydrates are classified according to their degree of polymerization into sugars, oligosaccharides and polysaccharides, the latter consisting of starches with different degrees of resistance to digestion, and dietary fibers or nonstarch polysaccharides.
- Glycemic carbohydrates are digested (hydrolyzed by enzymes) to sugars (monosaccharides) in the small bowel and absorbed and metabolized.
- Nonglycemic carbohydrates are fermented in varying degrees to short-chain fatty acids (SCFA), carbon dioxide,

hydrogen and methane in the large bowel. Absorbed SCFA are metabolized in colonic epithelial, hepatic and muscle cells.
- For optimum function of the nervous system and other cells, blood glucose concentrations are tightly controlled by a group of hormones (insulin in the absorptive phase; glucagon, adrenaline and cortisol in the postabsorptive phase), utilizing several possible metabolic pathways for glucose anabolism and catabolism.
- Intakes of optimum amounts of different types of carbohydrates are associated with good health through effects on energy balance, digestive functions, blood glucose control and other risk factors for several chronic diseases.

5.1 Introduction: carbohydrates in foods

Carbohydrates are one of the four major classes of biomolecules and play several important roles in all life forms including:

- sources of metabolic fuels and energy stores
- structural components of cell walls in plants and of the exoskeleton of arthropods
- parts of RNA and DNA in which ribose and deoxyribose, respectively, are linked by N-glycosidic bonds to purine and pyrimidine bases
- integral features of many proteins and lipids (glycoproteins and glycolipids), especially in cell membranes where they are essential for cell–cell recognition and molecular targeting.

Carbohydrates are very diverse molecules that can be classified by their molecular size (degree of polymerization or DP) into sugars (DP 1–2), oligosaccharides (DP 3–9) and polysaccharides (DP > 9). The physicochemical properties of carbohydrates and their fates within the body are also influenced by their monosaccharide composition and the type of linkage between sugar residues. Examples of food carbohydrates and an overview of their digestive fates are given in Table 5.1.

From birth, carbohydrate provides a large part of the energy in human diets, with approximately 40% of the energy in mature breast milk being supplied as lactose. After weaning, carbohydrates are the largest source (40–80%) of the energy in many human diets, with most of this derived from plant material except where

Table 5.1 Classes of food carbohydrates and their likely fates in the human gut

Class	DP	Example	Site of digestion	Absorbed molecules
Monosaccharides	1	Glucose	Small bowel	Glucose
	1	Fructose	Small bowel[a]	Fructose
	2	Sucrose	Small bowel	Glucose + fructose
	2	Lactose[b]	Small bowel	Glucose + galactose
Oligosaccharides	3	Raffinose	Large bowel	SCFA
	3–9	Inulin	Large bowel	SCFA
Polysaccharides	>9	Starches	Predominantly small bowel[c]	Glucose
	>9	Nonstarch polysaccharides	Large bowel	SCFA

[a] Except where very large doses are consumed in a single meal.
[b] Except in lactose-intolerant subjects, where lactose flows to the large bowel.
[c] Some starch escapes small bowel digestion (resistant starch). In all these cases, the carbohydrate entering the large bowel
becomes a substrate for bacterial fermentation to short-chain fatty acids (SCFA).
DP: degree of polymerization.

milk or milk products containing lactose are consumed. The carbohydrate contents of some vegetable dishes are summarized in Table 5.2.

5.2 Digestive fate of dietary carbohydrates

As with other food components, the digestive fate of particular carbohydrates depends on their inherent chemical nature and on the supramolecular structures within foods of which they are a part. To be absorbed from the gut, carbohydrates must be broken down to their constituent monosaccharide units, and a battery of hydrolytic enzymes capable of splitting the bonds between sugar residues is secreted within the mouth, from the pancreas and on the apical membrane of enterocytes. While these carbohydrases ensure that about 95% of the carbohydrate in most human diets is digested and absorbed within the small intestine, there is considerable variation in bioavailability between different carbohydrate classes and between different foods. Carbohydrates that are digested to sugars and absorbed as such in the small bowel are called "glycemic" carbohydrates.

Hydrolysis in the mouth and small bowel

The major carbohydrase secreted by the salivary glands and by the acinar cells of the pancreas is the endo-glycosidase α-amylase, which hydrolyzes (digests) internal α-1,4-linkages in amylose and amylopectin molecules to yield maltose, maltotriose and dextrins. These oligosaccharides, together with the food di-

saccharides sucrose and lactose, are hydrolyzed by specific oligosaccharidases expressed on the apical membrane of the epithelial cells that populate the small intestinal villi. Sucrase–isomaltase is a glycoprotein anchored via its amino-terminal domain in the apical membrane which hydrolyzes all of the sucrose and most of the maltose and isomaltose. The resulting monomeric sugars are then available for transport into the enterocytes.

Absorption and malabsorption in the small bowel

Glucose and galactose are transported across the apical membrane by the sodium-glucose transport protein-1 (SGLT1), a process that is powered by Na^+/K^+-ATPase on the basolateral membrane (see Figure 5.1). In contrast, fructose is absorbed by facilitated transport via the membrane-spanning GLUT5 protein. A member of the same family of transporter proteins, GLUT2, is the facilitated transporter on the basolateral membrane which shuttles all three monosaccharides from the enterocyte towards the blood vessels linking with the portal vein for delivery to the liver.

The capacity of the human intestine for transport of glucose, galactose and fructose is enormous – estimated to be about 10 kg per day – so that this does not limit absorption in healthy individuals. Carbohydrate malabsorption is usually caused by an inherited or acquired defect in the brush border oligosaccharidases. More than 75% of human adults are lactose intolerant because of a loss (possibly genetically determined) of lactase activity after weaning (primary lactose intolerance). In such individuals, ingestion of more

Table 5.2 Carbohydrate composition (g/100 g) of some vegetable dishes

Dish	Water	Carbohydrate	Starch	Total sugars	Glucose	Fructose	Galactose	Sucrose	Maltose	Lactose	Oligosaccharides	NSP	Cellulose
Bhaji, okra	77.7	7.6	0.4	5.5	1.9	1.7	0	1.9	0	Tr	1.7	3.2	1.0
Cannelloni, spinach	73.4	12.6	10.4	2.2	0.1	0.1	0	0.1	0.1	1.7	Tr	1.2	0.8
Chili, bean and lentil	72.6	13.1	7.9	4.3	1.3	1.4	0	1.6	0	0	0.8	3.6	1.1
Curry, chickpea	52.7	21.3	18.7	1.2	Tr	0.1	0	1.0	0	0	1.4	4.5	1.1
Flan, cheese and mushroom	49.1	18.7	16.4	2.3	0.2	0.2	0	0.1	Tr	1.8	Tr	0.9	0.1
Pizza, cheese and tomato	51.0	25.2	23.0	2.2	0.6	0.6	0	0.9	0.1	Tr	0	1.4	0.2
Shepherd's pie, vegetable	71.7	15.8	14.0	1.4	0.5	0.4	0	0.6	0	0	0.4	2.4	0.8

Data from Holland et al. (1992). Reproduced with permission from HMSO.
NSP: nonstarch polysaccharides (Englyst method).
Tr: trace.

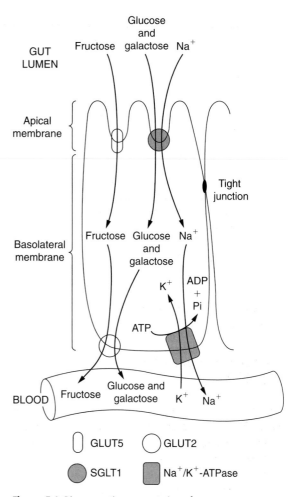

Figure 5.1 Diagrammatic representation of sugar transporters on enterocytes, showing the transport of glucose and galactose across the apical membrane.

than very small amounts of lactose leads to the passage of the sugar to the large bowel, where it is fermented to produce short-chain fatty acids (SCFA) and gases as end-products. The appearance of hydrogen in the breath after ingestion of lactose is the basis for diagnosis of malabsorption of this carbohydrate. Diseases of the intestinal tract, such as protein-energy malnutrition, intestinal infections and celiac disease, which reduce expression of lactase on the enterocyte apical membrane, can result in secondary lactase insufficiency. Sucrase– isomaltase activity, which rises rapidly from the pylorus towards the jejunum and then declines, is inducible by sucrose feeding. About 10% of Greenland Eskimos and 0.2% of North Americans have sucrase– isomaltase deficiency. A missense mutation in SGLT1 is responsible for the very rare glucose–galactose malabsorption syndrome, but such individuals absorb fructose well. In up to 60% of adults, the capacity for facilitated diffusion of fructose appears to be limited, resulting in symptoms of "intestinal distress" when challenged by consumption of 50 g fructose.

5.3 Glycemic carbohydrates

The rate of uptake of glucose (and other sugars) from the gut is determined by the rate of hydrolysis of oligo-saccharides and polysaccharides that are susceptible to pancreatic and brush border enzymes. In addition to the primary structure of the polymers, many factors intrinsic to the ingested foods and to the consumer influence these rates, including:

- food factors:
  - particle size
  - macrostructure and microstructure of food, especially whether cell walls are intact
  - amylose : amylopectin ratio of starches
  - lipid content of food
  - presence (or otherwise) of enzyme inhibitors
- consumer factors:
  - degree of comminution in the mouth
  - rate of gastric emptying
  - small bowel transit time.

All three main sugars absorbed from the gut (glucose, galactose and fructose) are transported via the portal vein to the liver (glucose concentrations in the portal vein after a meal can rise to almost 10 mM), but only glucose appears in significant concentrations in the peripheral circulation. Most of the galactose and fructose is removed during first pass through the liver via specific receptors on hepatocytes, so that the blood concentration of these sugars rarely exceeds 1 mM. Within the hepatocytes, galactose is converted to galactose-1-phosphate by the enzyme galactokinase and then to glucose-1-phosphate in three further steps. Fructose is also phosphorylated in hepatocytes (by fructokinase) to fructose-1-phosphate, which is subsequently split by aldolase B to yield one molecule of each of the glycolytic intermediates dihydroxyacetone phosphate and glyceraldehyde. Although the liver removes some glucose, using the bidirectional transporter GLUT2, most is transported in the peripheral circulation for utilization by muscle, adipose and other tissues.

Metabolic utilization of carbohydrate

Peripheral tissues utilize glucose and the above-mentioned intermediates from fructose and galactose via glycolysis and the citric acid or Krebs cycle pathways. Glycolysis, a sequence of reactions in which glucose is converted to pyruvate, with concomitant production of ATP, is the prelude to the citric acid cycle and electron transport chain, which together release the energy contained in glucose. Under aerobic conditions pyruvate enters mitochondria, where it is completely oxidized to carbon dioxide and water. If the supply of oxygen is limited, as in actively contracting muscle, pyruvate is converted to lactate. Therefore, complete oxidation of glucose to carbon dioxide and water occurs under aerobic conditions through the reactions of the glycolytic pathway (in the cell's cytoplasm), the Krebs cycle and oxidative phosphorylation (in the mitochondrion). The overall reaction can be summarized stoichiometrically as:

$$C_6H_{12}O_6 + 6O_2 \rightarrow 6CO_2 + 6H_2O$$

Approximately 40% of the free energy (ΔG) released by this transformation is captured by the production of ATP (38 moles of ATP per mole of glucose oxidized), which is used for a wide variety of purposes including powering muscle contraction, transporting substances across membranes against a concentration gradient and synthesis of cell macromolecules. The remainder of the free energy is released as heat.

When the demand for oxygen exceeds supply, as in muscle during intense exercise, anaerobic glycolysis produces lactic acid as a major end-product. The relative lack of oxygen means that oxidative phosphorylation cannot keep up with the supply of reduced dinucleotides and, for glycolysis to proceed, NADH must be recycled back to NAD^+. This is achieved by the reaction:

$$\text{Pyruvate} + \text{NADH} + H^+ \rightarrow \text{Lactate} + NAD^+$$

which is catalyzed by the enzyme lactate dehydrogenase. Anaerobic glycolysis provides some or all of the ATP needs for some cells and tissues, for example erythrocytes, white blood cells, lymphocytes, the kidney medulla and eye tissues. The lactate released from tissues undergoing anaerobic glycolysis is taken up by other tissues that have a high number of mitochondria per cell, such as heart muscle, in which the lactate is converted back to pyruvate and then enters the Krebs cycle via acetyl coenzyme A.

In hepatic and muscle cells some glucose is converted to glycogen in the glycogenesis pathway. Glycogen is a readily mobilized storage form of glucose residues linked with α-1,4-glycosidic bonds into a large, branched polymer. Glycogen is a reservoir of glucose for strenuous muscle activity and its synthesis and degradation are important for the regulation of blood glucose concentrations.

Regulation of blood glucose concentration

The exocrine pancreas (and other tissues) is primed to expect a rise in blood glucose concentration by peptide hormones such as gastric inhibitory peptide (GIP) which are secreted from enteroendocrine cells within the mucosa of the small bowel. As the glucose concentration in blood rises above 5 mM after a meal, these peptide hormones amplify the response of the β-cells of the endocrine pancreas, resulting in the discharge of the hormone insulin from secretory granules which fuse with the cell membrane. Insulin has several effects on metabolism, including facilitating the transport, by GLUT4, of glucose into adipocytes and muscle cells.

In healthy people, blood glucose concentration (glycemia) is homeostatically controlled within a fairly narrow range. It seldom falls below about 5 mM, even after a prolonged fast, and returns to this value within a couple of hours of a meal. In the absence of uptake from the gut (the postabsorptive state), about 8 g glucose/h is provided for those tissues with an obligatory demand for glucose, namely the brain, red blood cells, mammary gland and testis, by breakdown of stores of glycogen in the liver and muscle and by gluconeogenesis. The brain of an adult has a glucose requirement of about 120 g/day. The amount readily available in glycogen approximates 190 g. In long periods of fasting and starvation glucose must be formed from noncarbohydrate sources by a process known as gluconeogenesis. Gluconeogenesis occurs in the liver (responsible for about 90% of gluconeogenesis) and kidney and is the synthesis of glucose from a range of substrates including pyruvate, lactate, glycerol and amino acids. Amino acids are derived by catabolism of the body's proteins. All amino acids, with the exceptions of lysine and leucine, are glucogenic. Triacylglycerols (from adipose tissue) are catabolized to release glycerol. These gluconeogenic processes are triggered by a fall in blood glucose concentration below about 5 mM and are signaled to the tissues by the secretion of glucagon and the glucocorticoid hormones.

Diabetes and its consequences

Diabetes may be diagnosed as an exaggerated response in blood glucose concentration following ingestion of a fixed amount of glucose (glucose tolerance test). The most common forms of diabetes are insulin-dependent diabetes mellitus (IDDM or type I diabetes) and noninsulin-dependent diabetes mellitus (NIDDM or type II diabetes). IDDM results from the autoimmune destruction of the β-cells of the endocrine pancreas (possibly following viral exposure), the consequence of which is insulin insufficiency. Control of blood glucose concentrations in IDDM requires the exogenous supply of insulin by injection. Implanted insulin minipumps or pancreatic β-cells may offer alternative forms of treatment in the future. Symptoms of type I diabetes include the presence of glucose in urine, passage of large volumes of urine, body weight loss and, in extreme cases, ketosis (excess production of acetone, acetoacetate and β-hydroxybutyrate). Although there is good evidence of genetic predisposition to NIDDM, expression of the disease is due mainly to lifestyles (excess energy intakes and low physical activity) resulting in obesity, especially where the extra fat is accumulated on the trunk. The early stages of NIDDM are characterized by insulin insensitivity/resistance, that is, failure of the tissues to produce a normal response to insulin release which can be seen as relatively wide swings in blood glucose concentrations following a carbohydrate-containing meal. Raised blood glucose concentration sustained for several years is believed to be fundamental to the spectrum of complications including macrovascular (atherosclerosis) and microvascular diseases and problems with the kidneys (nephropathy), nerves (neuropathy) and eyes (retinopathy and cataract) experienced by diabetics.

Dietary management of blood glucose concentration

Glycemic index

As an aid to the dietary management of blood glucose concentrations in diabetics, Jenkins and colleagues introduced the concept of the glycemic index (GI), which provides a means of comparing quantitatively the blood glucose responses (determined directly by *in vivo* experiments) following ingestion of equivalent amounts of digestible carbohydrate from different foods. When a range of carbohydrate-containing foods was ranked according to their GI values, there was a strong linear relationship with the rapidly available glucose (RAG) from similar foods determined *in vitro* as the sum of free glucose, glucose from sucrose and glucose released from starches over a 20 min period of hydrolysis with a battery of enzymes under strictly controlled conditions (Englyst method). This offers the possibility of assaying foods *in vitro* for their RAG content, which will be quicker and cheaper than the current approach based on GI measurements *in vivo*.

Studies with glucose and starches enriched with the stable isotope carbon-13 have demonstrated that glucose absorption from the gut following a meal continues for several hours after blood concentrations have returned to fasting levels. In this later postprandial period, insulin secretion is sufficient to ensure that the rate of glucose absorption is matched by the rate of glucose removal from the circulation. ^{13}C-Labeled substrates are being used increasingly to investigate the kinetics of digestion, absorption and metabolic disposal of glucose and other sugars from a range of foods. When continued over several years, high rates of glucose absorption and the subsequent challenge to the capacity of the pancreatic β-cells to secrete insulin may be the primary determinants of insulin resistance and eventual pancreatic failure which contribute strongly to the aetiology of diabetes and cardiovascular disease. Such kinetic studies are likely to be helpful in identifying foods with slower rates of intestinal hydrolysis, information that can be used in public health advice or in counseling of individuals.

Fructose

When glucose and fructose are available simultaneously after a meal containing sucrose, how does the body select which fuel to use first for oxidative purposes? This question has been resolved by experiments in which volunteers consumed, on two separate occasions, high sucrose test meals which were identical except that one or other of the constituent monomeric sugars was ^{13}C-labeled in each meal. The volunteers blew into tubes at intervals after the meals to provide breath samples for measurement of enrichment of expired CO_2 with ^{13}C. The results showed that after the high sucrose meal, fructose was oxidized much more rapidly and extensively than was glucose (Figure 5.2).

This rapid oxidation of fructose may be explained by the fact that, because it is phosphorylated in hepatocytes, it bypasses 6-phosphofructokinase, one of the key regulatory enzymes in glycolysis.

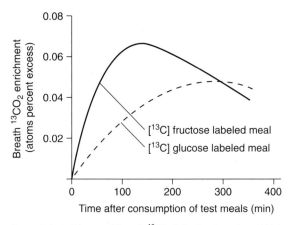

Figure 5.2 Enrichment of breath $^{13}CO_2$ following ingestion of high sucrose test meals labeled with [^{13}C]fructose and [^{13}C]glucose. (Redrawn from Daly *et al.*, 2000.)

5.4 Nonglycemic carbohydrates

Carbohydrates that are not absorbed in the small intestine enter the large bowel, where they are partially or completely broken down by bacteria in the colon by a process called fermentation. McCance and Lawrence in 1929 were the first to classify carbohydrates as "available" and "unavailable". They realized that not all carbohydrates provide "carbohydrates for metabolism" to the body. They called these carbohydrates "unavailable". This was a very useful concept because it drew attention to the fact that some carbohydrate is not digested and absorbed in the small intestine, but rather reaches the large bowel where it is fermented. However, it is now realized that it is misleading to talk of carbohydrate as unavailable because some indigestible carbohydrate can provide the body with energy through fermentation in the colon. Thus, "unavailable carbohydrates" are not really unavailable. For this reason, it has been suggested by the Food and Agriculture Organization (FAO) of the United Nations and World Health Organization that the term "nonglycemic carbohydrates" is more appropriate.

Nature of carbohydrates that enter the colon

Carbohydrates that enter the colon can be classified either physiologically or chemically. Neither of these classifications is entirely satisfactory because it is difficult to measure the physiologically indigestible carbohydrate and this varies in different people. Further, the chemical structure of carbohydrates does not always predict their physiological behavior.

Physiological classification of carbohydrates entering the colon

Carbohydrates enter the colon either because: (1) monosaccharide transporters do not exist in the intestinal mucosa or do not function at a high enough rate; (2) the enzymes needed to digest the carbohydrates are not present in the small intestine; (3) the enzymes are present but cannot gain access to the carbohydrates; or (4) the enzymes do not digest the carbohydrates rapidly enough for them to be completely absorbed. In addition, a small amount of carbohydrate entering the colon consists of carbohydrate residues occurring on mucopolysaccharides (mucus) secreted by the small and large intestinal mucosal cells.

Some carbohydrates are always nonglycemic because the human species lacks the enzymes necessary for their digestion. However, a significant proportion (perhaps up to half) of all carbohydrates that escape digestion in the small intestine have a chemical structure which is such that they could potentially be digested or absorbed in the small intestine, but they are variably absorbed for various reasons, examples of which are given below.

First, some monosaccharides and sugar alcohols are only partially absorbed because of low affinity for intestinal transporters. Xylose is taken up by the glucose transporter, but is only partly absorbed because of a low affinity. Fructose is poorly absorbed on its own, but readily absorbed in the presence of glucose. The surface area of the small intestine available for absorption is reduced by diseases that cause atrophy of the intestinal mucosa, such as tropical sprue or celiac disease, or surgical resection of a portion of the intestine (e.g. for Crohn's disease). An increased rate of intestinal transit (e.g. high osmotic load in the small intestinal lumen from undigested sugars) reduces the time available for absorption to occur.

Secondly, some individuals have a low or absent intestinal lactase activity, thus lactose is partly or completely nonabsorbed in these individuals. The availability of pancreatic amylase may be reduced in cystic fibrosis or in individuals whose pancreatic mass has been destroyed by, for example, recurrent pancreatitis.

Thirdly, although starch (amylopectin or amylose) is potentially digested in the small intestine, if it is trapped inside intact cell walls or other plant cell structures, intestinal enzymes may not be able to gain access to it, and therefore it remains undigested. The digestibility of the carbohydrates in banana depends on the degree of ripeness. The starch in green banana is very indigestible, but as the banana ripens, the starch is converted to digestible sugars.

Finally, there are many reasons why carbohydrates may not be digested rapidly enough to be completely absorbed. Some forms of retrograded or resistant starch, or foods with a large particle size, are digested so slowly that the time spent in the small intestine is not long enough for their complete digestion. Digestion of these carbohydrates can be altered by factors that affect transit time. The presence of osmotically active and unabsorbed molecules (such as unabsorbed sugars) will draw water into the intestine and speed the rate of transit. Substances that increase bulk, such as wheat bran, will have similar effects. Transit rate is slowed in old age and in the presence of viscous fibers. Drugs may increase or decrease the rate of transit. Certain disorders can also affect transit time, such as gastroparesis, a complication of type I diabetes.

Chemical classification of carbohydrates entering the colon

The chemical classification of carbohydrates entering the colon is as follows:

- *Monosaccharides:* all except for glucose, fructose and galactose are partly or completely unabsorbed. Fructose in the absence of a source of glucose (mono-, di- or polysaccharide) is partly unabsorbed.
- *Sugar alcohols:* all are partly or completely unabsorbed.
- *Disaccharides:* all except for maltose, sucrose and lactose are unabsorbed. Lactose is completely or partly unabsorbed in individuals with low intestinal lactase activity.
- *Oligosaccharides:* all are unabsorbed except for maltodextins.
- *Polysaccharides:* all nonstarch polysaccharides are unabsorbed.
- *Resistant starch.*

Amount of carbohydrate entering the colon

It is difficult to measure the amount of carbohydrate entering the human colon. However, it has been estimated that at least 30 g of carbohydrate is required to support the growth of the bacterial population in the colon of an individual on a typical Western diet producing about 100 g stool/day. About half of that amount will come from nonstarch polysaccharide (NSP, also known as dietary fiber), 1–2 g from indigestible oligosaccharides and probably about 1–2 g from intestinal mucopolysaccharides. These components add up to only 18–20 g. Where does the other 10–12 g come from? It is believed to come from starch, because experiments in humans show that about 5–15% of the starch in foods enters the colon. Typical Western diets contain about 120–150 g starch per day, and if 8% of this enters the colon, this will provide the additional 10–12 g carbohydrate. The amount of carbohydrate entering the colon, however, can be increased several-fold, up to 100 g/day or more, by changes in diet such as increased intake of NSP, non-digestible or partially digestible carbohydrates (ingredients in functional foods), total starch, resistant starch or slowly digested, low GI foods.

Resistant starch

Resistant starch is starch that escapes digestion in the small intestine and enters the colon. However, there is controversy over the amounts of resistant starch in foods because there is no universally accepted method for measuring it (different methods yield different results). The amount of resistant starch measured chemically is generally less than that observed to enter the colon (or leave the small intestine) in experiments in human volunteers.

In the 1970s and early 1980s it first became apparent that appreciable amounts of starch are not digested in the small bowel, from experiments showing that breath hydrogen increased after eating normal starchy foods. The only source of hydrogen gas in the human body is as a product of the anaerobic fermentation of carbohydrates by colonic bacteria (see below). If a person consumed a load of an absorbable sugar such as glucose, breath hydrogen did not go up. In contrast, if lactulose (an unabsorbed disaccharide of fructose and galactose) was consumed, breath hydrogen increased rapidly, and the area under the breath hydrogen curve over an 8–12 h period was directly proportional to the amount of lactulose consumed. If subjects ate common starchy foods such as white bread or potato, breath hydrogen levels increased to an extent that suggested that 5–10% of the starch was fermented in the colon. Subsequently, other ways of measuring carbohydrate entering the colon were developed. In one technique,

subjects swallowed a tube that was passed through the stomach and along to the end of small intestine so that the material leaving the small intestine and about to enter the colon could be sampled. Another method was to study people who have had their colons removed surgically and in whom the end of the ileum was sutured to a stoma in the body wall. In this way, the material leaving their small intestine could be collected quantitatively in a bag attached to their abdomen. With the latter methods, the amount of carbohydrate leaving the small intestine can be measured directly. These methods confirmed that a substantial amount of starch enters the colon.

The main forms of resistant starch (RS) are: physically enclosed starch, for example within intact cell structures (known at RS_1), raw starch granules (RS_2) and retrograded amylose (RS_3). These kinds of starch can be identified chemically using methods developed by Englyst and colleagues.

Dietary fiber

Major interest in dietary fiber began in the early 1970s with the proposal by Burkitt and Trowell that many Western diseases were due to a lack of fiber in the diet. However, the definition of dietary fiber has been, and continues to be, a source of scientific controversy. Indeed, two consecutive reports from the FAO (1979 and 1997) recommended that the term "dietary fiber" be phased out. Nevertheless, the term appears to be here to stay because it is accepted by consumers, the food industry and governments.

A definition and method of measuring fiber is important for scientific studies and for food labeling purposes. The student must be aware that the definitions and methods of measuring fiber have changed over time, and differ in different parts of the world. Knowledge of what is meant by the term "fiber" and what is included in the measurement is essential for proper interpretation of the scientific literature (but often is not given in the methods section of papers and reports).

Originally, Burkitt and Trowell defined fiber as the components of plant cell walls that are indigestible in the human small intestine. Later, the definition was expanded to include storage polysaccharides within plant cells (e.g. the gums in some legumes). Many different methods were developed to measure dietary fiber, but they measured different things. All of the methods start with the drying and grinding of the food and extraction of the fat using an organic solvent.

If the remaining material is treated with strong acid, the chemical bonds in starch and many (but not all) polysaccharides will be broken down to release their component sugars. If these are filtered away, the residue is "crude fiber". For many years this was the way in which fiber was measured for food tables. However, acid hydrolysis breaks down many carbohydrates that would not be digested in the small intestine. So, in more modern methods, the food residue is digested with amylase to hydrolyze the starch to soluble sugars and oligosaccharides. The latter are removed by filtration or by centrifugation to leave a residue containing mainly dietary fiber, proteins and inorganic materials.

The two main methods used to determine dietary fiber are chemical and gravimetric. In the chemical method (used in the UK), the residue is subjected to acid hydrolysis and the resultant sugars are measured colorimetrically, by gas chromatography or by high-performance liquid chromatography. The sum of all these sugars comprises NSP. The chemical method includes only carbohydrates in NSP. In the gravimetric method (used in the USA and elsewhere), the residue is dried and weighed, and the amounts of protein and mineral materials present are subtracted (after separate analyses). The gravimetric method includes the NSP, plus other noncarbohydrate components such as lignin and waxes. Recently, all countries in Europe have recognized the gravimetric method as an approved method for measuring fiber in foods.

The main areas of disagreement now with respect to fiber are whether indigestible oligosaccharides and sugars and nonplant compounds should be included and whether the definition of fiber should include a physiological component. In Japan, fructo-oligosaccharides (FOS) are classified as dietary fiber for food labeling purposes. However, FOS and similar compounds, being soluble in water, are not included in the dietary fiber methods, because they are filtered out along with the sugars resulting from the starch hydrolysis. Specific methods exist for FOS and related compounds, and they could be included as fiber. Certain animal-derived compounds, such as chitin and chitosan, derived from the shells of shrimp and crabs, are indigestible, would be included in the gravimetric fiber analysis and could be classified as fiber. Chitin has some physiological properties, such as cholesterol lowering, which are associated with dietary fiber. There are many other indigestible carbohydrate and non-carbohydrate compounds, both natural and artificial, that could be classified as "fiber" (e.g. polydextrose, sucrose polyester, styrofoam). Should these be included in dietary fiber? In favor of this is the argument that some of these materials have physiological properties associated with fiber, such as stool bulking, or effects on satiety or blood glucose and cholesterol. Against this is the feeling that dietary fiber should include only plant materials that are normally present in the diet. These are not easy issues and they have not been resolved.

Intakes of dietary fiber, oligosaccharides and other indigestible sugars

Vegetarians tend to have higher fiber intakes than omnivores. The typical intake of dietary fiber in North America and northern and central Europe is about 15 g/day. In Scandinavia and Italy, fiber consumption is 20–30 g/day, while in African countries such as Uganda, Kenya, Malawi and Nigeria intakes may be as high as 50 g/day or more. Naturally occurring oligosaccharides are consumed in legumes, onions, fennel, chicory and similar foods. Intakes in Western countries are probably up to 2–4 g/day. Fructo- and galacto-oligosaccharides are now being added to certain "functional foods" in a number of countries, and intakes from such sources may increase substantially (up to 10–20 g/day). Many kinds of indigestible or partially digested carbohydrates are entering the food supply in dietetic, diabetic or functional foods, including sugar alcohols (polyols, e.g. sorbitol, mannitol, lactitol), polydextrose, resistant starch, hydrogenated starch and other chemically modified starches and carbohydrates. Thus, the total amount of carbohydrate entering the colon could become very substantial for people using these foods. Individually, these ingredients are generally recognized as safe, and evidence from populations consuming 50 g and more NSP per day suggests that the colon has the capacity to adapt to large increases in the load of carbohydrate. However, safe upper limits of intake are unknown and the health implications of an increased supply of a wide range of carbohydrates to the colon are currently based on inference rather than scientific data.

Fermentation in the colon

The colon contains a complex ecosystem consisting of over 400 known species of bacteria that exist in a symbiotic relationship with the host. The bacteria obtain the substrates that they require for growth from the

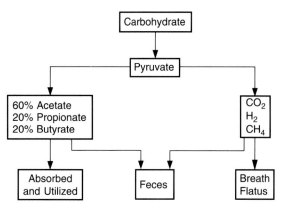

Figure 5.3 Overview of carbohydrate fermentation in the human colon.

host, and return to the host the by-products of their metabolism. The major substrate that the bacteria receive from the host is carbohydrate, mostly in the form of polysaccharides. They obtain nitrogen from urea (which diffuses into the colon from the blood) and undigested amino acids and proteins. Fermentation is the process by which microorganisms break down monosaccharides and amino acids to derive energy for their own metabolism. Fermentation reactions do not involve respiratory chains that use molecular oxygen or nitrate as terminal electron acceptors. Most of the fermentation in the human colon is anaerobic, that is, it proceeds in the absence of a source of oxygen. Different bacteria use different substrates via different types of chemical reaction. However, as a summary of the overall process, fermentation converts carbohydrates to energy, plus various end-products, which include the gases carbon dioxide, hydrogen and methane, and the SCFA acetic (C2), propionic (C3) and butyric (C4) acids. Acetate, propionate and butyrate appear in colonic contents in approximate molar ratios of 60:20:20, respectively. Most of the SCFA produced are absorbed and provide energy for the body (Figure 5.3).

The roles of SCFA in metabolism are discussed later in this chapter. Formic acid (C1) and minor amounts of longer chain SCFA and branched-chain SCFA may also be produced. In addition, lactic and succinic acids and ethanol or methanol may be intermediate or end-products depending on the conditions of the fermentation. For example, rapid fermentation in an environment with a low pH results in the accumulation of lactic and succinic acids.

The first step in fermentation is the breakdown of polysaccharides, oligosaccharides and disaccharides to their monosaccharide subunits. This is achieved either by the secretion of hydrolytic enzymes by bacteria into the colonic lumen or, more commonly, by expression of such enzymes on the bacterial surface so that the products of hydrolysis are taken up directly by the organism producing the enzyme. To degrade the NSP of dietary fiber, the bacteria may need to attach themselves to the surface of the remnants of the plant cell walls or other particulate material.

Once the monosaccharide is internalized, the majority of carbohydrate-fermenting species in the colon use the glycolytic pathway to metabolize carbohydrate to pyruvate. This pathway results in the reduction of NAD^+ to NADH. Fermentation reactions are controlled by the need to maintain redox balance between reduced and oxidized forms of pyridine nucleotides. The regeneration of NAD^+ may be achieved in a number of different ways (Figure 5.4).

Electron sink products such as ethanol, lactate, hydrogen and succinate are produced by some bacteria to regenerate oxidized pyridine nucleotides. These fermentation intermediates are subsequently fermented to SCFA by other gut bacteria, and are important factors in maintaining species diversity in the ecosystem.

Fate of short-chain fatty acids

Colonic fermentation can be viewed as a way in which the human host can recover part of the energy of malabsorbed carbohydrates. The amount of energy recovered from fermentation depends on the fermentability of the carbohydrate (which can range from 0 to 100%) and the nature of the products of fermentation. On a typical Western diet, about 40–50% of the energy in carbohydrate that enters the colon is available to the human host as SCFA. The rest of the energy is unavailable to the host, being lost as heat or unfermented carbohydrate, or used to produce gases or for bacterial growth (Figure 5.5).

SCFA are almost completely absorbed and, while some butyrate is oxidized by colonocytes (the epithelial cells lining the colon), most arrives at the liver via the portal vein. Propionate and butyrate are removed in first pass through the liver, but increased concentrations of acetate can be observed in peripheral blood several hours after consumption of indigestible but fermentable carbohydrates. These absorbed SCFA are readily oxidized and contribute modestly (up to 10%) to the body's energy supply.

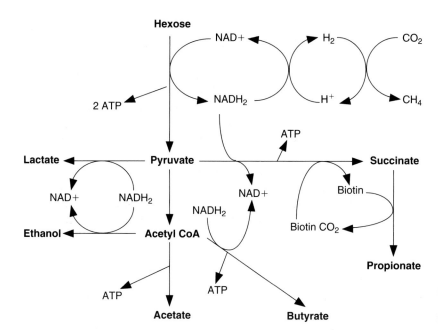

Figure 5.4 Summary of biochemical pathways used by the anaerobic bacteria in the colon.

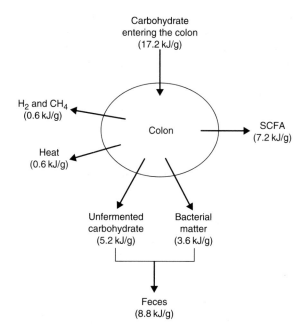

Figure 5.5 Quantitative fate of carbohydrate in the colon.

There is considerable interest in possible effects of individual SCFA on the health of the colon and the whole body. The strongest evidence to date is for an anti-cancer effect of butyrate, which may be due to butyrate's ability to induce differentiation and apoptosis (pro-grammed cell death) of colon cancer cells. There is some support for the hypothesis that propionate may help to reduce the risk of cardiovascular disease by lowering blood cholesterol concentration and/or by an effect on hemostasis, but the evidence so far is not conclusive.

5.5 Carbohydrates and dental caries

The resident bacteria in the mouth ferment carbo-hydrates to yield acidic end-products (mainly lactic acid but also some formic, acetic and propionic acids), which result in a drop in dental plaque pH. When the pH falls below 5.5, the dental enamel dissolves in the plaque fluid and repeated exposure to periods of very low pH can lead to caries. Not all carbohydrates are equally cariogenic. The sugars found commonly in human foods, e.g. sucrose, fructose, glucose and mal-tose, are all readily fermented by bacteria in the mouth. Lactose, galactose and starches are less cariogenic, while sugar alcohols such as xylitol (used as a sweetener in some confectionery and chewing gums) are non-cariogenic. Eating sugars with meals reduces the risk of caries, as does the consumption of cheese, which provides phosphates to prevent demineralization and to encourage demineralization of the enamel. Fluoride ingestion in foods and drinking water or topical application via toothpastes and mouth rinses prevents dental caries. Too much fluoride in drinking water can cause fluorosis, which damages the skeleton and teeth. The optimum concentration of fluoride in temperate areas of the world is 1 mg/l, falling to 0.6 mg/l in tropical climates where fluid intake is likely to be greater.

5.6 Perspectives on the future

The carbohydrate structure and amounts in many foods and ingredients can be manipulated to achieve specific physicochemical properties of benefit for food structure and organoleptic effects and to produce a diverse range of physiological effects. It can be expected that many functional foods of the future will contain such specially selected or modified carbohydrates, but the metabolic and health consequences of these carbohydrates should be examined in more detail before health claims can be justified.

Future research on carbohydrate nutrition should also focus on the physiological and biochemical (metabolic) effects of the SCFA produced from non-glycemic carbohydrates.

To provide a sound evidence base for recommendations for intakes of specific carbohydrates, the relationships between intakes of different types and quantities of carbohydrate with health and disease, for example during transition of traditional people and consequent lowering of intakes, should be a fruitful area for research.

Further reading

Asp N-G. In: Advanced Dietary Fibre Technology. (BV McCleary, L Prosky, eds), pp. 77–88. Oxford: Blackwell Science, 2001.
Brody T. Nutritional Biochemistry, 2nd edn. San Diego, CA: Academic Press, 1999.
Daly ME, Vale C, Walker M et al. Am J Clin Nutr 2000; 71: 1516–1524.
Holland B, Unwin ID, Buss DH. Vegetable dishes. Second supplement to McCance and Widdowson's The Composition of Foods, 5th edn. Cambridge: Royal Society of Chemistry, 1992.
Johnson LR. Gastrointestinal Physiology, 5th edn. St Louis, MO: Mosby, 1997.
Rugg-Gunn AJ. Nutrition and Dental Health. Oxford: Oxford University Press, 1993.

6
Nutrition and Metabolism of Lipids

Stephen C Cunnane and Bruce A Griffin

Key messages

- Lipids are organic compounds composed of a carbon skeleton with hydrogen and oxygen substitutions. The most abundant lipids are sterols or esters of fatty acids with various alcohols such as glycerol and cholesterol.
- Fatty acids are the densest dietary source of energy, but lipids also have important structural roles in membranes. The processes controlling the synthesis, modification and degradation of fatty acids contribute to the fatty acid profile of membrane and storage lipids.
- By enhancing the taste of cooked foods, some dietary lipids are potentially significant risk factors for obesity and other chronic, degenerative diseases that influence human morbidity and mortality.

- Dietary lipids are emulsified, lypolized (hydrolyzed) and solubilized in the upper small gut before they are absorbed in the ileum, entering enterocytes with the help of fatty acid binding proteins.
- Lipids are precursors to hormones such as steroids and eicosanoids, and dietary lipids are carriers for fat-soluble vitamins.
- Lipids are transported in the blood circulation as lipoprotein particles; the chylomicrons, very low-density, low-density and high-density lipoproteins.
- Some polyunsaturated fatty acids are vitamin like because they cannot be synthesized de novo (linoleate, α-linolenate).

6.1 Introduction: the history of lipids in human nutrition

The term "lipid" was introduced by Bloor in 1943, by which time the existence of cholesterol had been known for nearly 200 years and individual fats for 130 years. Cholesterol was named "cholesterine" (Greek for bile-solid) by Chevreul in 1816, although he did not discover it. Cholesterol's association with aortic plaques dates at least to Vogel's work in 1843. Chevreul isolated a mixture of 16–18 carbon saturated fatty acids in 1813 that was called margarine because he thought it was a single 17 carbon fatty acid, margarate. The mixed triglyceride of palmitate (16:0) and stearate (18:0) was also called margarine, while the triglyceride of oleate, stearate and palmitate became known as oleomargarine. Phospholipids were discovered by Thudicum, who isolated and named sphingosine in 1884 and also lecithin (phosphatidylcholine) and kephalin (phosphatidylethanolamine). The difference in polarity across phospholipids

is a key attribute of these molecules and was termed "amphipathic" by Hartley in 1936 and renamed "amphiphilic" by Winsor in 1948.

The first understanding of how fat was absorbed emerged in 1879 when Munk studied fat emulsions and showed that lymph contained triglycerides after a fatty meal, and even after a meal not containing triglycerides. In 1905, Knoop deduced that fatty acid β-oxidation probably occurred by stepwise removal of two carbons from the fatty acid. The probable role of two carbon units as building blocks in synthesis of fatty acids was recognized by Raper in 1907, but it took until the 1940s for Schoenheimer, Rittenberg, Bloch and others to confirm this using tracers such as deuterated water and carbon-13. The late 1940s was a seminal period for developing an understanding of how fatty acid oxidation occurs. Green and colleagues discovered that ketones were fatty acid oxidation products, and Lehninger demonstrated the role of mitochondria as the cellular site of fatty acid oxidation. Microsomal desaturases

Table 6.1 Classification of lipids

Simple lipids (fatty acids esterified with alcohols)	Fats (fatty acids esterified with glycerol)
	Waxes (true waxes, sterol esters, vitamin A and D esters)
Complex lipids (fatty acids esterified with alcohols plus other groups)	Phospholipids (contain phosphoric acid and, usually, a nitrogenous base)
	Glycolipids (lipids containing a carbohydrate and nitrogen but no phosphate and no glycerol)
	Sulfolipids (lipids containing a sulfur group)
	Lipoproteins (lipids attached to plasma or other proteins)
	Lipopolysaccharides (lipids attached to polysaccharides)
Derived lipids (obtained by hydrolysis of simple or complex lipids)	Fatty acids (saturated, monounsaturated or polyunsaturated)
	Monoglycerides and diglycerides
	Alcohols (include sterols, steroids, vitamin D, vitamin A)
Miscellaneous lipids	Straight-chain hydrocarbons
	Carotenoids
	Squalene
	Vitamins E and K

were shown to introduce an unsaturated bond into long-chain fatty acids by Bloomfield and Bloch in 1960.

In 1929, Mildred and George Burr discovered that the absence of fat in a diet otherwise believed to contain all essential nutrients impaired growth and caused hair loss and scaling of the skin of rats. This led to the isolation of the two primary "essential" polyunsaturated fatty acids, linoleate (18:2n-6) and α-linolenate (18:3n-3). The prostaglandins are a subclass of eicosanoids that were discovered in the early 1930s by Von Euler, who mistakenly believed that they originated from the prostate gland. The link between the eicosanoids and polyunsaturates, principally arachidonate, was established in the 1960s.

6.2 Terminology of dietary fats

Lipids

Like other organic compounds, all lipids are composed of a carbon skeleton with hydrogen and oxygen substitutions. Nitrogen, sulfur and phosphorus are also present in some lipids. Water insolubility is a key but not absolute characteristic distinguishing most lipids from proteins and carbohydrates. There are some exceptions to this general rule, since short- to medium-chain fatty acids, soaps and some complex lipids are soluble in water. Hence, solubility in a "lipid solvent" such as ether, chloroform, benzene or acetone is a common, but circular definition of lipids.

As classified by Bloor, there are four categories of lipids: simple, compound (complex), derived and miscellaneous (Table 6.1). Simple lipids are esters of

fatty acids with various alcohols such as glycerol or cholesterol. They include triglycerides, also known as triacylglycerols (neutral fats and oils), waxes, cholesteryl esters, and vitamin A and D esters. Compound lipids are esters of fatty acids in combination with both alcohols and other groups. They include phospholipids, glycolipids, cerebrosides, sulfolipids, lipoproteins and lipopolysaccharides. Derived lipids are hydrolysis products of simple or compound lipids, including fatty acids, monoglycerides and diglycerides, straight-chain and ring-containing alcohols, sterols and steroids. Miscellaneous lipids include some wax lipids, carotenoids, squalene and vitamins E and K.

Saturated and unsaturated fatty acids

The main components of dietary lipids are fatty acids varying in length from one to greater than 30 carbons. They are carboxylic acids with the structure RCOOH, where R is hydrogen in formic acid, CH_3 in acetic acid, or else a chain of one to over 30 CH_2 groups terminated by a CH_3 group. The various names for individual fatty acids (common, official) and their abbreviations are complicated and the use of one or other form is somewhat arbitrary. The basic rule for the abbreviations is that there are three parts: number of carbons, number of double bonds and position of the first double bond. Thus, the common dietary saturated fatty acid palmitate is 16:0 because it has 16 carbons and no double bonds. The common dietary polyunsaturated fatty acid linoleate is 18:2n-6 because it has 18 carbons and two double bonds, and the first double bond is at the sixth carbon from the methyl-terminal. Beyond six carbons in length, most fatty acids have an even number of

Table 6.2 Nomenclature of common fatty acids

Saturated	Monounsaturated	Polyunsaturated
Formic (1 : 0)	Lauroleic (12 : 1n-3)	Linoleic (18 : 2n-6)
Acetic (2 : 0)	Myristoleic (14 : 1n-5)	γ-Linolenic (18 : 3n-6)
Propionic (3 : 0)	Palmitoleic (16 : 1n-7)	Dihomo-γ-linolenic (20 : 3n-6)
Butyric (4 : 0)	Oleic (18 : 1n-9)	Arachidonate (20 : 4n-6)
Valeric (5 : 0)	Elaidic (*trans*-18 : 1n-9)	Adrenate (22 : 4n-6)
Caproic (6 : 0)	Vaccenic (18 : 1n-7)	n-6 Docosapentaenoic (22 : 5n-6)
Caprylic (8 : 0)	Petroselinic (18 : 1n-12)	α-Linolenic (18 : 3n-3)
Capric (10 : 0)	Gadoleic (20 : 1n-11)	Stearidonic (18 : 4n-3)
Lauric (12 : 0)	Gondoic (20 : 1n-9)	Eicosapentaenoic (20 : 5n-3)
Myristic (14 : 0)	Euricic (22 : 1n-9)	n-3 Docosapentaenoic (22 : 5n-3)
Palmitic (16 : 0)	Nervonic (24 : 1n-9)	Docosahexaenoic (22 : 6n-3)
Margeric (17 : 0)		
Stearic (18 : 0)		
Arachidic (20 : 0)		
Behenic (22 : 0)		
Lignoceric (24 : 0)		

carbons (Table 6.2). Older fatty acid terminology referring to saturated or unsaturated carbons in lipids that still occasionally appears includes: aliphatic (a saturated carbon), olefinic (an unsaturated carbon), allylic (a saturated carbon adjacent to an unsaturated carbon) and doubly allylic carbon (a saturated carbon situated between two unsaturated carbons).

Lengthening of the chain and the introduction of additional double bonds beyond the first one occur from the carboxyl-terminal. The presence of one or more double bonds in a fatty acid defines it as "unsaturated", compared with a saturated fatty acid which contains no double bonds. A saturated fatty acid generally occupies less space than an equivalent chain length unsaturated fatty acid (Figure 6.1). Double bonds allow for isomerization or different orientation (*cis* or *trans*) of the adjoining carbons across the double bond (Figure 6.2). In longer chain fatty acids, double bonds can also be at different positions in the molecule. Hence, unsaturation introduces a large amount of structural variety in fatty acids and the resulting lipids. Further details about the features of the different families of fatty acids are given in Sections 6.6 and 6.8.

Short- and medium-chain fatty acids

Short-chain fatty acids (<8 carbons) are water soluble. Except in milk lipids, they are not commonly esterified into body lipids. Short-chain fatty acids are found primarily in dietary products containing ruminant milk fat. Hence, although they are produced in relatively large quantities by fermentation of nondigested

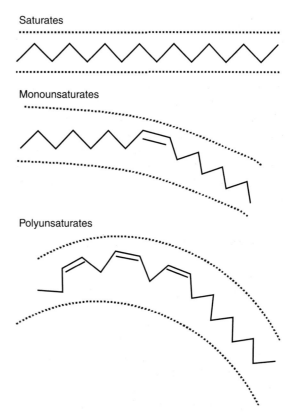

Saturates

Monounsaturates

Polyunsaturates

Figure 6.1 Stick models illustrating the basic structural differences between saturated, *cis*-monounsaturated and *cis*-polyunsaturated fatty acids. As shown in two dimensions, the increasing curvature caused by inserting one or more double bonds increases the area occupied by the fatty acid. The physical area occupied by unsaturated fatty acids is further accentuated in three dimensions because esterified fatty acids rotate around the anchored terminal.

cis-Monounsaturates

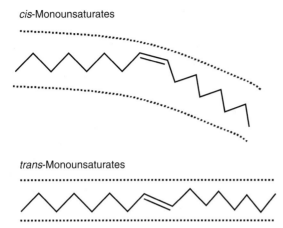

trans-Monounsaturates

Figure 6.2 Stick models comparing a *cis*- to a *trans*-unsaturated fatty acid. A *cis*-unsaturated double bond creates a U-shaped space and confers curvature to the molecule because, relative to the longitudinal axis of the fatty acid, the two hydrogens at the double bond are on the same side of the molecule. A *trans*-unsaturated double bond does not confer curvature to the molecule because the hydrogens are on opposite sides of the double bond. A *trans*-double bond therefore tends to give the fatty acid physicochemical properties more like that of a saturated fatty acid.

carbohydrate in the colon, as such, they do not become part of the body lipid pools. Medium-chain fatty acids (8–14 carbons) arise as intermediates in the synthesis of long-chain fatty acids or by the consumption of coconut oil or medium-chain triglyceride derived from it. Like short-chain fatty acids, medium-chain fatty acids are present in milk but they are also rarely esterified into body lipids, except when consumed in large amounts in clinical situations requiring alternative energy sources. Medium-chain fatty acids (8–14 carbons) are rare in the diet except for coconut and milk fat.

Long-chain saturated and monounsaturated fatty acids

Long-chain fatty acids (>14 carbons) are the main constituents of dietary fat. The most common saturated fatty acids in the body are palmitate and stearate. They originate from three sources: directly from the diet, by complete synthesis from acetyl-coenzyme A (CoA), or by lengthening (chain elongation) of a pre-existing shorter-chain fatty acid. Hence, dietary or newly synthesized palmitate can be elongated within the body to form stearate and on to arachidate (20:0), behenate (22:0) and lignocerate (24:0). In practice, little stearate present in the human body appears to be derived by chain elongation of pre-existing palmitate.

In humans, saturates longer than 24 carbons do exist but usually only arise during genetic defects in fatty acid oxidation, as will be discussed later.

Palmitate and stearate are important membrane constituents, being found in most tissue phospholipids at 20–40% of the total fatty acid profile. Brain membranes contain 20–24 carbon saturates that, like palmitate and stearate, are synthesized within the brain and have little or no access to the brain from the circulation. The normal membrane content of long-chain saturates can probably be sustained without a dietary source of these fatty acids. Compared with all other classes of dietary fatty acid, especially monounsaturated or polyunsaturated fatty acids, excess intake or synthesis of long-chain saturates is associated with an increased risk of cardiovascular disease.

The most common long-chain *cis*-monounsaturated fatty acids in diet and in the body are oleate (18:1n-9) and palmitoleate (16:1n-7), with the former predominating by far in both the body's storage and membrane lipids. As with stearate, most oleate in the human body appears to be of dietary origin. Hence, although humans have the capacity to desaturate stearate to oleate, dietary oleate is probably the dominant source of oleate in the body. Only plants can take oleate and further desaturate it to linoleate and again to α-linolenate. As with saturates >18 carbons in length, 20-, 22- and 24-carbon monounsaturates derived from oleate are present in specialized membranes such as myelin.

Polyunsaturates (essential fatty acids)

Linoleate and α-linolenate are the primary dietary *cis*-polyunsaturated fatty acids in most diets. Neither can be synthesized *de novo* (from acetate) in animals, but they can be made by chain elongation from the two respective 16-carbon precursors, hexadecadienoate (16:2n-6) and hexadecatrienoate (16:3n-3), which are found in common edible green plants at up to 13% of total fatty acids. Hence, significant consumption of green vegetables will provide 16-carbon polyunsaturates that contribute to the total available linoleate and α-linolenate.

Linoleate is the predominant polyunsaturated fatty acid in the body, commonly accounting for 12–15% of adipose tissue fatty acids. In the body's lean tissues there are at least three polyunsaturates present in amounts >5% of the fatty acid profile (linoleate, arachidonate, docosahexaenoate). In addition, at least two other biologically active polyunsaturates are present in body lipids [dihomo-γ-linolenate (20:3n-6) and eicosapentaenoate (20 : 5n-3)], although usually in amounts between 1 and 3% of total fatty acids. Marine fish are the richest source of 20–22-carbon polyunsaturates. α-Linolenate and its precursor, hexadecatrienoate (16 : 3n-3), are the only n-3 polyunsaturates in common terrestrial plants.

Hydrogenated and conjugated fatty acid isomers

The introduction of unsaturation with one double bond creates the possibility of both positional and geometric isomers in fatty acids. Among long-chain unsaturated fatty acids, positional isomers exist because the double bond can be introduced into several different locations, i.e. 18 : 1n-7, 18 : 1n-9, 18 : 1n-11, etc. Geometric isomers exist because the two remaining hydrogens at each double bond can be opposite each other (*trans*) or on the same side of the molecule (*cis*; Figure 6.2). Thus, there is *cis*-18 : 1n-9 (oleate) and *trans*-18 : 1n-9 (elaidate), and so on for all unsaturated fatty acids, with the combinations mounting exponentially as the number of double bonds increases.

Trans isomers of monounsaturated or polyunsaturated fatty acids arise primarily from partial hydrogenation during food processing of oils, but some also occur naturally in ruminants. The number of *trans* isomers increases with the number of double bonds, so there is only one *trans* isomer of oleate but there are three *trans* isomers of linoleate and seven of α-linolenate. Virtually all naturally occurring polyunsaturated fatty acids have double bonds that are methylene interrupted, i.e. have a CH_2 group between the two double bonds. Again, through food processing, however, methylene interruption between double bonds can be lost and the bonds move one carbon closer together, becoming conjugated. Thus, the double bonds in linoleate are at the 9–10 and 11–12 carbons, but in conjugated linoleate they are at the 9–10 carbons and the 11–12 carbons. Some degree of further desaturation and chain elongation can occur in conjugated fatty acids, but much less than with methylene-interrupted polyunsaturates. Thus, conjugated linoleate is the main conjugated fatty acid and its nutritional and health implications have raised considerable recent interest.

Fats and oils

Fats are esters of fatty acids with glycerol (Table 6.1). They usually occur as triesters or triglycerides, although monoglycerides and diglycerides occur during fat digestion and are used in food processing. Most common dietary fats contain a mixture of 16–18-carbon saturated and unsaturated fatty acids. By convention, fats that are liquid at room temperature are called oils, a feature arising from their lower proportion of saturated (straight-chain) and higher proportion of unsaturated (bent-chain) fatty acids. Unsaturated fatty acids usually have a lower melting point, thereby more easily liquefying the fats of which they are a component. Triglycerides of animal origin are commonly fats, while those of fish or plant origin are usually oils. Animal fats and fish oils frequently contain cholesterol, whereas plant oils do not contain cholesterol but usually contain other "phyto" sterols.

Triglycerides are primarily used as fuels, so dietary fats (mostly triglycerides) are commonly associated with energy metabolism rather than with structural lipids found in membranes. However, membrane lipids as well as triglycerides are extracted with lipid solvents used to determine the fat content of foods, tissues or plant material. Hence, because organs such as brain are rich in membrane phospholipids, when the total lipids are extracted to determine the organ's chemical composition, these organs are said to have a certain fat content. On a chemical basis this is true, but this description often misconstrues the nature of the lipid because the brain in particular contains virtually no triglyceride.

Phospholipids

Phospholipids contain two nonpolar, hydrophobic acyl tail groups and a single functional head group that is polar and hydrophilic. Hence, they are relatively balanced amphiphilic lipids and, in this capacity, are crucial components of biological membranes. The head groups contain phosphorus and amino acids (choline, serine, ethanolamine), sugars (inositol) or an alcohol (glycerol). Phosphatidylcholine is the most abundant phospholipid in animal tissues but phosphatidylglycerols (glycosides) predominate in plant lipids. Phospholipids containing a fatty acid amide are sphingolipids. Various phospholipases can hydrolyze the acyl groups or head group during digestion or metabolism.

One of the outstanding characteristics that make phospholipids suitable as major constituents of biological membranes is that, in water, they naturally aggregate into spherical or rod-like liposomes or vesicles, with the hydrophilic portion facing outwards and the hydrophobic portion facing inwards (Figure 6.3). Changing the constituent acyl groups from saturated

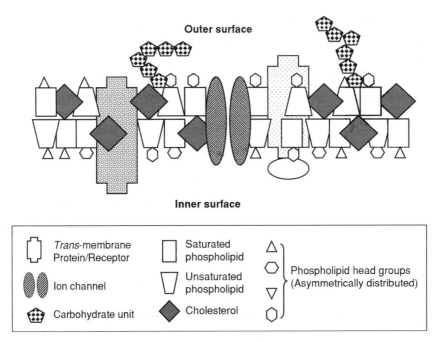

Figure 6.3 Simplified schematic view of a membrane bilayer. The main components are proteins, free cholesterol, phospholipids and carbohydrates. There are many different proteins with a myriad of shapes, membrane distribution and functions, of which three are illustrated. Membrane phospholipids principally help to create the bilayer. They have four types of "head groups" (choline, ethanolamine, serine and inositol) which are located at or near the membrane's two surfaces. The two fatty acids in phospholipids are mixtures of 16–22 carbon saturates, monounsaturates and polyunsaturates in all combinations, with those rich in unsaturated fatty acids occupying more space, hence their trapezoid shape compared with the narrower, rectangular shape of the more saturated phospholipids. Free cholesterol represents 30–40% of the lipid in most membranes. The many different carbohydrates are on the membrane's surfaces and are bound to lipids and/or proteins in the membrane.

to polyunsaturated changes the fluidity of these aggregates because of the greater amount of space occupied by more unsaturated fatty acids. At interfaces between nonmiscible polar and nonpolar solvents, phospholipids also form a film or monolayer.

Sterols

The main sterol of importance in human nutrition is cholesterol. It has multiple roles including being:

- a vital component of biological membranes
- a precursor to bile salts used in fat digestion
- a precursor to steroid hormones.

Sterols are secondary alcohols belonging to the polyisoprenoids or terpinoids (terpenes), which have a common precursor, isopentenyl diphosphate. Other members of the terpinoids include squalene, carotenoids and dolichols. Bacteria appear to be the only life forms not containing cholesterol. Sterols have a common cyclopentano(a)perhydrophenanthrene skeleton with different substitutions giving rise to the multiple sterols and steroids.

6.3 Lipid components of the diet

Food or dietary sources of lipids are listed in Table 6.3. Cholesterol is found only in animal lipids, while a variety of other phytosterols occur in plants. Soyabeans, leafy plants and lean animal meat are rich in dietary phospholipids. Animal fat and plant oils from seeds or nuts are rich in triglycerides.

The leafy and fruit components of plants contain phospholipids and sterols, whereas seeds contain triglycerides. With rare exceptions such as flaxseed (linseed), edible green leaves are proportionally much richer in α-linolenate than are seeds. Seed oils are usually rich in either linoleate or oleate. Common plant sterols include β-sitosterol, β-sitostanol and campesterol. One of the main nutritional uses of plant sterols is inhibition of cholesterol absorption.

Table 6.3 Common food sources of lipids

Cholesterol	Eggs, organ meats
Phytosterols	Soya products, olive oil
Short-chain fatty acids (1–6 carbons)	Milk fat
Medium-chain fatty acids (8–14 carbons)	Milk fat, coconut fat
Long-chain fatty acids (16–20 carbons)	Saturates: animal fat, shortening, butter, palm oil, peanuts
	Monounsaturates: olive, canola oils
	Linoleate: sunflower, safflower, corn oils, soyabean
	α-Linolenate: flaxseed oil, canola, soyabean oil, walnuts
	γ-Linolenate: evening primrose oil, borage oil, blackcurrant seed oil
	Stearidonate: blackcurrant seed oil
	Arachidonate: lean meat and organ lipids
	Eicosapentaenoate: marine cold-water fish, shellfish, some seaweeds
	Docosahexaenoate: marine cold-water fish, shellfish
	Trans fatty acids: partially hydrogenated fats and oils

Phospholipids and cholesterol comprise the majority of lipids in tissues (gut, kidney, brain, skeletal muscle, etc.) of lean, undomesticated animals. By contrast, in domesticated animals, triglycerides or nonmembrane lipids present in subcutaneous and intramuscular adipose tissue deposits are the dominant form of lipid on a weight basis. This is because domestication usually involves rearing animals with minimal exercise and on higher energy intakes, leading to more subcutaneous and visceral triglycerides obtained through both fat synthesis and deposition of dietary fat. Animal meat lipids are the main dietary source of arachidonate (20:4n-6), although it can also be obtained from tropical marine fish.

Lipoproteins are the main form of lipid in the blood (see Section 6.5). Like lipoproteins, milk lipids also occur as globules comprised of a combination of a mainly triglyceride core surrounded by a membrane containing proteins, cholesterol and phospholipids.

Phospholipids and cholesterol comprise the main lipids of undomesticated edible fish, which usually have low amounts of triglyceride or stored body fat. As in domesticated animals, it is likely that subcutaneous and intramuscular fat deposits of triglyceride will increase in commercially farmed fish. Cold-water marine fish are the main dietary source of eicosapentaenoate (20:5n-3) and docosahexaenoate (22:6n-3), but the former is also found in several types of edible seaweed. Tropical fish generally have higher arachidonate than do cold-water fish.

Partial hydrogenation is a common feature of unsaturated fatty acids in processed foods. Complete hydrogenation makes fats very hard and is more expensive than partial hydrogenation. Depending on the applications and the source of the original oil or fat, partial hydrogenation is an economical way to control the properties of fats or oils used in food production. Dietary diglycerides and monoglycerides are used by the food industry for emulsification of water- and oil-based components in foods such as ice cream and mayonnaise.

6.4 Digestion, absorption and transport of dietary fat

The average daily intake of fat in a Western diet ranges from between 50 to 100 g and provides between 35 and 40% of total energy. It consists mainly of triglycerides, also known as triacylglycerols (TAG), which form the principal component of visible oils and fats, and minor quantities of phospholipids and cholesterol esters (CE). The physical properties of dietary fat, such as their hardness at room temperature (melting point) and subsequent metabolic properties once in the body, are determined by the number of double bonds in their constituent fatty acids (degree of saturation or unsaturation) and length of the fatty acid carbon chain (see Tables 6.2 and 6.3). As mentioned in Section 6.2, fats that are solid at room temperature tend to consist of long-chain saturated fats (>12 carbons, no double bonds), while oils consist of long-chain unsaturated fats with several double bonds. It has become conventional to refer to dietary fats as "lipids" once they have been absorbed into the body via the small intestine, although it is not incorrect to refer to dietary fat as "dietary lipid".

Reception, emulsification, lipolysis, solubilization and absorption

The digestion of dietary fat takes place in three phases, known as the gastric, duodenal and ilial phases. These involve crude emulsification in the stomach, lipolytic breakdown by lipases and solubilization with bile salts in the duodenum and, finally, absorption into the epithelial cells or enterocytes lining the walls of the small intestine or ileum. Digestion may actually be initiated in the mouth under the influence of a lingual lipase secreted by the palate, although its contribution to lipolysis in adults is questionable and thought to be more important in young suckling infants, in which its release is stimulated by suckling and the presence of milk. It is possible that this lingual lipase is carried into the stomach, where it acts as a human gastric lipase (HGL) which has been shown to degrade up to 10% of ingested fat. Although these early products of fat digestion, fatty acids and monoglycerols, represent a relatively minor component of fat digested their entry into the duodenum is believed to supply a major stimulus for the production of the hormone cholecystokinine (CCK), which inhibits gut motility.

The stomach serves mainly as an organ of mechanical digestion and by churning its contents produces a coarse creamy emulsion known as chyme. The circular pyloric sphincter muscle that separates the stomach from the duodenum and, with other factors, controls the rate of gastric emptying, opens twice a minute to release approximately 3 ml of chyme. Since emulsified fat in chyme is less dense than the aqueous material, the two fractions separate with the fat collecting above the aqueous layer. As a result, the entry of emulsified fat into the duodenum is delayed, allowing sufficient time for the minor breakdown products to act on CCK.

The duodenal phase involves the breakdown of the emulsified fat by a process known as lipolysis and the solubilization of the products of lipolysis. The entry of chyme containing minor lipolytic products into the duodenum stimulates the following:

- release of CCK, which inhibits gut motility
- secretion of bile acids from the gallbladder
- release of pancreatic juice containing a battery of lipases.

Lipolysis is an enzyme-catalyzed hydrolysis that releases fatty acids from lipids (TAG, phospholipids and CE). It involves the hydrolytic cleavage of bonds between a fatty acid and the glycerol backbone of TAG and phospholipids, and cholesterol in CE, and occurs not only in the digestive tract but also in circulating and intracellular lipids (Figure 6.4). The lipolysis of emulsified dietary fat entering the duodenum is catalyzed by a battery of pancreatic enzymes including a pancreatic lipase that acts chiefly on TAG, phospholipase A_2 and cholesterol ester hydrolase acting on phospholipids and CE, respectively. The hydrolysis of TAG by pancreatic lipase occurs in a sequential fashion with the initial removal of a fatty acid from position 1 and then position 3 from the glycerol backbone, generating a 2,3-diacylglycerol, followed by 2-monoacylglycerol (2-MAG).

Solubilization of emulsified fat

Fats by definition are insoluble in water and must be rendered soluble before they can be absorbed in the gut, and transported within cells and in the circulation. In each of these situations this is achieved by the hydrophobic fat or lipid associating with molecules that are capable of interfacing with both hydrophobic and hydrophilic environments. Molecules with these characteristics are called amphipathic molecules, examples of which are phospholipids, bile salts and specialized proteins known as apoproteins (Figure 6.5). In the small intestine emulsified fats are solubilized by associating with bile salts produced in the liver and stored and released from the gallbladder, and phospholipids to form complex aggregates known as mixed micelles. Lipids within cells and in the circulation are solubilized by combining with specific proteins known as fatty acid binding proteins (FABP) and apolipoproteins (ApoA, B, C, E), respectively. Further details of the structure and function of these specialized proteins are given in Section 6.5.

The action of pancreatic lipase on TAG yields free fatty acids and 2-MAG. Fatty acids of short and medium chain length (<12 carbons) are absorbed directly into the portal circulation with free glycerol and transported bound to albumin to the liver, where they are rapidly oxidized. In contrast, long-chain fatty acids (LCFA; >12 carbons) associate with bile salts in bile juice from the gallbladder and are absorbed into the enterocyte for further processing and packaging into transport lipoproteins. The primary bile salts, cholic and chenodeoxycholic acids are produced from cholesterol in the liver under the action of the rate-limiting enzyme 7-α-hydroxylase. These bile salts act effectively

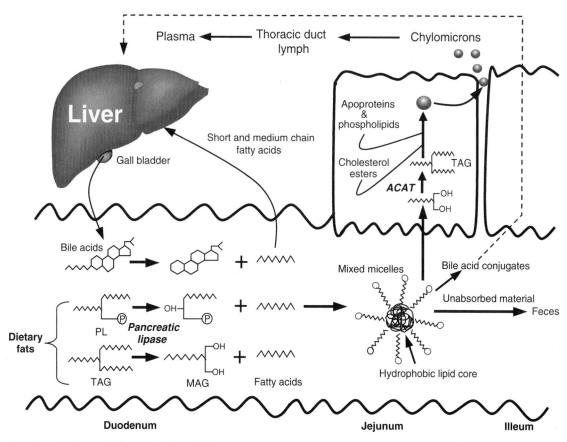

Figure 6.4 Reception, emulsification, lipolysis, solubilization and absorption of fats.

as detergents, solubilizing lipids by the formation of mixed micelles. These are spherical associations of amphipathic molecules (with hydrophobic and hydrophilic regions) with a hydrophilic surface of bile salts and phospholipids that encapsulate a hydrophobic core of more insoluble LCFA and 2-MAG (see Figure 6.4). The micelle core will also contain some lipid-soluble vitamins including tocopherols and carotenoids. The formation of mixed micelles increases the solubility of fat by 100–1000-fold. They create an acidic microenvironment for the lipid core which, through protonation, facilitates the dissociation of LCFA and 2-MAG from the micelle and diffusion into the enterocyte.

Absorption of solubilized fat

The ilial or absorptive phase involves the transit of dietary fats from mixed micelles into the enterocyte. Although originally believed to be a purely passive process,

dependent on factors such as the rate of gastric emptying, extent of mixing and gut motility, the translocation of LCFA and 2-MAG from the micelle into the enterocyte is now known to be assisted by the presence of FABP within the cell membrane and the cell. These maintain a diffusion gradient down which LCFA and MAG can flow into the cell. FABP have numerous roles within cells and specificity for different types of LCFA. Thus, the absorption of LCFA and 2-MAG derived from dietary TAG occurs by facilitated diffusion via FABP, which increases membrane permeation and promotes cellular uptake of LCFA and monoglycerides. An additional factor that drives the diffusion gradient is the rapid re-esterification of LCFA into 2-MAG and 2-MAG into TAG within the enterocyte by the enzyme acyl-CoA-cholesterol acyltransferase (ACAT). The absorption of dietary TAG in the small intestine is extremely efficient, with up to 90% being absorbed. Dietary cholesterol also associates within mixed micelles and is absorbed in a similar manner by specific sterol-carrying proteins resident in the enterocyte membrane. Thus, cholesterol is also absorbed by a protein-facilitated mechanism but, in contrast to dietary

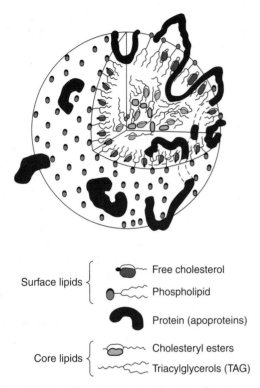

Figure 6.5 General lipoprotein structure. (Reproduced from Durrington, 1995 with permission of Elsevier Science.)

TAG, only about 40% of dietary cholesterol will be absorbed directly.

Enterohepatic circulation

The absorption of fat in the small intestine is dependent on the availability of bile acids from biliary secretions which also contain free cholesterol. Both bile acids (>95%) and biliary cholesterol are salvaged by an energy-dependent process in the terminal ileum. This active process of reabsorption via the enterohepatic circulation is tightly controlled by a feedback mechanism that is sensitive to hepatic levels of cholesterol. Thus, the reabsorption of cholesterol downregulates the activity of 7-α-hydroxylase, shutting down the further production of bile acids. Substances in the lumen of the gut that are capable of binding or competing with bind bile acids such as naturally occurring plant sterols or soluble nonstarch polysaccharides (NSP) prevent their reabsorption which, in effect, interrupts the enterohepatic circulation. This depletes the supply of cholesterol and accelerates the production of bile acids, depleting the liver of cholesterol (Figure 6.6). To replenish this loss, liver cells respond by increasing their uptake of cholesterol from circulating lipoproteins in the blood, with the result of a decrease in blood cholesterol. Interruption of the enterohepatic circulation helps to explain the cholesterol-lowering action of some of the earliest known cholesterol-lowering drugs, but also such dietary constituents as the phytosterols (sitosterol and

Figure 6.6 Interruption of the entero-hepatic circulation.

stanol esters) and soluble fiber or NSP. For further details of the control mechanism see Section 6.5.

Re-esterification of triacylglycerols in the enterocyte

Once LCFA have entered the cell they are activated by acyl-CoA and are re-esterified with glycerol back into TAG and phospholipids by two distinct biochemical pathways, the 2-MAG and glycerol-3-phosphate (G-3-P) pathways. The difference between these two pathways lies in:

- their substrates of activation
- the former using 2-MAG and the latter α-glycero-3-phosphate
- their location within different cellular organelles: the 2-MAG reside in the smooth endoplasmic reticulm and the G-3-P in the rough endoplasmic reticulum
- the periods during which they are most active.

The 2-MAG pathway is quantitatively of greater importance in the enterocyte of the intestine and thus predominates in the postprandial period, whereas the G-3-P is more active in the postabsorptive phase in tissues such as liver, muscle and adipose tissue. Following the absorption of a fatty meal and uptake of 2-MAG into the enterocyte, up to 90% of these molecules are rapidly acylated back to 1,2-diacylglycerol and finally TAG by the sequential actions of three enzymes: CoA ligase, monoglycerol acyltransferase and diacylglycerol acyltransferase. In a similar fashion, lysophosphatidyl-choline, produced by the action of pancreatic phospho-lipase A on dietary phospholipids, is absorbed by the enterocyte and re-esterified back to phosphatidylcholine in the enterocyte by direct acetylation (Figure 6.7). The bulk of free cholesterol absorbed from the intestinal lumen is also re-esterified in the enterocyte by the enzyme ACAT.

Lipoprotein assembly and secretion

Plasma lipoproteins are a family of spherical, macro-molecular complexes of lipid and protein, the principal function of which is to transport endogenous lipids (synthesized in the liver) and exogenous lipids (synthesized in the gut from dietary fats) from these sites of production and absorption to peripheral sites of utilization (e.g. oxidation in muscle, incorporation in membranes or as precursors of biologically active metabolites) and storage (e.g. adipose tissue).

In the small intestine, the newly re-esterified TAG and CE associate with specific amphipathic proteins and phospholipids in the enterocyte to form the largest and most TAG-rich lipoproteins, known as chylomicrons.

Figure 6.7 Re-esterification of triacylglycerides in enterocytes. (Reproduced from Mangiapane and Salter, 1999, with permission of the publisher.)

The enterocyte is capable of synthesizing three different apoproteins (apo): apoA-I, apoA-IV and apoB (B-48). The latter apoprotein is expressed in two isoforms, the arbitrarily named apoB-100, which is synthesized in the liver, and a shorter relative of B-100, which is produced by the enterocyte and is approximately 48% of the size of B-100 and thus appropriately named apoB-48. While both apoproteins are products of the same gene, the mRNA undergoes post-transcriptional editing in the enterocyte to produce a truncated polypeptide. ApoB-48 is produced in the rough endoplasmic reticulum and transferred to the smooth endoplasmic reticulum, where it combines with a lipid droplet, or nascent chylomicron, and then migrates to the Golgi apparatus. Here, the apoproteins (A-I, A-IV and B-48) are glycosylated before the chylomicrons eventually leave the enterocyte by exocytosis through the basement membrane, across the intracellular space between the enterocyte and the lacteal, and are finally discharged into the lymphatic vessels.

Postprandial lipemia

The turbidy or milkiness of serum or plasma following the ingestion of fat marks the arrival of dietary fat now contained in chylomicrons in the blood. The milky appearance of plasma or serum after the ingestion of fat arises from the chylomicrons, which are of a sufficient size physically to scatter light and create the milky appearance of serum or plasma after a meal. The size and composition of the chylomicrons produced after a fatty meal are determined by the fat content of the meal. Hence, the nature of fatty acids in chylomicron TAG reflects the nature of fatty acid in the meal. Each chylomicron particle carries a single molecule of apoB-48 which, unlike its other smaller counterparts A-I and A-IV, remains with the chylomicron throughout its life in the circulation. There is little evidence to suggest that the production of apoB-48, and thus the number of particles, increases in response to an increased flux of dietary fat. Instead, the enterocyte packs more TAG into each chylomicron and expands the size of each chylomicron to facilitate the transport of larger amounts of absorbed dietary fat. There is evidence to suggest that chylomicrons containing lipids enriched with polyunsaturated fatty acids (PUFA) are larger than chylomicrons enriched with saturated fat, since the former occupy more space when packaged into a lipoprotein. This has implications for the subsequent metabolism and fate of these lipoproteins in the circulation, because TAG associated with larger chylomicrons is known to be hydrolyzed more rapidly. It is thought that apoB-48 is produced continuously in the enterocyte-forming pools of apoB-48 in readiness for the sudden reception of dietary fat and production of chylomicrons. Nevertheless, small chylomicrons can be detected throughout the postabsorptive phase.

The onset, duration and magnitude of postprandial lipemia can be monitored in the laboratory after a standard fat-containing meal by making serial measurements of serum TAG or more specifically TAG associated with TAG-rich lipoproteins over a postprandial period of up to 8 or 9 h (remnants of chylomicrons can be detected 12 h after a meal). Alternatively, the levels of apoB-48 or retinyl esters in serum act as useful markers or tracer molecules for following the metabolism of chylomicrons in the postprandial period. In normal subjects postprandial lipemia peaks between 3 and 4 h and subsides to baseline concentration after 5–6 h. In some cases postprandial TAG (chylomicrons) can appear in the blood within 30 min and peak as early as 1 h after the ingestion of fat. So rapid is this rise in TAG that it is believed to represent preformed lipid in the enterocyte from the previous meal which is shunted into the circulation by the incoming fat load. Note that in addition to the time taken to emulsify, hydrolyze and absorb dietary fat, re-esterification of TAG in the enterocyte and lipoprotein assembly alone takes about 15 min, although shunting means that the first TAG can appear within 30 min, with the first peak after 1 h. This shunting is particularly noticeable during the day and gives rise to two or even more peaks, whereas postprandial peaks following an overnight fast are usually monophasic.

Chylomicrons are not the only TAG-rich lipoproteins in the postprandial phase. Chylomicrons clearly contribute significantly to the extent of postprandial lipemia, and the rate at which the TAG in these lipoproteins is hydrolyzed is known to be a critical determinant of the extent and time-course of postprandial lipemia. The TAG in circulating chylomicrons is lipolyzed by a rate-limiting lipase known as lipoprotein lipase (LPL). LPL is tethered to the endothelial lining of blood vessels in peripheral tissues, most notably muscle and adipose tissue, by proteoglycan fibers, and as such is known as an endothelial lipase. Several molecules of LPL can interact and lipolyze the TAG from a single chylomicron particle to generate a chylomicron remnant which is removed by specific receptors in the liver. The situation is complicated by the fact that TAG-rich lipoproteins

Table 6.4 Plasma lipoproteins: classes, composition and distribution

	Chylomicrons	VLDL	LDL	HDL
Mass (10^6 Dal)	0.4–3.0	10–100	2–3.5	0.2–0.3
Density (g/ml)	>0.95	<1.006	1.02–1.063	1.063–1.210
Particle diameter (nm)	>90	30–90	22–28	5–12
Apoproteins	B-48, A-I, C-I, C-II, C-III, E	B-100, E	B-100	A-I, A-II
Lipids % mass (molecules/particle)				
Cholesterol	8 (60 000)	22 (10 000)	48 (2000)	20 (100)
Triacylglycerol	83 (500 000)	50 (24 000)	10 (300)	8 (20)
Ratio of particles				
Postabsorptive	1	40	1000	10 000
Postprandial	1	25	250	250 000

VLDL: very low-density lipoprotein; LDL: low-density lipoprotein; HDL: high-density lipoprotein.

from the liver, known as very low-density lipoproteins (VLDL), also contribute to this postprandial lipemia to variable extents in health and disease states. These endogenous VLDL are similar in lipid composition to chylomicrons but considerably smaller (Table 6.4). While chylomicrons carry up to 80% of the TAG during the postprandial period they are significantly outnumbered by the smaller VLDL particles at all times. VLDL are also metabolized by LPL, which creates competition for clearance between endogenous and exogenous lipoproteins.

Postprandial lipemia: relevance to atherosclerosis

It was suggested by Zilversmit in 1979 that atherosclerosis was a postprandial phenomenon. This concept was based on the finding that patients either with or at high risk of developing coronary heart disease (CHD) showed an impaired capacity to remove TAG-rich lipoproteins from the circulation after a meal. This resulted in enhanced postprandial lipemia, which also became known as the TAG intolerance hypothesis. At about the same time, evidence emerged that TAG-rich lipoproteins (remnants of chylomicrons) were directly atherogenic, meaning that they can damage the endothelial lining of arteries and promote the deposition of cholesterol in coronary arteries. For this reason, there is considerable research interest in the metabolic determinants of postprandial lipemia. This includes the mechanisms that underlie the production and removal of TAG-rich lipoproteins, not only in the intestine but also in the liver, since the production and removal of VLDL can clearly influence postprandial

events. The quality and, to a lesser extent, quantity of dietary fat are extremely important in this respect and have a major role to play in modulating lipid-mediated atherosclerosis.

6.5 Circulating lipids: lipoprotein structures and metabolism

By definition, circulating blood fats (lipids) are insoluble in water and must be solubilized for transportation in serum by combining with bipolar molecules with charged and noncharged regions (apoproteins and phospholipids). This property, known as amphipathicity, enables these molecules to associate with aqueous (hydrophilic) and nonaqueous (hydrophobic) environments and are thus perfect for wrapping up insoluble lipids, chiefly TAG and CE, in macromolecular lipid–protein complexes called lipoproteins. It is worth remembering that in the absence of lipoproteins, TAG would exist in aqueous blood as immiscible oil droplets, while free fatty acids liberated from TAG and phospholipids in the absence of the serum protein albumin would act as detergents and dissolve cell membranes.

Lipoprotein structure: a shopping bag and groceries

The general structure of a lipoprotein consists of a central core of hydrophobic, neutral lipid (TAG and CE) surrounded by a hydrophilic coat of phospholipids, free cholesterol and apoproteins. A useful analogy for this arrangement of molecules is that of a shopping bag and groceries, with the lipid core representing the lipid groceries and the outer coat the fabric of the bag. The apoproteins weave in and out of the lipid core and outer surface layer and form the thread of the fabric which holds the bag together (Figure 6.5). This clever arrangement of molecules renders the hydrophobic lipids soluble for the purpose of transport in blood. In addition to conferring structural integrity on the lipoprotein particle, apoproteins have a vital role in controlling the metabolism of lipoproteins by acting as ligands for cell membrane receptors and cofactors for key enzymes.

Serum lipoproteins can be subdivided into distinct classes on the basis of their physical properties and/or composition, both of which reflect the physiological role in the transport of lipids from sites of synthesis (endogenous lipids) and absorption (exogenous lipids, absorbed in the gut) to sites of storage (adipose tissue) and utilization (skeletal muscle). The principal classes of lipoproteins are traditionally defined by density, which is determined by the ratio of lipid to protein in the lipoprotein particle. Since lipids tend to occupy a greater molecular volume than proteins they are lighter and less dense. Thus, particles with high lipid content are larger and less dense (carry more lipid groceries!) than lipoproteins enriched with protein. This property relates directly to the transport function and metabolic interrelationships between lipoprotein classes in blood. It can also be used to separate lipoproteins of different densities, since lipoproteins of different density have different flotation characteristics in the ultracentrifuge. (Note that lipoproteins will float when subjected to centrifugal force, whereas pure proteins sink.) Alternative schemes of lipoprotein classification include separation on the basis of net charge (electrophoretic mobility), particle size (exclusion chromatography, gradient gel electrophoresis) and variable immunological characteristics conferred upon the lipoprotein by the types of apoproteins in each lipoprotein subclass (Table 6.4). Some of these techniques permit the further resolution of VLDL, low-density lipoproteins (LDL) and high-density lipoproteins (HDL) into discrete subclasses, the distribution of which relates to CHD risk and is determined by genetic and lifestyle factors.

Lipoprotein transport pathways

Lipoprotein transport can be described in terms of the production, transport and removal of cholesterol or TAG from the circulation. In reality, these two processes are inseparable because both TAG and cholesterol are transported together in lipoproteins. Lipoproteins are in a constant state of change, with lipids and apoproteins constantly shuttling between different lipoproteins which interrelate through integrated metabolic pathways. A useful comparison here is to think of lipoproteins as tube trains, with passengers representing lipid and apoprotein molecules being transported on a complex network of lines, with a constant movement of passengers between trains in different stations. Metabolic control is imposed on this system by the rate at which the lipoproteins and their contents enter and leave the system and by their physicochemical properties, in other words, the number of trains and types of passenger.

All lipoproteins, with the notable exception of HDL, begin life as particles packed full of TAG. Their principal transport function in the first instance is to deliver fatty acids liberated from the TAG to tissues. The enterocytes in the gut are the producers of lipoproteins which deliver dietary fats into the blood as chylomicrons (exogenous lipid), whereas the liver is the central terminus for the production of VLDL and removal of its cholesterol-rich end-products, LDL. VLDL, although smaller than a chylomicron, resembles the latter in many ways and is often referred to as the liver's chylomicron. While the rate at which the gut produces chylomicrons depends largely on the amount of absorbed dietary fat, the rate of production of VLDL is determined by the supply of fatty acids in the liver which can be re-esterified back to TAG for VLDL production. These fatty acids are derived chiefly from the uptake of circulating lipoproteins and nonesterified fatty acids. Note that although the liver has the capacity to synthesize fatty acids, the amount of *de novo* synthesis in humans on mixed Western diets is negligible and may only become significant on extremely low-fat (high-carbohydrate) diets.

Metabolic determinants of lipoprotein metabolism

The metabolism of serum lipoproteins and fate of their transport lipids is controlled by:

- the physical and chemical characteristics of the lipoprotein, such as its size and lipid and apoprotein content
- the activity of the endothelial LPL and hepatic lipase (HL), so called because they are attached to the surface of endothelial cells lining blood vessels in

peripheral tissues, such as adipose tissue and skeletal muscle, and the liver, respectively
- lipid transfer proteins (CE) and phospholipid transfer proteins (CETP and PLTP)
- apoproteins which act as activators of enzymes and ligands for specific lipoprotein receptors on the surfaces of cells (apoB-100 and apoE as ligands for the LDL and remnant receptors in the liver, respectively)
- the activity of specific lipoprotein receptors on cell surfaces.

Lipoprotein transport is traditionally described in terms of the forward and reverse transport of cholesterol. Forward transport encompasses the exogenous and endogenous pathways, that is arrival of cholesterol in the blood from either the gut or the liver and carriage back to the liver for processing; the liver has the unique capacity to secrete cholesterol either as free cholesterol or as bile acids. In contrast, reverse transport describes the HDL pathway and the efflux of cholesterol out of peripheral tissues back to the liver. This directionality can be misleading, since all pathways direct cholesterol back to the liver. Both the exogenous and endogenous pathways share a common saturable lipolytic pathway which consists of a delipidation cascade in which the TAG-rich lipoproteins (chylomicrons and VLDL), after receiving apoC from HDL, an essential cofactor for the activation of LPL, are progressively depleted of their TAG in a stepwise fashion by LPL to become cholesterol-rich remnants which are removed by specific, high-affinity receptors found chiefly in the liver. Several molecules of LPL may bind to a single chylomicron or VLDL particle, although LPL shows greater affinity for chylomicrons in preference to VLDL. This situation leads to competition between these TAG-rich lipoproteins and provides a mechanism to explain how VLDL can influence the clearance of TAG in the postprandial period.

Lipolyzed chylomicrons form chylomicron remnants which, during passage through the liver, bind to specific receptors on the surface of hepatocytes that recognize apoE, an apoprotein that is also acquired at an early stage from HDL. Remnant receptors are maintained at a very high level of activity and are not down-regulated through a feedback mechanism (see LDL receptor). This is fortunate since chylomicron remnants have been shown to be the only native circulating lipoprotein capable of depositing their cholesterol in artery walls, thus promoting coronary atherosclerosis. The secretion of VLDL from the liver is again followed by the sequential lipolysis of TAG by LPL and generation of VLDL remnants or, in this case, the further lipolysis of these remnants into LDL. The remnants and LDL bind to another receptor in the liver that recognizes both apoE exclusively in VLDL remnants and apoB-100 in LDL, namely the LDL receptor. Approximately 60% of LDL is removed by the LDL receptor. The remainder is internalized into cells via scavenger receptors. This latter route has been associated with the development of atherosclerotic lesions.

Whether a VLDL particle is removed as a remnant or transcends to LDL largely depends on its pedigree, that is its size and lipid composition. Experiments with radioactively labeled VLDL have shown that larger, TAG-rich VLDL particles are less likely to be converted into LDL and are removed as partially delipidated VLDL remnants, whereas smaller VLDL is a precursor of LDL.

The low-density lipoprotein receptor pathway

The relationship between cholesterol and CHD is directly responsible for the rapid growth, and occasional quantum leaps, in our understanding of cholesterol homeostasis in relation to diet and disease, the most prolific of which was the discovery of the LDL receptor pathway by the Nobel Prize winners Goldstein and Brown (Figure 6.8). All cells, most notably those in the liver, have a highly developed and sensitive mechanism for regulating the intracellular and intravascular levels of cholesterol. Cells in the liver synthesize approximately 500 mg of cholesterol a day but import the same quantity from the blood in the form of LDL. When stressed, cells will always import cholesterol in preference to synthesizing it themselves in order to save energy. Cholesterol is acquired by the cell through the uptake and degradation of LDL particles. As the requirement for cholesterol increases within the cell it increases the activity of LDL, more LDL is removed from the blood and serum cholesterol falls. Conversely, if the cell becomes overloaded with cholesterol, the activity of receptors falls and LDL levels in the blood increase. In the complete absence of LDL, cells have the capacity to manufacture sufficient cholesterol to meet their metabolic needs. The activity of the LDL receptor is regulated by the intracellular level of free cholesterol. Thus, anything that increases free cholesterol within the cell will inadvertently lower serum LDL-cholesterol. Intracellular free cholesterol represses the activity of a sterol regulatory

Figure 6.8 Low-density lipoprotein receptor pathway.

element binding protein (SREBP), which acts as positive nuclear transcription factor (promotes the transcription of a specific gene). The gene in this case is the one coding for LDL receptor protein. The metabolic effects of intracellular free cholesterol are:

- it increases the production of LDL receptors
- it inhibits the synthesis of cholesterol by the enzyme 3-hydroxy-3-methylglutaryl (HMG)-CoA reductase
- it increases the re-esterification of cholesterol for storage as cholesterol esters.

Goldstein and Brown were aided in the discovery of this pathway by the condition known as familial hypercholesterolemia, a genetic abnormality that arises from a mutation in the LDL receptor gene, leading to a deficiency of LDL receptors and considerably elevated serum cholesterol concentrations in early (15–20 mmol/l) and premature cardiovascular disease. These workers also initiated pioneering studies on the influence of dietary fats on the activity of the LDL pathway, which led to a coherent explanation for the hypercholesterolemic effect of saturated fats.

Reverse cholesterol transport

The removal of cholesterol from tissues back to the liver via HDL represents the only route of elimination for cholesterol from the body. This function of HDL underlies the cardioprotective role of HDL, as indicated by the strong inverse relationship between serum HDL cholesterol and CHD risk. The HDL

pathway is influenced by dietary factors that either enhance or compromise the efficiency of cholesterol removal, as reflected by changes in the concentration of serum HDL.

HDL is synthesized in the gut and liver and increases its particle size in the circulation as a result of the acquisition of cholesterol from two principal sources: from surface material released from TAG-rich lipoproteins during lipolysis, and from peripheral tissues. The particles responsible for removing cholesterol from cells are very small pre-HDL particles composed of phospholipid and apoA-I. (ApoA-I is capable of this function on its own.) The efflux of free cholesterol from tissue sites, including deposits of cholesterol in the coronary arteries, is facilitated by the formation of a free cholesterol gradient from the cell across the cell membrane to pre-HDL. The gradient is generated by the re-esterification of free cholesterol by the enzyme lecithin: cholesterol acyltransferase (LCAT) and the migration of these newly formed cholesterol esters into the hydrophobic core of what becomes mature HDL. The newly acquired cholesterol is transported back to the liver either directly by HDL or indirectly by transfer to apoB-containing lipoproteins VLDL and LDL. Blood vessels in the liver contain a close relative of LPL, called hepatic lipase (HL). This enzyme acts on smaller lipoproteins and especially the surface phospholipid of HDL, where it effectively punches a hole in the surface coat to facilitate access to the lipid core and delivery of CE to the hepatocyte (Figure 6.9).

LCAT = Lecithin: cholesterylacyltransferase
CETP = Cholesteryl ester transfer protein
CE = Cholesterol esters

Figure 6.9 Reverse cholesterol transport.

Interrelationships among serum triacylglycerols and low- and high-density lipoproteins

Lipids are constantly moving between lipoprotein particles. This movement is not totally random but influenced by the relative lipid composition of the lipoproteins and by specific lipid transfer proteins (LTP) which act as lipid shuttles. In a normal, healthy individual, TAG-rich lipoproteins transfer TAG to LDL and HDL in equimolar exchange for CE. This is mediated through an LTP called cholesteryl transfer protein (CETP). In this way, CE are transferred from HDL to VLDL for passage back to the liver. Conversely, when the concentration of serum TAG and thus TAG-rich lipoproteins is increased, for example by either the overproduction of TAG in the liver or the impaired removal of TAG by LPL, the result is a net transfer of TAG into LDL and HDL. As LDL and HDL are overloaded with TAG they become favored substrates for the action of HL and are remodeled into smaller and denser particles. Small, dense HDL is catabolized rapidly in the liver. This lowers serum HDL, and results in a reduced capacity to perform reverse cholesterol transport. In contrast, small, dense LDL is removed less effectively by LDL receptors and accumulates in serum.

Small, dense LDL has a much greater potential to infiltrate the artery wall and deposit its cholesterol. Even moderately raised serum TAG ($>$1.5 mmol/l) can be inversely associated with HDL-cholesterol and a predominance of small, dense LDL. This collection of findings is known as the atherogenic lipoprotein phenotype (ALP) and is a very common but modifiable source of increased CHD risk in free-living populations.

Endocrine control of lipoprotein metabolism

All hormones exert an influence on lipoprotein metabolism. However, with respect to diet and the control of postprandial lipid metabolism, insulin has by far the greatest impact. Although classically associated with carbohydrate metabolism and the uptake of glucose into cells, the actions of insulin are central to the control of postprandial lipid metabolism. Insulin is secreted in response to the reception of food in the gut and exerts the following effects:

- it stimulates LPL in adipose tissue
- it suppresses the intracellular lipolysis of stored TAG in adipose tissue by inhibiting hormone-sensitive lipase
- it suppresses the release of VLDL from the liver.

Insulin co-ordinates the lipolysis of dietary TAG and uptake of nonesterified fatty acids (NEFA) into adipose tissue. It achieves this by minimizing the release of NEFA from TAG stores in adipose tissue and TAG produced in the liver by suppressing the secretion of VLDL. The sensitivity of the target tissues, liver and adipose tissue, to insulin is critical to the maintenance of these effects. Failure of insulin action, insulin resistance, in conditions such as obesity and diabetes, results in dyslipidemia characterized by an impaired capacity to lipolyze TAG-rich lipoproteins (TAG intolerance or enhanced postprandial lipemia). This effect is compounded by the failure of insulin to suppress the mobilization of NEFA from adipose tissue TAG, which increases the flux of NEFA to the liver and stimulates the overproduction of VLDL. The suppression on the secretion of VLDL is also abolished and VLDL is free to compete with chylomicrons, enhancing postprandial lipemia still further. This series of events gives rise to insulin-resistant dyslipidemia, which presents with the same picture of lipoprotein abnormalities found in an ALP. Insulin also stimulates the synthesis of cholesterol by activating HMG-CoA reductase and the activity of LDL receptors, although the overall effect on cholesterol homeostasis is very small.

Sex hormones

The effect of sex hormones on serum lipoproteins is best illustrated by the pronounced differences between adult male and premenopausal females. Males present with higher total serum and LDL-cholesterol, higher serum TAG and lower HDL-cholesterol concentrations than females. This difference in lipid profiles confers protection against CHD on premenopausal females up until estrogen failure at the menopause. Estrogen was the first compound shown to stimulate LDL receptor activity and this effect accounts for the lower LDL level in females, but also the sharp increase in LDL-cholesterol after the menopause, to levels above those of males. Estrogens stimulate the production of TAG and VLDL but any adverse effect is clearly outweighed by the efficient removal mechanisms that maintain lower serum TAG levels than males until the menopause. In addition to these actions, estrogen selectively inhibits the activity of HL, which contributes to the significant elevation in HDL. In direct contrast, the androgenic male hormone testosterone suppresses LDL receptor activity and is a powerful stimulant of HL activity, which lowers HDL-cholesterol in males. (Note that anabolic steroids promote acute decreases in HDL-cholesterol through stimulation of HL.)

The triacylglycerol hypothesis

The ability of an organism to protect itself against the overaccumulation of cholesterol through diet depends to a large extent on increasing the efficiency of utilization of TAG-rich lipoproteins, which represent the precursors of potentially harmful cholesterol-rich chylomicron remnants and LDL. Dietary effects on serum cholesterol or LDL alone do not provide an adequate basis on which to explain the relationship between diet and CHD within populations. The effects of diet, and in particular dietary fats, in modulating the clearance of TAG-rich lipoproteins in the postprandial period is of paramount importance in preventing the accumulation of atherogenic remnants and development of proatherogenic abnormalities in LDL and HDL. The actions of insulin co-ordinate the metabolism of TAG-rich lipoproteins but can become defective through energy imbalance, weight gain and ultimately obesity. As a consequence, the most common abnormalities in lipoproteins to increase risk in populations arise from a primary defect in the metabolism of TAG, induced through insulin resistance and not cholesterol per se. Equally important is the fact that these defects originate, in part, through diet–gene interactions and are thus highly amenable to dietary modification.

6.6 Body lipid pools

Lipids in the human body exist in two major pools: structural lipids in membranes and storage lipids in body fat. The lipid composition and metabolic fate of these two pools are quite distinct, although many of the fatty acids occupying both pools are the same. The main components of both membrane and storage lipids are the long-chain (16–24 carbon) saturated, monounsaturated and polyunsaturated fatty acids. Although several of the major long-chain fatty acids in the body are common to both membrane and storage lipids, namely palmitate, stearate, oleate and linoleate, three important distinctions exist between membrane and storage lipids.

- Membrane lipids are not usually hydrolyzed to release free fatty acids for energy metabolism.
- Membrane lipids contain a much higher proportion of long-chain PUFA.

- Membrane lipids are more diverse and rarely include triglycerides, which are the main component of storage lipids.

Structural lipid pool

Biological membranes surrounding cells and subcellular organelles exist primarily as lipid bilayers (Figure 6.3). The lipids in both the inner and outer surfaces of membranes are composed mainly of phospholipids and free cholesterol, which interface with a myriad of proteins functioning as receptors, transporters, enzymes, ion channels, etc. Some lipids, i.e. PUFA, confer the feature of "fluidity" to membranes, while others, i.e. cholesterol and saturated fatty acids, have the opposite rigidifying effect. Membranes have extraordinarily diverse fatty acid profiles and phospholipid composition depending on their tissue and subcellular location. They are also the body's reservoir of both fat-soluble vitamins and eicosanoid precursors such as arachidonate.

Most of the body's cholesterol is present in the unesterified form in membranes, where it represents 35–45% of total lipids. Skin, plasma and adrenal cortex contain 55–75% of cholesterol in the esterified form. Bile also contains free cholesterol and bile salts derived from cholesterol.

Storage lipid pool

Triglycerides are the main energy storage form of lipids and they are the principal component of body fat. Triglycerides containing fatty acids destined for oxidation are also present in measurable but much lower amounts in all tissues that can oxidize long-chain fatty acids, i.e. muscle and heart. Triglycerides are synthesized by the intestine and liver, where they are subsequently incorporated into lipoproteins (see Section 6.4) for the transport of lipids to and from other tissues.

The main fatty acids in the triglycerides of adult human body fat are palmitate (20–30%), stearate (10–20%), oleate (45–55%) and linoleate (10–15%). The fatty acid profile of adult body fat always reflects the profile of dietary fat. Only rarely would this result in other fatty acids being more prevalent in body fat than the four listed here. At birth, the fatty acid profile of body fat is unusual in having very low linoleate (<3%) and α-linolenate (<1%) but a higher proportion of long-chain polyunsaturates than later in life. Body fat occupies several discrete sites that expand and contract as needed. Body fat is about 82% by weight triglyceride,

making it by far the main body pool of palmitate, sterate, oleate and linoleate.

The main sites of body fat are subcutaneous and intravisceral and they have different rates of response to stimuli for accumulation or release of fatty acids. Within a given site, growing evidence suggests that PUFA are more easily released from fat triglycerides than are saturated fatty acids, especially during fasting or longer term energy deficit.

Plasma and milk lipids

In a way, plasma and milk lipids are an exception to the general rule distinguishing membrane and storage lipids. Plasma and milk lipids are present mostly as lipoproteins, comprising mostly phospholipids and cholesterol in the surrounding membrane and triglycerides in the core (see Section 6.5). Plasma lipids contain the only significant pool of free fatty acids or NEFA in the body. Free fatty acids are not components of lipoproteins but are transported bound to albumin. They are liberated mostly from adipose tissue when plasma glucose and insulin are low. Plasma also contains proportionally more fatty acids esterified to cholesterol (cholesteryl esters) than are found in tissues.

Whole body content and organ profile of fatty acids

An estimate of the whole body content of lipids in a healthy adult human is given in Table 6.5. Additional body fat is deposited during pregnancy, but the fatty acid composition remains similar to that of nonpregnant adults and reflects dietary fat intake. The total lipid

Table 6.5 Body fat content of major fatty acids in humans

Fatty acid	Content (g)
Palmitic acid	3320
Stearic acid	550
Oleic acid	6640
Linoleic acid	1560
Arachidonic acid	80
α-Linolenic acid	130
Eicosapentaenoic acid	<10
Docosahexaenoic acid	<10
Total	12 300

Data are based on a 70 kg adult human with 20% (14 kg) body fat. Fat tissue contains about 88% actual fatty acids by weight, yielding about 12.3 kg fatty acids in this example.

content of plasma rises in the third trimester, with a proportionally greater increase in saturated than poly-unsaturated fatty acids. This downward trend in the percentage of polyunsaturates towards term has led to some concern about the possible adverse consequences for the fetus of deficiency of polyunsaturates. However, the actual amount of polyunsaturates in blood lipids rises but less so than for saturated fatty acids, hence the proportional decrease for polyunsaturates.

Soon after birth, body lipid composition starts to change. Brain cholesterol rises moderately from under 40% to nearly 50% of brain lipids. Docosahexaenoate also rises rapidly in brain lipids, followed a little later by an increasing content of long-chain saturates and monounsaturates as myelin develops. Adipose tissue contains very little linoleate or α-linolenate at birth but their content increases rapidly with milk feeding. Plasma cholesterol is relatively low at birth and in infancy, but usually rises by some two-fold into adulthood.

In general, regardless of the profile of dietary fatty acids, saturated and monounsaturated fatty acids predominate in adipose tissue, whereas there is a closer balance between saturates, monounsaturates and poly-unsaturates in structural lipids. Long-chain PUFA such as docosahexaenoate are present in high concentrations in specialized membranes including those of the retina photoreceptor, in synapses of the brain and in sperm.

6.7 Long-chain fatty acid metabolism

Synthesis

Synthesis of fatty acids occurs in the cytosol. It begins with acetyl-CoA being converted to malonyl-CoA by acetyl-CoA carboxylase, an enzyme dependent on biotin. Malonyl-CoA and a second acetyl-CoA then condense via β-ketothiolase. This is subsequently reduced, dehydrated and then hydrogenated to yield a four-carbon product that recycles through the same series of steps until the most common long-chain fatty acid product, palmitate, is produced (Figure 6.10). Acetyl-CoA is primarily an intramitochondrial product. Thus, the transfer of acetyl-CoA to the cytosol for fatty acid synthesis appears to require its conversion to citrate to exit the mitochondria before being reconverted to acetyl-CoA in the cytosol.

There are three main features of long-chain fatty acid synthesis in mammals:

• inhibition by starvation

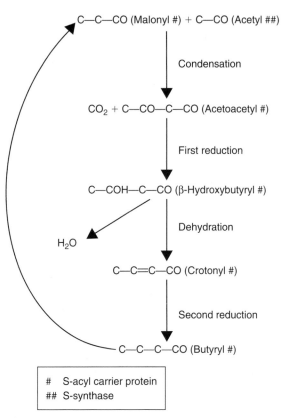

Figure 6.10 Principal steps in fatty acid synthesis. The individual steps occur with the substrate being anchored to the acyl carrier protein.

• stimulation by feeding carbohydrate after fasting
• general inhibition by dietary fat.

Carbohydrate is an important source of carbon for generating acetyl-CoA and citrate used in fatty acid synthesis. Enzymes of carbohydrate metabolism also help to generate the NADPH needed in fatty acid synthesis. Acetyl-CoA carboxylase is a key control point in the pathway and is both activated and induced to polymerize by citrate. Acetyl-CoA carboxylase is inhibited by long-chain fatty acids, especially polyunsaturates such as linoleate. This is probably one important negative feedback mechanism by which both starvation and dietary fat decrease fatty acid synthesis. High amounts of free long-chain fatty acids would also compete for CoA, leading to their β-oxidation. Elongation of palmitate to stearate, etc., can occur in mitochondria using acetyl-CoA, but is more commonly associated with the endoplasmic reticulum where malonyl-CoA is the substrate.

Humans consuming >25% dietary fat synthesize relatively low amounts of fat (<2 g/day). Compared with other animals, humans also appear to have a relatively low capacity to convert stearate to oleate and linoleate or α-linolenate to the respective longer chain polyunsaturates. Hence, the fatty acid profiles of most human tissues generally reflect the intake of dietary fatty acids; when long-chain n-3 polyunsaturates are present in the diet, this is evident in both free-living humans as well as in experimental animals. Nevertheless, fatty acid synthesis is stimulated by fasting/refeeding or weight cycling, so these perturbations in normal food intake can markedly alter tissue fatty acid profiles.

Oxidation

β-Oxidation is the process by which fatty acids are utilized for energy. Saturated fatty acids destined for β-oxidation are transported as CoA esters to the outer leaflet of mitochondria by FABP. They are then translocated inside the mitochondria by carnitine acyltransferases. The β-oxidation process involves repeated dehydrogenation at sequential two-carbon steps and reduction of the associated flavoproteins (see Figure 6.11). Five ATP molecules are produced during production of each acetyl-CoA. A further 12 ATP molecules are produced after the acetyl-CoA condenses with oxaloacetate to form citrate and goes through the tricarboxylic acid cycle.

The efficiency of fatty acid oxidation depends on the availability of oxaloacetate and, hence, concurrent carbohydrate oxidation. β-Oxidation of saturated fatty acids appears to be simpler than oxidation of unsaturated fatty acids because, before the acetyl-CoA cleavage, it involves the formation of a *trans* double bond two carbons from the CoA. In contrast, β-oxidation of unsaturated fatty acids yields a double bond in a different position that then requires further isomerization or hydrogenation. From a biochemical perspective, this extra step appears to make the oxidation of unsaturated fatty acids less efficient than that of saturated fatty acids. However, abundant *in vivo* and *in vitro* research in both humans and animals clearly shows that long-chain *cis*-unsaturated fatty acids with one to three double bonds (oleate, linoleate, α-linolenate) are more readily β-oxidized than saturated fatty acids of equivalent chain length, such as palmitate and stearate. Oxidizing polyunsaturates and monounsaturates more easily than saturates has potential implications for chronic diseases such as coronary artery disease because their slower oxidation

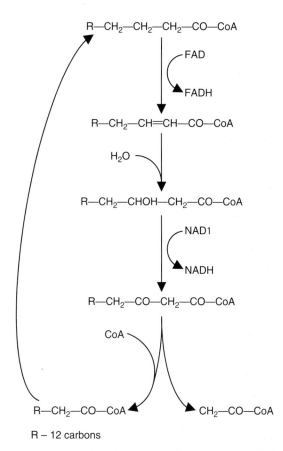

Figure 6.11 Principal steps in β-oxidation of a saturated fatty acid. The steps shown follow fatty acid "activation" (binding to coenzyme A) and carnitine-dependent transport to the inner surface of the mitochondria. Unsaturated fatty acids require additional steps to remove the double bonds before continuing with the pathway shown.

implies slower clearance from the blood, thereby providing more opportunity for esterification to cholesterol and subsequent deposition in the vessel wall.

In peroxisomes, fatty acid β-oxidation is a truncated process by which long-chain PUFA are chain-shortened. This peroxisomal detour has been identified as an obligatory step in the endogenous synthesis of docosahexanoate from eicosapentaenoate.

Odd-carbon long-chain fatty acids are relatively uncommon but, when β-oxidized, yield propionyl-CoA, the further β-oxidation of which requires biotin and vitamin B_{12} as coenzymes.

Ketogenesis and ketosis

Large amounts of free fatty acids inhibit glycolysis and the enzymes of the tricarboxylic acid cycle, thereby impairing production of oxaloacetate. When insufficient oxaloacetate is available to support the continued oxidation of acetyl-CoA, two acetyl-CoA molecules condense to form a ketone, acetoacetate. Acetoacetate can be spontaneously decarboxylated to form acetone, a volatile ketone, or converted to a third ketone, β-hydroxybutyrate. When glucose is limiting, ketones are an alternative source of energy for certain organs, particularly the brain. They are also efficient substrates for lipid synthesis during early postnatal development. Conditions favoring ketogenesis include starvation, diabetes and a very high-fat, low-carbohydrate "ketogenic" diet.

Carbon recycling

Carbon recycling is the process by which acetyl-CoA derived from β-oxidation of one fatty acid is incorporated into another lipid instead of completing the β-oxidation process to carbon dioxide. In principle, all fatty acids undergo this process to some extent but it is most clearly evident for two polyunsaturated fatty acids, linoleate and α-linolenate. Carbon recycling captures the overwhelming majority of α-linolenate carbon, i.e. about 10 times more than is incorporated into docosahexaenoate, which remains in the body of suckling rats 48 h after dosing with uniformly ^{13}C-labeled α-linolenate. Carbon recycling of linoleate in the rat captures similar amounts of the linoleate skeleton compared with that of arachidonate, the main desaturation and chain-elongation product of linoleate. Hence, carbon recycling appears to be a ubiquitous feature of the metabolism of polyunsaturates, although its biological significance is still unclear.

Peroxidation

Peroxidation (auto-oxidation) is the nonenzyme catalyzed reaction of molecular oxygen with organic compounds to form peroxides and related breakdown products. PUFA are particularly vulnerable to peroxidation at the double bonds. Initiating agents such as pre-existing peroxides, transition metals, or ultraviolet or ionizing radiation produce singlet oxygen. Singlet oxygen can then abstract hydrogen at the double bonds of polyunsaturates to produce free (peroxy) radicals, which abstract further hydrogens from the same or different fatty acids and propagate the peroxidation process. Eventually, this leads to termination by the formation of stable degradation products or hydro-

Figure 6.12 Principal steps in peroxidation of a polyunsaturated fatty acid.

peroxides (Figure 6.12). *Trans* isomers are frequently formed during the process. Hydroperoxides can form further hydroperoxy radicals or can be reduced by antioxidants, which contain thiol groups, i.e. glutathione and cysteine. Peroxidation of dietary fats gives rise to aldehydes, i.e. 2-undecenal, 2-decenal, nonanal or octanal, which have a particular odor commonly known as rancidity.

Since peroxidation is a feature of polyunsaturates, it is a potential hazard facing most membranes and dietary lipids. Antioxidants such as vitamin E are usually present in sufficient amounts to prevent or block peroxidation in living tissues. Humans and animals readily detect peroxidized fats in foods by their disagreeable odor and avoid them. Modeling the relevance of effects of peroxides observed *in vivo* and *in vitro*, however, is particularly challenging because lipid peroxidation undoubtedly is an important part of several necessary biological processes such as activating the immune response.

Desaturation, chain elongation and chain shortening

One important characteristic of long-chain fatty acid metabolism in both plants and animals is the capacity to convert one to another via the processes of desaturation, chain elongation and chain shortening.

Plants and animals use desaturases to insert a double bond into long-chain fatty acids. There are several desaturases, depending on the position in the acyl chain into which the double bond will be inserted. Although myristate (14:0) and palmitate can be converted to their monounsaturated derivatives, myristoleate (14:1n-5) and palmitoleate (16:1n-7) respectively, commonly, it is only the fatty acids of 18 or more carbons that undergo desaturation. The Δ^9 desaturases in all organisms except for anaerobic bacteria use oxygen and NADPH to introduce a *cis* double bond at carbons 9 and 10 of stearate. This is accomplished by an enzyme complex consisting of a series of two cytochromes and the terminal desaturase itself. The acyl-CoA form of fatty acids is the usual substrate for the desaturases, but fatty acids esterified to phospholipids can also be desaturated *in situ*.

All mammals that have been studied can convert stearate to oleate via Δ^9 desaturase. However, in the absence of dietary oleate, young rats may have insufficient capacity to sustain normal tissue oleate levels. Normal values depend on the reference, which can vary widely depending on the source and amount of oleate in the diet. Nevertheless, it is important to distinguish between the existence of a given desaturase and the capacity of that pathway to make sufficient of the necessary product fatty acid. Hence, as with the long-chain polyunsaturates and, indeed, with other nutrients such as amino acids (see Chapter 4), it is important to keep in mind that the existence of a pathway to make a particular fatty acid or amino acid does not guarantee sufficient capacity of that pathway to make that product. This is the origin of the concept of conditional essentiality or indispensability. Both plants and animals are capable of desaturating at the 9–10 carbon (Δ^9 desaturase) of stearate, resulting in oleate. However, only plants are capable of desaturating oleate to linoleate and then to α-linolenate. Once linoleate and α-linolenate are consumed by animals, their conversion to the longer chain polyunsaturates of their respective families proceeds primarily by an alternating series of desaturation (Δ^6 and Δ^5 desaturases) and chain-elongation steps (Figure 6.13). Sequential desaturations or chain-elongations are also a possibility, resulting in a large variety although low abundance of other polyunsaturates.

During dietary deficiency of linoleate or α-linolenate, oleate can also be desaturated and chain elongated to the polyunsaturated fatty acid eicosatrienoate (20:3n-9). Hence, most but not all polyunsaturates are derived from linoleate or α-linolenate.

Chain elongation of saturated and unsaturated fatty acids occurs primarily in the endoplasmic reticulum, although it has also been demonstrated to occur in mitochondria. Unlike the desaturation steps immediately before and after, the elongation steps do not appear to be rate limiting in the metabolism of linoleate or α-linolenate.

Despite the capacity to insert at least three double bonds in both n-3 and n-6 polyunsaturates, there is no proof that a Δ^4 desaturase exists to insert the final double bond in docosapentaenoate (22:5n-6) or docosahexaenoate (Figure 6.13). Rather, it appears that the precursors to these two fatty acids undergo a second elongation, repeated Δ^6 desaturation followed by chain shortening in peroxisomes. This unexpectedly convoluted series of steps is corroborated by the docosahexaenoate deficiency observed in disorders of peroxisomal biogenesis such as Zellweger syndrome.

Hydrogenation

Opposite to the desaturation process is hydrogenation or removal of unsaturated bonds in lipids. Rumen bacteria are the only organisms known to have this capability. As in chemical hydrogenation practiced by the food industry, biohydrogenation in the rumen can be incomplete, resulting in the formation of small amounts of *trans* isomers, particularly of oleate, linoleate and α-linolenate, which are found in milk fat.

Eicosanoids

Eicosanoids are 20-carbon, oxygen-substituted cyclized metabolites of dihomo-γ-linolenate, arachidonate or eicosapentaenoate. They are produced via a cascade of steps starting with the cyclo-oxygenase or lipoxygenase enzymes present in microsomes. The main cyclo-oxygenase products comprise the classical

ω6 Polyunsaturates

Linoleic

γ-Linolenic

Dihomo-γ-Linolenic

Arachidonic

Adrenic

ω6-Docosapentaenoic

Δ⁶-Desaturation

Chain elongation

Δ⁵-Desaturation

Chain elongation

Chain elongation, peroxisomal chain shortening

ω3 Polyunsaturates

α-Linolenic

Stearidonic

ω3-Eicosatrienoic

Eicosapentaenoic

ω3-Docosapentaenoic

Docosahexaenoic

Figure 6.13 Conversion of linoleic (18:2n-6) and α-linolenic (18:3n-3) acids to their respective longer chain, more unsaturated polyunsaturates. In membranes, linoleic and arachidonic acids are the principal n-6 polyunsaturates, while docosahexaenoic acid is the principal n-3 polyunsaturate. Hence, these two families of fatty acids have different affinities for the desaturation and chain-elongation enzymes. This pathway is principally based in the endoplasmic reticulum but appears to depend on peroxisomes for the final chain shortening, which involves 24 carbon intermediates that are not illustrated.

prostaglandins, prostacyclin and the thromboxanes. The main lipoxygenase products are the leukotrienes (slow-reacting substances of anaphylaxis) and the non-cyclized hydroperoxy derivatives of arachidonate that give rise to the hepoxilins and lipoxins (Figure 6.14).

Eicosanoids are considered to be fast-acting local hormones, the presence of which in the plasma and urine is largely a spillover from localized production, usually in response to an injury or a stimulus that releases the free precursor, most commonly arachidonate. The site of highest eicosanoid concentration appears to be the seminal fluid, although some species have no detectable eicosanoids in semen. Eicosanoids are second messengers modulating, among other pathways, protein phosphorylation. The lung is a major site of eicosanoid inactivation.

Four important characteristics of eicosanoid action should be noted. First, individual eicosanoids often have biphasic actions as one moves from very low through to higher, often pharmacological, concentrations. Thus, effects can vary dramatically depending not only on the experimental system but also on the eicosanoid concentration used. Secondly, several of the more abundant

eicosanoids arising from the same precursor fatty acid have opposite actions to each other. For instance, prostacyclin and thromboxane A_2 are both derived from arachidonate but the former originates primarily from the endothelium and inhibits platelet aggregation, while the latter originates primarily from platelets and is a potent platelet aggregating agent. Thirdly, competing eicosanoids derived from dihomo-γ-linolenate (1 series) and from eicosapentaenoate (3 series) often have effects that oppose those derived from arachidonate (2 series) (Figures 6.14, 6.15). Thus, unlike prostaglandin E_2, prostaglandin E_1 has anti-inflammatory actions, reduces vascular tone and inhibits platelet aggregation. Fourthly, varying the ratio of the precursor fatty acids in the diet is an effective way to modify eicosanoid production. Thus, eicosapentaenoate and dihomo-γ-linolenate inhibit the synthesis of 2 series eicosanoids derived from arachidonate. This occurs by inhibiting arachidonate release from membranes by phospholipase A_2 and its cascade through the cyclooxygenases and lipoxygenases. The overproduction of 2 series eicosanoids is associated with higher blood pressure, increased platelet aggregation and inflammatory processes, and

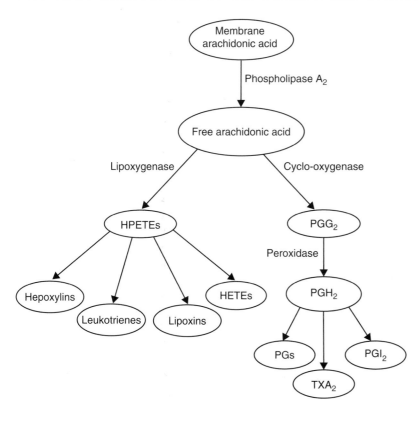

Figure 6.14 The arachidonic acid cascade is a fundamental component of cell signaling during injury. Phospholipase A_2 is immediately activated and the free arachidonic acid thus released is accessible to a controlled peroxidation process involving several cyclo-oxygenases (constitutive or inducible) and lipoxygenases. Over 50 metabolically active products are potentially produced, depending on the tissue involved, the type of cell that has been stimulated and the type of injury. Only the main classes of these metabolites are shown. Before excretion, they are further metabolized to stable products that are not shown. Several of the cyclo-oxygenase products are competitive with each other, such as the platelet aggregating and blood vessel wall constricting effects of thromboxane A_2 (TXA_2) produced in platelets, versus the opposite effects of prostacyclin (PGI_2) derived from the blood vessel wall. HPETE: hydroperoxyeicosatetraenoic acid; PG: prostaglandin; HETE: hydroxyeicosatetraenoic acid; TX: thromboxane.

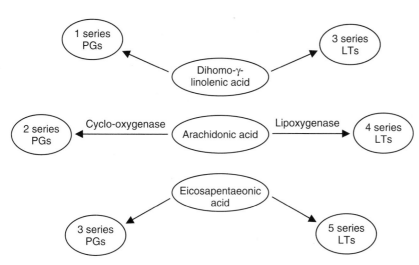

Figure 6.15 Arachidonic acid is not the only 20-carbon polyunsaturated fatty acid that can be metabolized via the cyclo-oxygenases and lipoxygenases; both dihomo-γ-linolenic acid (20 : 3n-6) and eicosapentaenoic acid (20 : 5n-3) are well-established precursors as well, and produce prostaglandins (PG) and leukotrienes (LT) that are frequently competitive with those produced from arachidonate, thereby neutralizing the effects of the arachidonate cascade (see Figure 6.14). This provides a critical balance in the overall reaction to cell injury.

can be effectively inhibited by dietary approaches using oils rich in eicosapentaenoate and γ-linolenate (18 : 3n-6), the precursor to dihomo-γ-linolenate.

Stable analogues of some classical prostaglandins have specialized medical applications, including the termination of pregnancy and the closing of a patent ductus arteriosus shortly after birth. Many anti-inflammatory and antipyretic drugs are inhibitors of eicosanoid synthesis. One potentially dangerous side-effect of inhibiting eicosanoid synthesis is gastric erosion and bleeding. Receptor antagonists of leukotrienes are effective in reducing the symptoms of asthma.

6.8 Nutritional regulation of long-chain fatty acid profiles and metabolism

Phospholipids of all cellular and subcellular membranes contain a diverse range of long-chain fatty acids, the profile of which is subject to both dietary influence and endogenous control. A few organs, notably the brain, maintain extraordinarily strict control of their membrane composition. Usually, however, the fatty acid profile of most organs is responsive to the influence of changes in dietary fatty acid composition and other nutritional variables, yet maintains the vital "gatekeeper" functions of all membranes. Hence, when changes in dietary fat change membrane fatty acid profiles, appropriate membrane fluidity can be maintained by the addition or removal of other lipids such as cholesterol. Insufficient energy intake and the presence of disease have important consequences for fatty acid synthesis, desaturation and chain elongation and, consequently, tissue fatty acid profiles.

Saturates and monounsaturates

Inadequate energy intake increases macronutrient oxidation, including fatty acids. Short-term fasting followed by refeeding a carbohydrate-rich meal is the classic way to stimulate fatty acid synthesis. Insulin is implicated in this process. When repeated, fasting/refeeding or weight cycling induces a gradual increase in the proportion of saturated and monounsaturated compared with polyunsaturated fatty acids in tissues, especially body fat. This shift occurs because of the increase in fatty acid synthesis, the easier oxidation of polyunsaturates and the inhibition of desaturation and chain elongation by fasting. The implications of such an alteration in tissue fatty acid profiles have not yet been extensively studied, but probably involve changes in insulin sensitivity and other hormone effects. Protein deficiency also inhibits desaturation and chain elongation of PUFA.

Copper supplementation increases Δ^9 desaturase activity in animals, resulting in higher oleate levels. This effect was first observed when copper was used to reduce gastrointestinal infection in pigs, but also led to softer back fat. Opposite to the effects of copper supplementation, copper deficiency inhibits synthesis of both oleate and docosahexaenoate.

Polyunsaturated fatty acids

There are four key features of the nutritional regulation of the profiles and metabolism of PUFA. These attributes govern the effects of deficiency or excess of one or more of these families of fatty acids almost as much as their level in the diet. These key features are:

- specificity within families
- competition between families
- substrate and end-product inhibition
- cofactor nutrients.

Specificity

An n-6 PUFA cannot be converted to an n-3 or n-9 polyunsaturated fatty acid. Thus, deficiency of one family of polyunsaturates cannot be corrected by excess of those in a different family and, indeed, is exacerbated by excess intake of the other families.

Competition

The three families of polyunsaturates appear to use a common series of desaturases and chain elongases. The preference of these enzymes is for the more unsaturated fatty acids so, everything else being equal, more α-linolenate will be desaturated than linoleate or oleate. In practice, more linoleate is consumed than α-linolenate and, as a result, more arachidonate is produced endogenously than eicosapentaenoate. Furthermore, this competition for desaturation and chain elongation between linoleate and α-linolenate can lead to exacerbation of symptoms of deficiency of one or other fatty acid family. Thus, as has been demonstrated both clinically and experimentally, excess linoleate intake using sunflower oil is a common way to accelerate deficiency of n-3 polyunsaturates.

Inhibition

Excess linoleate or α-linolenate intake appears to inhibit production of the respective long-chain products in the same fatty acid family, i.e. high α-linolenate intake inhibits synthesis of docosahexaenoate. Likewise, the main end-products of desaturation and chain elongation tend to inhibit further metabolism through this pathway, so arachidonate inhibits its own synthesis. Similarly, dietary deficiency of linoleate increases activity of the Δ^6 and Δ^5 desaturases, presumably to restore depleted levels of long-chain n-6 polyunsaturates such as arachidonate.

Cofactors

The cofactor requirements of the desaturation-chain-elongation enzymes are not yet well understood, but a few relationships are known. The desaturases are metalloenzymes containing iron, and iron deficiency therefore inhibits desaturase activity. Magnesium is needed for microsomal desaturase activity *in vitro*. Zinc deficiency inhibits Δ^6 and Δ^5 desaturation, apparently by interrupting the flow of electrons from NADH. This effect is severe enough that inherited forms of zinc deficiency such as acrodermatitis enteropathica cause a precipitous decline in plasma arachidonate, greater than usually observed with dietary deficiency of n-6 polyunsaturates.

6.9 Nutritional and metabolic effects of dietary fatty acids

Two types of issue exist in relation to the nutritional and health implications of individual dietary lipids.

- Whether synthesized endogenously or only obtained from the diet, what are the specific membrane, precursor or metabolic effects of dietary lipids beyond that of providing energy?
- Whether synthesized endogenously or obtained from the diet, does an excess amount of a dietary lipid have beneficial or deleterious implications for health?

Short- and medium-chain fatty acids

Short-chain fatty acids (1–6 carbons) are mostly derived from carbohydrate fermentation in the large bowel and appear to mainly be used for energy, although they are also substrates in several pathways. Butyrate may have an important role as an energy substrate for enterocytes. Medium-chain fatty acids (8–14 carbons) naturally appear in mammalian milk and are almost exclusively used as energy substrates. They may also be chain elongated to palmitate.

Saturated fatty acids

Palmitate and stearate comprise a major proportion of the acyl groups of membrane phospholipids and all mammals have the capacity to synthesize them. Hence, empirically, they presumably have an important function in energy metabolism, cell structure, normal development and growth. The 20–24-carbon saturates are important constituents of myelin. However, in any

of these functions, it is unlikely that a dietary source of saturates is necessary. In fact, the brain is unable to acquire saturated fatty acids from the circulation and relies on its own endogenous synthesis for these fatty acids. Furthermore, chronic excess intake and/or synthesis of palmitate and stearate is associated with an increased risk of diabetes and coronary artery disease.

Monounsaturated fatty acids

Little is known about the nutritional or health implications of palmitoleate (16 : 1n-7), but there is a burgeoning interest in the main dietary monounsaturated fatty acid, oleate, and the health implications of olive oil. In the context of the same total fat intake, the main benefit of higher oleate intake seems to be that the reduced intake of palmitate and stearate helps to lower serum cholesterol.

Partially hydrogenated fatty acids

Partially hydrogenated fatty acids contain a large proportion of *trans* fatty acids that are not naturally occurring but arise directly from food processing. Hence, unlike saturates and *cis*-unsaturated fatty acids, they are not a necessary component of the diet except in the small amounts found in cow's milk. Their physical characteristics make them economically suitable for inclusion in a wide variety of baked, fried and oil-based foods, from which they can easily contribute up to 10% of dietary fat depending on food selection. Epidemiological evidence and some experimental studies show that common dietary *trans* fatty acids raise LDL-cholesterol in healthy adults, so the main nutritional concern is that they may contribute to an increased risk of cardiovascular disease.

Trans fatty acids have also been experimentally shown to compete with and impair the metabolism of other dietary long-chain fatty acids, but the relevance of these observations in humans is unclear. *Trans* fatty acids can be present in baby foods at relatively high concentrations but, so far, there is no evidence of deleterious effects on growth or development. Some information on the metabolism of *trans* fatty acids in humans has been gained from tracer studies, but fundamental information, such as the rate at which they are oxidized, is still unknown.

Polyunsaturated fatty acids

Unlike saturates and monounsaturates, a dietary source of n-6 and n-3 polyunsaturates is a necessity for normal growth and development. As with other essential nutrients, this has given rise to assessment of the dietary requirements for polyunsaturates and the implications of inadequate dietary intake of them.

It has been accepted for over 50 years that n-6 polyunsaturates, particularly linoleate, are required in the diet of all mammals, including humans. Official dietary guidelines generally recommend a dietary source of linoleate at 1–2% of energy intake. It has taken much longer to demonstrate that n-3 polyunsaturates are required by humans. Although this now seems widely accepted among nutrition researchers, some countries, including the USA, still do not yet officially recognize that, as a minimum, α-linolenate is a required nutrient. As with other nutrients, the requirement for polyunsaturates varies according to the stage of the life cycle, with pregnancy, lactation and infancy being the most vulnerable. Symptoms of linoleate deficiency are virtually impossible to induce in healthy adult humans, so the concept of "conditional indispensability or dispensability" of polyunsaturates has recently emerged to replace the older but ambiguous term, "essential fatty acid". Linoleate appears to be conditionally dispensable in healthy nonpregnant adults, but is not in pregnancy, lactation or infancy.

Because of the competition between the two families of polyunsaturates, deficiency of n-3 polyunsaturates is commonly induced by an excess of dietary linoleate. Hence, discussion of the requirements for linoleate and α-linolenate often focuses on their ratio in the diet. The ratio of n-6 to n-3 polyunsaturates in human milk (5 : 1 to 10 : 1) has been widely viewed as a suitable reference for this ratio in the general diet. In most affluent countries, this ratio remains much higher, at about 20 : 1, and is implicated in subclinical deficiency of n-3 polyunsaturates.

Essential fatty acid deficiency

The first experimental model of deficiency of polyunsaturates was total fat deficiency. The elimination of dietary fat had to be extreme because the traces of fat found in starch and dietary proteins were sufficient to prevent reproducible symptoms of fat deficiency. The deficiency symptoms are now well known and involve dry, scaly skin, growth retardation and reproductive failure. Most of these gross symptoms are relieved by linoleate and arachidonate. Although α-linolenate cannot be synthesized *de novo*, it has little effect on these gross symptoms. However, careful studies using a diet

that is not only extremely deficient in n-3 polyunsaturates but contains an excess of n-6 polyunsaturates led to deficiency of n-3 polyunsaturates, characterized by delayed and impaired neuronal development and impaired vision. These symptoms have been traced in many species to inadequate accumulation of docosahexaenoate in the brain and eye, respectively. Hence, the main function of n-3 polyunsaturates appears to hinge on synthesis of docosahexaenoate. In contrast, the function of n-6 polyunsaturates involves independent roles of at least linoleate and arachidonate.

Human cases of deficiency of polyunsaturates usually involve a clinical disorder, often involving weight loss, trauma such as surgery, or a disease requiring parenteral nutrition. However, reports of these cases are uncommon and describe dissimilar characteristics, leading one to question whether the same deficiency exists. Recent investigations into the amount of polyunsaturates in the whole body and the rate at which they can be oxidized suggest that traumatic or disease-related processes leading to weight loss affect metabolism of polyunsaturates more severely than simple dietary deficiency in a weight-stable, healthy individual. For example, deficiency of linoleate has been long suspected but difficult to demonstrate in cystic fibrosis. Despite poor fat digestion, intake levels of linoleate may not be inadequate but its β-oxidation could well be abnormally high owing to the chronic infectious challenge.

Clinical importance of polyunsaturates

Infant brain and visual development is dependent on adequate accumulation of docosahexaenoate. The 1990s saw intense clinical and experimental assessment of the role of docosahexaenoate in early brain development and a widespread concern that many infant formulae do not yet contain docosahexaenoate. Several clinical studies and extensive use of formula containing docosahexaenoate and arachidonate have shown that they are safe. Many but not all such studies show an improvement in visual and cognitive scores compared with matched formulae containing no docosahexaenoate or arachidonate. The infant brain and body as a whole clearly acquire less docosahexaenoate when only α-linolenate is given. As a whole, these data suggest that docosahexaenoate is a conditionally indispensable fatty acid.

Aside from questionable deficiency of polyunsaturates in cystic fibrosis (see above), one of the most graphic examples of their deficiency being caused by an inherited disease is Zellweger syndrome. This condition causes severe mental retardation and early death. It is a disorder of peroxisomal biogenesis and one outcome is markedly impaired synthesis of docosahexaenoate. Dietary supplements with docosahexaenoate appear partially to restore neurological development.

Epidemiological evidence shows that chronic degenerative diseases of affluence are directly associated with the deficiency of n-3 polyunsaturated fatty acids. Indeed, countries with relatively high rates of these diseases usually have an adequate to perhaps unnecessarily higher intake of linoleate. Perhaps the high linoleate is part of the problem, because considerable epidemiological and experimental evidence suggests that deaths from coronary artery disease and several types of cancer are associated with low intakes of n-3 polyunsaturates. Mental illnesses such as schizophrenia may also be associated with low intake of n-3 polyunsaturates and respond to supplements of n-3 polyunsaturates. A more balanced ratio of intake of n-6 and n-3 polyunsaturates might achieve a reduction in the rate of these degenerative diseases but has not yet been widely investigated.

Diets in Palaeolithic times contained no processed food and probably had a more balanced ratio of n-3 to n-6 polyunsaturates and a lower level of saturates. Such diets would be predicted to lead to a lower incidence of degenerative disease. Since the brain has a very high energy requirement, it has also been speculated that human brain evolution beyond that of other primates was dependent on a reliable and rich source of dietary energy and a direct source of long-chain polyunsaturates, particularly docosahexaenoate.

6.10 Cholesterol synthesis and regulation

Cholesterol and the brain
Mammalian brain function is dependent on specialized membranes designed for signal transmission. Greater cognitive sophistication in humans appears to depend on the much higher number of connections and, consequently, greater potential for signal processing. Like the membrane lipids of most other mammalian organs, brain lipids contain a relatively high proportion of cholesterol, which increases from about 40% of the lipid content in neonates to nearly 50% in adults.

Unlike other organs, the mammalian brain is probably unique in being unable to acquire appreciable amounts of cholesterol from the circulation, i.e. from the diet or from synthesis outside the brain. This has been extensively studied in the young rat and supporting, although inconclusive, evidence is also available for the pig. The brain has sufficient capacity to synthesize cholesterol from acetyl-CoA derived primarily from either glucose or ketones. Hence, it achieves the required level of cholesterol apparently entirely by endogenous synthesis. In neonates, ketones appear to play a greater role as brain cholesterol substrates than in adults, where their main function seems to be as an alternative fuel to glucose. Among the common dietary long-chain fatty acids that would give rise to ketones during fat oxidation, PUFA, particularly linoleate and α-linolenate, appear to be the best substrates for ketogenesis, since carbon from them readily appears in brain cholesterol in suckling rats.

6.11 Effect of diet on serum lipids and lipoproteins

Diet and serum cholesterol
Diet exerts a profound influence on blood lipids and lipoproteins and as such should always be a major component of strategies for the primary prevention of diseases in which lipids play an aetiological role, such as CHD. Nevertheless, despite convincing epidemiological evidence and the existence of credible biochemical mechanisms to support a relationship between dietary fat and serum cholesterol, the outcome of prospective intervention trials designed to test this relationship within populations has been disappointing.

Over 30 years ago Keys and Hegsted made the landmark observation that variation in the concentration of serum cholesterol across seven different countries was positively related to the amount of energy derived from saturated fat. Conversely, they found that intake of dietary PUFA was inversely related to serum cholesterol. From this finding they were able to formulate equations that enabled them to predict the quantitative effect of saturated and polyunsaturated fat on serum cholesterol (Figure 6.16). In simpler terms, the ratio of PUFA to saturated fatty acids (SFA), the P:S ratio, was used with effect to predict changes in serum cholesterol. Although still effective today, the equations and ratio are slowly being superseded by advanced knowledge of the biological effects of individual fatty acids. It is now established that saturated

Figure 6.16 Influence of dietary fatty acids on serum cholesterol.

fats with between 12 and 16 carbon atoms, namely lauric, myristic and palmitic acids, are particularly hypercholesterolemic, whereas stearic acid, an extremely abundant SFA in most diets, is relatively neutral in its effects on serum cholesterol. [Note that stearic acid is desaturated to monounsaturated fatty acids (MUFA) by Δ^9 desaturase.] The cholesterol-raising effect of SFA arises chiefly from an increase in LDL-cholesterol and is about twice as potent as the hypocholesterolemic effect of dietary PUFA. Paradoxically, SFA actually increase serum HDL-cholesterol. The polyunsaturates are divisible into two main series on the basis of the position of the first double bond from the methyl end of the fatty acid chain, the parent fatty acids being linoleic (C18-2n-6) and α-linolenic (C18-3n-3) acids. The cholesterol-lowering effects of dietary PUFA are largely attributable to linoleic acid and are also believed to act through effects on LDL. Historically, monounsaturated fat was considered to be neutral with respect to its effects on lipids and lipoproteins and was omitted from the predictive formula. However, further studies, prompted by interest in the role of MUFA in the Mediterranean diet, have shown that MUFA decreases LDL-cholesterol, although possibly to a lesser extent than linoleic acid, and increases HDL-cholesterol. An additional benefit of MUFA is thought to be conferred by the presence of a single double bond in MUFA, which when incorporated in membrane phospholipids of LDL protects this lipoprotein from oxidative modification, an essential prerequisite step in the deposition of cholesterol in the artery wall. In this regard, there is presently some concern that increasing dietary PUFA will impose additional oxidative stress on LDL. While this idea

forms part of the rationale for limiting the amount of dietary PUFA to less than 10% energy intake, there is as yet no convincing evidence of adverse effects from increasing the level of PUFA in tissues and circulating lipoproteins.

Trans *fatty acids*

Saturated fats are comprised of straight chains of carbon atoms which pack together tightly in the phospholipids of cell membranes and lipoproteins. In contrast, carbon double bonds in the *cis* configuration in MUFA and PUFA introduce a bend or kink into the carbon chain which alters the physical properties of the phospholipids containing these fatty acids as, for example, by increasing their packing volume, a physical property that contributes to an increase in membrane fluidity. The partial hydrogenation of MUFA and PUFA, most notably during the industrial processing of foods for the purpose of solidifying unsaturated oils, results in a loss of this kink as the fatty acid assumes a straighter, *trans* configuration that resembles that found in SFA. This likeness in chemical structure is thought to account for the SFA-like effects of *trans* fatty acids such as elaidic acid (*trans* isomer of oleic acid) on serum lipids (see Figs 6.1 and 6.2). The results of prospective cohort studies such as the Nurses' Health Study showed that high levels of *trans* fats in excess of 7% energy increased serum LDL and reduced HDL. However, despite the continued and extensive use of partially hydrogenated fats in products such as cakes, biscuits and spreads, the average intake in most Western diets does not exceed 3–4% energy intake and at this level of intake *trans* fats are unlikely to exert adverse effects on serum lipids.

Plant sterols and soluble nonstarch polysaccharides

These compounds may be grouped together as they share a similar mode of action on LDL cholesterol, which is to reduce the availability of dietary and biliary cholesterol for absorption in the gut. This action interrupts the enterohepatic circulation and up-regulates the activity of LDL receptors (see Section 6.5). Plant sterols and their esters such as those incorporated into margarines (stanols and stanol esters), despite being nearly identical in structure to cholesterol, are poorly absorbed and interfere with the reabsorption of cholesterol originating from bile and dietary sources by either coprecipitation or competition. Margarines or spreads (30–40 g/day) containing plant sterols or their derivatives have been shown to reduce LDL-cholesterol by up to 14% in controlled trials. Soluble NSP such as that found in gums and gelling agents from fruit (gum arabic and pectins) act in a similar way and have been shown to be equally efficacious in reducing serum LDL-cholesterol.

Dietary cholesterol

There is a popular misconception that dietary cholesterol correlates directly with serum cholesterol, when in fact dietary cholesterol, within a range of normal dietary consumption (100–400 mg/day), has only a very small impact on serum cholesterol levels. Eggs represent the principal source of dietary cholesterol in most diets (1 egg yolk = 150–250 mg cholesterol); in their absence most Western diets would contain considerably less than 100 mg cholesterol/day. The classic but extreme egg-feeding studies showed that feeding of up to six eggs a day (900 mg cholesterol) increased LDL-cholesterol acutely. However, the body effectively counters this effect with sensitive compensatory mechanisms to deal with an increasing load of dietary cholesterol, one of which is to reduce the amount of cholesterol absorbed in the gut. This compensation effectively abolishes any dose–response relationship between dietary cholesterol, over a practically realistic range of intakes, and serum cholesterol. Two factors that may influence the variability in response to dietary cholesterol are dietary SFA, which have been shown to augment the cholesterol-raising effects of dietary cholesterol, and a phenomenon of increased susceptibility to dietary cholesterol in some individuals for some, as yet, unknown reason.

To give perspective to these dietary influences on serum cholesterol in relation to CHD, a meta-analysis of dietary intervention trials undertaken by the World Health Organization (WHO) revealed that dietary modification could only achieve reductions in serum cholesterol of between 4 and 5%. This finding is in sharp contrast with the potent effects of cholesterol-lowering drugs, which can reduce serum cholesterol by 30–40% and have been shown, unequivocally, to reduce the incidence of death from CHD. It also highlights the need to address other risk factors which are more responsive to dietary change.

Fat quantity versus quality: importance of the ratio of n-6 : n-3 PUFA

The underlying principle for a reduction in total fat intake is to reduce energy intake from the consumption of the most energy-dense macronutrient in order to prevent weight gain and ultimately obesity. The current recommendation for the UK is to reduce energy derived from fat to 35% or less. Since weight gain is associated with raised serum TAG and abnormalities in circulating lipoproteins, reducing total fat intake should, in theory, reduce blood lipids. However, in practice there is little evidence to support such an effect within populations. Meta-analyses have revealed that little benefit is to be gained, at least in terms of changes in blood lipids, by reducing total fat without altering the composition of dietary fatty acids. Meta-analyses have also helped to resolve the issue of what represents the most appropriate replacement nutrient for SFA. Since PUFA, and specifically linoleic acid, was shown to counter the actions of SFA and was abundant in natural sources such as sunflower and corn oils, it was an obvious first choice. The alternative was to substitute fat with dietary carbohydrate. There have been problems associated with both of these approaches. First, increasing dietary linoleic acid excludes the lesser abundant, but more metabolically active n-3 PUFA, and especially the longer chain members of this series derived from marine oils [C20 : 5, eicosapentaenoic acid (EPA) and C22 : 6, docosahexaenoic acid (DHA)]. Overemphasis on linoleic acid in the food industry, together with a widespread resistance to the consumption of fish, has led to the development of a serious imbalance in the ratio of n-6 to n-3 PUFA in northern Europe and the USA since the 1970s. This situation has major implications for the development of abnormalities in circulating lipoproteins, since deficiency in EPA and DHA could give rise to increased serum TAG through the overproduction of endogenous TAG (VLDL) in the liver and intolerance to dietary (exogenous) fat and an ALP. The frequency of this dyslipidemia is believed to be very rare in Mediterranean countries that have a high intake of dietary n-3 PUFA and an n-6:n-3 ratio closer to 1. Dietary carbohydrates also incur the problem of having the potential to increase serum TAG. Carbohydrate-induced hypertriacylglycerolemia is not, as was originally thought, a short-term adaptive response in the liver to a change in the pattern of oxidation of fat to carbohydrate, but represents a real phenomenon associated, in particular, with the consumption of sucrose in individuals with insulin-resistant dyslipidemia. An emerging consensus of opinion based on several meta-analyses of dietary intervention trials swings in favor of dietary MUFA as the most favored substitute for dietary SFA, and even linoleic acid in areas of high intake.

Effects of n-3 PUFA from plants and fish

In 1994 the dietary recommendation for long-chain n-3 PUFA (EPA/DHA) in the UK was to double intake by consuming two portions of oily fish per week, taking intake from approximately 0.1 to 0.2 g/day This advice was based on evidence from the DART study, which showed that eating fish could prevent the risk of a second heart attack. Since this end-point was associated with an acute manifestation of CHD, i.e. coronary thrombosis, and fish oil produced no effects on serum and LDL-cholesterol, the benefits were assumed to arise solely from the capacity of these fatty acids to reduce the tendency of the blood to clot. The potent TAG-lowering effect of fish oil was largely ignored at this stage because the role of TAG as a risk factor for CHD was still very contentious. This view was soon to change. Serum TAG is now widely recognized as a major risk factor for CHD and there is also conclusive evidence to show that fish oil supplementation (1 g/day for 3 years) reduces the incidence of death from CHD in healthy, free-living subjects. Long-chain n-3 PUFA exert multiple effects on lipid metabolism, the most notable of which is the capacity to decrease postabsorptive serum TAG levels by 20–30%. Fish oil-enriched diets have also been shown to attenuate the magnitude and duration of postprandial lipemia following the ingestion of a fat-containing meal. These effects are frequently accompanied by beneficial changes in circulating LDL and HDL, and the correction of an ALP. Increased awareness

of these favorable lipid effects has raised the need to increase intakes of EPA and DHA and to redress the imbalance in the ratio of n-6:n-3 PUFA. Unfortunately, it has been impossible to achieve this aim through the consumption of even greater amounts of oily fish, and alternative strategies have had to be devised. One approach has been to increase the level of the shorter chain precursor of EPA/DHA, α-linolenic acid (C18:3n-3). The latter is derived from plant seeds such as flax and rapeseed, and is desaturated and elongated to its longer chain relatives in the body. The efficiency of this conversion is reduced by high levels of linoleic acid, which competes more effectively than α-linolenic acid for desaturation. There is, as yet, little evidence to suggest that the rate of conversion of dietary α-linolenic acid to EPA and DHA is sufficient to achieve fish oil-like effects on blood lipids (Table 6.6).

How do dietary fatty acids influence serum cholesterol and triacylglycerols?

In common with other physiological systems, lipoprotein metabolism is co-ordinated by an interplay between the activity of specific genes and hormones that determine the production and activity of functional proteins (enzymes, receptors, lipid transfer and apoproteins). Effects on these functional proteins ultimately regulate the quantity and quality of circulating lipids and lipoproteins. While there have been significant advances in knowledge of the modulatory effects of dietary fatty acids on hormones and gene expression, evidence for the effects of dietary fats on functional proteins is by far the most well defined.

Saturated fatty acids and low-density lipoprotein cholesterol

The most well-elucidated mechanism to explain how different dietary fats produce variable effects on LDL-cholesterol is through the LDL receptor pathway, the control of which has already been described (see Section 6.5). The ability of the cell to regulate its pool of free cholesterol depends to a large extent on the nature of the fatty acids available for esterification by the enzyme ACAT, an intracellular relative of LCAT. ACAT favors unsaturated fatty acids (MUFA and PUFA) as substrates for esterification, which utilizes free cholesterol within the cell. The resulting reduction in intracellular free cholesterol stimulates the transcription of the LDL receptor gene and production of new LDL receptors through the SREBP mechanism

Table 6.6 Effects on plasma lipids of substituting dietary saturated fats with PUFA, MUFA, and carbohydrates

	LDL-C	HDL-C	TAG	TC:HDL
SFA (C12–C16)	⇑⇑	↗	↗	⇑
n-6 PUFA Linoleic acid (sunflower/corn)	⇓	⬌[a]	↘	⇓
n-3 PUFA LC = EPA/DHA (fish oil) SC = linolenic acid (flax/soyabean/rape)	⬌[b]	⬌	⇓⇓	⬌
n-9 MUFA Oleic acid (olive oil/rape)	↘	↗	⇒	⇓
Carbohydrate Sucrose/fructose?	↘	⇓	⇑	⇑

[a]n-6 PUFA in excess of 10% energy.
[b]Increase in response to redistribution of LDL subclasses.
PUFA: polyunsaturated fatty acids; MUFA: monounsaturated fatty acids;
SFA: saturated fatty acids; LC: long chain; EPA: eicosapentaenoic acid; DHA: docosahexaenoic acid; SC: short chain;
LDL-C: low-density lipoprotein cholesterol; HDL-C: high-density lipoprotein cholesterol; TAG: triacylglycerols; TC: total cholesterol.

already described, and fall in circulating LDL. Conversely, SFA are poor substrates for ACAT and their presence in the cell exerts the opposite effect on free cholesterol levels, thus increasing circulating LDL-cholesterol and total serum cholesterol (Figure 6.8). Fatty acids may also exert direct effects on the activity of LDL receptors by altering the composition of membrane phospholipids and thus membrane fluidity. Alternatively, there is evidence to suggest that dietary PUFA could up-regulate LDL receptors indirectly by increasing the cholesterol content (lithogenicity) of bile and in this way accelerate the excretion of cholesterol.

Long-chain n-3 PUFA and serum triacylglycerols

Long chain n-3 PUFA have potent effects in the liver, where they suppress the production of endogenous TAG by inhibiting the enzymes phosphatidic acid phosphatase and diacylglycerol acyltransferase. This effectively reduces the production of TAG-rich VLDL. (Note that apoB-100 is produced constitutively, so that

the production of VLDL is driven by the supply of substrates for the synthesis of TAG.) In addition, long-chain n-3 PUFA accelerate the clearance of TAG-rich lipoproteins from the circulation in the postprandial phase by stimulating the activity of LPL. Together, these effects are thought to underlie the ability of these fatty acids to correct the lipoprotein abnormalities associated with an ALP. In this respect, it is possible that many of their dramatic effects on serum lipids arise from an increase in the sensitivity of tissues to the action of insulin. This would apply to skeletal muscle, adipose tissue and the liver.

Diet–gene interactions

It has been estimated that diet could account for up to 50% of the variation in blood lipids and lipoprotein levels between individuals. This would mean that genetic differences must explain the remaining 50%. In real terms, interactions between diet and genes represent a sizeable proportion of each of these unrealistically discrete fractions.

Table 6.7 Effect of apoprotein E phenotype on serum cholesterol

Phenotype (gene frequency)	Receptor binding affinity	Hepatic free cholesterol	LDL receptor activity	LDL-C
E4 ($\varepsilon_4$15%)	+++	↑ (feedback)	↓	↑
E3 ($\varepsilon_3$77%)	++	→	→	→
E2 ($\varepsilon_2$8%)	+	↓ (feedback)	↑	↓

Carriage of ε_4 allele associated with increased risk of coronary heart disease and greater changes in low-density lipoprotein cholesterol (LDL-C) in response to increased dietary fat and cholesterol in men.

Fixed genetic polymorphisms

Variation in the structure of specific genes between individuals (genetic heterogeneity) has been shown to give rise to differences in dietary responsiveness. A few common polymorphisms have been identified in genes associated with lipoprotein metabolism, the best example of which is apoE. ApoE facilitates the uptake of TAG-rich lipoproteins (chylomicron remnants and VLDL) via the remnant and LDL receptors and, thus, in part, determines the removal of TAG from the circulation. The gene for apoE is polymorphic, which means that it exists in multiple forms between individuals. This polymorphism generates several isoforms of the protein that express variable affinities for their receptors and thus variable potential to remove TAG-rich lipoproteins from the circulation. In this way, apoE genotype can modulate the response of an individual to any dietary fat that exerts an influence on TAG-rich lipoproteins, giving rise to the concept of genetic susceptibility to diet (Table 6.7).

Modulation of gene expression

Dietary fatty acids and their intracellular (eicosanoid) derivatives can also influence the expression of genes (rate of gene transcription) by interacting with specific nuclear receptors within the nucleus of cells. These nuclear receptors control the rate of gene transcription by binding to specific regions of DNA known as responsive elements. Genes associated with the production of functional proteins can be either stimulated or repressed according to the nature of the nuclear transcription factor and its binding substrate (PUFA or derivative). Peroxisome proliferator activated receptors (PPAR) represent examples of nuclear receptors that may utilize long-chain PUFA as substrates. PPAR can be found in all tissues of the body, but notably in the liver, where they control the synthesis of lipid and apoproteins (PPAR-α), and in adipose tissue (PPAR-γ) where they control the differentiation of adipocytes and insulin-sensitive mobilization and synthesis of TAG.

6.12 Perspectives on the future

Future research on fatty acids and their role in health and disease will be largely dictated by progress in intervention studies using fatty acid supplements in chronic diseases of inflammation, brain degeneration, cancer and heart disease. Some of these studies will be based on yet to be discovered effects of dietary fats on gene expression; others will be based on information that we already have. No doubt the search for the "ideal" fat intake will continue, but this seems misguided because humans in good health in different cultures and geographical locations ultimately consume a wide range of total fat and fatty acid ratios; their overall health is based on much more than their fat intake. Nevertheless, pursuit of an ideal fat intake or composition will satisfy the thirst of many researchers, consumers and government agencies but, in all likelihood, will not greatly alter the impact of fats on disease processes. These would include:

- the role of the quantity and quality of dietary fat on postprandial lipemia, specific lipoproteins and the risk of CHD
- the metabolic roles of the short-chain fatty acids (1–6 carbons)

- the effect of *trans* fatty acids in baby foods, and the level of intake of *trans* fatty acids that will increase the risk of CHD in adults
- suitable ratios of n-3 to n-6 polyunsaturates to prevent, reverse and/or treat chronic degenerative diseases
- the requirements of docosahexanoate and other long-chain polyunsaturates in infant and enteral feeding
- the conditional indispensability of particular fatty acids throughout the life cycle (especially during pregnancy and lactation, and in the aged)
- the effects of particular dietary fatty acids and combinations of fatty acids on hormone and gene expression.

More knowledge in all of these areas will lead to a better understanding of the mechanisms through which dietary lipids influence serum lipids and lipoproteins and therefore the risk of chronic diseases. It will also lead to improved recommendations regarding the quantity and quality of dietary fats that are commensurate with optimum health and development.

Further reading

Cunnane SC. Alpha-linolenate acid in human nutrition. In: Flaxseed in Human Nutrition (SC Cunnane, LU Thompson, eds), pp. 99–127. Champaign, IL: AOCS Press, 1995.

Dolecek TA. Epidemiological evidence of relationships between dietary polyunsaturated fatty acids and mortality in the Multiple Risk Factor Intervention Trial. Proc Soc Exp Biol Med 1992; 200: 177, 182.

Durrington PN. Hyperlipidaemia Diagnosis and Management, 2nd edn. Oxford: Elsevier Science, 1995.

Lands WEM. Impact of daily food choices on health promotion and disease prevention. In: Fatty Acids and Lipids – New Findings (H Hamazaki, H Okuyama, eds), pp. 1–5. Basel: Karger, 2001.

Mangiapane EH, Salter AM. In: Diet, Lipoproteins and Coronary Heart Disease. A Biochemical Perspective. Nottingham: Nottingham University Press, 1999.

Simopoulos AP. Evolutionary aspects of diet and essential fatty acids. In: Fatty Acids and Lipids – New Findings (T Hamazaki, H Okuyama, eds), pp. 18–27. Basel: Karger, 2001.

Willett WC. Eat, Drink and Be Healthy: The Harvard Medical School Guide to Healthy Eating. New York: Simon and Schuster, 2001.

7
Dietary Reference Standards

Kate M Younger

Key messages

- This chapter discusses the development of terminology and the change in conceptual approaches to setting nutrient recommendations from adequate to optimum nutrition.
- The interpretation and uses of dietary recommendations are discussed.
- It describes how reference values can be used to assess the adequacy of the nutrient intakes of population groups.
- Methods used to determine requirements are discussed. These include: deprivation studies, radioactive tracer studies, balance studies, factorial methods, measurement of nutrient level in biological tissues, biochemical and biological markers, and animal experiments.

7.1 Introduction

The first attempt to set standards for nutrient intakes was by the Food and Nutrition Board of the National Research Council of the USA in 1941, which published recommended daily allowances (RDA) in 1943 to "provide standards to serve as a goal for good nutrition". The first UK RDA followed in 1950, published by the British Medical Association, and many other countries and international agencies now publish dietary standards that are intended to allow the adequacy of the nutrient intakes of groups or populations to be assessed by comparison with the standards.

As the amount known about human requirements and nutrient functions has increased, so too has the size of the documents describing the recommendations, from a mere six pages dealing with 10 nutrients in 1943, to the series of weighty books, each dealing with the dietary reference intakes (DRI) of only a few of more than 30 nutrients, currently being published by the US Food and Nutrition Board. Furthermore, continuing research and the development of more informed interpretations of the expanding body of data available necessitate the regular revision and updating of the recommendations; thus, the "standards" of the past become obsolete as they are replaced by new

figures based on new data or new interpretations of existing data.

7.2 Terminology and conceptual approaches to setting nutrient recommendations

From the time of their first issue in the 1940s and throughout the next 50 years, the concepts and terminology of RDA remained unchanged. The basis on which these RDA were built was the statistical distribution of individual requirements to prevent deficiency criteria for the target nutrient. The peak of the curve of the Gaussian distributions of such requirements is the "average requirement", with half the population having requirements above this value and the other half having lower requirements. The RDA was taken to be a point on that distribution that was equal to the mean or "average requirements" plus 2 standard deviations (SD) (Figure 7.1). By setting the recommendation close to the upper end of the distribution of individual requirements, the needs of most of the population would be met. If the standard were set to meet the apparent needs of almost everyone, the resultant value would be so high as to be unattainable at population level. If the

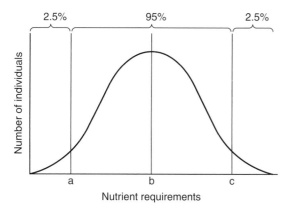

Figure 7.1 Frequency distribution of individual requirements for a nutrient. (a) The mean minus a notional 2 SD: intakes below this will be inadequate for nearly all of the population; (b) the mean: the mid-point of the population's requirement; (c) the mean plus a notional 2 SD: the intake that is adequate for nearly all of the population. Note: In practice, because insufficient data exist to establish reliable means and SDs for many nutrient requirements, the reference intakes describing the points a and c on the curve are generally set, in the case of a: at the level that is judged to prevent the appearance of signs of deficiency (biochemical or clinical), and in the case of c: at the level above which all individuals appear to be adequately supplied. Thus, it is unlikely that even 2.5% of the population would not achieve adequacy at intake level c.

standard were set at the point of the average of all individual requirements, then half the population would have requirements in excess of the standard. In a normal distribution, some 2.5% of points lie at the upper and lower tails outside that range of the mean plus or minus 2 SD. Thus, by setting the RDA to this point of the mean plus 2 SD, we are setting the standard for 97.5% of the population. The consumption of most nutrients at levels somewhat greater than actually required is generally not harmful, hence setting recommendations at the population average requirement plus a notional 2 SD is logical if the aim is to describe an intake that is adequate for almost everyone. However, this is spectacularly inappropriate in the case of recommendations for energy intake, since even relatively small imbalances in energy intake over expenditure will lead, over time, to overweight and ultimately obesity, an increasing problem in most populations. Recommendations for energy intake are therefore given only as the estimated population average requirement.

Thus, for almost half a century, these were the terms used and the underlying conceptual approaches. However, since the 1980s, changes have occurred in both of these areas.

Changes in terminology

Two basic changes occurred with regard to terminology. The first was that the term "recommended dietary allowance" was altered and the second was that new terms were introduced so that the adequacy of diets could be evaluated from several perspectives. The reason for changing the terminology was in effect to re-emphasize some of the basic concepts underlying the term RDA. "Recommended" has a prescriptive air about it and there were concerns that consumers might see this as something that had to be met daily and met precisely. The term "allowance" reinforces the perception of a prescriptive approach. Thus, the UK adopted the term dietary reference value (DRV), the EU introduced the term population reference intake (PRI) and the USA introduced the term dietary reference intakes (DRI). All are precisely equivalent to the original concept of the RDA, a term that many countries prefer to continue to use.

Two new terms were introduced: a minimum requirement and a safe upper level. The minimum requirement represents the average requirement minus 2 SD [see point (a) in Figure 7.1]. A definition describing this point is given in the caption to Figure 7.1 along with the various terms used to define this point (see Box 7.1). The concept of an upper safe limit of intake has gained importance in view of the increased opportunity for people to consume high levels of nutrients from fortified foods or supplements. The recently revised US DRI set "tolerable upper intake" levels (UL) which are judged to be the highest level of nutrient intake that is likely to pose no risk of adverse health effects in almost all individuals in a group. The current European and UK recommendations also address this concern in the case of those nutrients for which toxic levels have been reported. The terms used by different recommending bodies to describe the various points on the distribution of individual requirements for a nutrient are given in Box 7.2, while precise definitions may be found in the relevant publications referred to.

The World Health Organization (WHO) has taken a rather different approach, defining population safe ranges of intake. "Normative requirement" is now used to describe the population mean normative requirement (which would allow the maintenance of or a desirable body store or reserve); "maximum" to refer to the upper limit of safe ranges of population mean intakes; and "basal" for the lower such limit, below which clinically detectable signs of inadequacy would be expected to appear. These WHO requirements are

Box 7.1 Terms used to describe points a, b and c on the frequency distribution

	a	b	c
European Communities Scientific Committee for Food **Population Reference Intakes** (1993)	Lowest threshold intake (**LTI**)	Average requirement (**AR**)	Population reference intake (**PRI**)
US Food and Nutrition Board, National Academy of Sciences, National Research Council **Recommended Daily Allowances** (1989)			Recommended daily allowance (**RDA**)
US Food and Nutrition Board, Institute of Medicine, National Academies and Health, Canada **Dietary Reference Intakes** (1999–)		Estimated average requirement (**EAR**)	Recommended daily allowance (**RDA**)
British Committee on Medical Aspects of Food Policy (COMA) **Dietary Reference Values** (1991)	Lower reference nutrient intake (**LRNI**)	Estimated average requirement (**EAR**)	Reference nutrient intake (**RNI**)

Box 7.2 Additional terms used

European PRI (1993)	Acceptable range of intakes
US RDA (1989)	Safe intake and adequate intake
US DRI (1999–)	Adequate intake (**AI**) and tolerable upper intake level (**UL**)
British DRV (1991)	Safe and adequate intake
WHO (1974–1996)	Recommended intake
WHO (1996)	Basal, normative and maximum population requirement ranges

revised in groups of nutrients at different times (see Further reading), and in those that date from 1974 to 1996 the term "recommended intake" is used to describe the average requirement plus an amount that takes into account interindividual variability and hence is considered to be sufficient for the maintenance of health in nearly all people.

Changes in conceptual approach

When a committee sits to make a recommendation for a standard in relation to nutrient intakes, it begins with a distribution of requirements. In the past, although the choice of criteria for requirement might vary between committees, the orientation was always the same: requirements were set at a level that should prevent deficiency symptoms. More recently, the concern for health promotion through diet has led to the introduction of the concept of optimal nutrition, where the optimal intake of a nutrient could be defined as that intake that maximizes physiological and mental function and minimizes the development of degenerative diseases. It should be borne in mind that

while this may appear simple enough to define in the case of single nutrients, things clearly become more complex when considering all nutrients together, in all possible physiological situations.

It is now recognized that there are several levels for considering the concept of optimal nutrition:

- the level that prevents deficiency symptoms, traditionally used to establish reference nutrient intakes
- the level that optimizes body stores of a nutrient
- the level that optimizes some biochemical or physiological function
- the level that optimizes a risk factor for some chronic disease
- the level that minimizes the incidence of a disease.

In the USA, the reference value for calcium is based on optimizing bone calcium levels, which is a move away from the traditional approach of focusing on preventing deficiency symptoms. An example of attempts to set the reference standard for optimizing a biochemical function is a level of folic acid that would minimize the plasma levels of homocysteine, a potential risk factor for cardiovascular disease. Another might be the level of zinc to optimize cell-mediated immunity. An example of a possible reference standard to optimize a risk factor for a disease is the level of sodium that would minimize hypertension or the level of n-3 polyunsaturated fatty acids (PUFA) to lower plasma triacylglycerols (TAG). The amount of folic acid to minimize the population burden of neural tube defect would be an example of a reference value to minimize the incidence of a disease. At present, there is much debate as to the best approach to choosing criteria for setting reference standards for minerals and vitamins, and this is an area that is likely to continue to court controversy. An important point to note in this respect is that while minimizing frank deficiency symptoms of micronutrients is an acute issue in many developing countries, any evolution of our concepts of desirable or optimal nutrient requirements must lead to a revision of the estimate of the numbers of those with inadequate nutrition.

7.3 Interpretation and uses of dietary recommendations

When using dietary recommendations, several important points need to be considered.

The nutrient levels recommended are per person per day. However, in practice this will usually be achieved as an average over a period of time (days, weeks or months) owing to daily fluctuations in the diet. As stated above, the setting of a range of dietary recommendations should encourage appropriate interpretation of dietary intake data, rather than the inappropriate assumption that the value identified to meet the needs of practically all healthy people is a minimum requirement for individuals. If an individual's nutrient intake can be averaged over a sufficient period then this improves the validity of the comparison with dietary recommendations. However, in the case of energy intakes, such a comparison is still inappropriate: dietary reference values for energy are only intended for use with groups, and it is more useful to compare an individual's energy intake with some measure or calculation of their expenditure in order to assess adequacy.

In the case of a group, the assumption can be made that the quality of the diet can be averaged across the group at a given time-point, and therefore that apparently healthy individuals within a group may compensate for a relative deficiency on one day by a relative excess on another. It should also be remembered that allowances may need to be made for body size, activity level and perhaps other characteristics of the individual or group under consideration, since the recommended intakes are designed for "reference" populations.

Another assumption made when setting recommendations for a particular nutrient is that the intake of all other nutrients is adequate, which in an apparently healthy population eating a varied diet is probably a reasonable assumption.

Recommendations are not intended to address the needs of people who are not healthy: no allowance is made for altered nutrient requirements due to illness or injury. For example, patients confined to bed may require less energy owing to inactivity, and may require higher micronutrient intakes because of an illness causing malabsorption by the gut. Certain nutrients may also be used as therapeutic agents, for example n-3 fatty acids can have anti-inflammatory effects. These clinical aspects are considered elsewhere in these texts.

One complication arising in the formulation of dietary recommendations is caused by the fact that various groups of people within a population may have different nutrient requirements. Therefore, the population is divided into subgroups: children and adults by age bands, and by gender. For women, allowances are also made for pregnancy and lactation.

Infants are recommended to be fully breast-fed for the first few months of life and this poses a problem for the bodies setting the dietary recommendations, who have to set standards for those infants who are not breast-fed. The dietary recommendations for formula-fed infants are based on the energy and nutrients supplied in breast milk, but because the bioavailability of some nutrients is lower in formulae than in breast milk, the amounts stated appear higher than those that might be expected to be achieved by breast-feeding. This should not therefore be interpreted as an inadequacy on the part of human (breast) milk compared with formula milks, but rather the reverse.

The dietary recommendations for infants postweaning, and for children and adolescents are generally based on less robust scientific evidence than those for adults, for whom much more good information is available. In the absence of reliable data, values for children are usually derived by extrapolation from those of young adults. The calculation of nutrient requirements is generally based on energy expenditure because metabolic requirements for energy probably go hand in hand with those for nutrients in growing children. In the case of infants postweaning on mixed diets, values are obtained by interpolation between values known for infants younger than 6 months and those calculated for toddlers aged 1–3 years. Thus, the dietary recommendations for children and adolescents need to be approached with some caution, being more suitable for planning and labeling purposes than as a description of actual needs.

Finally, assessment of the dietary adequacy of people at the other end of the population age range is made difficult by the lack of data on healthy elderly people. One of the normal characteristics of agng is that various body functions deteriorate to some extent, and disease and illness become more common as people age. Until more data are available, the assumption is made that, except for energy and a few nutrients, the requirements of the elderly (usually defined as those over 65 years old) are no different from those of younger adults.

Bearing the above points in mind, dietary recommendations can be useful at various levels:

- by governments and nongovernment organizations (NGOs) to identify the energy and nutrient requirements of populations and hence allow informed decisions on food policy. This could include the provision of food aid or supplements (or rationing) where the diet is inadequate, fortification of foods, providing appropriate nutrition education, introducing legislation concerning the food supply, influencing the import and export of food, subsidies on certain foods or for producers of food, and so on;
- by the food industry in the development and marketing of products. The industry is aware of consumers' increasing interest in the nutritional quality of the food that they buy, and has responded by providing foods to address particular perceived needs, and more informative food labels;
- by researchers and the health professions to assess the nutritional adequacy of the diets of groups (or, cautiously, of individuals) by comparing dietary intake survey data with the dietary reference values (see below). Once the limitations of the dietary assessment data have been taken into account (see Chapter 10), this information can be used to attempt to improve people's nutrient intakes by bringing them more into line with the dietary recommendations. The formulation of dietary advice or guidelines depends on an appreciation of the existing situation: the solution can only be framed once the problem is characterized;
- by institutions and caterers to assess the requirements of groups and devise nutritionally adequate menus. This is a great deal more easily said than done, mainly because of the financial constraints involved and, often, the food preferences of the population being catered for;
- by the public to help in the interpretation of nutrition information on food labels that may describe nutrient content in both absolute terms (g, mg, etc.)

and as a percentage of the recommended dietary intake (RDA) for that nutrient (usually per 100 g or per "serving"). It is thought that the latter is more meaningful to consumers, even though the concepts involved in setting the dietary recommendations are rather complex (making it difficult to judge which level of recommendation should be used as the standard) and they can be open to misinterpretation (see above). Unless consumers are provided with nutrition information in the most appropriate form on food labels, they cannot make informed choices as to what foods to buy and eat to meet their own perceived needs. At the very least, consumers should be able to compare products to get their money's worth.

7.4 The use of reference values to assess the adequacy of the nutrient intakes of population groups

Ideally, this is accomplished by discovering the distribution of intakes of a nutrient in the population group (e.g. by carrying out a dietary survey), and comparing these intakes with the distribution of requirements for that nutrient within the same population. In practice, reliable data with which to plot the second of these distributions have rarely been collected, and therefore what must be used is an estimation of the average requirement together with an estimation of the variance in that requirement, i.e. the standard deviation (based on whatever scientific evidence is available), which is used to plot the population distribution of requirements as shown in Figure 7.1.

When considering how to assess the adequacy of nutrient intakes of populations it is important to compare the intakes with the most appropriate level of requirement as defined in dietary recommendations.

It is not useful to compare usual intakes with the RDA (PRI, RNI, i.e. the average requirement plus a notional 2 SD) at the population level since this approach leads to overestimates of the prevalence of inadequacy. (It may, however, be justified to compare an individual's intake with the RDA.) Furthermore, this approach might be seen to encourage the consumption of higher intakes, which could be toxic in the case of certain nutrients.

Comparison of the population intake with the average requirement (AR, EAR) is now considered to be the best estimation of dietary adequacy; if the average intake is less than the average requirement, then it is clear that there could be a problem in that population. Accordingly, using the average requirement as a cut-off point, the proportion of individuals in the group whose usual intakes are not meeting their requirements can be calculated, allowing the problem to be quantified. However, this approach cannot be used in the case of energy since energy intakes and requirements are highly correlated (the effects of an imbalance being quickly obvious to the individual).

The lowest defined intake level (LTI, LRNI, i.e. the average requirement minus a notional 2 SD) is not regarded as being useful in the context of assessing the adequacy of population nutrient intakes, since it would identify only those individuals who were almost certainly not meeting their requirement, and by the same token omitting to include many in the population who would be at appreciable risk of nutrient inadequacy (in other words, those whose intake was below the average requirement).

Finally, the tolerable upper levels of intake defined for certain nutrients can also be used as cut-off points to identify those individuals at risk of consuming toxic levels of a nutrient.

7.5 Methods used to determine requirements and set dietary recommendations

In order to derive the most accurate and appropriate dietary recommendations, committees of experts are established, which look at the scientific evidence and use their judgement to decide which nutrients to consider and then, for each nutrient, make decisions in respect of:

- the criterion by which to define adequacy
- the estimation of the average amount required to meet that criterion of adequacy
- the estimated standard deviation of requirement in the population under consideration (i.e. the shape of the frequency distribution over the range of requirements: broad, narrow, skewed, etc.).

The problem of different committees identifying different criteria of adequacy is illustrated by vitamin C (ascorbic acid). Experimental evidence (the Sheffield and Iowa studies) has shown that an intake of approximately 10 mg/day is required to prevent the deficiency disease scurvy in adult men. At intakes below 30 mg/day, serum levels are negligible, rising steeply between intakes of 30 and 70 mg/day, after which they begin to plateau (and urinary excretion of the unmetabolized vitamin increases). The question facing the committees drafting dietary reference values is whether to choose a level of intake that allows some storage of the vitamin in the body pool (e.g. EU AR 30 mg/day for adults), or one that more nearly maximizes plasma and body pool levels (e.g. US EAR 60 and 75 mg/day for women and men, respectively). Similarly, variations in calcium recommendations exist because some committees choose to use zero calcium balance as the criterion of adequacy, while others use maximum skeletal calcium reserves.

In some cases, one recommending body will include a nutrient among its dietary recommendations while others will not, for example vitamin E, the requirement for which depends directly on the dietary intake and tissue levels of PUFA, which are highly skewed. The vitamin E requirement corresponding to the highest levels of PUFA intake would be much higher than that needed by those with much lower (but adequate) intakes. To set the high value as the recommendation might suggest to those with lower polyunsaturate intakes that they should increase their intake of vitamin E (unnecessarily). Thus, in Britain and Europe, only "safe and adequate" intakes have been set, based on actual intakes in healthy populations, which should be at least 3 mg/day for women and 4 mg/day for men. In contrast, the US RDA (DRI) has been raised to 15 mg/day as α-tocopherol, based on induced vitamin E deficiency studies in humans and measures of lipid peroxidation.

There are even some examples of dietary components that have not traditionally been regarded as essential nutrients having recommendations set for them, as in the case of choline. The US DRI defines an adequate intake for choline (of 450 and 550 mg/day for women and men, respectively), on the basis that endogenous synthesis of this compound is not always adequate to meet the demand for it (for the synthesis of acetylcholine, phospholipids and betaine). Dietary intake data for choline and the scientific evidence for inadequacy are limited, thus dose–response studies would need to be done before an average requirement could be derived. It is probable that further dietary components will be included in dietary recommendations as research data accumulate. Potential candidates include the flavonoids and some other antioxidant compounds.

7.6 Methods used to determine requirements

Deprivation studies

This is the most direct method and involves removing the nutrient from the diet, observing the symptoms of deficiency and then adding back the nutrient until the symptoms are cured or prevented. Difficulties with this approach are: first, that the experiment may need to continue for several years owing to the presence of body stores of the nutrient, and often requires a very limited and therefore boring dietary regimen; secondly, unpredicted long-term adverse consequences may result; and thirdly, such experiments are not ethical in vulnerable groups such as children (often the most relevant for study). In some cases, epidemiological data may be available, for example the deficiency disease beriberi occurs in populations whose average thiamin intake falls below 0.2 mg/4.2 MJ (1000 kcal).

Radioactive tracer studies

This approach makes use of a known amount of the radioactively labeled nutrient, which is assumed to disperse evenly in the body pool, allowing the estimation of the total pool size by dilution of the isotope in samples of, for instance plasma or urine (i.e. if the body pool is large, then the dilution will be greater than if the body pool is small). Specific activity, that is radioactivity per unit weight of the nutrient in the samples, can be used to calculate pool size as long as the total dose administered is known. The rate of loss can then be monitored by taking serial samples, allowing calculation of the depletion rate. In the case of vitamin C, the average body pool size of a healthy male was found to be 1500 mg which, on a vitamin C-free diet, depleted at a rate of approximately 3% (of the body pool) per day. This fractional catabolic rate was independent of body pool size, and symptoms of scurvy appeared when the body pool fell below 300 mg. The estimated replacement intake needed to maintain the body pool above 300 mg was therefore 3% of 300 mg, i.e. 9 mg (similar to the 10 mg found to be needed to prevent scurvy in the earlier Sheffield experiment).

Balance studies

These rely on the assumption that in healthy individuals of stable body weight, the body pool of some nutrients (e.g. nitrogen, calcium and sodium) remains constant. Compensation mechanisms equalize the intake and output of the nutrient over a wide range of intakes, thereby maintaining the body pool. Thus, day-to-day variations of intake are compensated for by changes in either the rate of absorption in the gut (generally in the case of those nutrients of which the uptake is regulated) or the rate of excretion in the urine (in the case of very soluble nutrients) or feces, or both. However, there comes a point beyond which balance cannot be maintained, therefore it can be proposed that the minimum intake of a nutrient at which balance can be maintained is the subject's minimum required intake of that nutrient. However, this approach would need to be extended over time to investigate possible adaptive responses to reduced intakes, for example absorption could eventually be increased. In the case of calcium, the European consensus is that average daily losses are assumed to be 160 mg/day in adults, and absorption is assumed to be 30%, thus around 530 mg would need to be consumed to balance the losses. Adding or subtracting 30% to allow for individual variation (the notional 2 SD explained above) gives (rounded) dietary reference values of 400, 550 and 700 mg/day (LTI, AR and PRI, respectively).

Factorial methods

These are predictions, rather than measurements, of the requirements of groups or individuals, taking into account a number of measured variables (factors, hence "factorial") and making assumptions where measurements cannot be made. For example, the increased requirements during growth, pregnancy or lactation are calculated by this method; this approach is necessitated by the lack of experimental data in these physiological situations owing to ethical problems. The idea is that the rate of accumulation of nutrients can be calculated and hence the amount required in the diet to allow that accumulation can be predicted. In the case of pregnancy, the requirement is estimated to be the amount of the nutrient needed to achieve balance when not pregnant plus the amount accumulated daily during the pregnancy, all multiplied by a factor accounting for the efficiency of absorption and assimilation (e.g. 30% for calcium). For lactation, the calculation for energy is based on the amount in the milk secreted daily, which is increased by a factor accounting for the efficiency of conversion from dietary energy to milk energy (reckoned to be 95%), from which total is subtracted an allowance for the contribution from the extra fat stores laid down during pregnancy, which it is desirable to reduce in this way. The difficulty with this approach is that the theoretical predictions do not necessarily take account of physiological adaptations (e.g. increased efficiency of absorption in the gut) that may reduce the predicted requirement. This would apply particularly in the case of pregnancy, as shown by the ability of women to produce normal babies even in times of food shortage.

Measurement of nutrient levels in biological tissues

Some nutrient requirements can be defined according to the intakes needed to maintain a certain level of the nutrient in blood or tissue. For many water-soluble nutrients, such as vitamin C, blood levels reflect recent dietary intake, and the vitamin is not generally measurable in plasma at intakes less than about 40 mg/day. This level of intake has therefore been chosen as the basis for the reference in some countries such as the UK. This approach is not, however, suitable for those nutrients of which the plasma concentration is homeostatically regulated, such as calcium. In the case of the fat-soluble vitamin retinol, the dietary intake required to maintain a liver concentration of 20 μg/g has been used as the basis of the reference intake. To do this, the body pool size needed to be estimated; assumptions were made as to the proportion of body weight represented by the liver (3%) and the proportion of the body pool of retinol contained in the liver (90%). The fractional catabolic rate has been measured as 0.5% of the body pool per day, so this would be the amount needing to be replaced daily. The efficiency of conversion of dietary vitamin A to stored retinol was taken to be 50% (measured range 40–90%), giving an EAR of around 500 μg/day for a 74 kg man.

Biochemical markers

In many respects, biochemical markers represent the most satisfactory measure of nutrient adequacy since they are specific to the nutrient in question, are sensitive enough to identify subclinical deficiencies, and may be measured precisely and accurately. However, such markers are only available for a few nutrients, mostly vitamins, at present. One well-established example of a biochemical marker is the erythrocyte glutathione reductase activation test for riboflavin status. Erythrocytes are a useful cell to use for enzyme assays since they are easily obtainable and have a known lifespan in the circulation (average 120 days), aiding the interpretation of results. Glutathione reductase depends on riboflavin and when activity is measured in both the presence and absence of excess riboflavin, the ratio of the two activities (the erythrocyte glutathione reductase activation coefficient, EGRAC) reflects riboflavin status: if perfectly sufficient, the ratio would be 1.0, whereas deficiency gives values greater than 1.0.

Biological markers

These are measures of some biological function that is directly dependent on the nutrient of interest; again, not always easy to find, hence the recent suggestion that some functional indices be considered that are not necessarily directly dependent on the nutrient. Iron status is assessed according to a battery of biological markers, including plasma ferritin (which reflects body iron stores), serum transferrin saturation (the amount of plasma transferrin in relation to the amount of iron transported by it is reduced in deficiency), plasma soluble transferrin receptor (an index of tissue iron status) and the more traditional tests such as blood hemoglobin (now considered to be a rather insensitive and unreliable measure of iron status since it only indicates frank anemia, and also changes as a normal response to altered physiological states such as pregnancy).

Vitamin K status is assessed by measuring prothrombin time (the length of time taken by plasma to clot), which is increased when vitamin K levels fall since the synthesis of prothrombin in the liver depends on vitamin K as a cofactor. This test is clinically useful in patients requiring anticoagulant therapy (e.g. using warfarin, which blocks the effect of vitamin K), in whom the drug dosage must be closely monitored.

Animal experiments

These are of limited use in defining human nutrient requirements because of species differences (e.g. rats can synthesize vitamin C, so it is not a "vitamin" for them), differences in metabolic body size (i.e. the proportions of metabolically active tissue, e.g. muscle, and less active tissue, e.g. adipose tissue, gut contents) and differences in growth rates (young animals generally grow far more rapidly than humans, e.g. cattle reach adult size in about 1 year). However, animals have provided much of the information on the identification of the essential nutrients, and their physiological and biochemical functions. Furthermore, animals can be used in experiments that would not be possible in humans, for example lifelong modifications in nutrient intake; it is merely the setting of human requirements for which they are inappropriate.

7.7 Perspectives on the future

As the amount known about human requirements and nutrient functions increases, so too will the complexity of dietary recommendations. It is probable that further dietary components will be included in dietary recommendations as research data accumulate. Potential candidates include the flavonoids and some other antioxidant compounds. Furthermore, continuing research and the development of more informed interpretations of the expanding body of data available necessitate the regular revision and updating of the recommendations.

The general conclusion that can be drawn here is that no single criterion of nutrient status can be used to define human requirements for all nutrients. This is not surprising when one considers the range of roles that the different essential nutrients play in humans.

Further reading

Department of Health. Report on Health and Social Subjects 41. Dietary reference values for food energy and nutrients for the United Kingdom. Committee on Medical Aspects of Food Policy. London: HMSO, 1991.

Department of Health. Report on Health and Social Subjects 49. Nutrition and bone health: with particular reference to calcium and vitamin D. Committee on Medical Aspects of Food and Nutrition Policy. London: The Stationery Office, 1998.

EC Scientific Committee for Food Report. 31st Series. Nutrient and energy intakes for the European Community. Luxembourg: Director General, Industry, 1993.

FAO/WHO. Requirements for vitamin A, iron, folate and vitamin B_{12}. Report of a Joint FAO/WHO Expert Consultation. Food and Nutrition Series. Rome: Food and Agriculture Organization, 1988.

FAO/UNU/WHO. Energy and protein requirements. Report of a Joint FAO/WHO/UNU Expert Consultation. Technical Report Series 724. Geneva: World Health Organization, 1985.

Institute of Medicine (USA). Dietary reference intakes. Calcium, phosphorus, magnesium, vitamin D and fluoride. Washington DC: National Academy Press, 1997.

Institute of Medicine (USA). Dietary reference intakes. Thiamin, riboflavin, niacin, vitamin B6, folate, vitamin B12, pantothenic acid, biotin and choline. Washington DC: National Academy Press, 1998.

Institute of Medicine (USA). Dietary reference intakes. Vitamin C, vitamin E, selenium and carotenoids. Washington DC: National Academy Press, 2000.

http://www.nap.edu/catalog/9810.html

National Research Council, Food and Nutrition Board, Commission on Life Sciences. Recommended dietary allowances, 10th edition. Washington DC: National Academy Press, 1989

WHO. Handbook on human nutritional requirements. Monograph series no 61. Geneva: World Health Organization, 1974.

WHO. Diet, nutrition and the prevention of chronic diseases. Technical Report Series 797. Geneva: World Health Organization, 1990.

WHO. Trace elements in human nutrition and health. Geneva: World Health Organization, in collaboration with FAO, AEA, 1996.

8
The Vitamins

David A Bender

Key messages

- The vitamins are a chemically disparate group of compounds with a variety of functions in the body.
- What they have in common is that they are organic compounds that are required for the maintenance of normal health and metabolic integrity.
- Vitamins are required in very small amounts, of the order of milligrams or micrograms per day, and thus can be distinguished from the essential fatty acids and the essential amino acids, which are required in larger amounts of grams per day.

- Where relevant, this chapter will deal with each of the vitamins under the following headings:

  – Vitamers
  – Absorption and metabolism
  – Metabolic functions and other uses
  – Deficiency
  – Requirements
  – Assessment of status
  – Toxicity and drug interactions.

8.1 Introduction

In order to demonstrate that a compound is a vitamin, it is necessary to demonstrate both that deprivation of experimental subjects will lead to the development of a more or less specific clinical deficiency disease and abnormal metabolic signs, and that restoration of the missing compound will prevent or cure the deficiency disease and normalize metabolic abnormalities. It is not adequate simply to demonstrate that a compound has a function in the body, since it may normally be synthesized in adequate amounts to meet requirements, or that a compound cures a disease, since this may simply reflect a pharmacological action and not indicate that the compound is a dietary essential.

The vitamins, and their principal functions and deficiency signs, are shown in Table 8.1; the curious nomenclature is a consequence of the way in which they were discovered at the beginning of the twentieth century, initially as unidentified factors that were found to be dietary essentials. The first studies showed that there was something in milk that was essential, in very small amounts, for the growth of animals fed on a diet consisting of purified fat, carbohydrate, protein and mineral salts. Two factors were found to be essential: one was found in the cream and the other in the watery part of milk. Logically, they were called factor A (fat-soluble, in the cream) and factor B (water-soluble, in the watery part of the milk). Factor B was identified chemically as an amine, and in 1913 the name "vitamin" was coined for these "vital amines".

Further studies showed that "vitamin B" was a mixture of a number of compounds, with different actions in the body, and so they were given numbers as well: vitamin B_1, vitamin B_2, and so on. There are gaps in the numerical order of the B vitamins. When what might have been called vitamin B_3 was discovered, it was found to be a chemical compound that was already known, nicotinic acid. It was therefore not given a number. Other gaps are because compounds that were assumed to be vitamins and were given numbers, such as B_4 and B_5, were later shown either not to be vitamins, or to be vitamins that had already been described by other workers and given other names.

Vitamins C, D and E were named in the order of their discovery. The name "vitamin F" was used at one

Table 8.1 The vitamins, their principal functions and deficiency diseases

Vitamin		Functions	Deficiency disease
A	Retinol β-Carotene	Visual pigments in the retina; cell differentiation; β-carotene is an antioxidant	Night blindness, xerophthalmia; keratinization of skin
D	Calciferol	Maintenance of calcium balance; enhances intestinal absorption of Ca^{2+} and mobilizes bone mineral	Rickets (poor mineralization of bone); osteomalacia (demineralization of bone)
E	Tocopherols Tocotrienols	Antioxidant, especially in cell membranes	Extremely rare: serious neurological dysfunction
K	Phylloquinone Menaquinones	Coenzyme in formation of γ-carboxy-glutamate in enzymes of blood clotting and bone matrix	Impaired blood clotting, hemorrhagic disease
B_1	Thiamin	Coenzyme in pyruvate and 2-keto-glutarate dehydrogenases, and transketolase; poorly defined function in nerve conduction	Peripheral nerve damage (beriberi) or central nervous system lesions (Wernicke–Korsakoff syndrome)
B_2	Riboflavin	Coenzyme in oxidation and reduction reactions; prosthetic group of flavoproteins	Lesions of corner of mouth, lips and tongue, sebhorreic dermatitis
Niacin	Nicotinic acid Nicotinamide	Coenzyme in oxidation and reduction reactions, functional part of NAD and NADP	Pellagra: photosensitive dermatitis, depressive psychosis
B_6	Pyridoxine Pyridoxal Pyridoxamine	Coenzyme in transamination and decarboxylation of amino acids and glycogen phosphorylase; role in steroid hormone action	Disorders of amino acid metabolism, convulsions
Folic acid		Coenzyme in transfer of one-carbon fragments	Megaloblastic anemia
B_{12}	Cobalamin	Coenzyme in transfer of one-carbon fragments and metabolism of folic acid	Pernicious anemia (megaloblastic anemia with degeneration of the spinal cord)
	Pantothenic acid	Functional part of coenzyme A and acyl carrier protein	Peripheral nerve damage (burning foot syndrome)
H	Biotin	Coenzyme in carboxylation reactions in gluconeogenesis and fatty acid synthesis	Impaired fat and carbohydrate metabolism, dermatitis
C	Ascorbic acid	Coenzyme in hydroxylation of proline and lysine in collagen synthesis; antioxidant; enhances absorption of iron	Scurvy: impaired wound healing, loss of dental cement, subcutaneous hemorrhage

time for what we now call the essential fatty acids; "vitamin G" was later found to be what was already known as vitamin B_2. Biotin is still sometimes called vitamin H. Vitamin K was discovered by Henrik Dam, in Denmark, as a result of studies of disorders of blood coagulation, and he named it for its function: *koagulation* in Danish, hence vitamin K.

As the chemistry of the vitamins was elucidated, so they were given names as well, as shown in Table 8.1. Where only one chemical compound has the biological activity of the vitamin, this is quite easy. Thus, vitamin B_1 is thiamin, vitamin B_2 is riboflavin, etc. With several of the vitamins, a number of chemically related compounds found in foods can be interconverted in the body, and all show the same biological activity. Such chemically related compounds are called vitamers, and a general name (a generic descriptor) is used

to include all compounds that display the same biological activity.

Some compounds have important metabolic functions, but are not considered to be vitamins, since they can be synthesized in the body, as far as is known in adequate amounts to meet requirements. These include carnitine, choline, inositol, taurine and ubiquinone.

Two compounds that are generally considered to be vitamins can be synthesized in the body, normally in adequate amounts to meet requirements: vitamin D, which is synthesized from 7-dehydrocholesterol in the skin in sunlight, and niacin, which is synthesized from the essential amino acid tryptophan. However, both were discovered as a result of studies of deficiency diseases that were, during the early twentieth century, significant public health problems: rickets (due to vitamin D deficiency and inadequate sunlight exposure) and pellagra (due to deficiency of both tryptophan and preformed niacin).

8.2 Vitamin A

Vitamin A was the first vitamin to be discovered, initially as an essential dietary factor for growth. It has a role in vision, as the prosthetic group of the light-sensitive proteins in the retina, and a major role in the regulation of gene expression and tissue differentiation. Deficiency

is a major problem of public health in large areas of the world.

Vitamers and international units

Two groups of compounds, shown in Figure 8.1, have vitamin A activity: retinol, retinaldehyde and retinoic acid (preformed vitamin A); and a variety of carotenes and related compounds (collectively known as carotenoids) that can be cleaved oxidatively to yield retinaldehyde, and hence retinol and retinoic acid. Those carotenoids that can be cleaved to yield retinaldehyde are known as pro-vitamin A carotenoids.

Figure 8.1 The major vitamin A vitamers and vitamin A active carotenoids.

Preformed vitamin A (mainly as retinyl esters) is found only in foods of animal origin. The richest source by far is liver, which may indeed contain sufficient vitamin A to pose a potential problem for pregnant women, since retinol is teratogenic in excess. Carotenes are found in green, yellow and red fruits and vegetables, as well as in liver, margarine and milk and milk products. In addition to their role as precursors of vitamin A, carotenoids have potentially useful antioxidant action, and there is epidemiological evidence that diets that are rich in carotenoids (both those that are vitamin A active and those that are not) are associated with a lower incidence of cancer and cardiovascular disease. However, intervention studies with β-carotene have been disappointing, and it is not possible to determine levels of carotene that are desirable in the diet, other than as a precursor of vitamin A.

Retinoic acid is a metabolite of retinol; it has important biological activities in its own right and will support growth in vitamin A-deficient animals. The oxidation of retinaldehyde to retinoic acid is irreversible, and retinoic acid cannot be converted *in vivo* to retinol, and does not support either vision or fertility in deficient animals.

Some 50 or more dietary carotenoids are potential sources of vitamin A; α-, β- and γ-carotenes and cryptoxanthin are quantitatively the most important. Although it would appear from its structure that one molecule of β-carotene will yield two of retinol, this is not so in practice, as discussed below, and a considerable amount is absorbed as carotene. Nutritionally, 6 μg of β-carotene is equivalent to 1 μg of preformed retinol. For other carotenes with vitamin A activity, 12 μg is equivalent to 1 μg of preformed retinol.

The total amount of vitamin A in foods is expressed as μg retinol equivalents, calculated from the sum of: μg preformed vitamin A + 1/6 × μg β-carotene + 1/12 × μg other provitamin A carotenoids.

Before pure vitamin A was available for chemical analysis, the vitamin A content of foods was determined by biological assays and the results were expressed in standardized international units (IU): $1\,IU = 0.3\,\mu g$ retinol, or 1 μg of retinol = 3.33 IU. Although obsolete, IU are sometimes still used in food labeling.

Metabolism and storage of vitamin A and pro-vitamin A carotenoids

Retinol is absorbed from the small intestine dissolved in lipid. About 70–90% of dietary retinol is normally absorbed, and even at high levels of intake this falls only slightly. However, in people with a very low fat intake (less than about 10% of energy from fat), absorption of both retinol and carotene is impaired, and low-fat diets are associated with vitamin A deficiency.

Dietary retinyl esters are hydrolyzed by lipases in the intestinal lumen and mucosal brush border membrane, then re-esterified to form retinyl palmitate before release into the circulation in chylomicrons.

Tissues can take up retinyl esters from chylomicrons, but most is in the chylomicron remnants that are taken up by the liver. Here retinyl esters are hydrolyzed, and the vitamin may either be secreted from the liver bound to retinol binding protein, or be transferred to stellate cells in the liver, where it is stored as retinyl esters in intracellular lipid droplets. Some 50–80% of the total body content of retinol is in the stellate cells of the liver, but a significant amount may also be stored in adipose tissue.

The main pathway for catabolism of retinol is oxidation to retinoic acid (which, as discussed below, has important biological activities in its own right, distinct from the activities of retinol). The main excretory product of both retinol and retinoic acid is retinoyl glucuronide, which is secreted in the bile.

As the intake of retinol increases, and the liver concentration rises above 70 μmol/kg, a different pathway becomes increasingly important for the catabolism of retinol in the liver. This is a microsomal cytochrome P_{450}-dependent oxidation, leading to a number of polar metabolites that are excreted in the urine and bile. At high intakes this pathway becomes saturated, and excess retinol is toxic since there is no further capacity for its catabolism and excretion.

Carotene dioxygenase

Like retinol, carotenoids are absorbed dissolved in lipid micelles; the biological availability and absorption of dietary carotene varies between 5 and 60%, depending on the nature of the food, whether it is cooked or raw, and the amount of fat in the meal.

As shown in Figure 8.2, β-carotene and other provitamin A carotenoids are cleaved in the intestinal mucosa by carotene dioxygenase, yielding retinaldehyde, which is reduced to retinol, then esterified and secreted in chylomicrons together with retinyl esters formed from dietary retinol.

Only a proportion of carotene undergoes oxidation in the intestinal mucosa, and a significant amount

Figure 8.2 The reaction of carotene dioxygenase. Carotene dioxygenase (EC 1.13.11.21), retinol dehydrogenase (EC 1.1.1.105), retinaldehyde oxidase (EC 1.2.3.11).

of carotene enters the circulation in chylomicrons. Carotene in the chylomicron remnants is cleared by the liver; it is assumed that some is cleaved by hepatic carotene dioxygenase, again giving rise to retinaldehyde and retinyl esters; the remainder is secreted in very low-density lipoproteins (VLDL), and may be taken up and cleaved by carotene dioxygenase in a variety of tissues.

Central oxidative cleavage of β-carotene, as shown in Figure 8.2, should rise to two molecules of retinaldehyde, which can be reduced to retinol. However, as noted above, the biological activity of β-carotene, on a molar basis, is considerably lower than that of retinol, not two-fold higher as might be expected. In addition to the relatively poor absorption of carotene from the diet, three factors may account for this.

- The intestinal activity of carotene dioxygenase is relatively low, so that a relatively large proportion of ingested β-carotene may appear in the circulation unchanged. This has confounded attempts to prevent vitamin A deficiency by increasing intakes of dark green leafy vegetables in developing countries.
- Other carotenoids in the diet may inhibit carotene dioxygenase and reduce the formation of retinol.
- While the principal site of carotene dioxygenase attack is the central bond of β-carotene, there is evidence that asymmetric cleavage also occurs, leading to the formation of 8′-, 10′- and 12′-apo-carotenals, which are oxidized to yield retinoic acid, but cannot be used as sources of retinol or retinaldehyde.

Plasma retinol binding protein

Retinol is released from the liver bound to an α-globulin, retinol binding protein (RBP); this serves to maintain the vitamin in aqueous solution, protects it against oxidation and delivers the vitamin to target tissues. RBP is secreted from the liver as a 1 : 1 complex with the thyroxine-binding prealbumin, transthyretin. This is important to prevent urinary loss of retinol bound to the relatively small RBP, which would otherwise be filtered by the kidney, with a considerable loss of vitamin A from the body.

Cell-surface receptors on target tissues take up retinol from the RBP–transthyretin complex, transferring it onto an intracellular RBP. The receptors also remove the carboxy-terminal arginine residue from RBP, so inactivating it by reducing its affinity for both transthyretin and retinol. As a result, apo-RBP is filtered at the glomerulus; most is reabsorbed in the proximal renal tubules and hydrolyzed. The apoprotein is not recycled.

During the development of vitamin A deficiency in experimental animals, the plasma concentration of RBP falls, while the liver content of apo-RBP rises. The administration of retinol results in release of holo-RBP from the liver. This provides the basis of the relative dose–response (RDR) test for liver stores of vitamin A (see below).

Metabolic functions of vitamin A and carotenes

The best known function of vitamin A, and historically the first to be defined, is in vision. More recently, retinoic acid has also been shown to have a major function in regulation of gene expression and tissue differentiation.

Vitamin A in vision

In the retina, retinaldehyde functions as the prosthetic group of the light-sensitive opsin proteins, forming rhodopsin (in rods) and iodopsin (in cones). Any one cone cell contains only one type of opsin, and hence is sensitive to only one color of light. Color blindness results from loss or mutation of one or other of the cone opsins.

In the pigment epithelium of the retina, all-*trans*-retinol is isomerized to 11-*cis*-retinol and then oxidized to 11-*cis*-retinaldehyde. This reacts with a lysine residue in opsin, forming the holoprotein rhodopsin. As shown in Figure 8.3, the absorption of light by rhodopsin causes isomerization of the retinaldehyde bound to opsin from 11-*cis* to all-*trans*, and a conformational change in opsin. This results in the release of retinaldehyde from the protein and the initiation of a nerve impulse. The overall process is known as bleaching, since it results in the loss of the color of rhodopsin.

The all-*trans*-retinaldehyde released from rhodopsin is reduced to all-*trans*-retinol, and joins the pool of retinol in the pigment epithelium for isomerization to 11-*cis*-retinol and regeneration of rhodopsin. The key to initiation of the visual cycle is the availability of 11-*cis*-retinaldehyde, and hence vitamin A. In deficiency both the time taken to adapt to darkness and the ability to see in poor light will be impaired.

The excited form of rhodopsin (metarhodopsin II) initiates a G-protein cascade leading to hyperpolarization of the outer section membrane of the rod or cone, caused by the closure of sodium channels through the membrane, and the initiation of a nerve impulse.

Retinoic acid and the regulation of gene expression

The main function of vitamin A in the body is in the control of cell differentiation and turnover. All-*trans*-retinoic acid and 9-*cis*-retinoic acid are active in the regulation of growth, development and tissue differentiation; they have different actions in different tissues. Like the steroid hormones and vitamin D, retinoic acid binds to nuclear receptors that bind to response elements (control regions) of DNA, and regulate the transcription of specific genes.

There are two families of nuclear retinoid receptors: the retinoic acid receptors (RAR) bind all-*trans*-retinoic acid or 9-*cis*-retinoic acid, and the retinoid X receptors (RXR) bind 9-*cis*-retinoic acid, and some of the other physiologically active retinoids as well. RXR can form active dimers with: RAR, RXR (homodimers) and the receptors for calcitriol (vitamin D), thyroid hormone, long-chain polyunsaturated fatty acid (PUFA) derivatives [the peroxisome proliferation activation (PPAR) receptor] and one for which the physiological ligand has not yet been identified (the COUP receptor).

The result of this is that a very large number of genes are sensitive to control by retinoic acid in different tissues, and at different stages in development, and retinoic acid is essential for the normal responses to vitamin D, thyroid hormone and long-chain PUFA derivatives.

The antioxidant function of carotenes

At least *in vitro*, and under conditions of low oxygen availability, carotenes can act as radical-trapping antioxidants. There is epidemiological evidence that high intakes of carotene are associated with a low incidence of cardiovascular disease and some forms of cancer, although the results of intervention trials with

Figure 8.3 Role of vitamin A and the cyclic AMP cascade in the visual cycle. Retinol isomerase (EC 5.2.1.3), phosphodiesterase (EC 3.1.4.35).

β-carotene have been disappointing, with an increased incidence of lung cancer among those taking carotene supplements.

Vitamin A deficiency: night blindness and xerophthalmia

Worldwide, vitamin A deficiency is a major public health problem and the most important preventable cause of blindness; the World Health Organization (WHO) estimates that some 256 million children under 5 years old show subclinical deficiency and 2.7 million have xerophthalmia.

The earliest signs of deficiency are associated with vision. Initially, there is a loss of sensitivity to green light; this is followed by impairment of the ability to adapt to dim light, then an inability to see at all in dim light: night blindness. More prolonged or severe deficiency leads to the condition called xerophthalmia: keratinization of the cornea, followed by ulceration – irreversible damage to the eye that causes blindness. At the same time there are changes in the skin, with excessive formation of keratinized tissue.

Vitamin A also plays an important role in the differentiation of immune system cells, and mild deficiency, not severe enough to cause any disturbance of vision, leads to increased susceptibility to a variety of infectious diseases. At the same time, the synthesis of RBP is reduced in response to infection (it is a negative acute-phase protein), so that there is a reduction in the circulating concentration of the vitamin, and hence further impairment of immune responses.

Signs of vitamin A deficiency also occur in protein–energy malnutrition, regardless of whether or not the intake of vitamin A is adequate. This is due to impairment of the synthesis of plasma RBP; functional vitamin A deficiency can occur secondary to protein–energy malnutrition.

Vitamin A requirements and reference intakes

There have been relatively few studies of vitamin A requirements in which subjects have been depleted of the vitamin for long enough to permit the development of clear deficiency signs. Current estimates of requirements are based on the intakes required to maintain a concentration in the liver of $70\,\mu$mol retinol/kg, as determined by measurement of the rate of metabolism of isotopically labeled vitamin A. This is adequate to maintain normal plasma concentrations of the vitamin, and people with this level of liver reserves can be maintained on a vitamin A-free diet for many months before they develop any detectable signs of deficiency.

The average requirement to maintain a concentration of $70\,\mu$mol/kg of liver is $6.7\,\mu$g retinol equivalents/kg body weight, and this is the basis for calculation of reference intakes.

Assessment of vitamin A status

The only direct assessment of vitamin A status is by liver biopsy and measurement of retinyl ester reserves. This is an invasive procedure that cannot be considered for routine investigations and population surveys. Status can also be assessed by clinical and functional tests, the plasma concentrations of retinol and RBP, and the response to a test dose of vitamin A, the RDR.

In field surveys, clinical signs of vitamin A deficiency, including Bitot's spots, corneal xerosis, corneal ulceration and keratomalacia, can be used to identify those suffering from vitamin A deficiency. The earliest signs of corneal damage are detected by conjunctival impression cytology (CIC); however, abnormalities only develop when liver reserves are seriously depleted.

The ability to adapt to dim light is impaired early in deficiency, and dark adaptation time is sometimes used to assess vitamin A status. However, the test is not suitable for use on children (the group most at risk of deficiency) and the apparatus is not suited to use in the field.

The fasting plasma concentration of retinol remains constant over a wide range of intakes and only falls significantly when liver reserves are nearly depleted. Therefore, while less sensitive to subtle changes within the normal range than some methods of assessing nutritional status, measurement of plasma retinol does provide a convenient and sensitive means of detecting people whose intake of vitamin A is inadequate to permit normal liver reserves to be maintained.

The RDR test is a test of the ability of a dose of retinol to raise the plasma concentration several hours later, after chylomicrons have been cleared from the circulation. It depends on the fact that apo-RBP accumulates in the liver in vitamin A deficiency. The RDR is the ratio of the rise in plasma retinol 5 h after the dose to the plasma concentration of retinol at the time. An RDR greater than 20% indicates depletion of liver retinol to less than $70\,\mu$mol/kg.

Toxicity of vitamin A

There is only a limited capacity to metabolize vitamin A. Excessively high intakes lead to accumulation in the liver and other tissues, beyond the capacity of normal binding proteins, so that free, unbound, vitamin A is present. This leads to liver and bone damage, hair loss, vomiting and headaches. Single doses of 60 mg of retinol are given to children in developing countries as a prophylactic against vitamin A deficiency: an amount adequate to meet the child's needs for 4–6 months. About 1% of children so treated show transient signs of toxicity, but this is considered an acceptable risk in view of the high prevalence and devastating effects of deficiency.

The chronic toxicity of vitamin A is a more general cause for concern; prolonged and regular intake of more than about 7.5–9 mg/day by adults (and significantly less for children) causes signs and symptoms of toxicity affecting:

- the central nervous system: headache, nausea, ataxia and anorexia, all associated with increased cerebrospinal fluid pressure
- the liver: hepatomegaly with histological changes in the liver, increased collagen formation and hyperlipidemia
- bones: joint pains, thickening of the long bones, hypercalcemia and calcification of soft tissues
- the skin: excessive dryness, scaling and chapping of the skin, desquamation and alopecia.

The recommended upper limits of habitual intake of retinol, compared with reference intakes, are shown in Table 8.2.

Teratogenicity of retinoids

The synthetic retinoids used in dermatology are highly teratogenic. After women have been treated with them, it is recommended that contraceptive precautions be continued for 12 months, because of the retention of retinoids in the body. By extrapolation, it has been assumed that retinol is also teratogenic, although there is little evidence. In case control studies, intakes between 2400–3300 µg/day during pregnancy have been associated with birth defects. Other studies have not demonstrated any teratogenic effect at this level of intake, and it has been suggested that the threshold plasma concentration associated with teratogenic effects is unlikely to be reached with intakes below 7500 µg/day. Nevertheless, pregnant women are advised not to consume more than 3000 µg/day (American Pediatric Association recommendation) or 3300 µg (UK Department of Health recommendation).

Table 8.2 Prudent upper levels of habitual vitamin A intake

Age group	Upper limit of intake (µg/day)	Reference intakes[a] (µg/day)
Infants	900	350–375
1–3 years	1800	400
4–6 years	3000	400–500
6–12 years	4500	500–700
13–20 years	6000	600–700
Adult men	9000	600–1000
Adult women	7500	600–800
Pregnant women	3300	700

[a] Reference intakes show range for the USA (RDA, 1989), UK (RNI, 1991) and EU (PRI, 1993).

Interactions of vitamin A with drugs and other nutrients

Historically, there was considerable confusion between vitamins A and D, and for many years it was not clear which acted in which system. By the 1950s it was believed that the problem had been solved, with clearly defined functions of vitamin A in vision, and vitamin D in calcium homeostasis and bone development. However, both have overlapping effects on a number of systems, including bone metabolism and immune system function. It is now known that this is the result of formation of retinoid–vitamin D receptor heterodimers, so that in some systems both are required for normal regulation of gene expression.

Chlorinated hydrocarbons, as contained in many agricultural pesticides, deplete liver retinol. Metabolites of polychlorinated biphenyls bind to the thyroxine binding site of transthyretin, and in doing so impair the binding of RBP. As a result there is free RBP-bound retinol in plasma, which is filtered at the glomerulus and hence lost in the urine.

In a number of studies of post-mortem tissue, between 5 and 10% of people in north America showed undetectably low liver reserves of retinol, although similar studies in Britain did not show any significant proportion of the population with very low liver reserves of vitamin A. These abnormally low liver reserves of retinol may be due not only to prolonged low intake, but also to the induction by barbiturates of cytochrome P_{450}, which catalyzes the catabolism of retinol.

8.3 Vitamin D

Vitamin D is not strictly a vitamin, since it can be synthesized in the skin, and indeed under most conditions endogenous synthesis is the major source of the vitamin: it is only when sunlight exposure is inadequate that a dietary source is required. Its main function is in the regulation of calcium absorption and homeostasis; most of its actions are mediated by way of nuclear receptors which regulate gene expression. Deficiency, leading to rickets in children and osteomalacia in adults, continues to be a problem in northern latitudes, where sunlight exposure is poor.

There are relatively few sources of vitamin D, mainly oily fish, with eggs, liver and butter providing modest amounts; fortified milk, containing ergocalciferol, is available in some countries. As a result, strict vegetarians are at risk of deficiency, especially in northern latitudes with little sunlight exposure.

Although meat provides apparently negligible quantities of vitamin D, it may be an important source, since what is present is largely the final active metabolite, calcitriol, which is many times more potent on a molar basis than is cholecalciferol.

Vitamers and international units

The normal dietary form of vitamin D is cholecalciferol (also known as calciol). This is also the compound that is formed in the skin by ultraviolet (UV) irradiation of 7-dehydrocholesterol. Some foods are enriched or fortified with (synthetic) ergocalciferol, which undergoes the same metabolism as cholecalciferol and has the same biological activity. Early studies assigned the name vitamin D_1 to an impure mixture of products derived from the irradiation of ergosterol; when ergocalciferol was identified it was called vitamin D_2, and when the physiological compound was identified as cholecalciferol it was called vitamin D_3.

Like vitamin A, vitamin D was originally measured in international units of biological activity before the pure compound was isolated: 1 IU = 25 ng of cholecalciferol; 1 μg of cholecalciferol = 40 IU.

Absorption and metabolism

Vitamin D is absorbed in lipid micelles and incorporated into chylomicrons; therefore, people on a low-fat diet will absorb little of such dietary vitamin D as is available. Indeed, it is noteworthy that at the time that rickets was a major public health problem in

Scotland, herrings (a rich source) were a significant part of the diet: it can only be assumed that the diet was also sufficiently low in fat to impair absorption of the vitamin.

Synthesis of vitamin D in the skin

As shown in Figure 8.4, the steroid 7-dehydrocholesterol (an intermediate in the synthesis of cholesterol that accumulates in the skin but not other tissues) undergoes a nonenzymic reaction on exposure to UV light, yielding previtamin D, which undergoes a further reaction over a period of hours to form cholecalciferol, which is absorbed into the bloodstream.

In temperate climates there is a marked seasonal variation in the plasma concentration of vitamin D; it is highest at the end of summer and lowest at the end of winter. Although there may be bright sunlight in winter, beyond about 40° N or S there is very little UV radiation of the appropriate wavelength for cholecalciferol synthesis when the sun is low in the sky. By contrast, in summer, when the sun is more or less overhead, there is a considerable amount of UV light even on a moderately cloudy day, and enough can penetrate thin clothes to result in significant formation of vitamin D.

In northerly climates, and especially in polluted industrial cities with little sunlight, people may well not be exposed to enough UV light to meet their vitamin D needs, and they will be reliant on the few dietary sources of the vitamin.

Metabolism to calcitriol

Cholecalciferol, either synthesized in the skin or taken in from foods, undergoes two hydroxylations to yield the active metabolite, 1,25-dihydroxyvitamin D or calcitriol, as shown in Figure 8.4. Ergocalciferol from fortified foods undergoes similar hydroxylation to yield ercalcitriol. The nomenclature of the vitamin D metabolites is shown in Table 8.3.

The first stage in vitamin D metabolism occurs in the liver, where it is hydroxylated to form the 25-hydroxy-derivative calcidiol. This is released into the circulation bound to a vitamin D binding globulin. There is no tissue storage of vitamin D; plasma calcidiol is the main storage form of the vitamin, and it is plasma calcidiol that shows the most significant seasonal variation in temperate climates.

The second stage of vitamin D metabolism occurs in the kidney, where calcidiol undergoes either

Figure 8.4 Vitamin D synthesis and metabolism.

Table 8.3 Nomenclature of vitamin D metabolites

Trivial name	Recommended name	Abbreviation
Vitamin D_3		
Cholecalciferol	Calciol	–
25-Hydroxycholecalciferol	Calcidiol	$25(OH)D_3$
1α-Hydroxycholecalciferol	1(S)-Hydroxycalciol	$1α(OH)D_3$
24,25-Dihydroxycholecalciferol	24(R)-Hydroxycalcidiol	$24,25(OH)_2D_3$
1,25-Dihydroxycholecalciferol	Calcitriol	$1,25(OH)_2D_3$
1,24,25-Trihydroxycholecalciferol	Calcitetrol	$1,24,25(OH)_3D_3$
Vitamin D_2		
Ergocalciferol	Ercalciol	–
25-Hydroxyergocalciferol	Ercalcidiol	$25(OH)D_2$
24,25-Dihydroxyergocalciferol	24(R)-Hydroxyercalcidiol	$24,25(OH)_2D_2$
1,25-Dihydroxyergocalciferol	Ercalcitriol	$1,25(OH)_2 D_2$
1,24,25-Trihydroxyergocalciferol	Ercalcitetrol	$1,24,25(OH)_3D_2$

The abbreviations shown in column 3 are not recommended, but are frequently used in the literature.

1-hydroxylation to yield the active metabolite 1,25-dihydroxyvitamin D (calcitriol) or 24-hydroxylation to yield an apparently inactive metabolite, 24,25-dihydroxyvitamin D (24-hydroxycalcidiol).

Regulation of vitamin D metabolism

The main function of vitamin D is in the control of calcium homeostasis and, in turn, vitamin D metabolism is regulated, at the level of 1- or 24-hydroxylation, by factors that respond to plasma concentrations of calcium and phosphate:

- Calcitriol acts to reduce its own synthesis and increase formation of 24-hydroxycalcidiol, by regulating the expression of the genes for the two hydroxylases.
- Parathyroid hormone is secreted in response to a fall in plasma calcium. In the kidney it acts to increase the activity of calcidiol 1-hydroxylase and decrease that of 24-hydroxylase. In turn, both calcitriol and high concentrations of calcium repress the synthesis of parathyroid hormone; calcium also inhibits the secretion of the hormone from the parathyroid gland.
- Calcium exerts its main effect on the synthesis and secretion of parathyroid hormone. However, calcium ions also have a direct effect on the kidney, reducing the activity of calcidiol 1-hydroxylase.
- Phosphate also affects calcidiol metabolism; throughout the day there is an inverse fluctuation of plasma phosphate and calcitriol, and feeding subjects on a low-phosphate diet results in increased circulating concentrations of calcitriol.

Metabolic functions of vitamin D

The principal function of vitamin D is to maintain the plasma concentration of calcium; calcitriol achieves this in three ways:

- increased intestinal absorption of calcium
- reduced excretion of calcium by stimulating resorption in the distal renal tubules (due to increased calbindin D synthesis)
- mobilization of bone mineral.

In addition, calcitriol has a variety of permissive or modulatory effects, in which it is a necessary, but not sufficient, factor in:

- insulin secretion
- synthesis and secretion of parathyroid and thyroid hormones
- inhibition of production of interleukin by activated T-lymphocytes and of immunoglobulin by activated B-lymphocytes
- differentiation of monocyte precursor cells
- modulation of cell proliferation.

In all of these actions, the role of calcitriol seems to be in the induction or maintenance of synthesis of calbindin D (and other calcium binding proteins), and the physiological effects are secondary to increased calcium uptake into the target cells.

Calcitriol acts like a steroid hormone, binding to a nuclear receptor protein. The calcitriol–receptor complex then binds to the enhancer site of the gene coding for a calcium binding protein, increasing its transcription and so increasing the amount of calcium binding protein in the cell.

The best studied actions of vitamin D are in the intestinal mucosa, where the intracellular calcium binding protein induced by vitamin D is essential for the absorption of calcium from the diet. Vitamin D also acts to increase the transport of calcium across the mucosal membrane by an effect on preformed calcium transport proteins in the cell membrane.

Calcitriol also raises plasma calcium by stimulating the mobilization of calcium from bone. It achieves this by activating osteoclast cells. However, it acts later to stimulate the laying down of new bone to replace the loss, by stimulating the differentiation and recruitment of osteoblasts.

Vitamin D deficiency: rickets and osteomalacia

Historically, rickets is a disease of toddlers, especially in northern industrial cities. Their bones are under-mineralized as a result of poor absorption of calcium in the absence of adequate amounts of calcitriol. When the child begins to walk, the long bones of the legs are deformed, leading to bow-legs or knock knees. More seriously, rickets can also lead to collapse of the ribcage and deformities of the bones of the pelvis. Similar problems may also occur in adolescents who are deficient in vitamin D during the adolescent growth spurt, when there is again a high demand for calcium for new bone formation.

Osteomalacia is the adult equivalent of rickets. It results from the demineralization of bone, rather than the failure to mineralize it in the first place, as is the case with rickets. Women who have little exposure to sunlight are especially at risk from osteomalacia after several pregnancies, because of the strain that pregnancy places on their marginal reserve of calcium.

Osteomalacia also occurs in the elderly. Here again the problem may be inadequate exposure to sunlight, but there is also evidence that the capacity to form 7-dehydrocholesterol in the skin decreases with advancing age, so that the elderly are more reliant on the few dietary sources of vitamin D.

Although vitamin D is essential for prevention and treatment of osteomalacia in the elderly, there is little evidence that it is beneficial in treating or preventing the other common degenerative bone disease of advancing age, osteoporosis, which is due to a loss of bone matrix, rather than enhanced release of calcium from bone with no effect on the organic matrix, as is seen in osteomalacia. The result is negative calcium balance and loss of bone mineral, but secondary to the loss of organic matrix, owing to progressive loss of estrogens and androgens, rather than failure of the vitamin D system.

Vitamin D requirements and reference intakes

It is difficult to determine requirements for dietary vitamin D, since the major source is synthesis in the skin. Before the development of methods for measurement of calcidiol the diagnosis of subclinical rickets was by detection of elevated alkaline phosphatase in plasma; nowadays, the main criterion of adequacy is the plasma concentration of calcidiol.

In elderly subjects with little sunlight exposure a dietary intake of $10\,\mu g$ of vitamin D/day results in a plasma calcidiol concentration of 20 nmol/l, the lower end of the reference range for younger adults at the end of winter. Therefore, the reference intake for the elderly is $10\,\mu g$/day, while average intakes of vitamin D from unfortified foods are less than $4\,\mu g$/day.

Vitamin D toxicity

During the 1950s, rickets was more or less totally eradicated in Britain and other temperate countries. This was due to enrichment of a large number of infant foods with vitamin D. However, a small number of infants suffered from vitamin D poisoning, the most serious effect of which is an elevated plasma concentration of calcium. This can lead to contraction of blood vessels, and hence dangerously high blood pressure, and calcinosis, that is the calcification of soft tissues, including the kidney, heart, lungs and blood vessel walls.

Some infants are sensitive to intakes of vitamin D as low as $50\,\mu g$/day. To avoid the serious problem of vitamin D poisoning in these susceptible infants, the extent to which infant foods are fortified with vitamin D has been reduced considerably. Unfortunately, this means that a small proportion, who have relatively high requirements, are now at risk of developing rickets. The problem is to identify those who have high requirements and provide them with supplements.

The toxic threshold in adults is not known, but all those patients suffering from vitamin D intoxication who have been investigated were taking more than $250\,\mu g$ of vitamin D/day.

Although excess dietary vitamin D is toxic, excessive exposure to sunlight does not lead to vitamin D poisoning. There is a limited capacity to form the precursor, 7-dehydrocholesterol, in the skin, and a limited capacity to take up cholecalciferol from the skin. Furthermore, prolonged exposure of previtamin D to UV light results in further reactions to yield biologically inactive compounds.

Interactions with drugs and other nutrients

As discussed above, vitamin D receptors form heterodimers with vitamin A receptors (RXR), so that many of the functions of vitamin D will require that vitamin A status is also adequate. A number of drugs, including barbiturates and other anticonvulsants, induce cytochrome P_{450}, resulting in increased catabolism of calcidiol, and hence drug-induced osteomalacia. The antituberculosis drug isoniazid inhibits cholecalciferol 25-hydroxylase in the liver, and again prolonged administration can lead to the development of osteomalacia.

Strontium is a potent inhibitor of the kidney 1-hydroxylase, and strontium intoxication can lead to the development of vitamin D-resistant rickets or osteomalacia. While there is normally little exposure to potentially toxic intakes of strontium, its salts are sometimes used to treat chronic lead intoxication.

8.4 Vitamin E

Although vitamin E was identified as a dietary essential for animals in the 1920s, it was not until 1983 that it was clearly demonstrated to be a dietary essential for human beings. Unlike other vitamins, no unequivocal physiological function for vitamin E has been defined; it acts as a lipid-soluble antioxidant in cell membranes, but many of its functions can be replaced by synthetic antioxidants. There is epidemiological evidence that high intakes of vitamin E are associated with lower incidence of cardiovascular disease.

Vegetable oils are rich sources of vitamin E, but significant amounts are also found in nuts and seeds, most green leafy vegetables and a variety of fish.

Vitamers and units of activity

Vitamin E is the generic descriptor for two families of compounds, the tocopherols and the tocotrienols (see Figure 8.5). The different vitamers have different

Figure 8.5 The vitamin E vitamers, tocopherols and tocotrienols.

biological potency. The most active is α-tocopherol, and it is usual to express vitamin E intake in terms of mg α-tocopherol equivalents. This is the sum of mg α-tocopherol + 0.5 × mg β-tocopherol + 0.1 × mg γ-tocopherol + 0.3 × mg α-tocotrienol. The other vitamers have negligble vitamin activity.

The obsolete international unit of vitamin E activity is still sometimes used: 1 IU = 0.67 mg α-tocopherol equivalent; 1 mg α-tocopherol = 1.49 IU.

Synthetic α-tocopherol does not have the same biological potency as the naturally occurring compound. This is because the side-chain of tocopherol has three centers of asymmetry and when it is synthesized chemically the result is a mixture of the various isomers. In the naturally occurring compound all three centers of asymmetry have the R-configuration, and naturally occurring α-tocopherol is called all-R, or RRR-α-tocopherol.

Absorption and metabolism

Tocopherols and tocotrienols are absorbed unchanged from the small intestine, in micelles with other dietary lipids, and incorporated into chylomicrons. The major route of excretion is in the bile, largely as unidentified metabolites, including glucuronides and other conjugates.

There are two mechanisms for tissue uptake of vitamin E. Lipoprotein lipase releases the vitamin by hydrolyzing the triacylglycerols in chylomicrons and VLDL, while separately there is uptake of low-density lipoprotein (LDL)-bound vitamin E by means of LDL receptors. Retention within tissues depends on binding proteins, and it is likely that the differences in biological activity of the vitamers are due to differential protein binding.

Metabolic functions of vitamin E

The main function of vitamin E is as a radical-trapping antioxidant in cell membranes and plasma lipoproteins. It is especially important in limiting radical damage resulting from oxidation of PUFA, by reacting with the lipid peroxide radicals before they can establish a chain reaction. The tocopheroxyl radical formed from vitamin E is relatively unreactive and persists long enough to undergo reaction to yield nonradical products. Commonly, the vitamin E radical in a membrane or lipoprotein is reduced back to tocopherol by reaction with vitamin C in plasma. The resultant

monodehydroascorbate radical then undergoes enzymic or nonenzymic reaction to yield ascorbate and dehydroascorbate, neither of which is a radical.

The stability of the tocopheroxyl radical means that it can penetrate further into cells, or deeper into plasma lipoproteins, and potentially propagate a chain reaction. Therefore, although it is regarded as an antioxidant, vitamin E may, like other antioxidants, also have pro-oxidant actions at high concentrations. This may explain why, although epidemiological studies have shown a clear association between high blood concentrations of vitamin E and lower incidence of atherosclerosis, the results of intervention studies with relatively high doses of vitamin E have generally been disappointing.

The tocotrienols have lower vitamin activity than tocopherols, and indeed it is conventional to consider only γ-tocotrienol as a significant part of vitamin E intake. However, because of their unsaturated side-chain, the tocotrienols also have a hypocholesterolemic action not shared by the tocopherols. They act to reduce the activity of 3-hydroxy-3-methylglutaryl-coenzyme A (HMG CoA) reductase, the rate-limiting enzyme in the pathway for synthesis of cholesterol, by repressing synthesis of the enzyme.

Vitamin E deficiency

In experimental animals vitamin E deficiency results in a number of different conditions.

- Deficient female animals suffer the death and reabsorption of the fetuses. This provided the basis of the original biological assay of vitamin E.
- In male animals deficiency results in testicular atrophy and degeneration of the germinal epithelium of the seminiferous tubules.
- Both skeletal and cardiac muscle are affected in deficient animals. This is sometimes called nutritional muscular dystrophy; an unfortunate term, since there is no evidence that human muscular dystrophy is related to vitamin E deficiency, and it is better called necrotizing myopathy.
- The integrity of blood vessel walls is affected, with leakage of blood plasma into subcutaneous tissues and accumulation under the skin of a green fluid: exudative diathesis.
- The nervous system is affected, with the development of central nervous system necrosis and axonal dystrophy. This is exacerbated by feeding diets rich in PUFA.

Dietary deficiency of vitamin E in humans is unknown, although patients with severe fat malabsorption, cystic fibrosis, some forms of chronic liver disease or (very rare) congenital lack of plasma β-lipoprotein suffer deficiency because they are unable to absorb the vitamin or transport it around the body. They suffer from severe damage to nerve and muscle membranes.

Premature infants are at risk of vitamin E deficiency, since they are often born with inadequate reserves of the vitamin. The red blood cell membranes of deficient infants are abnormally fragile, as a result of unchecked oxidative radical attack. This may lead to hemolytic anemia if they are not given supplements of the vitamin.

Experimental animals that are depleted of vitamin E become sterile. However, there is no evidence that vitamin E nutritional status is in any way associated with human fertility, and there is certainly no evidence that vitamin E supplements increase sexual potency, prowess or vigor.

Vitamin E requirements

It is difficult to establish vitamin E requirements, partly because deficiency is more or less unknown, and also because the requirement depends on the intake of PUFA. It is generally accepted, albeit with little experimental evidence, that an acceptable intake of vitamin E is 0.4 mg α-tocopherol equivalent/g dietary PUFA.

Indices of vitamin E status

The plasma concentration of α-tocopherol is used to assess vitamin E status; since most vitamin E is transported in plasma lipoproteins, it is the concentration per gram total plasma lipid, or better per mole cholesterol that is useful, rather than the simple concentration.

Erythrocytes are incapable of *de novo* lipid synthesis, so peroxidative damage resulting from oxygen stress has a serious effect, shortening red cell life and possibly precipitating hemolytic anemia in vitamin E deficiency. This has been exploited as a method of assessing status by measuring the hemolysis of red cells, induced by dilute hydrogen peroxide, expressed as a ratio of percentage of the hemolysis observed on incubation in water. This gives a means of assessing the functional adequacy of vitamin E intake, albeit one that will be affected by other, unrelated, factors. Plasma concentrations of α-tocopherol below 2.2 mmol/mol cholesterol or 1.1 μmol/g total plasma lipid are associated with

increased susceptibility of erythrocytes to induced hemolysis *in vitro*.

An alternative method of assessing functional antioxidant status, again one that is affected by both vitamin E and other antioxidants, is by measuring the exhalation of pentane arising from the catabolism of the products of peroxidation of n-6 PUFA or ethane arising from n-3 PUFA.

Higher levels of intake

There is good epidemiological evidence that high plasma concentrations of vitamin E are associated with a lower risk of atherosclerosis and ischemic heart disease. This is because high concentrations of vitamin E inhibit the oxidation of PUFA in plasma lipoproteins, and it is this oxidation that is responsible for the initiation of atherosclerosis. The levels that appear to be beneficial would require an intake of 17–40 mg α-tocopherol/day, which is above what could be achieved by eating ordinary foods. There is no known hazard from consuming even considerably higher amounts of vitamin E. However, intervention trials with α-tocopherol supplements have generally shown a decrease in nonfatal myocardial infarctions, with no change, or even a slight increase, in fatal infarctions. It is not clear whether this reflects the pro-oxidant action of tocopherol at high concentrations, or whether plasma α-tocopherol is simply a marker for some other protective factor in foods.

Interactions with other nutrients

Vitamin C in plasma and extracellular fluid is important in reducing the tocopheroxyl radical in membranes and lipoproteins back to tocopherol. There is also evidence that a variety of lipid-soluble antioxidants may be important in the antioxidant action of vitamin E in membranes and lipoproteins, including ubiquinone and synthetic antioxidants used in food processing, such as butylated hydroxytoluene and butylated hydroxyanisole. Synthetic antioxidants will prevent or cure a number of the signs of vitamin E deficiency in experimental animals.

There is a considerable overlap between the functions of vitamin E and selenium. Vitamin E reduces lipid peroxide radicals to yield unreactive fatty acids; the selenium-dependent enzyme glutathione peroxidase reduces hydrogen peroxide to water, thus lowering the intracellular concentration of potentially lipid-damaging peroxide. A membrane-specific isoenzyme of glutathione peroxidase will also reduce the tocopheroxyl radical back to tocopherol. Thus, vitamin E acts to remove the products of lipid peroxidation, while selenium acts both to remove the cause of lipid peroxidation and to recycle vitamin E.

8.5 Vitamin K

Vitamin K was discovered as a result of investigations into the cause of a bleeding disorder (hemorrhagic disease) of cattle fed on silage made from sweet clover and of chickens fed on a fat-free diet. The missing factor in the diet of the chickens was identified as vitamin K, while the problem in the cattle was that the feed contained dicumarol, an antagonist of the vitamin.

Since the effect of an excessive intake of dicumarol was severely impaired blood clotting, it was isolated and tested in low doses as an anticoagulant, for use in patients at risk of thrombosis. Although it was effective, it had unwanted side-effects, and synthetic vitamin K antagonists were developed for clinical use as anticoagulants. The most commonly used of these is warfarin, which is also used, in larger amounts, to kill rodents.

Vitamers

Three compounds have the biological activity of vitamin K (see Figure 8.6):

- phylloquinone, the normal dietary source, found in green leafy vegetables
- menaquinones, a family of related compounds synthesized by intestinal bacteria, with differing lengths of the side-chain
- menadione and menadiol diacetate, synthetic compounds that can be metabolized to phylloquinone.

Dietary sources, bacterial synthesis and metabolism

Phylloquinone has a role in photosynthesis, and therefore it is found in all green leafy vegetables; the richest sources are spring (collard) greens, spinach and Brussels sprouts. In addition, soyabean, rapeseed, cottonseed and olive oils are relatively rich in vitamin K, although other oils are not.

About 80% of dietary phylloquinone is normally absorbed into the lymphatic system in chylomicrons, and is then taken up by the liver from chylomicron remnants and released into the circulation in VLDL.

Intestinal bacteria synthesize a variety of menaquinones, which are absorbed to a limited extent from the

Figure 8.6 The vitamin K vitamers, phylloquinone (vitamin K_1), menaquinone (vitamin K_2) and menadione (a synthetic compound, vitamin K_3).

large intestine, again into the lymphatic system, cleared by the liver and released in VLDL. It is often suggested that about half of the requirement for vitamin K is met by intestinal bacterial synthesis, but there is little evidence for this, other than the fact that about half of the vitamin K in liver is phylloquinone and the remainder a variety of menaquinones. It is not clear to what extent the menaquinones are biologically active. It is possible to induce signs of vitamin K deficiency simply by feeding a phylloquinone-deficient diet, without inhibiting intestinal bacterial action.

The synthetic compound menadione is absorbed largely into the hepatic portal system, and undergoes alkylation in the liver to yield menaquinone-4, which is released together with phylloquinone and other menaquinones in VLDL.

Metabolic functions of vitamin K

Although it has been known since the 1920s that vitamin K was required for blood clotting, it was not until the 1970s that its precise function was established. It is the cofactor for the carboxylation of glutamate residues in the postsynthetic modification of proteins to form the unusual amino acid γ-carboxyglutamate, abbreviated to Gla (see Figure 8.7).

In the presence of warfarin, vitamin K epoxide cannot be reduced back to the active hydroquinone, but accumulates and is excreted as a variety of conjugates. However, if enough vitamin K is provided in the diet, the quinone can be reduced to the active hydroquinone by the warfarin-insensitive enzyme, and carboxylation can continue, with stoichiometric utilization of vitamin K and excretion of the epoxide. High doses of vitamin K are used to treat patients who have received an overdose of warfarin, and at least part of the resistance of some populations of rats to the action of warfarin is due to a high consumption of vitamin K from maram grass, although there are also genetically resistant populations of rodents.

Prothrombin and several other proteins of the blood clotting system (factors VII, IX and X, and proteins C and S) each contain between four and six γ-carboxyglutamate residues per mole. γ-Carboxyglutamate chelates calcium ions, and so permits the binding of the blood clotting proteins to lipid membranes. In vitamin K deficiency, or in the presence of an antagonist such as warfarin, an abnormal precursor of prothrombin (preprothrombin) containing little or no γ-carboxyglutamate is released into the circulation. Preprothrombin cannot chelate calcium or bind to phospholipid membranes, and so is unable to initiate blood clotting. Preprothrombin is sometimes known as PIVKA: the protein induced by vitamin K absence.

Bone vitamin K-dependent proteins

It has long been known that treatment of pregnant women with warfarin or other anticoagulants can lead to bone abnormalities in the child: the fetal warfarin syndrome. Two proteins in bone matrix contain γ-carboxyglutamate: osteocalcin and a less well characterized protein simply known as bone matrix Gla protein. Osteocalcin is interesting in that as well as γ-carboxyglutamate, it also contains hydroxyproline, so its synthesis is dependent on both vitamins K and C;

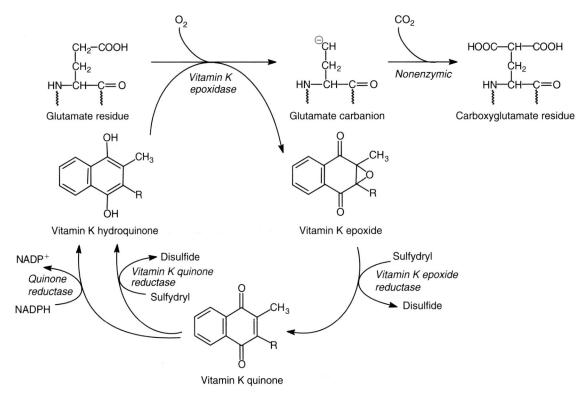

Figure 8.7 Role of vitamin K in the carboxylation of glutamate. Vitamin K epoxidase (EC 1.14.99.20), warfarin-sensitive epoxide/quinone reductase (EC 1.1.4.1), warfarin-insensitive quinone reductase (EC 1.1.4.2).

in addition, its synthesis is induced by vitamin D, and the release into the circulation of osteocalcin provides a sensitive index of vitamin D action. Osteocalcin comprises some 1–2% of total bone protein, and while it obviously functions as a calcium binding protein and modifies the crystallization of bone mineral, its precise function remains unclear.

Vitamin K deficiency and requirements

Apart from deliberate experimental manipulation, vitamin K deficiency is unknown, and determination of requirements is complicated by a lack of data on the importance of menaquinones synthesized by intestinal bacteria.

The main way of determining vitamin K status, and monitoring the efficacy of anticoagulant therapy, is by measuring the time required for the formation of a fibrin clot in citrated blood plasma after the addition of calcium ions and thromboplastin: the prothrombin time. A more sensitive index is provided by direct measurement of preprothrombin in plasma, most commonly by immunoassay using antisera against preprothrombin that do not react with prothrombin.

Based on determination of clotting time, and direct measurement of prothrombin and preprothrombin, an intake of 1 μg/kg body weight per day is considered adequate; this forms the basis of reference intakes of between 65 and 80 μg/day for adults.

A small number of newborn infants have very low reserves of vitamin K and are at risk of potentially fatal hemorrhagic disease. It is therefore generally recommended that all neonates should be given a single prophylactic dose of vitamin K.

Toxicity and drug interactions

There is no evidence that phylloquinone has any significant toxicity. However, the synthetic analogue menadione can undergo nonenzymic redox cycling, and injection of menadione in newborn infants has been implicated in the later development of leukemia. For this reason it is generally advised that prophylactic vitamin K given at birth should be as phylloquinone by mouth rather than menadione by injection. Menadione may also cause hemolytic anemia, hyperbilirubinemia and kernicterus in the newborn.

High intakes of vitamin K can overcome the effects of warfarin and other anticoagulants. This means that patients who are being treated with warfarin could overcome the beneficial effects of their medication if they took supplements of vitamin K. The danger is that if their dose of warfarin is increased to counteract the effects of the vitamin supplements and they then stop taking the supplements, they would be receiving considerably too much warfarin and would be at risk of hemorrhage.

It is unlikely that a normal diet could provide a sufficient excess of vitamin K to lead to problems, but habitual consumption of especially rich sources could result in intakes close to those that antagonize therapeutic warfarin. A diet containing relatively large amounts of foods prepared with vitamin K-rich oils may also pose a risk.

8.6 Vitamin B$_1$ (thiamin)

Historically, thiamin deficiency affecting the peripheral nervous system (beriberi) was a major public health problem in south-east Asia following the introduction of the steam-powered mill that made highly polished (and therefore thiamin-depleted) rice widely available. There are still sporadic outbreaks of deficiency among people whose diet is rich in carbohydrate and poor in thiamin. More commonly, thiamin deficiency affecting the heart and central nervous system is a problem in people with an excessive consumption of alcohol, to the extent that there was a serious suggestion in Australia at one time that thiamin should be added to beer.

The structures of thiamin and the coenzyme thiamin diphosphate are shown in Figure 8.8.

Thiamin is widely distributed in foods, with pork being an especially rich source; potatoes, whole-grain cereals, meat and fish are the major sources in most diets. Like other water-soluble vitamins, thiamin is readily lost

Figure 8.8 Thiamin (vitamin B$_1$) and the coenzyme thiamin diphosphate.

by leaching into cooking water; furthermore, it is unstable to light, and although bread and flour contain significant amounts of thiamin, much or all of this can be lost when baked goods are exposed to sunlight in a shop window.

Thiamin is also destroyed by sulfites, and in potato products that have been blanched by immersion in sulfite solution there is little or no thiamin remaining. Polyphenols, including tannic acid in tea and betel nuts, also destroy thiamin, and have been associated with thiamin deficiency.

Thiaminases that catalyze base exchange or hydrolysis of thiamin are found in microorganisms (including some that colonize the gut), a variety of plants and raw fish. The presence of thiaminase in fermented fish is believed to be a significant factor in the etiology of thiamin deficiency in parts of south-east Asia.

Absorption and metabolism of thiamin

Thiamin is absorbed in the duodenum and proximal jejunum, and then transferred to the portal circulation by an active transport process that is inhibited by alcohol. This may explain why alcoholics are especially susceptible to thiamin deficiency.

Tissues take up both free thiamin and thiamin monophosphate, then phosphorylate them further to yield thiamin diphosphate (the active coenzyme) and, in the nervous system, thiamin triphosphate.

Some free thiamin is excreted in the urine, increasing with diuresis, and a significant amount may also be lost in sweat. Most urinary excretion is as thiochrome, the result of nonenzymic cyclization, as well as a variety of products of side-chain oxidation and ring cleavage.

There is little storage of thiamin in the body, and biochemical signs of deficiency can be observed within a few days of initiating a thiamin-free diet.

Metabolic functions of thiamin

Thiamin has a central role in energy-yielding metabolism, and especially the metabolism of carbohydrates. Thiamin diphosphate (also known as thiamin pyrophosphate, see Figure 8.8) is the coenzyme for three oxidative decarboxylation reactions: pyruvate dehydrogenase in carbohydrate metabolism, α-ketoglutarate dehydrogenase in the citric acid cycle, and the branched-chain keto-acid dehydrogenase involved in the metabolism of leucine, isoleucine and valine. These three enzymes are multienzyme complexes that catalyze oxidative decarboxylation of the substrate linked to reduction of enzyme-bound lipoamide, and eventually reduction of NAD^+ to NADH.

Thiamin diphosphate is also the coenzyme for transketolase, in the pentose phosphate pathway of carbohydrate metabolism. This is the major pathway of carbohydrate metabolism in some tissues, and an important alternative to glycolysis in all tissues, being the source of half of the NADPH required for fatty acid synthesis.

In addition to its coenzyme role, thiamin, as the triphosphate, has a function in nerve conduction. Thiamin triphosphate is believed to act as a phosphate donor for phosphorylation of one of the proteins in the nerve membrane sodium transport channel.

Thiamin deficiency

Thiamin deficiency can result in three distinct syndromes:

- a chronic peripheral neuritis, beriberi, which may or may not be associated with heart failure and edema
- acute pernicious (fulminating) beriberi (shoshin beriberi), in which heart failure and metabolic abnormalities predominate, with little evidence of peripheral neuritis
- Wernicke's encephalopathy with Korsakoff's psychosis, a thiamin-responsive condition associated especially with alcohol and narcotic abuse.

In general, a relatively acute deficiency is involved in the central nervous system lesions of the Wernicke–Korsakoff syndrome, and a high energy intake, as in alcoholics, is also a predisposing factor. Dry beriberi is associated with a more prolonged, and presumably less severe, deficiency, with a generally low food intake, while higher carbohydrate intake and physical activity predispose to wet beriberi.

The role of thiamin diphosphate in pyruvate dehydrogenase means that in deficiency there is impaired conversion of pyruvate to acetyl-CoA, and hence impaired entry of pyruvate into the citric acid cycle. Especially in subjects on a relatively high carbohydrate diet, this results in increased plasma concentrations of lactate and pyruvate, which may lead to life-threatening lactic acidosis. The increase in plasma lactate and pyruvate after a test dose of glucose has been used as a means of assessing thiamin nutritional status.

Figure 8.9 Riboflavin (vitamin B_2) and the flavin coenzymes, riboflavin monophosphate and flavin adenine dinucleotide.

Dry beriberi

Chronic deficiency of thiamin, especially associated with a high carbohydrate diet, results in beriberi, which is a symmetrical ascending peripheral neuritis. Initially, the patient complains of weakness, stiffness and cramps in the legs, and is unable to walk more than a short distance. There may be numbness of the dorsum of the feet and ankles, and vibration sense may be diminished. As the disease progresses, the ankle jerk reflex is lost, and the muscular weakness spreads upwards, involving first the extensor muscles of the foot, then the muscles of the calf, and finally the extensors and flexors of the thigh. At this stage there is pronounced toe and foot drop: the patient is unable to keep either the toe or the whole foot extended off the ground. When the arms are affected there is a similar inability to keep the hand extended: wrist drop.

The affected muscles become tender, numb and hyperesthetic. The hyperesthesia extends in the form of a band around the limb, the so-called stocking and glove distribution, and is followed by anesthesia.

There is deep muscle pain, and in the terminal stages, when the patient is bed-ridden, even slight pressure, as from bed-clothes, causes considerable pain.

Wet beriberi

The heart may also be affected in beriberi, with dilatation of arterioles, rapid blood flow and increased pulse rate leading to right-sided heart failure and edema, so-called wet beriberi. The signs of chronic heart failure may be seen without peripheral neuritis. The arteriolar dilatation probably results from high circulating concentrations of lactate and pyruvate as a result of impaired activity of pyruvate dehydrogenase.

Acute pernicious (fulminating) beriberi: shoshin beriberi

Heart failure without increased cardiac output, and no peripheral edema, may also occur acutely, associated with severe lactic acidosis. This was a common presentation of deficiency in Japan, where it was called shoshin (meaning acute) beriberi; in the 1920s some 26 000 deaths a year were recorded.

With improved knowledge of the cause and improved nutritional status, the disease had become more or less unknown, although in the 1980s it reappeared among Japanese adolescents consuming a diet based largely on such high-carbohydrate, low-nutrient, foods as sweet carbonated drinks, "instant" noodles and polished rice. It also occurs among alcoholics, when the lactic acidosis may be life-threatening, without clear signs of heart failure. Acute beriberi has also been reported when previously starved subjects are given intravenous glucose.

Wernicke–Korsakoff syndrome

While peripheral neuritis, acute cardiac beriberi and lactic acidosis occur in thiamin deficiency associated with alcohol misuse, the more usual presentation is as the Wernicke–Korsakoff syndrome, due to central nervous system lesions.

Initially, there is a confused state, Korsakoff's psychosis, which is characterized by confabulation and loss of recent memory, although memory for past events may be unimpaired. Later, clear neurological signs develop: Wernicke's encephalopathy. This is characterized by nystagmus and extraocular palsy. Post-mortem examination shows characteristic brain lesions.

Like shoshin beriberi, Wernicke's encephalopathy can develop acutely, without the more gradual development of Korsakoff's psychosis, among previously starved patients given intravenous glucose and seriously ill patients given parenteral hyperalimentation.

Thiamin requirements

Because thiamin has a central role in energy-yielding, and especially carbohydrate, metabolism, requirements depend mainly on carbohydrate intake, and have been related to "nonfat calories". In practice, requirements and reference intakes are calculated on the basis of total energy intake, assuming that the average diet provides 40% of energy from fat. For diets that are lower in fat, and hence higher in carbohydrate, thiamin requirements may be somewhat higher.

From depletion/repletion studies, an intake of at least 0.2 mg of thiamin/1000 kcal is required to prevent the development of deficiency signs and maintain normal urinary excretion, but an intake of 0.23 mg/1000 kcal is required for a normal transketolase activation coefficient (see below).

Reference intakes are calculated on the basis of 100 μg/MJ (0.5 mg/1000 kcal) for adults consuming more than 2000 kcal/day, with a minimum requirement for people with a low energy intake of 0.8–1.0 mg/day to allow for metabolism of endogenous substrates.

Assessment of thiamin status

The impairment of pyruvate dehydrogenase in thiamin deficiency results in a considerable increase in the plasma concentrations of lactate and pyruvate. This has been exploited as a means of assessing thiamin status, by measuring changes in the plasma concentrations of lactate and pyruvate after an oral dose of glucose and mild exercise. The test not specific for thiamin deficiency since a variety of other conditions can also result in metabolic acidosis. While it may be useful in depletion/repletion studies, it is little used nowadays in assessment of nutritional status.

Whole blood total thiamin below 150 nmol/l is considered to indicate deficiency. However, the changes observed in depletion studies are small. Even in patients with frank beriberi the total thiamin concentration in erythrocytes is only 20% lower than normal, so whole blood thiamin is not a sensitive index of status.

Although there are several urinary metabolites of thiamin, a significant proportion is excreted either unchanged or as thiochrome, and therefore the urinary excretion of the vitamin (measured as thiochrome) can provide information on nutritional status. Excretion decreases proportionally with intake in adequately nourished subjects, but at low intakes there is a threshold below which further reduction in intake has little effect on excretion.

The activation of apo-transketolase in erythrocyte lysate by thiamin diphosphate added *in vitro* has become the most widely used and accepted index of thiamin nutritional status. Apotransketolase is unstable both *in vivo* and *in vitro*, so problems may arise in the interpretation of results, especially if samples have been stored for any appreciable time. An activation coefficient >1.25 is indicative of deficiency, and <1.15 is considered to reflect adequate thiamin nutrition.

8.7 Vitamin B$_2$ (riboflavin)

Riboflavin deficiency is a significant public health problem in many areas of the world. The vitamin has a central role as a coenzyme in energy-yielding metabolism, yet deficiency is rarely, if ever, fatal, since there is very efficient conservation and recycling of riboflavin in deficiency.

The structures of riboflavin and the riboflavin-derived coenzymes are shown in Figure 8.9.

Milk and dairy products are important sources, providing 25% or more of total riboflavin intake in most diets, and it is noteworthy that average riboflavin status in different countries reflects milk consumption to a considerable extent. Other rich sources are eggs, meat and fish. In addition, because of its intense yellow color, riboflavin is widely used as a food color.

Photolytic destruction

Photolysis of riboflavin leads to the formation of lumiflavin (in alkaline solution) and lumichrome (in acidic or neutral solution), both of which are biologically inactive. Exposure of milk in clear glass bottles to sunlight or fluorescent light can result in the loss of significant amounts of riboflavin. This is potentially nutritionally important. Lumiflavin and lumichrome catalyze oxidation of lipids (to lipid peroxides) and methionine (to methional), resulting in the development of an unpleasant flavor, known as the "sunlight" flavor.

Absorption and metabolism

Apart from milk and eggs, which contain relatively large amounts of free riboflavin bound to specific binding proteins, most of the vitamin in foods is as flavin coenzymes bound to enzymes, which are released when the protein is hydrolyzed. Intestinal phosphatases then hydrolyze the coenzymes to liberate riboflavin, which is absorbed in the upper small intestine. The absorption of riboflavin is limited and after relatively high doses only a small proportion is absorbed.

Much of the absorbed riboflavin is phosphorylated in the intestinal mucosa and enters the bloodstream as riboflavin phosphate, although this does not seem to be essential for absorption of the vitamin.

About 50% of plasma riboflavin is free riboflavin, which is the main transport form, with 44% as flavin adenine dinucleotide (FAD) and the remainder as riboflavin phosphate. The vitamin is largely protein-bound in plasma; free riboflavin binds to both albumin and α- and β-globulins; both riboflavin and the coenzymes also bind to immunoglobulins.

Uptake into tissues is by passive carrier-mediated transport of free riboflavin, followed by metabolic trapping by phosphorylation to riboflavin phosphate, and onward metabolism to FAD.

Riboflavin phosphate and FAD that are not bound to proteins are rapidly hydrolyzed to riboflavin, which diffuses out of tissues into the bloodstream. Riboflavin and riboflavin phosphate that are not bound to plasma proteins are filtered at the glomerulus; renal tubular resorption is saturated at normal plasma concentrations. There is also active tubular secretion of the vitamin; urinary excretion of riboflavin after relatively high doses can be two- to three-fold greater than the glomerular filtration rate.

Under normal conditions about 25% of the urinary excretion of riboflavin is as the unchanged vitamin, with a small amount as a variety of glycosides of riboflavin and its metabolites.

Riboflavin balance

There is no significant storage of riboflavin; apart from the limitation on absorption, any surplus intake is excreted rapidly, so that once metabolic requirements have been met urinary excretion of riboflavin and its metabolites reflects intake until intestinal absorption is saturated. In depleted animals, the maximum growth response is achieved with intakes that give about 75% saturation of tissues, and the intake to achieve tissue saturation is that at which there is quantitative excretion of the vitamin.

There is very efficient conservation of tissue riboflavin in deficiency, and almost the only loss of riboflavin from tissues will be the small amount that is covalently bound to enzymes and cannot be salvaged for reuse. There is only a four-fold difference between the minimum concentration of flavins in the liver in deficiency and the level at which saturation occurs. In the central nervous system there is only a 35% difference between deficiency and saturation.

Metabolic functions of the flavin coenzymes

The metabolic function of the flavin coenzymes is as electron carriers in a wide variety of oxidation and reduction reactions central to all metabolic processes, including the mitochondrial electron transport chain, and key enzymes in fatty acid and amino acid oxidation, and the citric acid cycle. The flavin coenzymes remain bound to the enzyme throughout the catalytic cycle. The majority of flavoproteins have FAD as the prosthetic group rather than riboflavin phosphate; some have both flavin coenzymes and some have other prosthetic groups as well.

Flavins can undergo a one-electron reduction to the semiquinone radical or a two-electron reduction to dihydroflavin. In some enzymes formation of dihydroflavin occurs by two single-electron steps, with intermediate formation of the semiquinone radical. Dihydroflavin can be oxidized by reaction with a substrate, $NAD(P)^+$, or cytochromes in a variety of dehydrogenases, or can react with molecular oxygen in oxygenases and mixed function oxidases (hydroxylases).

Flavins and oxidative stress

Reoxidation of the reduced flavin in oxygenases and mixed function oxidases proceeds by way of formation of the flavin radical and flavin hydroperoxide, with the intermediate generation of superoxide and perhydroxyl radicals and hydrogen peroxide. Because of this, flavin oxidases make a significant contribution to the total oxidant stress of the body. Overall, some 3–5% of the daily consumption of about 30 mol of oxygen by an adult is converted to singlet oxygen, hydrogen peroxide and the superoxide, perhydroxyl and hydroxyl radicals, rather than undergoing complete reduction to water in the electron transport chain. There is thus a total production of some 1.5 mol of reactive oxygen species daily, potentially capable of causing damage to membrane lipids, proteins and nucleic acids.

Riboflavin deficiency

Although riboflavin is involved in all areas of metabolism, and deficiency is widespread on a global scale, deficiency is not fatal. There seem to be two reasons why deficiency is not fatal. One is that, although deficiency is common, the vitamin is widespread in foods and most diets will provide minimally adequate amounts to permit maintenance of central metabolic pathways. The second, more important, reason is that in deficiency there is extremely efficient reutilization of the riboflavin that is released by the turnover of flavoproteins, so that only a very small amount is metabolized or excreted.

Riboflavin deficiency is characterized by lesions of the margin of the lips (cheilosis) and corners of the mouth (angular stomatitis), a painful desquamation of the tongue, so that it is red, dry and atrophic (magenta tongue), and a sebhorreic dermatitis, with filiform excrescences, affecting especially the nasolabial folds, eyelids and ears, with abnormalities of the skin around the vulva and anus and at the free border of the prepuce.

There may also be conjunctivitis with vascularization of the cornea and opacity of the lens. This last is the only lesion of ariboflavinosis for which the biochemical basis is known: glutathione is important in maintaining the normal clarity of crystallin in the lens, and glutathione reductase is a flavoprotein that is particularly sensitive to riboflavin depletion.

The main metabolic effect of riboflavin deficiency is on lipid metabolism. Riboflavin-deficient animals have a lower metabolic rate than controls and require a 15–20% higher food intake to maintain body weight. Feeding a high-fat diet leads to more marked impairment of growth and a higher requirement for riboflavin to restore growth.

Resistance to malaria in riboflavin deficiency

Several studies have noted that in areas where malaria is endemic, riboflavin-deficient subjects are relatively resistant and have a lower parasite burden than adequately nourished subjects. The biochemical basis of this resistance to malaria in riboflavin deficiency is not known, but two possible mechanisms have been proposed.

- The malarial parasites may have a particularly high requirement for riboflavin. Some flavin analogues have antimalarial action.
- As a result of impaired antioxidant activity in erythrocytes, there may be increased fragility of erythrocyte membranes or reduced membrane fluidity. As in sickle cell trait, which also protects against malaria, this may result in exposure of the parasites to the host's immune system at a vulnerable stage in their development, resulting in the production of protective antibodies.

Riboflavin requirements

Estimates of riboflavin requirements are based on depletion/repletion studies to determine the minimum intake at which there is significant excretion of the vitamin. In deficiency there is virtually no excretion of the vitamin; as requirements are met, so any excess is excreted in the urine. On this basis the minimum adult requirement for riboflavin is 0.5–0.8 mg/day. At intakes of 1.1–1.6 mg/day urinary excretion rises sharply, suggesting that tissue reserves are saturated.

A more generous estimate of requirements, and the basis of reference intakes, is the level of intake at which there is normalization of the activity of the red cell enzyme glutathione reductase; the activity of this flavoprotein is especially sensitive to riboflavin nutritional status. Normal values of the activation coefficient are seen in subjects whose habitual intake of riboflavin is between 1.2 and 1.5 mg/day.

Because of the central role of flavin coenzymes in energy-yielding metabolism, reference intakes are sometimes calculated on the basis of energy intake: 0.14–0.19 mg/MJ (0.6–0.8 mg/1000 kcal). However, in view of the wide range of riboflavin-dependent reactions, other than those of energy-yielding metabolism, it is difficult to justify this basis for the calculation of requirements.

Assessment of riboflavin nutritional status

The urinary excretion of riboflavin and its metabolites (either basal excretion or after a test dose) can be used as an index of status. However, riboflavin excretion is only correlated with intake in subjects who are maintaining nitrogen balance. In subjects in negative nitrogen balance there may be more urinary excretion than would be expected, largely as a result of the catabolism of tissue flavoproteins, and loss of their prosthetic groups. Higher intakes of protein than are required to maintain nitrogen balance do not affect the requirement for riboflavin or indices of riboflavin nutritional status.

Glutathione reductase is especially sensitive to riboflavin depletion. The activity of the enzyme in erythrocytes can therefore be used as an index of riboflavin status. Interpretation of the results can be complicated by anemia, and it is more usual to use the activation of erythrocyte glutathione reductase (EGR) by FAD added *in vitro*. An activation coefficient of 1.0–1.4 reflects adequate nutritional status, whereas >1.7 indicates deficiency.

Interactions with drugs and other nutrients

The phenothiazines such as chlorpromazine, used in the treatment of schizophrenia, and the tricyclic antidepressant drugs such as imipramine, are structural analogues of riboflavin, and inhibit flavokinase. In experimental animals administration of these drugs at doses equivalent to those used clinically results in an increase in the EGR activation coefficient and increased urinary excretion of riboflavin, with reduced tissue concentrations of riboflavin phosphate and FAD, despite feeding diets providing more riboflavin than is needed to meet requirements. While there is no evidence that

patients treated with these drugs for a prolonged period develop clinical signs of riboflavin deficiency, long-term use of chlorpromazine is associated with a reduction in metabolic rate.

Riboflavin deficiency is sometimes associated with hypochromic anemia as a result of impaired iron absorption. A greater proportion of a test dose of iron is retained in the intestinal mucosal cells bound to ferritin, and hence lost in the feces, rather than being absorbed, because the mobilization of iron bound to ferritin in mucosal cells for transfer to transferrin requires oxidation by a flavin-dependent enzyme.

Riboflavin depletion decreases the oxidation of dietary vitamin B_6 to pyridoxal; pyridoxine oxidase is a flavoprotein and is very sensitive to riboflavin depletion. It is not clear to what extent there is functional vitamin B_6 deficiency in riboflavin deficiency. This is partly because vitamin B_6 nutritional status is generally assessed by the metabolism of a test dose of tryptophan and kynurenine hydroxylase in the tryptophan oxidative pathway is a flavoprotein; riboflavin deficiency can therefore disturb tryptophan metabolism quite separately from its effects on vitamin B_6 nutritional status.

The disturbance of tryptophan metabolism in riboflavin deficiency, due to impairment of kynurenine hydroxylase, can also result in reduced synthesis of NAD from tryptophan, and may therefore be a factor in the etiology of pellagra.

8.8 Niacin

Niacin is not strictly a vitamin, since it can be synthesized in the body from the essential amino acid tryptophan. Indeed, it is only when tryptophan metabolism is deranged that dietary preformed niacin becomes important. Nevertheless, niacin was discovered as a nutrient during studies of the deficiency disease pellagra, which was a major public health problem in the southern USA throughout the first half of the twentieth century, and continued to be a problem in parts of India and sub-Saharan Africa until the 1990s.

Vitamers and niacin equivalents

Two compounds, nicotinic acid and nicotinamide, have the biological activity of niacin. When nicotinic acid was discovered to be a curative and preventive factor for pellagra, it was already known as a chemical compound, and was therefore never assigned a number

Nicotinic acid   Nicotinamide

Nicotinamide adenine dinucleotide (NAD)

Phosphorylated in NADP

Figure 8.10 The niacin vitamers, nicotinic acid and nicotinamide, and the coenzyme NAD.

among the B vitamins. The name niacin was coined in the USA when it was decided to enrich maize meal with the vitamin to prevent pellagra; it was considered that the name nicotinic acid was not desirable because of its the similarity to nicotine. In USA the term niacin is commonly used to mean specifically nicotinic acid, and nicotinamide is known as niacinamide; elsewhere "niacin" is used as a generic descriptor for both vitamers. Figure 8.10 shows the structures of nicotinic acid and niacin, as well as the nicotinamide nucleotide coenzymes, NAD and NADP.

The nicotinamide ring of NAD can be synthesized in the body from the essential amino acid tryptophan. In adults almost all of the dietary intake of tryptophan, apart from the small amount that is used for net new protein synthesis, is metabolized by this pathway, and hence is potentially available for NAD synthesis.

Several studies have investigated the equivalence of dietary tryptophan and preformed niacin as precursors of the nicotinamide nucleotides, generally by determining the excretion of niacin metabolites in response to test doses of the precursors, in subjects maintained on deficient diets. The most extensive such study was that of Horwitt et al. in 1956. They found that there was a considerable variation between subjects in the response to tryptophan and niacin, and it was in order to allow for this individual variation that they proposed the ratio of 60 mg of tryptophan equivalent to 1 mg of preformed niacin. Changes in hormonal

status may result in considerable changes in this ratio, with between 7 and 30 mg of dietary tryptophan being equivalent to 1 mg of preformed niacin in late pregnancy.

The niacin content of foods is generally expressed as mg niacin equivalents; 1 mg niacin equivalent = mg preformed niacin + 1/60 × mg tryptophan. Because most of the niacin in cereals is biologically unavailable (see below), it is conventional to ignore preformed niacin in cereal products.

Because endogenous synthesis from tryptophan is more important than preformed dietary niacin, the main dietary sources of niacin are generally those that are also rich sources of protein. It is only when the dietary staple is a cereal such as maize, which is remarkably lacking in tryptophan, that problems of deficiency occur. Trigonelline in coffee beans is demethylated to nicotinic acid during roasting, and moderate coffee consumption may meet a significant proportion of niacin requirements.

Unavailable niacin in cereals

Chemical analysis reveals niacin in cereals (largely in the bran), but this is biologically unavailable, since it is bound as niacytin – nicotinoyl esters to a variety of macromolecules. In wheat bran some 60% is esterified to polysaccharides, and the remainder to polypeptides and glycopeptides.

Treatment of cereals with alkali (e.g. by soaking overnight in calcium hydroxide solution, as is the traditional method for the preparation of tortillas in Mexico) and baking with alkaline baking powder releases much of the nicotinic acid. This may explain why pellagra has always been rare in Mexico, despite the fact that maize is the dietary staple.

Up to 10% of the niacin in niacytin may be biologically available as a result of hydrolysis by gastric acid.

Absorption and metabolism

Niacin is present in tissues, and therefore in foods, largely as the nicotinamide nucleotides. The postmortem hydrolysis of NAD(P) is extremely rapid in animal tissues, so it is likely that much of the niacin of meat (a major dietary source of the preformed vitamin) is free nicotinamide.

Nicotinamide nucleotides present in the intestinal lumen are not absorbed as such, but undergo hydrolysis to free nicotinamide. Many intestinal bacteria have high nicotinamide deamidase activity, and a significant proportion of dietary nicotinamide may be deamidated in the intestinal lumen. Both nicotinic acid and nicotinamide are absorbed from the small intestine by a sodium-dependent saturable process.

The nicotinamide nucleotide coenzymes can be synthesized from either of the niacin vitamers, and from quinolinic acid, an intermediate in the metabolism of tryptophan. In the liver, synthesis of the coenzymes increases with increasing intake of tryptophan, but not preformed niacin. The liver exports nicotinamide, derived from turnover of coenzymes, for uptake by other tissues.

Catabolism of NAD(P)

The catabolism of NAD^+ is catalyzed by four enzymes:

- NAD glycohydrolase, which releases nicotinamide and ADP-ribose
- NAD pyrophosphatase, which releases nicotinamide mononucleotide; this can be either hydrolyzed by NAD glycohydrolase to release nicotinamide, or reutilized to form NAD
- ADP-ribosyltransferases
- poly(ADP-ribose) polymerase.

The activation of ADP-ribosyltransferase and poly (ADP-ribose) polymerase by toxins, oxidative stress or DNA damage may result in considerable depletion of intracellular NAD(P), and may indeed provide a protective suicide mechanism to ensure that cells that have suffered very severe damage die, as a result of NAD(P) depletion. The administration of DNA-breaking carcinogens to experimental animals results in the excretion of large amounts of nicotinamide metabolites and depletion of tissue NAD(P); addition of the compounds to cells in culture has a similar effect. Chronic exposure to such carcinogens and mycotoxins may be a contributory factor in the etiology of pellagra when dietary intakes of tryptophan and niacin are marginal.

Urinary excretion of niacin and metabolites

Under normal conditions there is little or no urinary excretion of either nicotinamide or nicotinic acid. This is because both vitamers are actively resorbed from the glomerular filtrate. It is only when the concentration is so high that the resorption mechanism is saturated that there is any significant excretion of niacin.

Nicotinamide in excess of requirements for NAD synthesis is methylated by nicotinamide N-methyltransferase. N^1-Methylnicotinamide is actively secreted into the urine by the proximal renal tubules. N^1-Methylnicotinamide can also be metabolized further, to yield methylpyridone-2-carboxamide and methylpyridone-4-carboxamide.

Nicotinamide can also undergo oxidation to nicotinamide N-oxide when large amounts of nicotinamide are ingested. Nicotinic acid can be conjugated with glycine to form nicotinuric acid (nicotinoyl-glycine) or may be methylated to trigonelline (N^1-methylnicotinic acid). It is not clear to what extent urinary excretion of trigonelline reflects endogenous methylation of nicotinic acid, since there is a significant amount of trigonelline in foods, which may be absorbed, but cannot be utilized as a source of niacin, and is excreted unchanged.

Metabolic functions of niacin

The best defined role of niacin is in the metabolism of metabolic fuels, as the functional nicotinamide part of the coenzymes NAD and NADP, which play a major role in oxidation and reduction reactions. As shown in Figure 8.10, the oxidized coenzymes have a positive charge on the nicotinamide ring nitrogen and undergo a two-electron reduction. The oxidized forms are conventionally shown as $NAD(P)^+$ and the reduced forms either as $NAD(P)H_2$ or, more correctly, as $NAD(P)H + H^+$, since although it is a two-electron reduction, only one proton is incorporated into the ring, the other remaining associated with the coenzyme.

In general, NAD^+ is involved as an electron acceptor in energy-yielding metabolism, being oxidized by the mitochondrial electron transport chain, while the major coenzyme for reductive synthetic reactions is NADPH. An exception to this general rule is the pentose phosphate pathway of glucose metabolism, which results in the reduction of $NADP^+$ to NADPH, and is the principal metabolic source of reductant for fatty acid synthesis.

In addition to its coenzyme role, NAD has a function as the source of ADP-ribose for the ADP-ribosylation of a variety proteins and poly(ADP-ribosylation) and hence activation of nucleoproteins involved in the DNA repair mechanism.

In the nucleus, poly(ADP-ribose)polymerase is activated by binding to breakage points in DNA. The enzyme is involved in activation of the DNA repair mechanism in response to strand breakage caused by radical attack or UV radiation. In cells that have suffered considerable DNA damage, the activation of poly (ADP-ribose) polymerase may deplete intracellular

NAD to such an extent that ATP formation is impaired, leading to cell death.

The organic chromium compound known as the glucose tolerance factor, which enhances the binding of insulin to cell-surface receptors, is believed to be chromium nicotinate. While there is evidence of impaired glucose tolerance in chromium deficiency, there is no evidence that niacin deficiency has any such effect.

Pellagra: a disease of tryptophan and niacin deficiency

Pellagra became common in Europe when maize was introduced from the New World as a convenient high-yielding dietary staple, and by the late nineteenth century it was widespread throughout southern Europe, north and south Africa and the southern USA. The proteins of maize are particularly lacking in tryptophan, and as with other cereals little or none of the preformed niacin is biologically available.

Pellagra is characterized by a photosensitive dermatitis, like severe sunburn, typically with a butterfly-like pattern of distribution over the face, affecting all parts of the skin that are exposed to sunlight. Similar skin lesions may also occur in areas not exposed to sunlight, but subject to pressure, such as the knees, elbows, wrists and ankles. Advanced pellagra is also accompanied by dementia (more correctly a depressive psychosis), and there may be diarrhea. Untreated pellagra is fatal.

The depressive psychosis is superficially similar to schizophrenia and the organic psychoses, but clinically distinguishable by the sudden lucid phases which alternate with the most florid psychiatric signs. It is probable that these mental symptoms can be explained by a relative deficit of the essential amino acid tryptophan, and hence reduced synthesis of the neurotransmitter 5-hydroxytryptamine (serotonin), and not to a deficiency of niacin per se.

Additional factors in the etiology of pellagra

Pellagra also occurs in India among people whose dietary staple is jowar (*Sorghum vulgare*), even though the protein in this cereal contains more than enough tryptophan to permit adequate synthesis of NAD. Here the problem seems to be the relative excess of leucine in the protein, which can inhibit the synthesis of NAD from tryptophan. It is likely that leucine is a factor in the etiology of pellagra only when the dietary intakes of both tryptophan and niacin are extremely low, a condition that may occur when sorghum is the dietary staple, especially at times of food shortage.

Although the nutritional etiology of pellagra is well established, and tryptophan or niacin will prevent or cure the disease, additional factors, including deficiency of riboflavin or vitamin B_6, both of which are required for synthesis of NAD from tryptophan, may be important when intakes of tryptophan and niacin are only marginally adequate.

During the first half of the twentieth century, of the 87 000 people who died from pellagra in the USA there were twice as many women as men. Reports of individual outbreaks of pellagra, both in the USA and more recently elsewhere, show a similar gender ratio. This may well be the result of inhibition of tryptophan metabolism by estrogen metabolites, and hence reduced synthesis of NAD from tryptophan.

Several bacterial, fungal and environmental toxins activate ADP-ribosyltransferase or poly(ADP-ribose) polymerase, and it is possible that chronic exposure to such toxins will deplete tissue NAD(P) and hence be a contributory factor in the development of pellagra when intakes of tryptophan and niacin are marginal.

Niacin requirements

On the basis of depletion/repletion studies in which the urinary excretion of niacin metabolites was measured after feeding tryptophan or preformed niacin, the average requirement for niacin is 1.3 mg niacin equivalents/MJ energy expenditure, and reference intakes are based on 1.6 mg/MJ.

Average intakes of tryptophan in Western diets will more than meet requirements without the need for a dietary source of preformed niacin.

Assessment of niacin status

Although the nicotinamide nucleotide coenzymes function in a large number of oxidation and reduction reactions, this cannot be exploited as a means of assessing the state of the body's niacin reserves, because the coenzymes are not firmly attached to their apoenzymes, as are thiamin pyrophosphate, riboflavin and pyridoxal phosphate, but act as cosubstrates of the reactions, binding to and leaving the enzyme as the reaction proceeds. No specific metabolic lesions associated with NAD(P) depletion have been identified.

The two methods of assessing niacin nutritional status are measurement of the ratio of NAD:NADP in red blood cells and the urinary excretion of niacin metabolites, neither of which is wholly satisfactory.

Niacin toxicity

Nicotinic acid has been used to lower blood triacylglycerol and cholesterol in patients with hyperlipidemia. However, relatively large amounts are required (of the order of 1–6 g/day, compared with reference intakes of 18–20 mg/day). At this level of intake, nicotinic acid causes dilatation of blood vessels and flushing, with skin irritation, itching and a burning sensation. This effect wears off after a few days.

High intakes of both nicotinic acid and nicotinamide, in excess of 500 mg/day, also cause liver damage, and prolonged use can result in liver failure. This is especially a problem with sustained-release preparations of niacin, which permit a high blood level to be maintained for a relatively long time.

8.9 Vitamin B_6

Apart from a single outbreak in the 1950s, due to overheated infant milk formula, vitamin B_6 deficiency is unknown except under experimental conditions. Nevertheless, there is a considerable body of evidence that marginal status and biochemical deficiency may be relatively widespread in developed countries.

Vitamin B_6 is widely distributed in a variety of foods. However, a considerable proportion of the vitamin in plant foods may be present as glucosides, which are probably not biologically available, although a proportion may be hydrolyzed by intestinal bacteria.

When foods are heated, pyridoxal and pyridoxal phosphate can react with the ε-amino groups of lysine to form a Schiff base (aldimine). This renders both the vitamin B_6 and the lysine biologically unavailable; more importantly, the pyridoxyl-lysine released during digestion is absorbed and has antivitamin B_6 antimetabolite activity. Overall, it is estimated that some 70–80% of dietary vitamin B_6 is available.

Vitamers

The generic descriptor vitamin B_6 includes six vitamers: the alcohol pyridoxine, the aldehyde pyridoxal, the amine pyridoxamine and their $5'$-phosphates. There is some confusion in the literature, because at one time "pyridoxine" was used as a generic descriptor, with "pyridoxol" as the specific name for the alcohol. Since 1973 the official International Union of Pure and Applied Chemistry–International Union of Biochemistry (IUPAC – IUB) and International Union of Nutritional Sciences (IUNS) nomenclature has been as shown in Figure 8.11. The vitamers are metabolically interconvertible and, as far as is known, they have equal biological activity; they are all converted in the body to the metabolically active form, pyridoxal phosphate. 4-Pyridoxic acid is a biologically inactive end-product of vitamin B_6 metabolism.

Absorption and metabolism

The phosphorylated vitamers are dephosphorylated by membrane-bound alkaline phosphatase in the intestinal mucosa; pyridoxal, pyridoxamine and pyridoxine are all absorbed rapidly by passive diffusion. Intestinal mucosal cells have pyridoxine kinase, pyridoxine phosphate oxidase and phosphatases (see Figure 8.11), so that there is net accumulation of pyridoxal phosphate by metabolic trapping. Much of the ingested pyridoxine is released into the portal circulation as pyridoxal, after dephosphorylation at the serosal surface. Unlike other B vitamins, there seems to be no limit on the amount of vitamin B_6 that is absorbed.

Most of the absorbed vitamin is taken up by the liver by passive diffusion, followed by metabolic trapping as phosphate esters, which do not cross cell membranes, then oxidation to pyridoxal phosphate. The liver exports both pyridoxal phosphate (bound to albumin) and pyridoxal (which binds to both albumin and hemoglobin). Free pyridoxal remaining in the liver is rapidly oxidized to 4-pyridoxic acid, which is the main excretory product.

Extrahepatic tissues take up pyridoxal and pyridoxal phosphate from the plasma. The phosphate is hydrolyzed to pyridoxal, which can cross cell membranes, by extracellular alkaline phosphatase, then trapped intracellularly by phosphorylation. Tissue concentrations of pyridoxal phosphate are controlled by the balance between phosphorylation and dephosphorylation.

Some 80% of the body's total vitamin B_6 is pyridoxal phosphate in muscle, mostly associated with glycogen phosphorylase. This does not function as a reserve of the vitamin and is not released from muscle in times of deficiency; it is released into the circulation (as pyridoxal) in starvation, when glycogen reserves are exhausted and there is less requirement for phosphorylase activity. Under these conditions it is available for redistribution to other tissues, and especially the liver

Figure 8.11 Interconversion of the vitamin B_6 vitamers. Pyridoxal kinase (EC 2.7.1.38), pyridoxine phosphate oxidase (EC 1.1.1.65), pyridoxamine phosphate oxidase (EC 1.4.3.5).

and kidneys, to meet the increased requirement for gluconeogenesis from amino acids.

Metabolic functions of vitamin B_6

Pyridoxal phosphate is a coenzyme in three main areas of metabolism:

- in a wide variety of reactions of amino acids, especially transamination, in which it functions as the intermediate carrier of the amino group, and decarboxylation to form amines
- as the cofactor of glycogen phosphorylase in muscle and liver, where it is the phosphate group that is catalytically important
- in the regulation of the action of steroid hormones. Pyridoxal phosphate acts to remove the hormone–receptor complex from DNA binding, and so

terminate the action of the hormones. In vitamin B_6 deficiency there is increased sensitivity of target tissues to the actions of low concentrations of such hormones as the estrogens, androgens, cortisol and vitamin D.

Vitamin B_6 deficiency

Deficiency of vitamin B_6 severe enough to lead to clinical signs is extremely rare, and unequivocal deficiency has only been reported in one outbreak, during the 1950s, when babies were fed on a milk preparation that had been severely overheated during manufacture. Many of the affected infants suffered convulsions, which ceased rapidly following the administration of vitamin B_6.

The cause of the convulsions was severe impairment of the activity of the enzyme glutamate decarboxylase, which is a pyridoxal phosphate-dependent enzyme. The product of glutamate decarboxylase is γ-aminobutyric acid (GABA), a regulatory neurotransmitter in the central nervous system.

Moderate vitamin B_6 deficiency results in a number of abnormalities of amino acid metabolism, and especially of tryptophan and methionine. In experimental animals, a moderate degree of deficiency leads to increased sensitivity of target tissues to steroid hormone action. This may be important in the development of hormone-dependent cancer of the breast, uterus and prostate, and may therefore affect the prognosis. Vitamin B_6 supplementation may be a useful adjunct to other therapy in these common cancers; certainly, there is evidence that poor vitamin B_6 nutritional status is associated with a poor prognosis in women with breast cancer.

Vitamin B_6 requirements

Most studies of vitamin B_6 requirements have followed the development of abnormalities of tryptophan and methionine metabolism during depletion and normalization during repletion with graded intakes of the vitamin. While the tryptophan load test is unreliable as an index of vitamin B_6 nutritional status in field studies, under the controlled conditions of depletion/repletion studies it gives a useful indication of the state of vitamin B_6 nutrition.

Since the major role of vitamin B_6 is in amino acid metabolism it is likely that protein intake will affect vitamin B_6 requirements. Adults maintained on vitamin B_6-deficient diets develop abnormalities of tryptophan and methionine metabolism more quickly, and their blood vitamin B_6 falls more rapidly, when their protein intake is relatively high (80–160 g/day in various studies) than on low protein intakes (30–50 g/day). Similarly, during repletion of deficient subjects, tryptophan and methionine metabolism and blood vitamin B_6 are normalized more rapidly at low than at high levels of protein intake.

From such studies the mean requirement for vitamin B_6 is estimated to be 13 μg/g dietary protein, and reference intakes are based on 15–16 μg/g dietary protein.

Requirements of infants

Estimation of the vitamin B_6 requirements of infants presents a problem, and there is a clear need for further research. Human milk, which must be assumed to be adequate for infant nutrition, provides only some 2.5–3 μg of vitamin B_6/g protein. This is very much lower than the requirement for adults, although there is no reason why infants should have a lower requirement.

Based on the body content of 3.7 μg (15 nmol) of vitamin B_6/g body weight, and the rate of weight gain, a minimum requirement for infants over the first 6 months of life is 100 μg/day to establish tissue reserves, and an additional 20% to allow for metabolic turnover. Even if the mother receives daily supplements of 2.5 mg of vitamin B_6 throughout lactation, thus more than doubling her normal intake, the infant's intake ranges from 100 to 300 μg/day over the first 6 months of life. At 1 month this is only 8.5 μg/g protein, rising to 15 μg/g by 2 months.

Assessment of vitamin B_6 status

Fasting plasma total vitamin B_6 (measured microbiologically), or more specifically pyridoxal phosphate, is widely used as an index of vitamin B_6 nutritional status. Despite the fall in plasma pyridoxal phosphate in pregnancy, which has been widely interpreted as indicating vitamin B_6 depletion or an increased requirement, the plasma concentration of pyridoxal phosphate plus pyridoxal is unchanged. This suggests that determination of plasma pyridoxal phosphate alone may not be a reliable index of vitamin B_6 nutritional status.

About half of the normal dietary intake of vitamin B_6 is excreted as 4-pyridoxic acid. Urinary excretion of 4-pyridoxic acid will largely reflect recent intake of the vitamin rather than underlying nutritional status.

Coenzyme saturation of transaminases

The most widely used method of assessing vitamin B_6 status is by the activation of erythrocyte transaminases by pyridoxal phosphate added *in vitro*, expressed as either a percentage activation or, more commonly, an activation coefficient. An activation coefficient for alanine transaminase >1.25, or for aspartate transaminase >1.8, is considered to indicate deficiency.

The tryptophan load test

The tryptophan load test for vitamin B_6 nutritional status (the ability to metabolize a test dose of tryptophan) is one of the oldest metabolic tests for functional vitamin nutritional status. It was developed as a result of observation of the excretion of an abnormal colored compound, later identified as the tryptophan metabolite xanthurenic acid, in the urine of deficient animals.

Kynureninase (see Figure 8.12) is a pyridoxal phosphate-dependent enzyme, and its activity falls

Figure 8.12 Oxidative pathway of tryptophan: the basis of the tryptophan load test. Tryptophan dioxygenase (EC 1.13.11.11), formylkynurenine formamidase (EC 3.5.1.9), kynurenine hydroxylase (EC 1.14.13.9), kynureninase (EC 3.7.1.3).

markedly in vitamin B_6 deficiency, at least partly because it undergoes a slow mechanism-dependent inactivation that leaves catalytically inactive pyridoxamine phosphate at the active site of the enzyme. The enzyme can only be reactivated if there is an adequate supply of pyridoxal phosphate. This means that in vitamin B_6 deficiency there is a considerable accumulation of both hydroxykynurenine and kynurenine, sufficient to permit greater metabolic flux than usual through kynurenine transaminase, resulting in increased formation of kynurenic and xanthurenic acids.

Xanthurenic and kynurenic acids, and kynurenine and hydroxykynurenine, are easy to measure in urine, so the tryptophan load test [the ability to metabolize a test dose of 2–5 g (150–380 μmol/kg body weight) of tryptophan] has been widely adopted as a convenient and very sensitive index of vitamin B_6 nutritional status. However, because glucocorticoid hormones increase tryptophan dioxygenase activity, abnormal results of the tryptophan load test must be regarded with caution, and cannot necessarily be interpreted as indicating vitamin B_6 deficiency. Increased entry of tryptophan into the pathway will overwhelm the capacity of kynureninase, leading to increased formation of xanthurenic and kynurenic acids. Similarly,

estrogen metabolites inhibit kynureninase, leading to results that have been misinterpreted as vitamin B_6 deficiency.

The methionine load test

The metabolism of methionine includes two pyridoxal phosphate-dependent steps: cystathionine synthetase and cystathionase (see Figure 8.16). Cystathionase activity falls markedly in vitamin B_6 deficiency, and as a result there is an increase in the urinary excretion of homocysteine and cystathionine, both after a loading dose of methionine and under basal conditions. However, as discussed below, homocysteine metabolism is more affected by folate status than by vitamin B_6 status and, like the tryptophan load test, the methionine load test is probably not reliable as an index of vitamin B_6 status in field studies.

Nonnutritional uses of vitamin B_6

Several studies have suggested that oral contraceptives cause vitamin B_6 deficiency. As a result of this, supplements of vitamin B_6 of 50–100 mg/day, and sometimes higher, have been used to overcome the side-effects of oral contraceptives. Similar supplements have also been recommended for the treatment of the premenstrual syndrome, although there is little evidence of efficacy from placebo-controlled trials.

All of the studies that suggested that oral contraceptives cause vitamin B_6 deficiency used the metabolism of tryptophan as a means of assessing vitamin B_6 nutritional status. When other biochemical markers of status were also assessed, they were not affected by oral contraceptive use. Furthermore, most of these studies were performed using the now obsolete high-dose contraceptive pills.

Oral contraceptives do not cause vitamin B_6 deficiency. The problem is that estrogen metabolites inhibit kynureninase and reduce the activity of kynurenine hydroxylase. This results in the excretion of abnormal amounts of tryptophan metabolites, similar to what is seen in vitamin B_6 deficiency, but for quite a different reason.

Doses of 50–200 mg of vitamin B_6/day have an antiemetic effect, and the vitamin is widely used, alone or in conjunction with other antiemetics, to minimize the nausea associated with radiotherapy and to treat pregnancy sickness. There is no evidence that vitamin B_6 has any beneficial effect in pregnancy sickness, or that women who suffer from morning sickness have lower vitamin B_6 nutritional status than other pregnant women.

Doses of vitamin B_6 of 100 mg/day have been reported to be beneficial in the treatment of the carpal tunnel syndrome or tenosynovitis. However, most of the reports originate from one center and there appears to be little independent confirmation of the usefulness of the vitamin in this condition.

Vitamin B_6 toxicity

In experimental animals, doses of vitamin B_6 of 50 mg/kg body weight cause histological damage to dorsal nerve roots, and doses of 200 mg/kg body weight lead to the development of signs of peripheral neuropathy, with ataxia, muscle weakness and loss of balance. The clinical signs of vitamin B_6 toxicity in animals regress within 3 months after withdrawal of these massive doses, but sensory nerve conduction velocity, which decreases during the development of the neuropathy, does not recover fully.

The development of sensory neuropathy was reported in seven patients taking 2–7 g of pyridoxine/day. Although there was some residual damage, withdrawal of these extremely high doses resulted in a considerable recovery of sensory nerve function. Other reports have suggested that intakes as low as 50 mg/day are associated with neurological damage, although these studies were based on patients reporting symptoms rather than objective neurological examination.

8.10 Vitamin B_{12}

Dietary deficiency of vitamin B_{12} occurs only in strict vegans, since the vitamin is found almost exclusively in animal foods. However, functional deficiency (pernicious anemia, with spinal cord degeneration) as a result of impaired absorption is relatively common, especially in elderly people with atrophic gastritis.

Structure and vitamers

The structure of vitamin B_{12} is shown in Figure 8.13. The term corrinoid is used as a generic descriptor for cobalt-containing compounds of this general structure which, depending on the substituents in the pyrrole rings, may or may not have vitamin activity. The term "vitamin B_{12}" is used as a generic descriptor for the cobalamins, that is, those corrinoids having the biological activity of the vitamin. Some of the corrinoids that are growth factors for micro-organisms not only have no vitamin B_{12} activity, but may be antimetabolites of the vitamin.

Although cyanocobalamin was the first form in which vitamin B_{12} was isolated, it is not an important naturally occurring vitamer, but rather an artefact due to the presence of cyanide in the charcoal used in the extraction procedure. It is more stable to light than the other vitamers, and hence is commonly used in pharmaceutical preparations. Photolysis of cyanocobalamin in solution leads to the formation of aquo-cobalamin or hydroxocobalamin, depending on pH. Hydroxocobalamin is also used in pharmaceutical preparations, and is better retained after parenteral administration than is cyanocobalamin.

Vitamin B_{12} is found only in foods of animal origin, although it is also formed by some yeasts and bacteria. There are no plant sources of this vitamin. This means that strict vegetarians (vegans), who eat no foods of animal origin, are at risk of developing dietary vitamin B_{12} deficiency. The small amounts of vitamin B_{12} formed by bacteria on the surface of fruits may be adequate to meet requirements. Preparations of vitamin B_{12} made by bacterial fermentation that are ethically acceptable to vegans are readily available.

Figure 8.13 Vitamin B_{12}. Four coordination sites on the central cobalt atom are occupied by nitrogen atoms of the ring, and one by the nitrogen of the dimethylbenzimidazole side-chain. The sixth coordination site may be occupied by cyanide (cyanocobalamin), a hydroxyl ion (hydroxocobalamin), water (aquocobalamin) or a methyl group (methylcobalamin).

There are claims that yeast and some plants (especially some algae) contain vitamin B_{12}. This seems to be incorrect. The problem is that the officially recognized, and legally required, method of determining vitamin B_{12} in food analysis depends on the growth of micro-organisms for which vitamin B_{12} is an essential growth factor. However, these organisms can also use some corrinoids that have no vitamin activity. Therefore, analysis reveals the presence of something that appears to be vitamin B_{12}, but in fact is not the active vitamin and is useless in human nutrition. Biologically active vitamin B_{12} has been identified in some preparations of algae, but this seems to be the result of bacterial contamination of the lakes where the algae were harvested.

Absorption and metabolism of vitamin B_{12}

Absorption
Very small amounts of vitamin B_{12} can be absorbed by passive diffusion across the intestinal mucosa, but under normal conditions this is insignificant, accounting for less than 1% of large oral doses; the major route of vitamin B_{12} absorption is by way of attachment to a specific binding protein in the intestinal lumen.

This binding protein is intrinsic factor, so called because in the early studies of pernicious anemia it was

found that two curative factors were involved: an extrinsic or dietary factor, which is now known to be vitamin B_{12}, and an intrinsic or endogenously produced factor. Intrinsic factor is a small glycoprotein secreted by the parietal cells of the gastric mucosa, which also secrete hydrochloric acid.

Gastric acid and pepsin play a role in vitamin B_{12} nutrition, serving to release the vitamin from protein binding, and so make it available. Atrophic gastritis is a relatively common problem of advancing age; in the early stages there is failure of acid secretion but more or less normal secretion of intrinsic factor. This can result in vitamin B_{12} depletion due to failure to release the vitamin from dietary proteins, but the absorption of a test dose of free vitamin B_{12} is normal. In the stomach, vitamin B_{12} binds to cobalophilin, a binding protein secreted in the saliva.

In the duodenum cobalophilin is hydrolyzed, releasing the vitamin B_{12} for binding to intrinsic factor. Pancreatic insufficiency can therefore be a factor in the development of vitamin B_{12} deficiency, since failure to hydrolyze cobalophilin will result in the excretion of cobalophilin-bound vitamin B_{12} rather than transfer to intrinsic factor. Intrinsic factor binds the various vitamin B_{12} vitamers, but not other corrinoids.

Vitamin B_{12} is absorbed from the distal third of the ileum. There are intrinsic factor–vitamin B_{12} binding sites on the brush border of the mucosal cells in this region; neither free intrinsic factor nor free vitamin B_{12} interacts with these receptors.

In plasma, vitamin B_{12} circulates bound to transcobalamin I, which is required for tissue uptake of the vitamin, and transcobalamin II, which seems to be a storage form of the vitamin.

Enterohepatic circulation of vitamin B_{12}

There is a considerable enterohepatic circulation of vitamin B_{12}. A third plasma vitamin B_{12} binding protein, transcobalamin III, is rapidly cleared by the liver, with a plasma half-life of the order of 5 min. This provides a mechanism for returning vitamin B_{12} and its metabolites from peripheral tissues to the liver, as well as for clearance of other corrinoids without vitamin activity, which may arise from either foods or the products of intestinal bacterial action, and be absorbed passively across the lower gut.

These corrinoids are then secreted into the bile, bound to cobalophilins; 3–8 μg (2.25–6 nmol) of vitamin B_{12} may be secreted in the bile each day, about the same as the dietary intake. Like dietary vitamin B_{12} bound to salivary cobalophilin, the biliary cobalophilins are hydrolyzed in the duodenum, and the vitamin binds to intrinsic factor, so permitting reabsorption in the ileum. While cobalophilins and transcorrin III have low specificity, and will bind a variety of corrinoids, intrinsic factor binds only cobalamins, and so only the biologically active vitamin will be reabsorbed to any significant extent.

Metabolic functions of vitamin B_{12}

There are three vitamin B_{12}-dependent enzymes in human tissues: methylmalonyl-CoA mutase (discussed below under methylmalonic aciduria), leucine aminomutase and methionine synthetase (discussed in Section 8.11).

Vitamin B_{12} deficiency: pernicious anemia

Vitamin B_{12} deficiency causes pernicious anemia; the release into the bloodstream of immature precursors of red blood cells (megaloblastic anemia). As discussed below, vitamin B_{12} deficiency causes functional folate deficiency; this is what disturbs the rapid multiplication of red blood cells, causing immature precursors to be released into the circulation.

The other clinical feature of vitamin B_{12} deficiency, which is very rarely seen in folic acid deficiency, is degeneration of the spinal cord; hence the name "pernicious" for the anemia of vitamin B_{12} deficiency. The spinal cord degeneration is due to a failure of the methylation of one arginine residue on myelin basic protein, and occurs in about one-third of patients with anemia due to vitamin B_{12} deficiency, and in about one-third of patients who do not show signs of anemia.

The most common cause of pernicious anemia is failure of the absorption of vitamin B_{12}, rather than dietary deficiency. Classical pernicious anemia is due to failure of intrinsic factor secretion, commonly the result of autoimmune disease, with antibodies against either the gastric parietal cells or intrinsic factor. Atrophic gastritis with increasing age also leads to progressive failure of intrinsic factor secretion and vitamin B_{12} absorption.

Dietary deficiency of vitamin B_{12} does occur, rarely, in strict vegetarians (vegans). The rarity of vitamin B_{12} deficiency among people who have no apparent dietary source of the vitamin suggests that bacterial contamination of water and foods with vitamin B_{12}-producing organisms will provide minimally adequate amounts of the vitamin. The fruit bat develops vitamin B_{12} deficiency when fed on washed fruit under laboratory conditions, but in the wild microbial contamination of the outside of the fruit provides an adequate intake of the vitamin.

Vitamin B_{12} requirements

Most estimates of vitamin B_{12} requirements are based on the amounts given parenterally to maintain normal health in patients with pernicious anemia due to a failure of vitamin B_{12} absorption. This overestimates normal requirements, because of the enterohepatic circulation of vitamin B_{12}; in people with defective absorption, the vitamin that is excreted in the bile will be lost in the feces, whereas normally it is almost completely reabsorbed.

The total body pool of vitamin B_{12} is of the order of 2.5 mg (1.8 μmol), with a minimum desirable body pool of about 1 mg (0.3 μmol). The daily loss is about 0.1% of the body pool in subjects with normal enterohepatic circulation of the vitamin; on this basis requirements are about 1–2.5 μg/day and reference intakes for adults range between 1.4 and 2.0 μg.

Assessment of vitamin B$_{12}$ status

Measurement of plasma concentrations of vitamin B$_{12}$ is the method of choice, and several simple and reliable radioligand binding assays have been developed. A serum concentration of vitamin B$_{12}$ below 110 pmol/l is associated with megaloblastic bone marrow, incipient anemia and myelin damage. Below 150 pmol/l there are early bone-marrow changes, abnormalities of the dUMP suppression test (see Section 8.11) and methylmalonic aciduria after a valine load.

The Schilling test for vitamin B$_{12}$ absorption

The absorption of vitamin B$_{12}$ can be determined by the Schilling test. An oral dose of [^{57}Co] or [^{58}Co]vitamin B$_{12}$ is given with a parenteral flushing dose of 1 mg of nonradioactive vitamin to saturate body reserves, and the urinary excretion of radioactivity is followed as an index of absorption of the oral material. Normal subjects excrete 16–45% of the radioactivity over 24 h, while patients lacking intrinsic factor excrete less than 5%.

The test can be repeated, giving intrinsic factor orally together with the radioactive vitamin B$_{12}$; if the impaired absorption was due to a simple lack of intrinsic factor, and not to anti-intrinsic factor antibodies in saliva or gastric juice, then a normal amount of the radioactive material should be absorbed and excreted.

Methylmalonic aciduria

Methylmalonyl-CoA is formed as an intermediate in the catabolism of valine and by the carboxylation of propionyl-CoA arising in the catabolism of valine, cholesterol and (rare) fatty acids with an odd number of carbon atoms. Normally, it undergoes vitamin B$_{12}$-dependent rearrangement to succinyl-CoA, catalyzed by methylmalonyl-CoA mutase. Vitamin B$_{12}$ deficiency leads to an accumulation of methylmalonyl-CoA, some of which is hydrolyzed to yield methylmalonic acid, which is excreted in the urine. Urinary excretion of methylmalonic acid, especially after a loading dose of valine, provides a means of assessing vitamin B$_{12}$ nutritional status.

8.11 Folic acid

Folic acid functions in the transfer of one-carbon fragments in a wide variety of biosynthetic and catabolic reactions; it is therefore metabolically closely related to vitamin B$_{12}$. Deficiency of either vitamin has similar clinical effects, and the main effects of vitamin B$_{12}$ deficiency are exerted by effects on folate metabolism.

Apart from liver, the main dietary sources of folate are fruits and vegetables. Although folate is widely distributed in foods, dietary deficiency is not uncommon, and a number of commonly used drugs can cause folate depletion. More importantly, there is good evidence that intakes of folate considerably higher than normal dietary levels reduce the risk of neural tube defects, and pregnant women are recommended to take supplements. There is also evidence that high intakes of folate may be effective in reducing plasma homocysteine in subjects genetically at risk of hyperhomocystinemia (some 10–20% of the population), and hence reducing the risk of ischemic heart disease and stroke.

Vitamers and dietary equivalence

As shown in Figure 8.14, folic acid consists of a reduced pterin linked to p-aminobenzoic acid, forming pteroic acid. The carboxyl group of the p-aminobenzoic acid moiety is linked by a peptide bond to the α-amino group of glutamate, forming pteroylglutamate (PteGlu). The coenzymes may have up to seven additional glutamate residues linked by γ-peptide bonds, forming pteroyldiglutamate (PteGlu$_2$), pteroyltriglutamate (PteGlu$_3$), etc., collectively known as folate or pteroyl polyglutamate conjugates (PteGlu$_n$).

"Folate" is the preferred trivial name for pteroylglutamate, although both "folate" and "folic acid" may be used as a generic descriptor to include various polyglutamates. PteGlu$_2$ is sometimes referred to as folic acid diglutamate, PteGlu$_3$ as folic acid triglutamate, and so on.

Tetrahydrofolate can carry one-carbon fragments attached to N-5 (formyl, formimino or methyl groups), N-10 (formyl) or bridging N-5–N-10 (methylene or

Tetrahydrofolate (THF)

Figure 8.14 Tetrahydrofolate (folic acid).

methenyl groups). 5-Formyl-tetrahydrofolate is more stable to atmospheric oxidation than is folate, and is therefore commonly used in pharmaceutical preparations; it is also known as folinic acid, and the synthetic (racemic) compound as leucovorin.

The extent to which the different forms of folate can be absorbed varies; on average only about half of the folate in the diet is available, compared with more or less complete availability of the monoglutamate. To permit calculation of folate intakes, the dietary folate equivalent has been defined as 1 μg mixed food folates or 0.6 μg free folic acid. On this basis, total dietary folate equivalents = μg food folate + 1.7 × synthetic (free) folic acid.

Absorption and metabolism of folate

About 80% of dietary folate is as polyglutamates; a variable amount may be substituted with various one-carbon fragments or be present as dihydrofolate derivatives. Folate conjugates are hydrolyzed in the small intestine by conjugase (pteroylpolyglutamate hydrolase), a zinc-dependent enzyme of the pancreatic juice, bile and mucosal brush border; zinc deficiency can impair folate absorption.

Free folate, released by conjugase action, is absorbed by active transport in the jejunum. The folate in milk is mainly bound to a specific binding protein; the protein–tetrahydrofolate complex is absorbed intact, mainly in the ileum, by a mechanism that is distinct from the active transport system for the absorption of free folate. The biological availability of folate from milk, or of folate from diets to which milk has been added, is considerably greater than that of unbound folate.

Much of the dietary folate undergoes methylation and reduction within the intestinal mucosa, so that what enters the portal bloodstream is largely 5-methyl-tetrahydrofolate. Other substituted and unsubstituted folate monoglutamates, and dihydrofolate, are also absorbed; they are reduced and methylated in the liver, then secreted in the bile. The liver also takes up various folates released by tissues; again, these are reduced, methylated and secreted in the bile.

The total daily enterohepatic circulation of folate is equivalent to about one-third of the dietary intake. Despite this, there is very little fecal loss of folate; jejunal absorption of methyl-tetrahydrofolate is a very efficient process, and the fecal excretion of some 450 nmol (200 μg) of folates per day represents synthesis

by intestinal flora and does not reflect intake to any significant extent.

Tissue uptake of folate

Methyl-tetrahydrofolate circulates bound to albumin, and is available for uptake by extrahepatic tissues, where it is trapped by formation of polyglutamates, which do not cross cell membranes.

The main circulating folate is methyl-tetrahydrofolate, which is a poor substrate for polyglutamylation; demethylation by the action of methionine synthetase (see below) is required for effective metabolic trapping of folate. In vitamin B_{12} deficiency, when methionine synthetase activity is impaired, there will therefore be impairment of the uptake of folate into tissues.

Folate excretion

There is very little urinary loss of folate, only some 5–10 nmol/day. Not only is most folate in plasma bound to proteins (either folate binding protein for unsubstituted folate or albumin for methyltetrahydrofolate), and thus protected from glomerular filtration, but the renal brush border has a high concentration of folate binding protein which acts to reabsorb any filtered in the urine.

The catabolism of folate is largely by cleavage of the C-9–N-10 bond, catalyzed by carboxypeptidase G. The p-aminobenzoic acid moiety is amidated and excreted in the urine as p-acetamidobenzoate and p-acetamidobenzoyl-glutamate; pterin is excreted either unchanged or as a variety of biologically inactive compounds.

Metabolic functions of folate

The metabolic role of folate is as a carrier of one-carbon fragments, both in catabolism and in biosynthetic reactions. These may be carried as formyl, formimino, methyl or methylene residues. The major sources of these one-carbon fragments and their major uses, as well as the interconversions of the substituted folates, are shown in Figure 8.15.

The major point of entry for one-carbon fragments into substituted folates is methylene-tetrahydrofolate, which is formed by the catabolism of glycine, serine and choline. Serine is the most important source of substituted folates for biosynthetic reactions, and the activity of serine hydroxymethyltransferase is regulated by the state of folate substitution and the availability of folate. The reaction is freely reversible, and under

Sources of one-carbon fragments   **Uses of one-carbon fragments**

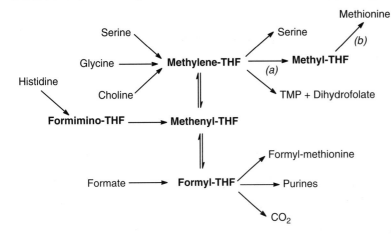

Figure 8.15 Interconversion of the principal one-carbon substituted folates; sources of one-carbon fragments are shown on the left, and pathways in which one-carbon units are used and free tetrahydrofolate is regenerated on the right. (a) Methylene-tetrahydrofolate reductase (EC 1.5.1.20); (b) methionine synthetase (EC 2.1.1.13).

appropriate conditions in liver it functions to form serine from glycine, as a substrate for gluconeogenesis.

Methylene-, methenyl- and 10-formyl-tetrahydrofolates are freely interconvertible. This means that when one-carbon folates are not required for synthetic reactions, the oxidation of formyl-tetrahydrofolate to carbon dioxide and folate provides a means of maintaining an adequate tissue pool of free folate.

By contrast, the reduction of methylene-tetrahydrofolate to methyl-tetrahydrofolate is irreversible, and the only way in which free folate can be formed from methyl-tetrahydrofolate is by the reaction of methionine synthetase (see below).

Thymidylate synthetase and dihydrofolate reductase
The methylation of deoxyuridine monophosphate (dUMP) to thymidine monophosphate (TMP), catalyzed by thymidylate synthetase, is essential for the synthesis of DNA, although preformed TMP can be reutilized by salvage from the catabolism of DNA.

The methyl donor is methylene-tetrahydrofolate; the reaction involves reduction of the one-carbon fragment to a methyl group at the expense of the folate, which is oxidized to dihydrofolate. Dihydrofolate is then reduced to tetrahydrofolate by dihydrofolate reductase.

Thymidylate synthase and dihydrofolate reductase are especially active in tissues with a high rate of cell division, and hence a high rate of DNA replication and a high requirement for thymidylate. Because of this, inhibitors of dihydrofolate reductase have been exploited as anticancer drugs such as methotrexate. Chemotherapy consists of alternating periods of administration of methotrexate and folate (normally as 5-formyl-tetrahydrofolate, leucovorin) to replete the normal tissues and avoid induction of folate deficiency; this is known as leucovorin rescue.

Methionine synthetase and the methyl-folate trap
In addition to its role in the synthesis of proteins, methionine, as the S-adenosyl derivative, acts as a methyl donor in a wide variety of biosynthetic reactions. As shown in Figure 8.16, the resultant homocysteine may be either metabolized to yield cysteine or remethylated to yield methionine.

Two enzymes catalyze the methylation of homocysteine to methionine.

- Methionine synthetase is a vitamin B_{12}-dependent enzyme, for which the methyl donor is methyl-tetrahydrofolate.
- Homocysteine methyltransferase utilizes betaine (an intermediate in the catabolism of choline) as the methyl donor, and is not vitamin B_{12} dependent.

Both enzymes are found in most tissues, but only the vitamin B_{12}-dependent methionine synthetase is found in the central nervous system.

The reduction of methylene-tetrahydrofolate to methyl-tetrahydrofolate is irreversible, and the major source of folate for tissues is methyl-tetrahydrofolate. The only metabolic role of methyl-tetrahydrofolate is the methylation of homocysteine to methionine, and

Figure 8.16 Methionine metabolism. Methionine synthetase (EC 2.1.1.13), methionine adenosyltransferase (EC 2.5.1.6), cystathionine synthetase (EC 4.2.1.22), cystathionase (EC 4.4.1.1).

this is the only way in which methyl-tetrahydrofolate can be demethylated to yield free folate in tissues. Methionine synthetase thus provides the link between the physiological functions of folate and vitamin B_{12}. Impairment of methionine synthetase activity in vitamin B_{12} deficiency will result in the accumulation of methyl-tetrahydrofolate, which can neither be utilized for any other one-carbon transfer reactions nor be demethylated to provide free folate.

This functional deficiency of folate is exacerbated by low tissue concentrations of methionine and an accumulation of homocysteine, since the transulfuration pathway from homocysteine to form cysteine is regulated by the availability of cysteine: it is a biosynthetic pathway rather than a pathway for disposal of methionine and homocysteine.

Methylene-tetrahydrofolate reductase and hyperhomocysteinemia

Elevated blood homocysteine is a significant risk factor for atherosclerosis, thrombosis and hypertension, independent of factors such as dietary lipids and plasma lipoproteins. About 10–15% of the population, and almost 30% of people with ischemic heart disease, have an abnormal variant of methylene-tetrahydrofolate reductase which is unstable, and loses activity more quickly than normal. The result of this is that people with the abnormal form of the enzyme have an impaired ability to form methyl-tetrahydrofolate (the main form in which folate is taken up by tissues) and suffer from functional folate deficiency. Therefore, they are unable to remethylate homocysteine to methionine adequately, and develop hyperhomocysteinemia.

People with the abnormal variant of methylene-tetrahydrofolate reductase do not develop hyperhomocysteinemia if they have a relatively high intake of folate. This seems to be due to the methylation of folate in the intestinal mucosa during absorption; intestinal mucosal cells have a rapid turnover (some 48 h between proliferation in the crypts and shedding at the tip of the villus), and therefore it is not important that methylene-tetrahydrofolate reductase is less stable than normal, as there is still an adequate activity of the enzyme in the intestinal mucosa to maintain a normal circulating level of methyl-tetrahydrofolate.

This has led to the suggestion that supplements of folate will reduce the incidence of cardiovascular disease; to date there is no evidence from intervention studies that the lowering of plasma homocysteine by folate supplements does reduce the risk, but mandatory enrichment of foods with folate has been introduced in some countries.

Folate deficiency: megaloblastic anemia

Dietary deficiency of folic acid is not uncommon and, as noted above, deficiency of vitamin B_{12} also leads to functional folic acid deficiency. In either case, it is cells that are dividing rapidly, and therefore have a large requirement for thymidine for DNA synthesis, that are most severely affected. These are the cells of the bone marrow which form red blood cells, the cells of the intestinal mucosa and the hair follicles. Clinically, folic acid deficiency leads to megaloblastic anemia, the release into the circulation of immature precursors of red blood cells.

Megaloblastic anemia is also seen in vitamin B_{12} deficiency, where it is due to functional folate deficiency as a result of trapping folate as methyl-tetrahydrofolate. However, the neurological degeneration of pernicious anemia is rarely seen in folate deficiency, and indeed a high intake of folate can mask the development of megaloblastic anemia in vitamin B_{12} deficiency, so that the presenting sign is irreversible nerve damage.

Folate requirements

Depletion/repletion studies to determine folate requirements using folate monoglutamate suggest a requirement

of the order of 80–100 μg (170–220 nmol)/day. The total body pool of folate in adults is some 17 μmol (7.5 mg), with a biological half-life of 101 days. This suggests a minimum requirement for replacement of 37 μg (85 nmol)/day. Studies of the urinary excretion of folate metabolites in subjects maintained on folate-free diets suggest that there is catabolism of some 80 μg (170 nmol) of folate/day.

Because of the problems in determining the biological availability of the various folate polyglutamate conjugates found in foods, reference intakes allow a wide margin of safety, and are based on an allowance of 3 μg (6.8 nmol)/kg body weight.

Folate in pregnancy
During the 1980s a considerable body of evidence accumulated that spina bifida and other neural tube defects (which occur in about 0.75–1% of pregnancies) were associated with low intakes of folate, and that increased intake during pregnancy might be protective. It is now established that supplements of folate begun periconceptually result in a significant reduction in the incidence of neural tube defects, and it is recommended that intakes be increased by 400 μg/day before conception. The studies were conducted using folate monoglutamate and it is unlikely that an equivalent increase in intake could be achieved from unfortified foods; therefore supplements are recommended. Closure of the neural tube occurs by day 28 of pregnancy, which is before the woman knows she is pregnant. The advice therefore is that all women who are, or may be about to become, pregnant, should take folate supplements.

Assessment of folate status

Measurement of the serum or red blood cell concentration of folate is the method of choice, and several simple and reliable radioligand binding assays have been developed. There are problems involved in radioligand binding assays for folate, and in some centers microbiological determination of plasma or whole blood folates is the preferred technique. Serum folate below 7 nmol/l or erythrocyte folate below 320 nmol/l indicates negative folate balance and early depletion of body reserves. At this stage the first bone-marrow changes are detectable.

Histidine metabolism: the FIGLU test
The ability to metabolize a test dose of histidine provides a sensitive functional test of folate nutritional

status; formiminoglutamate (FIGLU) is an intermediate in histidine catabolism, and is metabolized by the folate-dependent enzyme formiminoglutamate formimino-transferase. In folate deficiency the activity of this enzyme is impaired, and FIGLU accumulates and is excreted in the urine, especially after a test dose of histidine: the so-called FIGLU test.

Although the FIGLU test depends on folate nutritional status, the metabolism of histidine will also be impaired, and hence a positive result obtained, in vitamin B_{12} deficiency, because of the secondary deficiency of free folate. About 60% of vitamin B_{12}-deficient subjects show increased FIGLU excretion after a histidine load.

The dUMP suppression test

Rapidly dividing cells can either use preformed TMP for DNA synthesis, or synthesize it *de novo* from dUMP. Stimulated lymphocytes incubated with [^{3}H]TMP will incorporate label into DNA. In the presence of adequate amounts of methylene-tetrahydrofolate, the addition of dUMP as a substrate for thymidylate synthetase reduces the incorporation of [^{3}H]TMP as a result of dilution of the pool of labeled material by newly synthesized TMP and inhibition of thymidylate kinase by thymidine triphosphate.

In normal cells the incorporation of [^{3}H]thymidine into DNA after preincubation with dUMP is 1.4–1.8% of that without preincubation. By contrast, cells that are deficient in folate form little or no thymidine from dUMP, and hence incorporate nearly as much of the [^{3}H]thymidine after incubation with dUMP as they do without preincubation.

Either a primary deficiency of folic acid or functional deficiency secondary to vitamin B_{12} deficiency will have the same effect. In folate deficiency, addition of any biologically active form of folate, but not vitamin B_{12}, will normalize the dUMP suppression of [^{3}H]thymidine incorporation. In vitamin B_{12} deficiency, addition of vitamin B_{12} or methylene-tetrahydrofolate, but not methyl-tetrahydrofolate, will normalize dUMP suppression.

Drug–nutrient interactions of folate

Several folate antimetabolites are used clinically, as cancer chemotherapy (e.g. methotrexate), and as antibacterial (trimethoprim) and antimalarial (pyrimethamine) agents; they act as inhibitors of dihydrofolate reductase. Although drugs such as trimethoprim and pyrimethamine owe much of their clinical usefulness to considerably higher affinity for the dihydrofolate reductase of the target organism than the human enzyme, their prolonged use can result in folate deficiency.

A number of antiepileptic drugs, including diphenylhydantoin (phenytoin), and sometimes phenobarbital and primidone, can also cause folate deficiency. While overt megaloblastic anemia affects only some 0.75% of treated epileptics, there is some degree of macrocytosis in 40%. The megaloblastosis responds to folic acid supplements, but in about 50% of such patients treated with relatively high supplements for 1–3 years there is an increase in the frequency of epileptic fits.

Folate toxicity

Folate supplements of 400 μg/day reduce the incidence of spina bifida and neural tube defect; about 1% of pregnant women are at risk. Similar supplements lower plasma homocysteine in people with the abnormal variant of methylene-tetrahydrofolate reductase; between 10% and 20% of the population are homozygous for the abnormal gene.

There is some evidence that folate supplements in excess of 350 μg/day may impair zinc absorption. In addition, there are two potential problems that have to be considered when advocating either widespread use of folate supplements or enrichment of foods with folate for protection against heart disease and neural tube defect.

- Folate supplements will mask the megaloblastic anemia of vitamin B_{12} deficiency, and may hasten the development of the (irreversible) nerve damage. This is especially a problem of the elderly, who may suffer impaired absorption of vitamin B_{12} as a result of gastric atrophy with increasing age. It has been suggested that the addition of relatively large amounts of vitamin B_{12} to foods, as well as folate, would permit passive absorption of adequate amounts of vitamin B_{12} to prevent deficiency developing.
- Antagonism between folic acid and the anticonvulsants used in the treatment of epilepsy is part of their mechanism of action; about 2% of the population have (drug-controlled) epilepsy. Relatively large supplements of folic acid (in excess of 1000 μg/day) may antagonize the beneficial effects of the anticonvulsants and lead to an increase in the frequency of epileptic attacks. If enrichment of a food such as

bread with folate is to provide 400 μg/day to those who eat little bread, those who eat a relatively large amount may well have an intake in excess of 1000 μg/day.

8.12 Biotin

Biotin was originally discovered as part of the complex called *bios*, which promoted the growth of yeast and, separately, as vitamin H, the protective or curative factor in "egg white injury", the disease caused in humans and experimental animals by feeding diets containing large amounts of uncooked egg white. The structures of biotin, biocytin and carboxybiocytin (the active metabolic intermediate) are shown in Figure 8.17.

Biotin is widely distributed in many foods. It is synthesized by intestinal flora, and in balance studies the

Figure 8.17 Biotin, biotinyl-lysine (biocytin) and the role of biocytin as a carbon dioxide carrier.

total output of biotin in urine plus feces is three to six times greater than the intake, reflecting bacterial synthesis. It is not known to what extent this is available to the host.

Absorption and metabolism of biotin

Most biotin in foods is present as biocytin (ε-amino-biotinyllysine), which is released on proteolysis, then hydrolyzed by biotinidase in the pancreatic juice and intestinal mucosal secretions, to yield free biotin. The extent to which bound biotin in foods is biologically available is not known.

Free biotin is absorbed from the small intestine by active transport. Biotin circulates in the bloodstream both free and bound to a serum glycoprotein that has biotinidase activity, catalyzing the hydrolysis of biocytin.

Biotin enters tissues by a saturable transport system and is then incorporated into biotin-dependent enzymes as the ε-amino-lysine peptide, biocytin. Unlike other B vitamins, where concentrative uptake into tissues can be achieved by facilitated diffusion followed by metabolic trapping, the incorporation of biotin into enzymes is relatively slow, and cannot be considered part of the uptake process. On catabolism of the enzymes, biocytin is hydrolyzed by biotinidase, permitting reutilization.

Metabolic functions of biotin

Biotin functions to transfer carbon dioxide in a small number of carboxylation reactions. The reactive intermediate is 1-N-carboxy-biocytin (see Figure 8.17), formed from bicarbonate in an ATP-dependent reaction. A single enzyme acts on the apoenzymes of acetyl-CoA carboxylase, pyruvate carboxylase, propionyl-CoA carboxylase and methylcrotonyl-CoA carboxylase, to form the active holoenzymes from (inactive) apoenzymes and free biotin.

Biotin also has a role in the control of the cell cycle, by biotinylation of key nuclear proteins.

Biotin deficiency and requirements

Biotin is widely distributed in foods and deficiency is unknown, except among people maintained for many months on total parenteral nutrition, and a very small number of people who eat large amounts of uncooked egg. Avidin, a protein in egg white, binds biotin extremely tightly and renders it unavailable for absorption. Avidin is denatured by cooking and then loses its ability to bind biotin. The amount of avidin in uncooked egg white is relatively small, and problems of biotin deficiency have only occurred in people eating a dozen or more raw eggs a day, for some years.

The few early reports of human biotin deficiency are all of people who consumed large amounts of uncooked eggs. They developed a fine scaly dermatitis and hair loss (alopecia). Histology of the skin showed an absence of sebaceous glands and atrophy of the hair follicles. Provision of biotin supplements of 200–1000 μg/day resulted in cure of the skin lesions and regrowth of hair, despite continuing the abnormal diet providing large amounts of avidin. There have been no studies of provision of modest doses of biotin to such patients, and none in which their high intake of uncooked eggs was not either replaced by an equivalent intake of cooked eggs (in which avidin has been denatured by heat, and the yolks of which are a good source of biotin) or continued unchanged, so there is no information from these case reports of the amounts of biotin required for normal health. More recently, similar signs of biotin deficiency have been observed in patients receiving total parenteral nutrition for prolonged periods, after major resection of the gut. The signs resolve following the provision of biotin, but again there have been no studies of the amounts of biotin required; intakes have ranged between 60 and 200 μg/day.

Glucose metabolism in biotin deficiency

The impairment of pyruvate carboxylase in biotin deficiency results in impaired gluconeogenesis, and hence fasting hypoglycemia. In addition, biotin deficiency results in a lowering of the NADH : NAD ratio, and hence further reduction of gluconeogenesis by impairment of glyceraldehyde-3-phosphate dehydrogenase activity.

Rather than the expected hypoglycemia, biotin deficiency may sometimes be associated with hyperglycemia. This seems to be due to reduction of hepatic glucokinase to less than half the normal activity. Biotin induces glucokinase and also increases the activity of two other key enzymes of glycolysis, phosphofructokinase and pyruvate kinase.

Lipid metabolism in biotin deficiency

The skin lesions of biotin deficiency are similar to those seen in deficiency of essential fatty acids, and serum linoleic acid is lower than normal in biotin-deficient patients, owing to impairment of the elongation of PUFA as a result of reduced activity of acetyl-CoA carboxylase.

The impairment of lipogenesis also affects the tissue fatty acid composition, with an increase in the proportion of palmitoleic acid, mainly at the expense of stearic acid, apparently as a result of increased fatty acid desaturase activity in biotin deficiency. While dietary protein and fat intake also affect tissue fatty acid composition, the ratio of palmitoleic to stearic acid may provide a useful index of biotin nutritional status in some circumstances.

Biotin deficiency also results in an increase in the normally small amounts of odd-chain fatty acids (mainly C15:0 and C17:0) in triacylglycerols, phospholipids and cholesterol esters. This is a result of impaired activity of propionyl-CoA carboxylase, leading to an accumulation of propionyl-CoA, which can be incorporated into lipids in competition with acetyl-CoA.

Safe and adequate levels of intake

There is no evidence on which to estimate requirements for biotin. Average intakes are between 10 and 200 μg/day. Since dietary deficiency does not occur, such intakes are obviously more than adequate to meet requirements.

8.13 Pantothenic acid

Pantothenic acid (sometimes known as vitamin B_5, and at one time called vitamin B_3) has a central role in energy-yielding metabolism as the functional moiety of CoA and in the biosynthesis of fatty acids as the prosthetic group of acyl carrier protein. The structures of pantothenic acid and CoA are shown in Figure 8.18.

Pantothenic acid is widely distributed in all foodstuffs; the name derives from the Greek for "from everywhere", as opposed to other vitamins, which were originally isolated from individual especially rich sources. As a result, deficiency has not been unequivocally reported in humans except in specific depletion studies, which have generally used the antagonist ω-methyl-pantothenic acid.

Absorption, metabolism, and metabolic functions of pantothenic acid

About 85% of dietary pantothenic acid is as CoA and phosphopantetheine. In the intestinal lumen these are hydrolyzed to pantetheine; intestinal mucosal cells have a high pantetheinase activity and

Pantothenic acid   Coenzyme A (CoASH)

Figure 8.18 Pantothenic acid and coenzyme A.

rapidly hydrolyze pantetheine to pantothenic acid. The intestinal absorption of pantothenic acid seems to be by simple diffusion and occurs at a constant rate throughout the length of the small intestine; bacterial synthesis may contribute to pantothenic acid nutrition.

The first step in pantothenic acid utilization is phosphorylation. Pantothenate kinase is rate limiting, so that, unlike many vitamins which are accumulated by metabolic trapping, there can be significant accumulation of free pantothenic acid in tissues. It is then used for synthesis of CoA and the prosthetic group of acyl carrier protein. Pantothenic acid arising from the turnover of CoA and acyl carrier protein may be either reused or excreted unchanged in the urine.

Coenzyme A and acyl carrier protein

All tissues are capable of forming CoA from pantothenic acid. CoA functions as the carrier of fatty acids, as thio-esters, in mitochondrial β-oxidation. The resultant two-carbon fragments, as acetyl-CoA, then undergo oxidation in the citric acid cycle. CoA also functions as a carrier in the transfer of acetyl (and other fatty acyl) moieties in a variety of biosynthetic and catabolic reactions, including:

- cholesterol and steroid hormone synthesis
- long-chain fatty acid synthesis from palmitate and elongation of PUFA in mitochondria
- acylation of serine, threonine and cysteine residues on proteolipids, and acetylation of neuraminic acid.

Fatty acid synthesis is catalyzed by a cytosolic multienzyme complex in which the growing fatty acyl chain is bound by thio-ester linkage to an enzyme-bound 4′-phosphopantetheine residue, rather than to free CoA, as in β-oxidation. This component of the fatty acid synthetase complex is the acyl carrier protein.

Pantothenic acid deficiency and safe and adequate levels of intake

Prisoners of war in the Far East in the 1940s, who were severely malnourished, showed, among other signs and symptoms of vitamin deficiency diseases, a new condition of paresthesia and severe pain in the feet and toes, which was called the "burning foot syndrome" or nutritional melalgia. Although it was tentatively attributed to pantothenic acid deficiency, no specific trials of pantothenic acid were carried out, rather the subjects were given yeast extract and other rich sources of all vitamins as part of an urgent program of nutritional rehabilitation.

Experimental pantothenic acid depletion, commonly together with the administration of ω-methylpantothenic acid, results in the following signs and symptoms after 2–3 weeks:

- neuromotor disorders, including paresthesia of the hands and feet, hyperactive deep tendon reflexes and muscle weakness. These can be explained by the role of acetyl-CoA in the synthesis of the neurotransmitter acetylcholine, and impaired formation of threonine acyl esters in myelin. Dysmyelination may explain the persistence and recurrence of neurological problems many years after nutritional rehabilitation in people who had suffered from burning foot syndrome;

- mental depression, which again may be related to either acetylcholine deficit or impaired myelin synthesis;
- gastrointestinal complaints, including severe vomiting and pain, with depressed gastric acid secretion in response to gastrin;
- increased insulin sensitivity and a flattened glucose tolerance curve, which may reflect decreased antagonism by glucocorticoids;
- decreased serum cholesterol and decreased urinary excretion of 17-ketosteroids, reflecting the impairment of steroidogenesis;
- decreased acetylation of *p*-aminobenzoic acid, sulfonamides and other drugs, reflecting reduced availability of acetyl-CoA for these reactions;
- increased susceptibility to upper respiratory tract infections.

There is no evidence on which to estimate pantothenic acid requirements. Average intakes are between 3 and 7 mg/day, and since deficiency does not occur, such intakes are obviously more than adequate to meet requirements.

Nonnutritional uses of pantothenic acid

Blood levels of pantothenic acid have been reported to be low in patients with rheumatoid arthritis; some workers have reported apparently beneficial effects of supplementation, but these reports remain unconfirmed and there are no established pharmacological uses of the vitamin.

Pantothenic acid deficiency in rats leads to a loss of fur color and at one time pantothenic acid was known as the "anti-grey hair factor". There is no evidence that the normal greying of hair with age is related to pantothenic acid nutrition, or that pantothenic acid supplements have any effect on hair color. Its use in shampoo is not based on any evidence of efficacy.

Pantothenic acid has very low toxicity; intakes of up to 10 g of calcium pantothenate/day (compared with a normal dietary intake of 2–7 mg/day) have been given for up to 6 weeks with no apparent ill-effects.

8.14 Vitamin C (ascorbic acid)

Vitamin C is a vitamin for only a limited number of vertebrate species: humans and the other primates, the guinea-pig, bats, the passeriform birds and most fishes. Ascorbate is synthesized as an intermediate in the gulonolactone pathway of glucose metabolism; in those vertebrate species for which it is a vitamin, one enzyme of the pathway, gulonolactone oxidase, is absent.

The vitamin C deficiency disease, scurvy, has been known for many centuries and was described in the Ebers papyrus of 1500 BC and by Hippocrates. The Crusaders are said to have lost more men through scurvy than were killed in battle, while in some of the long voyages of exploration of the fourteenth and fifteenth centuries up to 90% of the crew died from scurvy. Cartier's expedition to Quebec in 1535 was struck by scurvy; the local Indians taught him to use an infusion of swamp spruce leaves to prevent or cure the condition.

Recognition that scurvy was due to a dietary deficiency came relatively early. James Lind demonstrated in 1757 that orange juice and lemon juice were protective, and Cook kept his crew in good health during his circumnavigation of the globe (1772–1775) by stopping frequently to take on fresh fruit and vegetables. In 1804 the British Navy decreed a daily ration of lemon or lime juice for all ratings, a requirement that was extended to the merchant navy in 1865.

The structure and metabolic interconversions of vitamin C are shown in Figure 8.19; both ascorbic acid and dehydroascorbic acid have vitamin activity.

Vitamin C is found in fruits and vegetables. Very significant losses of vitamin C occur as vegetables wilt, or when they are cut, as a result of release of ascorbate oxidase from the plant tissue. Significant losses of the vitamin also occur in cooking, both through leaching into the cooking water and also atmospheric oxidation, which continues when foods are left to stand before serving.

Absorption and metabolism of vitamin C

There is active transport of the vitamin at the intestinal mucosal brush border membrane. Both ascorbate and dehydroascorbate are absorbed across the buccal mucosa by carrier-mediated passive processes. Intestinal absorption of dehydroascorbate is carrier mediated, followed by reduction to ascorbate before transport across the basolateral membrane.

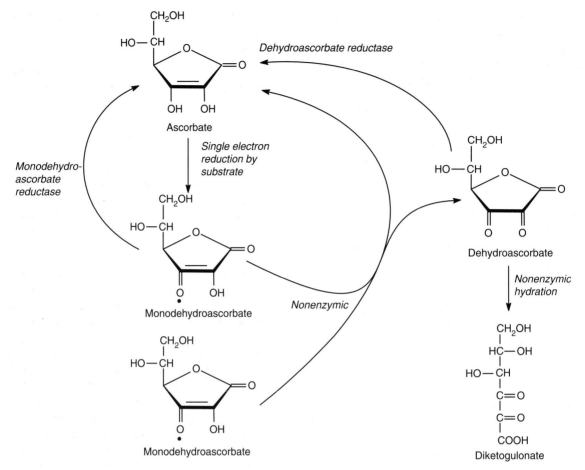

Figure 8.19 Oxidation of vitamin C (ascorbic acid). Monodehydroascorbate may undergo either enzymic reduction to ascorbate, or 2 moles may react together nonenzymically to form ascorbate and dehydroascorbate. Dehydroascorbate reductase (monodehydroascorbate reductase) (EC 1.6.5.4).

Some 80–95% of dietary ascorbate is absorbed at usual intakes (up to about 100 mg/day). The absorption of larger amounts of the vitamin is lower, and unabsorbed ascorbate from very high doses is a substrate for intestinal bacterial metabolism, causing gastrointestinal discomfort and diarrhea.

About 70% of blood ascorbate is in plasma and erythrocytes, which do not concentrate the vitamin from plasma. The remainder is in white cells, which have a marked ability to concentrate it.

Both ascorbate and dehydroascorbate circulate in free solution, and also bound to albumin. About 5% of plasma vitamin C is normally dehydroascorbate. Both vitamers are transported into cells by the glucose transporter, and concentrations of glucose of the order of those seen in diabetic hyperglycemia can inhibit ascorbate uptake significantly.

There is no specific storage organ for ascorbate; apart from leukocytes (which account for only 10% of total blood ascorbate), the only tissues showing a significant concentration of the vitamin are the adrenal and pituitary glands. Although the concentration of ascorbate in muscle is relatively low, skeletal muscle contains much of the body's pool of 900–1500 mg (5–8.5 mmol).

Dehydroascorbate can undergo metabolism to xylose, thus providing a route for entry into central carbohydrate metabolic pathways via the pentose phosphate pathway. However, oxidation to carbon dioxide is only a minor fate of ascorbate in humans. At usual intakes of the vitamin less than 1% of the radioactivity from [^{14}C]ascorbate is recovered as carbon dioxide. While more $^{14}CO_2$ is recovered from subjects receiving high intakes of the vitamin, this is the result of bacterial metabolism of unabsorbed vitamin in the intestinal lumen.

The fate of the greater part of ascorbic acid is excretion in the urine, either unchanged or as dehydroascorbate and diketogulonate. Both ascorbate and dehydroascorbate are filtered at the glomerulus, then reabsorbed. When glomerular filtration of ascorbate and dehydroascorbate exceeds the capacity of the transport systems, at a plasma concentration of ascorbate between 70 and 85 μmol/l, the vitamin is excreted in the urine in amounts proportional to intake.

Metabolic functions of vitamin C

Ascorbic acid has specific roles in two groups of enzymes: the copper-containing hydroxylases and the 2-oxoglutarate-linked iron-containing hydroxylases. It also increases the activity of a number of other enzymes *in vitro*, although this is a nonspecific reducing action rather than reflecting any metabolic function of the vitamin. In addition, it has a number of nonenzymic effects due to its action as a reducing agent and oxygen radical quencher.

Copper-containing hydroxylases
Dopamine β-hydroxylase is a copper-containing enzyme involved in the synthesis of the catecholamines noradrenaline and adrenaline from tyrosine in the adrenal medulla and central nervous system. The enzyme contains Cu^+, which is oxidized to Cu^{2+} during the hydroxylation of the substrate; reduction back to Cu^+ specifically requires ascorbate, which is oxidized to monodehydroascorbate.

Some peptide hormones have a carboxy-terminal amide that is hydroxylated on the α-carbon by a copper-containing enzyme, peptidylglycine hydroxylase. The α-hydroxyglycine residue then decomposes nonenzymically to yield the amidated peptide and glyoxylate. The copper prosthetic group is oxidized in the reaction, and as in dopamine β-hydroxylase, ascorbate is specifically required for reduction back to Cu^+.

Oxoglutarate-linked iron-containing hydroxylases
Several iron-containing hydroxylases share a common reaction mechanism, in which hydroxylation of the substrate is linked to decarboxylation of 2-oxoglutarate. Many of these enzymes are involved in the modification of precursor proteins to yield the final, mature, protein. This is a process of postsynthetic modification, that is,

modification of an amino acid residue after it has been incorporated into the protein during synthesis on the ribosome.

- Proline and lysine hydroxylases are required for the postsynthetic modification of procollagen in the formation of mature, insoluble, collagen, and proline hydroxylase is also required for the postsynthetic modification of the precursor proteins of osteocalcin and the C1q component of complement.
- Aspartate β-hydroxylase is required for the postsynthetic modification of the precursor of protein C, the vitamin K-dependent protease that hydrolyzes activated factor V in the blood-clotting cascade.
- Trimethyl-lysine and γ-butyrobetaine hydroxylases are required for the synthesis of carnitine.

Ascorbate is oxidized during the reaction of these enzymes, but not stoichiometrically with the decarboxylation of 2-oxoglutarate and hydroxylation of the substrate. The purified enzyme is active in the absence of ascorbate, but after some 5–10 s (about 15–30 cycles of enzyme action) the rate of reaction begins to fall. At this stage the iron in the catalytic site has been oxidized to Fe^{3+}, which is catalytically inactive; activity is restored only by ascorbate, which reduces it back to Fe^{2+}. The oxidation of Fe^{2+} is the consequence of a side-reaction rather than the main reaction of the enzyme, which explains how 15–30 cycles of enzyme activity can occur before there is significant loss of activity in the absence of ascorbate, and why the consumption of ascorbate is not stoichiometric.

Pro-oxidant and antioxidant roles of ascorbate
Ascorbate can act as a radical-trapping antioxidant, reacting with superoxide and a proton to yield hydrogen peroxide, or with the hydroxy radical to yield water. In each instance the product is the monodehydroascorbate radical. Thus, as well as reducing the tocopheroxyl radical formed by interaction of α-tocopherol in membranes with lipid peroxides, ascorbate acts to trap the oxygen radicals that would otherwise react to form lipid peroxides.

At high concentrations, ascorbate can reduce molecular oxygen to superoxide, being oxidized to monodehydroascorbate. At physiological concentrations of ascorbate, both Fe^{3+} and Cu^{2+} ions are reduced by ascorbate, yielding monodehydroascorbate. Fe^{2+} and Cu^+ are readily reoxidized by reaction with hydrogen peroxide to yield hydroxide ions and hydroxyl radicals.

Cu^+ also reacts with molecular oxygen to yield superoxide. Thus, as well as its antioxidant role, ascorbate has potential pro-oxidant activity, and the net result will depend on the relative rates of formation of superoxide and hydroxyl radicals by autoxidation and metal-catalyzed reactions of ascorbate, and the trapping of these radicals by ascorbate.

Vitamin C deficiency: scurvy

The vitamin C deficiency disease, scurvy, was formerly a common problem at the end of winter, when there had been no fresh fruits and vegetables for many months.

Although there is no specific organ for storage of vitamin C in the body, signs of deficiency do not develop in previously adequately nourished subjects until they have been deprived of the vitamin for 4–6 months, by which time plasma and tissue concentrations have fallen considerably. The earliest signs of scurvy in volunteers maintained on a vitamin C-free diet are skin changes, beginning with plugging of hair follicles by horny material, followed by enlargement of the hyperkeratotic follicles and petechial hemorrhage, with significant extravasation of red cells, presumably as a result of the increased fragility of blood capillaries.

At a later stage there is also hemorrhage of the gums, beginning in the interdental papillae and progressing to generalized sponginess and bleeding. This is frequently accompanied by secondary bacterial infection and considerable withdrawal of the gum from the necks of the teeth. As the condition progresses, there is loss of dental cement, and the teeth become loose in the alveolar bone and may be lost.

Wounds show only superficial healing in scurvy, with little or no formation of (collagen-rich) scar tissue, so that healing is delayed and wounds can readily be reopened. The scorbutic scar tissue has only about half the tensile strength of that normally formed.

Advanced scurvy is accompanied by intense pain in the bones, which can be attributed to changes in bone mineralization as a result of abnormal collagen synthesis. Bone formation ceases and the existing bone becomes rarefied, so that the bones fracture with minimal trauma.

The name scurvy is derived from the Italian *scorbutico*, meaning an irritable, neurotic, discontented, whining and cranky person. The disease is associated with listlessness and general malaise, and sometimes changes in personality and psychomotor performance and a lowering of the general level of arousal. These behavioral effects can be attributed to impaired synthesis of catecholamine neurotransmitters, as a result of low activity of dopamine β-hydroxylase.

Most of the other clinical signs of scurvy can be accounted for by the effects of ascorbate deficiency on collagen synthesis, as a result of impaired proline and lysine hydroxylase activity. Depletion of muscle carnitine, due to impaired activity of trimethyllysine and γ-butyrobetaine hydroxylases, may account for the lassitude and fatigue that precede clinical signs of scurvy.

Anemia in scurvy
Anemia is frequently associated with scurvy, and may be either macrocytic, indicative of folate deficiency, or hypochromic, indicative of iron deficiency.

Folate deficiency may be epiphenomenal, since the major dietary sources of folate are the same as those of ascorbate. However, some patients with clear megaloblastic anemia respond to the administration of vitamin C alone, suggesting that there may be a role of ascorbate in the maintenance of normal pools of reduced folates, although there is no evidence that any of the reactions of folate is ascorbate dependent.

Iron deficiency in scurvy may well be secondary to reduced absorption of inorganic iron and impaired mobilization of tissue iron reserves (see below). At the same time, the hemorrhages of advanced scurvy will cause a significant loss of blood.

There is also evidence that erythrocytes have a shorter half-life than normal in scurvy, possibly as a result of peroxidative damage to membrane lipids owing to impairment of the reduction of tocopheroxyl radical by ascorbate.

Vitamin C requirements

Vitamin C illustrates extremely well how different criteria of adequacy, and different interpretations of experimental evidence, can lead to different estimates of requirements, and to reference intakes ranging between 30 and 80 mg/day for adults.

The requirement for vitamin C to prevent clinical scurvy is less than 10 mg/day. However, at this level of intake wounds do not heal properly, because of the requirement for vitamin C for the synthesis of collagen in connective tissue. An intake of 20 mg/day is required for optimum wound healing. Allowing for individual variation in requirements, this gives a reference intake for adults of 30 mg/day, which was the British recommended daily allowance (RDA) until 1991, and is the

United Nations Food and Agriculture Organization (UNFAO)/World Health Organization (WHO) RDA.

The 1991 British reference nutrient intake (RNI) for vitamin C is based on the level of intake at which the plasma concentration rises sharply, showing that requirements have now been met, tissues are saturated and there is spare vitamin C being transported between tissues, available for excretion. This criterion of adequacy gives an RNI of 40 mg/day for adults.

The alternative approach to determining requirements is to estimate the total body content of vitamin C, then measure the rate at which it is metabolized, by giving a test dose of radioactive vitamin. This is the basis of both the US RDA of 60 mg/day for adults and the Netherlands RDA of 80 mg/day. Indeed, it also provides an alternative basis for the RNI of 40 mg/day adopted in Britain in 1991.

The problem lies in deciding what is an appropriate body content of vitamin C. The US studies were performed on subjects whose total body vitamin C was estimated to be 1500 mg at the beginning of a depletion study. However, there is no evidence that this is a necessary, or even a desirable, body content of the vitamin. It is simply the body content of the vitamin among a small group of young people eating a self-selected diet rich in fruit. There is good evidence that a total body content of 900 mg is more than adequate. It is three times larger than the body content at which the first signs of deficiency are observed, and will protect against the development of any signs of deficiency for several months on a completely vitamin C-free diet.

There is a further problem in interpreting the results of this kind of study. The rate at which vitamin C is metabolized varies with the amount consumed. This means that as the experimental subjects become depleted, so the rate at which they metabolize the vitamin decreases. Thus, calculation of the amount that is required to maintain the body content depends on both the way in which results obtained during depletion studies are extrapolated to the rate in subjects consuming a normal diet and the amount of vitamin C in that diet.

An intake of 40 mg/day is more than adequate to maintain a total body content of 900 mg of vitamin C (the British RNI). At a higher level of habitual intake, 60 mg/day is adequate to maintain a total body content of 1500 mg (the US RDA). Making allowances for changes in the rate of metabolism with different levels of intake, and allowing for incomplete absorption of the vitamin gives the Netherlands RDA of 80 mg/day.

Assessment of vitamin C status

Urinary excretion and saturation testing

Urinary excretion of ascorbate falls to undetectably low levels in deficiency, and therefore very low excretion will indicate deficiency. However, no guidelines for the interpretation of urinary ascorbate have been established.

It is relatively easy to assess the state of body reserves of vitamin C by measuring the excretion after a test dose. A subject who is saturated will excrete more or less the whole of a test dose of 500 mg of ascorbate over 6 h. A more precise method involves repeating the loading test daily until more or less complete recovery is achieved, thus giving an indication of how depleted the body stores were.

Blood concentrations of ascorbate

The plasma concentration of vitamin C falls relatively rapidly during experimental depletion studies, to undetectably low levels within 4 weeks of initiating a vitamin C-free diet, although clinical signs of scurvy may not develop for a further 3–4 months, and tissue concentrations of the vitamin may be as high as 50% of saturation. In field studies and surveys, subjects with plasma ascorbate below 11 μmol/l are considered to be at risk of developing scurvy, while anyone with a plasma concentration below 6 μmol/l would be expected to show clinical signs.

The concentration of ascorbate in leukocytes is well correlated with the concentrations in other tissues, and falls more slowly than plasma concentration in depletion studies. The reference range of leukocyte ascorbate is 1.1–2.8 mol/10^6 cells; a significant loss of leukocyte ascorbate coincides with the development of clear clinical signs of scurvy.

Without a differential white cell count, leukocyte ascorbate concentration cannot be considered to give a meaningful reflection of vitamin C status. The different types of leukocyte have different capacities to accumulate ascorbate. This means that a change in the proportion of granulocytes, platelets and mononuclear leukocytes will result in a change in the total concentration of ascorbate/10^6 cells, although there may well be no change in vitamin nutritional status. Stress, myocardial infarction, infection, burns and surgical trauma all result in changes in leukocyte distribution, with an increase in the proportion of granulocytes, and hence an apparent change in leukocyte ascorbate. This has been widely misinterpreted to indicate an increased requirement for vitamin C in these conditions.

Possible benefits of high intakes of vitamin C

At intakes above about 100 mg/day the body's capacity to metabolize vitamin C is saturated, and any further intake is excreted in the urine unchanged. Therefore, it would not seem justifiable to recommend higher levels of intake. However, in addition to its antioxidant role and its role in reducing the tocopheroxyl radical, and thus sparing vitamin E, vitamin C is important in the absorption of iron, and in preventing the formation of nitrosamines. Both of these actions depend on the presence of the vitamin in the gut together with food, and intakes totaling more than 100 mg/day may be beneficial.

Iron absorption

Inorganic dietary iron is absorbed as Fe^{2+} and not as Fe^{3+}; ascorbic acid in the intestinal lumen will both maintain iron in the reduced state and chelate it, thus increasing the amount absorbed. A dose of 25 mg of vitamin C taken together with a meal increases the absorption of iron by around 65%, while a 1 g dose gives a nine-fold increase. This occurs only when ascorbic acid is present together with the test meal; neither intravenous administration of vitamin C nor intake several hours before the test meal has any effect on iron absorption. Optimum iron absorption may therefore require significantly more than 100 mg of vitamin C/day.

Inhibition of nitrosamine formation

The safety of nitrates and nitrites used in curing meat, a traditional method of preservation, has been questioned because of the formation of nitrosamines by reaction between nitrite and amines naturally present in foods under the acid conditions in the stomach. In experimental animals nitrosamines are potent carcinogens, and some authorities have limited the amounts of these salts that are permitted, although there is no evidence of any hazard to humans from endogenous nitrosamine formation. Ascorbate can prevent the formation of nitrosamines by reacting nonenzymically with nitrite and other nitrosating reagents, forming NO, NO_2 and N_2. Again, this is an effect of ascorbate present in the stomach at the same time as the dietary nitrites and amines, rather than an effect of vitamin C nutritional status.

Pharmacological uses of vitamin C

Several studies have reported low ascorbate status in patients with advanced cancer, which is perhaps an unsurprising finding in seriously ill patients. With very little experimental evidence, it has been suggested that very high intakes of vitamin C (of the order of 10 g/day or more) may be beneficial in enhancing host resistance to cancer, and preventing the development of the acquired immunodeficiency syndrome (AIDS) in people who are human immunodeficiency virus (HIV) positive. In controlled studies with patients matched for age, gender, site and stage of primary tumors and metastases, and previous chemotherapy, there was no beneficial effect of high-dose ascorbic acid in the treatment of advanced cancer.

High doses of vitamin C have been recommended for the prevention and treatment of the common cold, with some evidence that the vitamin reduces the duration of symptoms. However, the evidence from controlled trials is unconvincing.

Toxicity of vitamin C

Regardless of whether or not high intakes of ascorbate have any beneficial effects, large numbers of people habitually take between 1 and 5 g/day of vitamin C supplements (compared with reference intakes of 30–80 mg/day) and some take considerably more. There is little evidence of any significant toxicity from these high intakes. Once the plasma concentration of ascorbate reaches the renal threshold, it is excreted more or less quantitatively with increasing intake, and there is no evidence that higher intakes increase the body pool above about 110 μmol/kg body weight. Unabsorbed ascorbate in the intestinal lumen is a substrate for bacterial fermentation, and may cause diarrhea and intestinal discomfort.

Up to 5% of the population are at risk from the development of renal oxalate stones. The risk is from both ingested oxalate and that formed endogenously, mainly from the metabolism of glycine. Some reports have suggested that people consuming high intakes of vitamin C excrete more oxalate in the urine. However, no pathway for the formation of oxalate from ascorbate is known, and it seems that the oxalate is formed nonenzymically under alkaline conditions either in the bladder or after collection, and hence high vitamin C intake is not a risk factor for renal stone formation.

8.15 Perspectives on the future

There are several compounds that have clearly defined functions in the body, but can be synthesized in apparently adequate amounts, so that they are not considered to be dietary essentials. These substances have been receiving increasing attention, and these, in addition to other compounds, are likely to continue to stimulate interest and discussion in the future.

Bioflavonoids

The most studied flavonoids are hesperitin and quercitin. Because they are biologically active, they are commonly called bioflavonoids. Most fruits and green leafy vegetables contain relatively large amounts of flavonoids; altogether some 2000 have been identified, and average intakes of flavonoids from a mixed diet are of the order of 1 g/day.

There is no evidence that the bioflavonoids are dietary essentials; indeed, it is not clear to what extent they are absorbed from the gastrointestinal tract. If they have any useful action it is as antioxidants; oxidation of flavonoids may serve to protect susceptible nutrients from damage in foods and the intestinal lumen, and also possibly act as antioxidants in plasma and tissues. There is epidemiological evidence that the intake of antioxidant flavonoids is inversely correlated with mortality from coronary heart disease.

Carnitine

Carnitine has a central role in the transport of fatty acids across the mitochondrial membrane. Tissues other than liver and skeletal muscle depend on active uptake from the bloodstream. Tissues with high rates of fatty acid oxidation have high rates of carnitine turnover, while in tissues with low rates of fatty acid oxidation it has a longer half-life. Deficiency of methionine or vitamin C may result in impaired synthesis of carnitine. In experimental animals, deficiency of lysine has little effect on plasma and tissue concentrations, but methionine deficiency can lead to carnitine depletion, and carnitine has a methionine-sparing effect in methionine-deficient animals. The administration of the anticonvulsant valproic acid can lead to carnitine depletion. This results in impaired β-oxidation of fatty acids and ketogenesis, and hence a nonketotic hypoglycemia, with elevated plasma nonesterified fatty acids and triglycerides. There may also be signs of liver dysfunction, with hyperammonemia and encephalopathy. The administration of carnitine supplements in these conditions has a beneficial effect.

Although carnitine is not generally nutritionally important, it may be required for premature infants,

since they have an inadequate capacity to synthesize it. There is some evidence that full-term infants may also have a greater requirement for carnitine than can be met by endogenous synthesis; infants fed on carnitine-free soya-milk formula have higher plasma concentrations of nonesterified fatty acids and triglycerides than those receiving carnitine supplements. Carnitine depletion, with disturbed lipid metabolism, has also been reported in adults maintained for prolonged periods on total parenteral nutrition. There is some evidence that supplements of carnitine may increase the ability of muscle to oxidize fatty acids, and so increase physical work capacity, although other studies have shown no effect.

Choline

Choline is important as a base in phospholipids: both phosphatidylcholine (lecithin) in all cell membranes and sphingomyelin in the nervous system. In addition, acetylcholine is a transmitter in the central and parasympathetic nervous systems and at neuromuscular junctions. There is some evidence that the availability of choline may be limiting for the synthesis of acetylcholine in the central nervous system under some conditions. In animals, deficiency of choline results in fatty infiltration of the liver, apparently as a result of impairment of the export of lipoproteins from hepatocytes; prolonged deficiency may result in cirrhosis. The kidney can also be affected, with tubular necrosis and interstitial hemorrhage, probably as a result of lysosomal membrane disruption.

There is no evidence that choline is a dietary requirement for humans, and no condition similar to the effects of choline deficiency in experimental animals has been reported. Since phosphatidylcholine is found in all biological membranes, dietary deficiency is unlikely to occur except when people are maintained on defined diets free from phospholipids. Plasma concentrations fall during long-term total parenteral nutrition, and it is possible that the impaired liver function seen in such patients is partly the result of choline depletion.

Inositol

Inositol's main function is in phospholipids; phosphatidylinositol constitutes some 5–10% of the total membrane phospholipids. In addition to its structural role in membranes, phosphatidylinositol has a major function in the intracellular responses to peptide hormones and neurotransmitters, yielding two intracellular second messengers, inositol trisphosphate and diacylglycerol.

There is no evidence that inositol is a dietary essential. Infants may have a higher requirement than can be met by endogenous synthesis. Untreated diabetics have high plasma concentrations of free inositol and high urinary excretion of inositol, associated with relatively low intracellular concentrations of inositol, suggesting that elevated plasma glucose may inhibit the uptake of inositol. There is some evidence that impaired nerve conduction velocity in diabetic neuropathy in both patients and experimental animals is associated with low intracellular concentrations of inositol, and inositol supplements may improve nerve conduction velocity. However, high intracellular concentrations of inositol also impair nerve conduction velocity, and supplements may have a deleterious effect.

Taurine

Until about 1976 it was assumed that taurine was a metabolic end-product, the only function of which was the conjugation of bile acids. The occurrence of changes in the electrical activity of the retina in children maintained on long-term total parenteral nutrition without added taurine have shown that it has physiological functions, and have raised the question of whether or not it should be regarded as a dietary essential.

Ubiquinone (coenzyme Q, "vitamin Q")

Ubiquinone is one of the electron carriers in mitochondria. Therefore, it has an essential function in all energy-yielding metabolism and may also have a general antioxidant role in membranes. Like vitamin E, it can be anchored in membranes by the hydrophobic tail, with the reactive quinone group at the membrane surface. Ubiquinone is readily synthesized in the body, and there is no evidence that it is a dietary essential, or that supplements serve any useful purpose, although they may have nonspecific antioxidant actions and so spare vitamin E.

"Phytoceuticals"

In addition to the compounds with clearly defined metabolic functions discussed above, a wide variety of compounds naturally present in foods, and especially in foods of plant origin, has potentially beneficial effects, although they are not nutrients. Collectively, they are known as phytoceuticals (substances of plant origin with potential pharmaceutical action) or nutraceuticals. The following compounds are examples of phytoceuticals.

- Many glucosinolates and glycosides either inhibit the enzymes of phase I metabolism of foreign compounds (the reactions that activate many potential carcinogens) or induce the reactions leading to conjugation, and hence excretion, of foreign compounds.
- Terpenes that are found in the volatile (essential) oils of herbs and spices are potentially active as lipid-soluble antioxidants, as are many of the carotenoids that are not active as precursors of vitamin A.
- Compounds such as squalene, which are precursors of cholesterol synthesis, have a hypocholesterolemic action, by reducing the activity of the rate-limiting enzyme of cholesterol synthesis, hydroxymethylglutaryl-CoA reductase.
- Various water-soluble compounds, including polyphenols, anthocyanins and flavonoids, have antioxidant action.
- Several plants (especially soyabeans) contain compounds with estrogenic action (phyto-estrogens) that also have antiestrogenic action and appear to be protective against the development of hormone-dependent cancer of the breast and uterus.

Further reading

Bender DA. Nutritional Biochemistry of the Vitamins, 2nd edn. Cambridge: Cambridge University Press, 2003.
Bender DA, Bender AE. Nutrition: A Reference Handbook. Oxford: Oxford University Press, 1997.

9
Minerals and Trace Elements

JJ Strain and Kevin D Cashman

Key messages

- This chapter defines the essential minerals and trace elements.
- It describes the functions and routes of metabolism within the body of each of the minerals and trace elements in turn.
- Dietary requirements and dietary sources are discussed for each mineral.
- Health effects and symptoms of both inadequate and toxic intakes are described.
- Methods of assessing the body status of each mineral and trace element are reviewed.

9.1 Introduction

Essential minerals, including the trace elements, are inorganic elements (see Figure 9.1) that have a physiological function within the body. These must be supplied in the diet (food and fluids) and vary from grams per day for the major (macro) minerals through milligrams to micrograms per day for the trace elements.

It has been proposed that the environment (most probably in the primordial sea around hydrothermal vents) in which living organisms evolved was a primary determinant of which elements became essential for life by providing structural integrity and catalytic ability to the first complex organic molecules. As life evolved from the oceans onto land, a natural selection process may have resulted in some elements becoming relatively more important because of superior catalytic abilities over other elements. In any event, the uneven distribution of elements in a land-based environment meant that efficient homeostatic mechanisms had to be in place to conserve essential elements and to eliminate excesses of essential and nonessential elements. The processes of absorption from the gastrointestinal tract and excretion with body fluids, therefore, are major ways in which the concentration and amount of an element can be controlled in the body. In addition, storage in inactive sites or in an unreactive form can

prevent an element from causing adverse effects in the body and release from storage can be important in times of dietary insufficiency.

All elements have the potential to cause toxic symptoms, whereas some, the known essential elements in Figure 9.1, have the potential to cause deficiency symptoms. Even so, deficiencies of only four of these inorganic elements are known to be prevalent in human populations. Two of these deficiencies, iodine and iron, are widespread in human populations while the other two, zinc and selenium, only occur in some population groups under specially defined conditions. Overt clinical signs of deficiency of any of the other inorganic elements are exceptional in humans and mainly occur secondary to other clinical conditions. Such observations do not preclude the possibility that suboptimum status of the great majority of the elements indicated in Figure 9.1 is important in human nutrition. Indeed, there is an increasing awareness of the potential role of suboptimal as well as supraoptimal nutritional status of minerals and trace elements in the development of degenerative age-related diseases, such as coronary heart disease, cancer and osteoporosis. Moreover, other elements, which currently have no published dietary recommendations but are highlighted in Figure 9.1, may prove to be essential for the optimum health and well-being of humans.

1a	2a	3a	4a	5a	6a	7a	8			1b	2b	3b	4b	5b	6b	7b	8b
1 H																	2 He
3 Li	4 Be											5 B	6 C	7 N	8 O	9 F	10 Ne
11 Na	12 Mg											13 Al	14 Si	15 P	16 S	17 Cl	18 Ar
19 K	20 Ca	21 Sc	22 Ti	23 V	24 Cr	25 Mn	26 Fe	27 Co	28 Ni	29 Cu	30 Zn	31 Ga	32 Ge	33 As	34 Se	35 Br	36 Kr
37 Rb	38 Sr	39 Y	40 Zr	41 Nb	42 Mo	43 Tc	44 Ru	45 Rh	46 Pd	47 Ag	48 Cd	49 In	50 Sn	51 Sb	52 Te	53 I	54 Xe
55 Cs	56 Ba	57 La	72 Hf	73 Ta	74 W	75 Re	76 Os	77 Ir	78 Pt	79 Au	80 Hg	81 Tl	82 Pb	83 Bi	84 Po	85 At	86 Rn
87 Fr	88 Ra	89 Ac	104	105	106												

Lanthanides	58 Ce	59 Pr	60 Nd	61 Pm	62 Sm	63 Eu	64 Gd	65 Tb	66 Dy	67 Ho	68 Er	69 Tm	70 Yb	71 Lu
Actinides	90 Th	91 Pa	92 U	93 Np	94 Pu	95 Am	96 Cm	97 Bk	98 Cf	99 Es	100 Fm	101 Md	102 No	103 Lr

Figure 9.1 The periodic table of the elements. The widely accepted or putative essential elements are encircled.

Major constraints to the elucidation of the potential roles of minerals and trace elements in the onset of degenerative diseases include difficulties in assessing status, and thereby defining requirements, and myriad interactions among minerals and other nutrient and nonnutrients in the diet. Sometimes, natural experiments of genetic disorders can throw light on the potential roles of minerals in disease processes and these will also be discussed as appropriate in the following sections.

9.2 Calcium

Calcium is a metallic element, fifth in abundance in the Earth's crust, of which it forms more than 3%. Calcium is never found in nature uncombined; it occurs abundantly as chalk, granite, eggshell, seashells, "hard" water, bone and limestone. The metal is used as a reducing agent in preparing other metals such as thorium, uranium and zirconium, and is used as a deoxidizer, disulfurizer or decarburizer for various ferrous and nonferrous alloys. It is also used as an alloying agent for aluminum, beryllium, copper, lead and magnesium alloys. Calcium was among the first materials known to be essential in the diet. All foods of vegetable origin contain small but useful amounts of calcium. Animals concentrate calcium in milk, and milk and dairy products are the most important food sources of calcium for many human populations.

Absorption, transport and tissue distribution

The adult human body contains about 1200 g of calcium, which amounts to about 1–2% of body weight. Of this, 99% is found in mineralized tissues, such as bones and teeth, where it is present as calcium phosphate (together with a small component of calcium carbonate), providing rigidity and structure. The remaining 1% is found in blood, extracellular fluid (ECF), muscle and other tissues.

Calcium is under close homeostatic control, with processes such as absorption, excretion and secretion and storage in bone being involved in maintaining the concentration of ionized calcium in the plasma within a tightly regulated range. This tight regulation of plasma calcium concentration is achieved through a complex physiological system comprising the interaction of the

Figure 9.2 Homeostatic regulation of serum calcium, showing the integration of hormone action at the tissue level. CT: calcitonin; PTH: parathyroid hormone; 1,25(OH)$_2$D: 1,25-dihydroxycholecalciferol (to convert from mg/day to mmol/day multiply by 40).

calcitropic hormones, such as parathyroid hormone (PTH), 1,25-dihydroxycholecalciferol [1,25(OH)$_2$D$_3$] and calcitonin, with specific target tissues (kidney, bone and intestine) that serve to increase or to decrease the entry of calcium into the extracellular space (plasma) (Figure 9.2). Only in extreme circumstances, such as severe malnutrition or hyperparathyroidism, is the serum ionized calcium concentration below or above the normal range. The secretion of these hormones is governed wholly, or in part, by the plasma concentration of ionized calcium, thus forming a negative feedback system. PTH and 1,25(OH)$_2$D$_3$ are secreted when plasma calcium is low, while calcitonin is secreted when plasma calcium is high.

Calcium in food occurs as salts or associated with other dietary constituents in the form of complexes of calcium ions. Calcium must be released in a soluble, and probably ionized, form before it can be absorbed. Calcium is absorbed in the intestine by two routes, transcellular and paracellular (Figure 9.3). The transcellular route involves active transport of calcium by the mucosal calcium transport protein, calbindin, and

is saturable and subject to physiological and nutritional regulation via vitamin D. The paracellular route involves passive calcium transport through the tight junctions between mucosal cells; it is nonsaturable, essentially independent of nutritional and physiological regulation, and concentration dependent. Most calcium absorption in humans occurs in the small intestine, but there is some evidence for a small colonic component. Transcellular calcium absorption responds to calcium needs, as reflected by changes in plasma calcium concentration, by hormone-mediated up- or down-regulation of calbindin in mucosal cells; for example, reduced plasma calcium evokes a PTH-mediated increase in plasma 1,25(OH)$_2$D$_3$, which stimulates increased calbindin synthesis in intestinal mucosal cells.

On average, between 10 and 30% of the calcium is absorbed from a mixed diet by healthy adults. However, the efficiency of intestinal calcium absorption is influenced by a variety of physiological factors (Table 9.1). Calcium absorption may also be influenced by a number of dietary factors (Table 9.1).

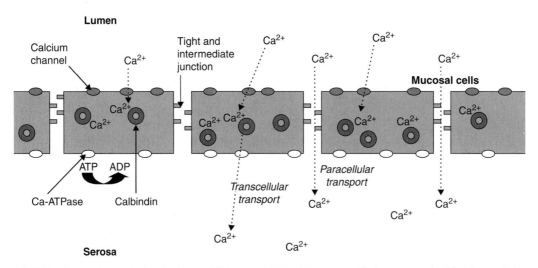

Figure 9.3 Calcium transport across the intestinal mucosal lining: paracellular calcium transport (between mucosal cells) and transcellular calcium transport (across the mucosal cell).

Table 9.1 Factors affecting calcium absorption

Increased absorption	Decreased absorption
Physiological factors	
Vitamin D adequacy	Vitamin D deficiency
Increased mucosal mass	Decreased mucosal mass
Calcium deficiency	Menopause
Phosphorus deficiency	Old age
Pregnancy	Decreased gastric acid (without a meal)
Lactation	Rapid intestinal transit time
Mucosal permeability disease states (e.g. hyperparathyroidism, sarcoidosis, idiopathic hypercalciuria)	Disease states (e.g. malabsorption syndrome, celiac disease, Crohn's disease, chronic renal failure diabetes, hypoparathyroidism, primary biliary cirrhosis)
Dietary factors	
Lactose (in infants)	Phytate
Casein phosphopeptides (?)[a]	Oxalate
Nondigestible oligosaccharides	Large calcium load
Small calcium load	High habitual calcium intake
Low habitual calcium intake	Ingestion without a meal
Ingestion with a meal	

[a] Conflicting data in the literature.

Metabolic function and essentiality

Calcium is required for normal growth and development of the skeleton. During skeletal growth and maturation, i.e. until the early twenties in humans, calcium accumulates in the skeleton at an average rate of 150 mg/day. During maturity, the body, and therefore the skeleton, is more or less in calcium equilibrium. From the age of about 50 years in men and from the menopause in women, bone balance becomes negative and bone is lost from all skeletal sites. This bone loss is associated with a marked rise in fracture rates in both sexes, but particularly in women. Adequate calcium intake is critical to achieving optimal peak bone mass (PBM) and modifies the rate of bone loss associated with agng. Extraskeletal calcium (representing around 1% of total body calcium) plays a role in mediating vascular contraction and vasodilatation, muscle contraction, nerve transmission and glandular secretion.

Deficiency symptoms

Because of the small metabolic pool of calcium (less than 0.1% in the ECF compartment) relative to the large skeletal reserve, for all practical purposes metabolic calcium deficiency probably never exists, at least not as a nutritional disorder. An inadequate intake or poor intestinal absorption of calcium causes the circulating ionized calcium concentration to decline acutely, which triggers an increase in PTH synthesis and release. PTH acts on three target organs to restore the circulating calcium concentration to normal (Figure 9.2). At the kidney, PTH promotes the reabsorption of calcium in the distal tubule. PTH affects the intestine indirectly by stimulating the production of $1,25(OH)_2D_3$, which in turn, leads to increased calcium absorption. PTH also induces bone resorption, thereby releasing calcium into blood. Owing to the action of PTH and $1,25(OH)_2D_3$ on the target tissues, plasma calcium concentrations are restored within minutes to hours.

If, however, there is a continual inadequate intake or poor intestinal absorption of calcium (e.g. because of vitamin D deficiency), circulating calcium concentration is maintained largely at the expense of skeletal mass, that is, from an increased rate of bone resorption. This PTH-mediated increase in bone resorption is one of several important causes of reduced bone mass and osteoporosis. The cumulative effect of calcium depletion (by whatever mechanism) on the skeleton over many years contributes to the increasing frequency of osteoporotic fractures with age. Prolonged inadequate calcium intake in younger people reduces the rate of accretion of the skeleton and may prevent the attainment of the genetically determined maximal PBM. This may increase the risk of osteoporosis as PBM in adulthood is predictive of bone mass in later life. Chronic inadequate intake or poor intestinal absorption of calcium may also play some role in the etiologies of hypertension, including pre-eclampsia and colon cancer.

Toxicity

The available data on the adverse effects of high calcium intakes in humans are primarily from the intake of calcium from nutrient supplements. The three most widely studied and biologically important are:

- kidney stone formation (nephrolithiasis)
- the syndrome of hypercalcemia and renal insufficiency, with or without alkalosis (referred to historically as milk alkali syndrome associated with peptic ulcer treatments)
- the effect on absorption of other essential minerals, e.g. iron, zinc, magnesium and phosphorus.

Based largely on the data on the association of high calcium intakes with hypercalcemia and renal insufficiency in adults, the US Food and Nutrition Board established a tolerable upper intake level (UL) of calcium of 2500 mg/day for children, adolescents and adults, as well as pregnant and lactating women.

Genetic diseases

Two rare inborn errors of vitamin D metabolism, vitamin D-dependent rickets types I and II, have an associated hypocalcemia that can impair the bone calcification process. Type I vitamin D-dependent rickets appears to be caused by mutations in the enzyme $25(OH)D_3$-1-α-hydroxylase [responsible for the synthesis of $1,25(OH)_2D_3$ from $25(OH)D_3$], leading to defective activity of this enzyme, whereas type I vitamin D-dependent rickets, which is associated with normal or elevated levels of $1,25(OH)_2D_3$, is thought to result from target tissue resistance to the action of $1,25(OH)_2D_3$. This resistance arises owing to changes in the vitamin D receptor molecule. Daily vitamin D_3 administration seems to be an effective therapy for both disorders.

A hypercalcemia has been noted in familial benign hypercalcemia (types I and III). Type I familial benign hypercalcemia, a renal tubular defect in calcium reabsorption, is caused by a mutation in the gene encoding the calcium-sensing receptor. Type III familial benign hypercalcemia represents a distinct genetic entity. However, the gene(s) responsible for this type of hypocalciuric hypercalcemia is still being mapped.

Assessing status

There is, as yet, no biochemical indicator that reflects calcium nutritional status. Blood calcium concentration, for example, is not a good indicator because it is tightly regulated. There are, however, some potential indicators of nutritional calcium adequacy, which are related to content or metabolism of the skeletal calcium reserve. Measures of bone mass may be used as indicators of body calcium status. These include bone mineral content (BMC, which is the amount of mineral at a particular skeletal site such as the femoral neck, lumbar spine or total body) and bone mineral density (BMD, which is BMC divided by the area of the scanned region). Besides their relationship to bone mass and strength, BMD and BMC are strong predictors of fracture risk and are thus functional indicators of calcium status. The US Food and Nutrition Board used data relating dietary calcium intake to BMD and BMC to establish the estimates of calcium intake requirements for pregnancy and lactation. Desirable calcium retention, which is based on balance data, may be considered a functional indicator of nutritional adequacy of calcium in population groups and was used by the US Food and Nutrition Board to establish recommendations for daily calcium intakes. This is based on the concept that to maximize skeletal strength, optimum bone mass must be attained through a maximum skeletal calcium reserve. Finally, recent research suggests that biochemical markers of bone turnover that predict bone mass changes and fracture risk may be functional indicators of the adequacy of calcium intake.

Requirements and dietary sources

Milk and milk products are the most important dietary sources of calcium for most people in Western countries, with cereal products and fruits and vegetables each making a much smaller contribution (Table 9.2). For example, the contribution of dairy products to total calcium intake has been estimated as 73% in the Netherlands, 51–52% in Germany, 51–52% in the USA, 57% in the UK and 52% in Ireland. Tinned fish, such as sardines, are rich sources of calcium but do not make a significant contribution to intake for most people. In general, foods of plant origin are not very rich sources of calcium. However, owing to the level of consumption, foods of plant origin make a significant contribution to total calcium intake. For example, in the USA, cereals contribute about 25–27% of total calcium intake, while in the UK cereals contribute about 25% of total calcium intake with about 14% from bread because of calcium fortification of white flour. Increased availability of calcium-fortified foods and dietary supplements containing calcium salts is leading to a wider range of rich dietary sources of calcium. Contributions from nutritional supplements or medicines may be significant for some people.

Given the high proportion of body calcium, which is present in bone, and the importance of bone as the major reservoir for calcium, development and maintenance of bone is the major determinant of calcium needs. Thus, unlike other nutrients, the requirement for calcium is considered to relate not to the maintenance of the metabolic function of the nutrient but to the maintenance of an optimal reserve and the support of the reserve's function (i.e. bone integrity). Calcium requirements, therefore, vary throughout an individual's life, with greater needs during the periods of rapid growth in childhood and adolescence, during pregnancy and lactation, and in later life. There are important genetic and environmental influences of calcium requirements. Genetic influences include such factors as bone architecture and geometry, and responsiveness of bone to hormones that mediate the function of bone as the body's calcium reserve. Environmental influences include factors such as dietary constituents and the degree of mechanical loading imposed on the skeleton in everyday life. Because of their effects on urinary

Table 9.2 Calcium and phosphorus contents of some common foods

Food source	Description	Range (mg/100 g)	
		Ca	P
Cheese	Hard, from milk	400–1200	400–810
Cheese	Soft, from milk	60–700	100–790
Sardines	Tinned, in oil	550	520
Milk	Cow's (3.9, 1.6 and 0.1% fat)	115–120	92–94
Yoghurt	Whole milk	160–200	130–170
Ice cream	Dairy	110–130	99–110
Eggs	Chicken, raw, whole	57	200
Chicken, duck, turkey	Raw	9–12	190–200
Beef, mutton, pork	Raw	7–10	60–200
Cod, plaice, whiting	Raw	16–51	170–180
Wheat flour	Whole flour	38	320
Wheat flour	White flour	15–140	110–120
Bread	White	100–180	79–120
Bread	Brown	100–140	150–180
Spinach	Raw	170	45
Watercress	Raw	170	52
Broccoli	Green, raw	56	87
Peas	Processed, canned	33	89
Rice	Raw, white, polished	18–25	54–67
Potatoes	Raw	5–6	34–37
Tofu	Soyabean, steamed or fried	510–1480	95–270

Data from Holland *et al.* (1995).

calcium losses, high intakes of both sodium and protein increase dietary calcium requirements.

There is considerable disagreement over human calcium requirements, and this is reflected in the wide variation in estimates of daily calcium requirements made by different expert authorities. For example, expert committees in the USA and the EU have established very different recommendations for calcium intake (Table 9.3). Much of this divergence arises because of different interpretations of available human calcium balance data. The higher recommendations in the USA derive from defining calcium requirements based on desirable calcium retention estimated from human calcium balance studies, i.e. that which results in the maximum skeletal calcium reserve.

Micronutrient interactions

There is considerable evidence from studies on experimental animals that excessive calcium intake can impair the nutritional status of other nutrients, particularly

Table 9.3 Recommended calcium intakes in the USA and UK

UK RNI (1998)[a]		US AI (1997)[b]	
Age group (years)	mg/day	Age group (years)	mg/day
0–1	525	0–0.5	210
1–3	350	0.5–1	270
4–6	450	1–3	500
7–10	550	4–8	800
11–14 M	1000	9–13	1300
15–18 M	1000	14–18	1300
11–14 F	800	19–30	1000
15–18 F	800	31–50	1000
19–50	700	51–70	1200
>50	700	>70	1200
		Pregnancy	
Pregnancy	NI	≤18	1300
		19–50	1000
Lactation	+550	Lactation	
		≤8	1300
		19–50	1000

[a] Reference nutrient intake (RNI); UK Department of Health (1991).
[b] Adequate intake (AI); US Institute of Medicine (1997). Estimates of Ca requirements refer to both males and females unless stated otherwise.
M: requirements for males; F: requirements for females; NI: no increment.

iron, zinc and magnesium, but data on humans are not clear. While calcium interacts with magnesium and phosphorus, and reduces their absorption, there is no evidence that high calcium intakes are associated with depletion of the affected nutrient. Calcium inhibits the absorption of iron in a dose-dependent and dose-saturable fashion. However, the available human data fail to show cases of iron deficiency or even decreased iron stores as a result of high calcium intake. There is some evidence that high dietary calcium intakes reduce zinc absorption and balance in humans and may increase the zinc requirement. Overall, the available data on the interaction of calcium with these nutrients do not show any clinically or functionally significant depletion of the affected nutrient in humans and, in the context of risk assessment, these interactions should probably not be considered adverse effects of calcium. However, such interactions deserve further investigation. It is well established that a deficiency of vitamin D (arising from a lack of exposure to sunlight, inadequate dietary intake, or both) can result in a reduced efficiency of intestinal calcium absorption which, in turn, can lead to a decrease in serum ionized calcium.

9.3 Magnesium

Like calcium, magnesium is an alkaline earth metal. Magnesium is the eighth most abundant element in the Earth's crust. It does not occur uncombined, but is found in large deposits in the form of magnesite, dolomite and other minerals. The metal is used in flashlight photography, flares and pyrotechnics. It is one-third lighter than aluminum, and in alloys is essential for aeroplane and missile construction. Magnesium is used in producing nodular graphite in cast iron and as an additive to conventional propellants. The hydroxide (milk of magnesia), chloride, sulfate (Epsom salts) and citrate are used in medicine.

Magnesium was first shown to be an essential dietary component for rats in 1932 and later for humans. This is a reflection of the role that magnesium plays in the stabilization of ATP and other molecules. Since then, nutritionists have come to realize that frank magnesium deficiency is rare and that it only occurs in clinical settings as a secondary consequence of another disease. More recently, moderate or marginal deficiency has been proposed as a risk factor for chronic diseases such as osteoporosis, cardiovascular disease and diabetes. These associations are controversial.

Absorption, transport and tissue distribution

Magnesium is the second most common cation found in the body (about 25 g). It is evenly distributed between the skeleton (50–60% of total) and the soft tissues (40–50% of total). In the skeleton, about one-third of the magnesium is on the surface of bone. This magnesium pool is thought to be exchangeable and thus may serve to maintain serum or soft-tissue magnesium concentrations in times of need. Body magnesium is most closely associated with cells; only 1% of total body magnesium is extracellular. Within the cell, magnesium is found in all of the compartments.

Magnesium homeostasis is maintained by controlling the efficiency of intestinal absorption and magnesium losses through the urine. The later process is a stronger regulatory control mechanism for magnesium. Magnesium absorption is presumed to occur throughout the small intestine of humans. In normal, healthy individuals, magnesium absorption is between 20 and 70% of magnesium in a meal. Magnesium crosses the intestinal epithelium by three different mechanisms: passive diffusion, solvent drag (i.e. following water movement) and active transport. Regulation of intestinal nutrient absorption is generally thought to occur only for the active component of absorption. The mechanisms controlling intestinal magnesium absorption are unclear at this time. Because of the chemical similarity of magnesium to calcium, scientists have examined whether vitamin D status regulates magnesium absorption. It appears that only large changes in vitamin D status lead to alterations in magnesium absorption. Only limited information is available on the influence of dietary components on magnesium in humans. Phosphate may be an inhibitor of magnesium absorption. Free phosphate may form insoluble salt complexes with magnesium; phosphate groups in phytate may also inhibit magnesium absorption. Fiber-rich foods have been shown to lower magnesium bioavailability. However, it is not clear whether this was an independent effect of fiber or a reflection of the phytate content of these foods. Protein and fructose may enhance magnesium absorption.

As mentioned above, the kidney is the principal organ involved in magnesium homeostasis. The renal handling of magnesium in humans is a filtration–reabsorption process. Approximately 70% of serum magnesium is ultrafiltrable, and the normal healthy kidney reabsorbs about 95% of filtered magnesium. When an individual is fed a low-magnesium diet, renal output of magnesium is reduced. Excessive magnesium loss via urine is a clinical condition contributing to magnesium depletion in patients with renal dysfunction.

Metabolic function and essentiality

Magnesium is essential for a wide range of fundamental cellular reactions, and is involved in at least 300 enzymic steps in intermediary metabolism, for example in the glycolytic cycle converting glucose to pyruvate, in β-oxidation of fatty acids and in protein synthesis. Magnesium plays an important role in the development and maintenance of bone; about 60% of total body magnesium is present in bone. Magnesium has also been demonstrated to enhance the condensation of chromatin, and given the role of chromosomal condensation in the regulation of gene activity, magnesium depletion could indirectly affect gene transcription.

Deficiency symptoms

Magnesium homeostasis can be maintained over a wide range of intakes in normal, healthy individuals. Thus, magnesium deficiency does not appear to be a problem in healthy people. Frank magnesium deficiency is only seen in humans under two conditions: as a secondary complication of a primary disease state (diseases of cardiovascular and neuromuscular function, endocrine disorders, malabsorption syndromes, muscle wasting) and resulting from rare genetic abnormalities of magnesium homeostasis. Symptoms of frank magnesium deficiency include:

- progressive reduction in plasma magnesium (10–30% below controls) and red blood cell magnesium (slower and less extreme than the fall in plasma magnesium)
- hypocalcemia and hypocalciuria
- hypokalemia resulting from excess potassium excretion and leading to negative potassium balance
- abnormal neuromuscular function.

All of these symptoms are reversible with dietary magnesium repletion. Disrupted calcium metabolism is also evident from the effect of magnesium depletion on serum PTH and vitamin D concentrations.

Scientists have attempted to demonstrate that suboptimal intake of magnesium [e.g. below the recommended dietary allowance (RDA) but not frank deficiency] is a contributor to the development of chronic maladies such as cardiovascular disease, diabetes mellitus, hypertension, eclampsia and pre-eclampsia and osteoporosis. However, the results of studies in this area are ambiguous. The lack of positive findings may reflect the lack of sensitive and reliable tools for assessing magnesium status, the failure to account for magnesium intake from water (in dietary studies) or the difficulty in attributing causality to a single nutrient owing to the apparent heterogeneity of causes arising from epidemiological data relating to most chronic diseases. The fact that the US RDA for magnesium was recently raised for most groups is a reflection that nutrition scientists believe that there is a negative consequence to suboptimal magnesium intake. Additional research is needed to justify this concern.

Toxicity

Magnesium, when ingested as a naturally occurring substance in foods, has not been demonstrated to exert any adverse effects in people with normal renal function. However, adverse effects of excess magnesium intake (e.g. diarrhea, nausea, abdominal cramping) have been observed with intakes from nonfood sources such as various magnesium salts used for pharmacological purposes. For this reason the US Food and Nutrition Board established the tolerable UL for adolescents and adults as 350 mg of nonfood magnesium.

Genetic diseases

Several disease states are associated with magnesium deficiency, some of which have genetic roots, for example hypomagnesemia with secondary hypocalcemia, primary hypomagnesemia with hypercalciuria, renal hypomagnesemia 2, Bartter's syndrome and Gitelman's syndrome.

Primary hypomagnesemia with hypercalciuria is caused by a mutation in the paracellin-1 (*PCLN1*) gene on chromosome 3. *PCLN1* is a component of the tight junction complex in nephrons and, therefore, has a role in renal magnesium ion reabsorption. Hypomagnesemia with secondary hypocalcemia is an autosomal recessive disorder and is determined by a mutation in a gene located on 9q12-q22.2.

Renal hypomagnesemia 2 is believed to be due to an autosomal dominant isolated renal magnesium loss, which is caused by misrouting of the $Na^+/K^{(+)}$-ATPase gamma-subunit. This small, type I membrane protein is localized on the basolateral membranes of nephron epithelial cells and is expressed in the distal convoluted tubule, the main site of active renal magnesium reabsorption.

It has been proposed that Bartter's syndrome is a heterogeneous entity with at least two subsets, Gitelman's syndrome and "true" Bartter's syndrome. True Bartter's syndrome, a hypokalemic alkalosis with hypercalciuria, is caused by mutation in the NaK2Cl cotransporter gene *SLC12A1* on chromosome 15. Bartter's syndrome is also caused by mutations in the $K^{(+)}$ channel gene *ROMK* on chromosome 11. Gitelman's syndrome, a hypokalemic alkalosis with hypocalciuria and hypomagnesemia, is caused by mutations in the thiazibe-sensitive NaCl cotransporter gene on 16q13.

Assessing status

Estimating magnesium requirements and establishing magnesium–disease relationships depend on accurate and specific indicators of magnesium status. Several such indicators have been described. All of these are based on measurement of the magnesium content in various body pools. Analysis of total magnesium in serum is often used as an indicator of magnesium status, although only about 1% of total body magnesium is present in ECF. It has been suggested that the concentration of ionized magnesium in serum may be a more reliable and relevant determinant of magnesium deficiency. In addition, intracellular magnesium concentration (usually measured in accessible tissues such as erythrocytes and lymphocytes) provides a more accurate assessment of body magnesium status than does the concentration of magnesium in serum. The dietary balance approach is considered to be the best available method for estimating magnesium requirements. While this method is a powerful research tool for the study of magnesium homeostasis, it is time, resource and labor intensive, and this limits its application to large populations. None of the currently available procedures is perfect for all circumstances.

Requirements and dietary sources

In 1997, the US RDA [the nutrient intake value that is sufficient to meet the requirement of nearly all (97–98%) individuals in a life-stage and sex group] for magnesium was revised upwards for most groups. The current RDA for adult women is now 320 mg/day and for adult men is 420 mg/day. An additional value is now part of the US Food and Nutrition Board's dietary reference intakes, the estimated average requirement (EAR; the nutrient intake value that is estimated to meet the requirement of 50% of the individuals in a life-stage and sex group). This was set to 265 and 350 mg/day for adult women and men, respectively. This value is similar to the mean magnesium intake reported for women and men in the USA (228 and 323 mg/day). Collectively, these data suggest that most Americans are not consuming enough magnesium in their diet. This also appears to be the case for several European populations. However, while the public health relevance of this observation is currently being debated, the fact that there is not a universally accepted reliable magnesium status assessment tool makes it difficult to determine the actual consequence of this apparent low intake.

For those who want to increase their magnesium intake, a number of high magnesium foods and dietary practices will lead to adequate intake. Foods with a high magnesium content include whole grains, legumes, green leafy vegetables and tofu; meat, fruits and dairy products have an intermediate magnesium content

Table 9.4 Magnesium content of some common foods

Food source	Description	Mg content (mg/100 g)
Beef	Lean (from six different cuts)	20
Lamb	Lean (from six different cuts)	24
Pork	Lean (from three different cuts)	22
Chicken	Raw, meat only	25
Cod, plaice, whiting	Raw	22–28
Eggs	Chicken, whole, raw	12
Cheese	Soft and hard varieties	8–45
Pulses	Raw	17–250
Wheat flour	Whole flour	120
Wheat flour	White flour	20–31
Milk	Cow's (3.9, 1.6 and 0.1% fat)	11–12
Yoghurt	Whole milk	19
Tofu	Soyabean, steamed	23–59
Green leafy vegetables	Raw	8–34
Rice	Raw, white, polished	32
Potatoes	Raw	14–17

Data from Holland *et al.* (1995).

(Table 9.4). The poorest sources of magnesium are refined foods. While high levels of calcium, phosphate or fiber may lead to reduced bioavailability of magnesium, differences in bioavailability of magnesium from various food sources does not appear to be a significant barrier to achieving adequate magnesium status. Thus, the current recommendations for a healthy diet based on the food pyramid are consistent with the goals of reaching the US RDA for magnesium.

Micronutrient interactions

As mentioned above, phosphorus as phosphate, especially in phytate, may decrease intestinal magnesium absorption. In general, calcium intake in the usual dietary range does not affect magnesium absorption, but calcium intakes in excess of 2.6 g have been reported to reduce magnesium balance. Magnesium intake in the usual dietary range does not appear to alter calcium balance.

9.4 Phosphorus

Phosphorus is never found free in nature, but is widely distributed in combination with minerals. Phosphate rock, which contains the mineral apatite, an impure tricalcium phosphate, is an important source of the element. Phosphorus is most commonly found in nature in its pentavalent form in combination with oxygen, as phosphate (PO_4^{3-}). Phosphorus (as phosphate) is an essential constituent of all known protoplasm and is uniform across most plant and animal tissues. A practical consequence is that, as organisms consume other organisms lower in the food chain (whether animal or plant), they automatically obtain their phosphorus.

Absorption, transport and tissue distribution

Phosphorus makes up about 0.65–1.1% of the adult body (~600 g). In the adult body 85% of phosphorus is in bone and the remaining 15% is distributed in soft tissues. Total phosphorus concentration in whole blood is 13 mmol/l, most of which is in the phospholipids of erythrocytes and plasma lipoproteins, with approximately 1 mmol/l present as inorganic phosphate. This inorganic component, while constituting only a minute percentage of body phosphorus (<0.1%), is of critical importance. In adults, this component makes up about 15 mmol in total and is located mainly in the blood and ECF. It is into the inorganic compartment that phosphate is inserted on absorption from the diet and resorption from bone, and from this compartment that most urinary phosphorus and hydroxyapatite mineral phosphorus are derived (Figure 9.4). This compartment is also the primary source from which the cells of all tissues derive both structural and high-energy phosphate.

Food phosphorus is a mixture of inorganic and organic forms. Intestinal phosphatases hydrolyze the organic forms contained in ingested protoplasm and, thus, most phosphorus absorption occurs as inorganic phosphate. On a mixed diet, absorption of total phosphorus ranges from 55 to 70% in adults. There is no evidence that this absorption varies with dietary intake. Furthermore, there appears to be no apparent adaptive mechanism that improves phosphorus absorption at low intakes. This is in sharp contrast to calcium, for which absorption efficiency increases as dietary intake decreases and for which adaptive mechanisms exist that improve absorption still further at habitual low intakes. While a portion of phosphorus absorption is by way of a saturable, active transport facilitated by $1,25(OH)_2D_3$ the fact that fractional phosphorus absorption is virtually constant across a broad range of intakes suggests that the bulk of phosphorus absorption occurs by passive, concentration-dependent processes.

Figure 9.4 Homeostatic regulation of serum phosphorus. PTH: parathyroid hormone.

Phosphorus absorption is reduced by ingestion of aluminum-containing antacids and by pharmacological doses of calcium carbonate. There is, however, no significant interference with phosphorus absorption by calcium at intakes within the typical adult range. Excretion of endogenous phosphorus is mainly through the kidneys. Inorganic serum phosphate is filtered at the glomerulus and reabsorbed in the proximal tubule. In the healthy adult, urine phosphorus is essentially equal to absorbed dietary phosphorus, minus small amounts of phosphorus lost in shed cells of skin and intestinal mucosa.

Metabolic function and essentiality

Structurally, phosphorus occurs as hydroxyapatite in calcified tissues and as phospholipids, which are a major component of most biological membranes, and as nucleotides and nucleic acid. Other functional roles of phosphorus include:

- buffering of acid or alkali excesses, hence helping to maintain normal pH
- the temporary storage and transfer of the energy derived from metabolic fuels

- by phosphorylation, and hence activation of many catalytic proteins.

As phosphorus is not irreversibly consumed in these processes and can be recycled indefinitely, the actual functions of dietary phosphorus are first to support tissue growth (either during individual development or through pregnancy and lactation), and secondly to replace excretory and dermal levels. In both processes, it is necessary to maintain a normal level of inorganic phosphate in the ECF, which would otherwise be depleted of phosphorus by growth and excretion.

Deficiency symptoms

Inadequate phosphorus intake is expressed as hypophosphatemia. Only limited quantities of phosphate are stored within cells, and most tissues depend on ECF inorganic phosphate for their metabolic phosphate. When ECF inorganic phosphate levels are low, cellular dysfunction follows. At a whole organism level, the effects of hypophosphatemia include anorexia, anemia, muscle weakness, bone pain, rickets and osteomalacia, general debility, increased susceptibility to infection, paresthesia, ataxia, confusion and even death. The skeleton will exhibit either rickets in children or osteo-malacia in adults. In both groups, the disorder consists of a failure to mineralize forming growth plate cartilage or bone matrix, together with impairment of chrondroblast and osteoblast function. These severe manifestations are usually confined to situations in which ECF phosphate falls below approximately 0.3 mmol/l. Phosphorus is so ubiquitous in various foods that near total starvation is required to produce dietary phosphorus deficiency.

Toxicity

Serum inorganic phosphate rises as total phosphorus intake increases. Excess phosphorus intake from any source is expressed as hyperphosphatemia and, essentially, all the adverse effects of phosphorus excess are owing to the elevated inorganic phosphate in the ECF. The principal effects that have been attributed to hyperphosphatemia are:

- adjustments in the hormonal control system regulating the calcium economy
- ectopic (metastatic) calcification, particularly of the kidney
- in some animal models, increased porosity of the skeleton
- a suggestion that high phosphorus intakes could decrease calcium absorption by complexing calcium in the chyme.

Concern about high phosphorus intake has been raised in recent years because of a probable population-level increase in phosphorus intake though such sources as cola beverages and food phosphate additives.

Genetic diseases

Several disease states are associated with phosphorus deficiency, some of which have genetic roots, for example X-linked hypophosphatemia, hypophosphatemic bone disease and Fanconi syndrome.

X-linked hypophosphatemia is, as the name implies, inherited as an X-linked dominant trait with the mutant gene located in Xp22.2-p.22.1. The classical triad, fully expressed in hemizygous male patients, consists of:

- hypophosphatemia
- lower limb deformities
- stunted growth rate.

Although low serum phosphate is evident early after birth, it is only at time of weight bearing that leg deformities and progressive departure from normal growth rate become sufficiently striking to attract attention and make parents seek medical opinion. It is generally accepted that hypophosphatemia is the consequence of a primary inborn error of phosphate transport, probably located in the proximal nephron.

Hypophosphatemic bone disease is characterized clinically by modest shortening of stature, bowing of the lower limbs and nonrachitic bone changes (somewhat resembling metaphyseal chondrodysplasia) and biochemically by hypophosphatemia. Although a defect in renal transport of phosphate was demonstrated, the defect appeared to be different from that of X-linked hypophosphatemia.

Fanconi syndrome is an autosomal dominant disorder. It is characterized by lactic aciduria and tubular proteinuria in childhood, with glycosuria and aminoaciduria developing in the second decade and osteomalacia from the start of the fourth decade. Glomerular function deteriorates slowly but is compatible with a normal lifespan. There has been reported linkage of the disorder to chromosome 15q15.3.

Assessing status, requirements and dietary sources

Until recently, dietary phosphorus recommendations have been tied to those for calcium, usually on an equimass or equimolar basis, and this approach was used in the USA, EU and UK in establishing recommended dietary allowances, population reference intakes and reference nutrient intakes, respectively, for phosphorus. However, the US Food and Nutrition Board recently suggested that a calcium:phosphorus concept of defining phosphorus requirements is of severely limited value, in that there is little merit in having the ratio "correct" if the absolute quantities of both nutrients are insufficient to support optimal growth. Therefore, because phosphorus intake directly affects serum inorganic phosphate, and because both hypophosphatemia and hyperphosphatemia directly result in dysfunction or disease, the US Food and Nutrition Board considered that the most logical indicator of nutritional adequacy of phosphorus intake in adults is inorganic phosphate. If serum inorganic phosphate is above the lower limits of normal for age, phosphorus intake may be considered adequate to meet cellular and bone formation needs of healthy individuals. Current US RDA for phosphorus are: infants 100 mg (first 6 months), 275 mg (7–12 months), children 460 mg (1–3 years), 500 mg (4–8 years), 1250 mg (9–18 years), adults 700 mg, pregnant women 1250 mg (<18 years), 700 mg (19–50 years), and lactating women 1250 mg (<18 years), 700 mg (19–50 years).

Phosphates are found in foods as naturally occurring components of biological molecules and as food additives in the form of various phosphate salts. The phosphorus density of cow's milk and other dairy produce is higher than of most other foods in a typical diet (Table 9.2). The same is true for diets high in colas and a few other soft drinks that use phosphoric acid as an acidulant.

Micronutrient interactions

It has been reported that intakes of polyphosphates, such as are found in food additives, can interfere with the absorption of iron, copper and zinc.

9.5 Sodium and chloride

Sodium is the sixth most abundant element in the Earth's crust and salt (sodium chloride) comprises about 80% of the dissolved matter in seawater. Although there is a wide variety of sodium salts, many of which are used as additives in food processing (e.g. sodium nitrate and monosodium glutamate), sodium chloride is the major source of sodium in foods. As sodium and chloride intakes in humans are so closely matched, both will be considered together in this text.

Salt was of major importance in early civilisations and in prehistory. Humans have special taste and salt appetite systems, which led to special culinary uses for salt and made it a much sought-after commodity. Nowadays, salt is still used widely to modify flavor, to alter the texture and consistency of food, and to control microbial growth (Table 9.5).

Absorption, transport and tissue distribution

Sodium is the major extracellular electrolyte and exists as the fully water-soluble cation. Chloride is also mainly found in ECF and is fully water soluble as the chloride anion. Both ions are readily absorbed from the digestive tract. Glucose and anions such as citrate, propionates and bicarbonate enhance the uptake of sodium. The

Table 9.5 Sodium-containing additives used in food processing

Additive	Use
Sodium citrate	Flavoring, preservative
Sodium chloride	Flavoring, texture, preservative
Sodium nitrate	Preservative, color fixative
Sodium nitrite	Preservative, color fixative
Sodium tripoliphosphate	Binder
Sodium benzoate	Preservative
Sodium eritrobate	Antioxidant
Sodium propionate	Preservative
Monosodium glutamate	Flavor enhancer
Sodium aluminosilicate	Anticaking agent
Sodium aluminum phosphate acidic	Acidity regulatory, emulsifier
Sodium cyclamate	Artificial sweetener
Sodium alginate	Thickener and vegetable gum
Sodium caseinate	Emulsifier
Sodium bicarbonate	Yeast substitute

"average" 70 kg male has about 90 g of sodium with up to 75% contained in the mineral apatite of bone. Plasma sodium is tightly regulated through a hormone system, which also regulates water balance, pH and osmotic pressure. Angiotensin and aldosterone both act to conserve sodium by increasing sodium reabsorption by the kidney. Sodium depletion stimulates the renal production of renin, which generates active angiotensin in the circulation. The latter stimulates vasoconstriction, which increases blood pressure, decreases water loss and stimulates aldosterone release from the adrenal cortex. Atrial natriuretic hormone counteracts the sodium retention mechanisms by suppressing renin and aldosterone release and by inducing water and sodium excretion. It also decreases blood pressure and antagonizes angiotensin. A raised plasma sodium concentration stimulates the renal reabsorption of water and decreases urinary output via antidiuretic hormone from the posterior pituitary. In contrast to sodium, chloride is passively distributed throughout the body and moves to replace anions lost to cells via other processes.

The main excretory route for both sodium and chloride is the urine. Sweat loss of these ions tends to be very low except with severe exertion in hot climates. Fecal losses are also low in healthy individuals.

Metabolic function and essentiality

Sodium cation is an active participant in the regulation of osmotic and electrolyte balances, while chloride anion is a passive participant in this regulatory system. Each ion, however, has other functions within the body.

Sodium is involved in nerve conduction, active cellular transport and the formation of mineral apatite of bone. Central to its role in water balance, nerve conduction and active transport is the plasma membrane enzyme sodium–potassium-ATPase (Na^+/K^+-ATPase). This enzyme pumps sodium out of the cell and at the same time returns potassium to the intracellular environment while ATP is hydrolyzed. Signal transmission along nerve cells, active transport of nutrients into the enterocyte and muscle contraction/relaxation all depend on the Na^+/K^+-ATPase pump. In the muscle there is an additional pump, the sodium–calcium system. The ATP utilized by the sodium pump comprises a substantial part of total metabolic activity and thermogenesis.

Among the main functions of chloride anion are as dissociated hydrochloric acid in the stomach and in the chloride shift in the erythrocyte plasma membrane, where it exchanges with the bicarbonate ion.

Deficiency symptoms

Obligatory losses of sodium are very low and low plasma sodium or chloride depletion is difficult to induce. Low plasma sodium or chloride is not diet related but rather caused by a variety of clinical conditions, including major trauma and cachexia and overuse of diuretics. Loss of sodium can also ensue as a result of excessive water intake, anorexia nervosa, ulcerative colitis, liver disease, congestive heart failure with edema, and severe infection and diarrhea. Acute diarrhea is the most common cause of sodium deficiency, and oral rehydration depends on the efficient enteric uptake of sodium from isotonic glucose/saline solutions and saves many lives worldwide. Vomiting, chronic renal disease, renal failure and chronic respiratory acidosis can result in chloride depletion.

Toxicity

Excessive salt intakes are usually excreted efficiently in healthy individuals, whereas high plasma sodium and chloride are commonly caused by diabetes insipidus, brainstem injury and dehydration through either excessive sweating or deficient water intake. The controversy with respect to excessive salt intake is its possible role in the degenerative diseases of coronary heart disease, stroke, gastric cancer, osteoporosis and bronchial hyperactivity. There are accumulating data

from epidemiological studies and controlled clinical trials to indicate an adverse effect of sodium intake on blood pressure, and that most people are sodium sensitive. The arguments arise in that it is still unclear whether lowering this intermediate or surrogate measure (blood pressure) of disease can be translated into reduced morbidity and mortality of the target conditions (stroke and coronary heart disease) and of unrelated conditions. The mechanism linking salt intake with blood pressure is also unclear but probably relates to sodium homeostasis, although some have suggested that chloride is the culprit. In any event, low sodium diets differ in nutrient composition from the prevailing diet and animal experimentation indicates that low potassium or calcium intake encourages a salt-induced increase in blood pressure, as does feeding simple carbohydrates (sucrose, glucose or fructose). Copper deficiency in rats has been demonstrated to increase blood pressure independently of sodium intake.

Nevertheless, efficient sodium conservation mechanisms mean that current sodium intakes in many populations are unnecessarily high and are probably much higher than the generally lower sodium diets eaten during the long period of human evolution. Clinical studies indicate that a high sodium diet increases calcium excretion and measures of bone resorption, thereby suggesting a possible role for high salt intakes in osteoporosis.

Cross-cultural epidemiology suggests that high salt intakes are associated with gastric cancer, whereas a low-salt diet is regarded as having a potentially favorable effect in asthma patients.

Genetic diseases

A number of rare genetic disorders has thrown some light on the pathological mechanisms linking sodium balance and hypertension (pathologically elevated blood pressure). Three candidate genes have been shown to cause monogenic forms of low renin salt-sensitive hypertension. These encode for enzymes involved in aldosterone biosynthesis or cortisol metabolism and for the epithelial sodium channel. These genetic defects decrease the ability of the renal tubules to excrete sodium. It is possible that similar genetic mechanisms operate in more common forms of hypertension such as essential hypertension and especially salt-sensitive hypertension. Moreover, molecular mechanisms associated with renin angiotensin–aldosterone are central to the pathophysiology of this condition. Common essential hypertension, however, is complex and heterogeneous and has a genetic heritability of about 30%. Moreover, a central role for sodium excretion in the pathophysiology of hypertension does not prove a causal role for high salt intakes per se.

Assessing status

The tight regulation of plasma sodium and, in turn, chloride ensures that fluctuations in the plasma concentration of these ions are minimized and changes only occur in certain pathological circumstances. Measurements of plasma sodium, therefore, are of little consequence as far as nutritional status is concerned. Total body (excluding bone) sodium, however, is increased in malnutrition and trauma and this total exchangeable sodium can be measured, with some technical difficulty, using radioisotopes.

Salt intakes are notoriously difficult to measure, and urinary sodium excretion is considered to be a valid measure of sodium intake under circumstances where little sodium is lost in sweat. Sodium in urine is easily measured, but the collection of complete 24 h urinary samples is difficult because of subject compliance, and the completeness of these collections should be validated using a marker such as para-amino benzoic acid. Lithium (as carbonate) fused with sodium chloride can act as a reliable tracer to estimate discretionary salt (cooking and table) intakes.

Requirements and dietary sources

Average requirements for sodium and chloride are estimated to be about 500 and 750 mg/day, respectively. Normal sodium (mostly from salt) intake varies from about 2 to 14 g/day, with chloride (mostly from salt) intakes generally slightly in excess of sodium (Table 9.6).

Table 9.6 Salt intake as NaCl (g/day)

Before 1982	Year	Intake	From 1988	Year	Intake
Communities not using added salt					
Brazil (Yanomamo Indian)	1975	0.06			
New Guinea (Chimbus)	1967	0.40			
Solomon Islands (Kwaio)		1.20			
Botswana (Kung bushmen)		1.80			
Polynesia (Pukapuka)		3.60			
Alaska (Eskimos)	1961	<4.00			
Marshall Islands in the Pacific		7.00			
Salt-using communities					
Kenya (Sambura nomads)		5–8	Mexico (Tarahumsa Indian)		3–10
Mexico (Tarahumsa Indian)	1978	5–8	Mexico, rural (Nalinalco)	1992	5.7
			Mexico, urban (Tlaplan)	1991	7.18
Denmark		9.8	Denmark	1988	8.00
Canada (Newfoundland)		9.9	Canada		8–10
New Zealand		10.1			
Sweden (Göteborg)		10.2			
USA (Evans Country, Georgia)		10.6	USA (Chicago)		7.7
Iran		10.9			
Belgium	1966	11.4	Belgium	1988	8.4
UK (Scotland)		11.5			
Australia		12.0			
India (north)		12–15	India		9–11.4
Federal Republic of Germany		13.1			
Finland (east)		14.3	Finland		10.6
Bahamas		15–30			
Kenya (Samburus, army)	1969	18.6			
Korea		19.9			
Japan					
Japan (farmers)	1955	60.3	Japan	1988	8–15
Japan (Akita)		27–30			
Japan	1964	20.9			

Table 9.7 Salting (g/100 g fresh weight) of foods in Western societies

	Na	K	Ca	Mg
Maize-based products				
Corn	4	284	55	41
Tortilla, rural	11	192	177	65
Breakfast cereals	866	101	3	11
Processed snacks	838	197	102	56
Wheat-based products				
Natural cereals	39	1166	94	343
Tortillas, wheat	622	73	11	17
Breakfast cereals	855	869	81	236
Processed bread (urban)	573	126	47	31
Salted bread, made locally (rural)	410	92	10	74
Sweet bread, made locally (rural)	97	93	87	18
Processed bread (rural)	344	79	213	18
Processed biscuits	582	80	16	17
Pulses				
Unprocessed, cooked	53	373	50	41
Processed, canned	354	371	27	79

Reproduced with permission from Sánchez-Castillo and James (1999).

Snack and processed foods have more added salt than unprocessed foods. The amount of discretionary salt added in cooking or at the table appears to vary greatly among individuals and among countries. Discretionary salt intakes can vary from less than 10% to 20–30% of total salt intake and these figures emphasize the major effect of processed foods on total salt intakes in most populations (Table 9.7).

Micronutrient interactions

The major interactions between sodium (and chloride) and other micronutrients are with respect to potassium and calcium. Data from animals (and some clinical studies) indicate that dietary potassium and calcium potentiate increases in blood pressure in salt-sensitive experimental models. There is evidence to suggest that the sodium to potassium ratio correlates more strongly with blood pressure than does either nutrient alone. As indicated previously, the metabolism of sodium, chloride and potassium is closely related, while sodium and calcium ions have a close metabolic relationship within cells.

9.6 Potassium

Potassium, sodium and chloride comprise the principal electrolytes within the body. In contrast to sodium and chloride, nutritional concerns with potassium are mainly concerned with the possibility of underconsumption.

Absorption, transport and tissue distribution

Potassium is the major intracellular electrolyte and exists as the fully water-soluble cation. More than 90% of dietary potassium is absorbed from the digestive tract.

Few dietary components affect absorption of potassium, although olive oil can increase, and dietary fiber decrease absorption to some extent. The "average" 70 kg male contains about 120 g of potassium, depending on muscle mass, with males having proportionally greater muscle mass, and hence potassium, than females. Almost all of the body potassium is exchangeable, intracellular concentration being more than 30 times the concentration of the ECF. Potassium is distributed within the body in response to energy-dependent sodium redistribution. Various hormonal and other factors regulate potassium homeostasis, both within cells and with the external environment. Hyperkalemia (too much potassium in the ECF) stimulates insulin, aldosterone and adrenaline secretions, which promote the uptake of potassium by body cells. The aldosterone hormone also stimulates potassium excretion by the kidney and, at the same time, conserves sodium. Hypokalemia has opposite effects, such that more potassium is released from cells. As with sodium, the kidney regulates potassium balance. Urine is the major excretory route in healthy people, with only small amounts lost in the feces and minimal amounts in sweat.

Metabolic function and essentiality

Potassium, sodium and chloride are the major determinants of osmotic pressure and electrolyte balance. The concentration difference of potassium and sodium across cell membranes is maintained by the Na^+/K^+-ATPase pump and is critical for nerve transmission and muscle function. The physiological importance of potassium in the body covers many systems including cardiovascular, respiratory, digestive, renal and endocrine. In addition, potassium is a cofactor for enzymes involved in *inter alia* energy metabolism, glycogenesis, and cellular growth and division.

Deficiency symptoms

The low concentration of potassium in plasma is tightly regulated. Hypokalemia, however, can result from either excessive uptake of potassium by cells or potassium depletion from the body. Insulin excess, catecholamine increases, Cushing's disease (excess steroids), diuretics that enhance potassium loss, chronic renal disease, diarrhea, vomiting and laxative abuse can result in hypokalemia. Low potassium intakes are unlikely to lead to clinical potassium depletion and hypokalemia except during starvation and anorexia nervosa.

The activity of nerves and muscles is affected in potassium depletion and other clinical sequelae involve cardiac (including cardiac arrest), renal and metabolic alterations. Potassium supplementation may have a role to play in chronic heart failure, and increased potassium intakes can decrease blood pressure via antagonistic metabolic interactions with sodium, resulting in increased sodium excretion, and also via a direct vasodilatory effect. Oral administration of potassium salts has been shown to improve calcium and phosphorous balance, reduce bone resorption and increase the rate of bone formation.

Toxicity

Hyperkalemia, as a result of either a shift of potassium from cells to the ECF or excessive potassium retention, can be caused by major trauma and infection, metabolic acidosis, Addison's disease (aldosterone insufficiency) and chronic renal failure. Overuse of potassium supplements can also result in potassium excess. As with potassium depletion, the most important clinical consequence of potassium excess is cardiac arrest.

Assessing status

The plasma concentration of potassium is not a reliable index of whole body potassium status. Total body potassium can be measured by ^{42}K dilution or by whole body counting of the naturally abundant ^{40}K to determine the amount of lean body tissue. More direct measures of tissue potassium can be obtained by muscle biopsies.

Requirement and dietary sources

Adult requirements for potassium are estimated to be about 2 g/day. Because of potential beneficial antagonistic effects against high salt intakes, higher intakes (around 3.5 g/day) of potassium are considered to be optimal, while chronic intakes above 5.9 g/day may be dangerous for individuals with impaired renal function. Potassium, like sodium and chloride, is naturally widely distributed in foods (see Table 9.8). Food pro-

Table 9.8 Sodium and potassium content of various foods (mg/100 g edible portion)

Food	Na	K
Legumes		
Red kidney beans	18	1370
Soyabeans	5	1730
Lentils	12	940
Dried fruit		
Raisins	60	1020
Figs	62	970
Nuts		
Walnuts	7	450
Almonds	14	780
Fruit and vegetables		
Banana	1	400
Melon	5–32	100–210
Potato	11	320
Spinach	140	500
Meat and fish		
Beef, veal, lamb	52–110	230–260
Chicken	81	320
Herring	120	320
Halibut	60	410
Tuna	47	400
Mussels	290	320
Miscellaneous		
Cow's milk	55	140
Chocolate	11	300

Reproduced with permission from Sánchez-Castillo and James (1999).

cessing (through leaching) may decrease potassium content as well as increasing salt content. Legumes, nuts, dried fruit and fresh fruit, especially bananas, melons, avocados and kiwi fruit, are rich sources of potassium. Major vegetable sources of potassium are potatoes and spinach, while cereal and dairy products, which have a lower potassium content but are consumed in large quantities, are also important dietary sources. In addition, meat and fish contain appreciable quantities of potassium. People who eat large quantities of fruit and vegetables may have dietary intakes of potassium exceeding 6 g/day.

Micronutrient interactions

As might be expected from the close metabolic interactions among the major electrolytes, potassium and sodium dietary interactions may be important in determining risk of coronary heart disease and stroke. Another potentially important interaction concerns calcium. Potassium appears to have positive effects on calcium balance by regulating acid–base balance and ameliorating any effects of sodium on calcium depletion.

9.7 Iron

Iron is a relatively abundant element in the universe. It is found in the sun and many types of stars in considerable quantity. The core of the Earth is thought to be largely composed of iron and it comprises 4.7% of the Earth's crust. The most common ore is hematite, which is frequently seen as black sands along beaches and streams. Taconite is becoming increasingly important as a commercial ore. Because iron is easy to obtain, its discovery is lost in the history of man, many thousands of years ago. The early Greeks were aware of the health-giving properties of iron. Iron has been used for centuries as a health tonic. It is therefore paradoxical that although the need for iron was discovered long ago and although it is the most common and cheapest of all metals, iron deficiency is probably the most frequent deficiency disorder in the world and the main remaining nutritional deficiency in Europe. Iron can exist in oxidation states ranging from -2 to $+6$. In biological systems, these oxidation states occur primarily as the ferrous (Fe^{2+}) and ferric (Fe^{3+}) forms and these are interchangeable.

Absorption, transport and tissue distribution

The iron content of a typical 70 kg adult man is approximately 4–5 g. Of this, approximately two-thirds is utilized as functional iron such as hemoglobin (60%), myoglobin (5%), and various heme (cytochromes and catalase) and nonheme (NADH hydrogenase, succinic dehydrogenase, aconitase) enzymes (5%). The remaining iron is found in body storage as ferritin (20%) and hemosiderin (10%), the two major iron-storage proteins. Only very minor quantities of iron (<0.1%) are found as a transit chelate with transferrin, the main iron-transport protein in the body.

The metabolism of iron differs from that of other minerals in one important respect: there is no physiological mechanism for iron excretion. The body has three unique mechanisms for maintaining iron balance and preventing iron deficiency and iron overload:

- storage of iron (with ferritin being an important reversible storage protein for iron)

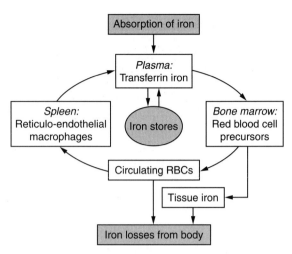

Figure 9.5 Metabolism of iron. There is a main internal loop with a continuous reutilization of iron and an external loop represented by iron losses from the body and absorption from the diet. Adapted from Hallberg *et al.* (1993).

- reutilization of iron (especially of iron in erythrocytes)
- regulation of iron absorption.

In theory, therefore, when the body needs more iron, absorption is increased, and when the body is iron sufficient, absorption is restricted. This control is not perfect but is still of great importance for the prevention of iron deficiency and excess. Iron from food is absorbed mainly in the duodenum by an active process that transports iron from the gut lumen into the mucosal cell. When required by the body for metabolic processes, iron passes directly through the mucosal cell into the bloodstream, where it is transported by transferrin, together with the iron released from old blood cells (i.e. the efficient iron recycling system, Figure 9.5), to the bone marrow (80%) and other tissues (20%). If iron is not required by the body, iron in the mucosal cell is stored as ferritin and is excreted in feces when the mucosal cell is exfoliated. Any absorbed iron in excess of needs is stored as ferritin or hemosiderin in the liver, spleen or bone marrow. Iron can be released from these iron stores for utilization in times of high need, such as during pregnancy.

Heme iron is absorbed by a different mechanism from nonheme iron. The heme molecule is absorbed intact into the mucosal cell, where iron is released by the enzyme, heme oxygenase. Its absorption is little influenced by the composition of the meal, and varies from 15 to 35% depending on the iron status of the consumer. Although heme iron represents only 10–15% of

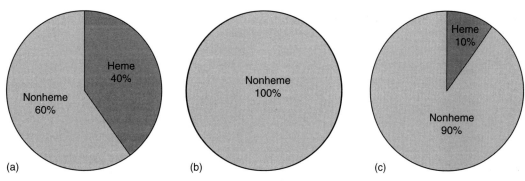

Figure 9.6 Heme and nonheme iron in foods: (a) foods of animal origin; (b) foods of plant origin; (c) dietary iron intake from all foods, daily average.

dietary iron intake in populations with a high meat intake, it could contribute 40% or more of the total absorbed iron (Figure 9.6). Many poorer regions of the world consume little animal tissue and rely entirely on nonheme iron. The absorption of nonheme iron is strongly influenced by dietary components, which bind iron in the intestinal lumen. The complexes formed can be either insoluble or so tightly bound that the iron is prevented from being absorbed. Alternatively, the complexes can be soluble and iron absorption is facilitated. Nonheme iron absorption can vary widely from less than 1% to more than 90%, but is usually in the region of 1–20%. The main inhibitory substances and enhancers of iron absorption are shown in Table 9.9.

Metabolic function and essentiality

Iron acts as a catalytic center for a broad spectrum of metabolic functions. As present in hemoglobin, iron is required for the transport of oxygen, critical for cell respiration. As myoglobin, iron is required for oxygen storage in muscle. Iron is also a component of various tissue enzymes, such as the cytochromes, that are critical for energy production, and enzymes necessary for immune system functioning. Therefore, these iron-containing molecules ensure that body fuels, such as carbohydrate, fat and protein are oxidized to provide the energy necessary for all physiological processes and movement. The importance of iron as an element necessary for life derives from its redox reactivity as it exists in two stable, interchangeable forms, ferrous (Fe^{2+}) and ferric (Fe^{3+}) iron. This reaction is an essential part of the electron transport chain, responsible for the generation of ATP during the oxidation of substances in intermediary metabolism and for the reductions necessary in the synthesis of larger molecules from their components.

Table 9.9 Factors affecting (a) heme and (b) nonheme iron absorption

Increased absorption	Decreased absorption
(a) Heme	
Physiological factors	
Low iron status	High iron status
Dietary factors	
Low heme iron intake	High heme iron intake
Meat	Calcium
(b) Nonheme	
Physiological factors	
Depleted iron status	Replete iron status
Pregnancy	Achlorhydria (low gastric acid)
Disease states (aplastic anemia, hemolytic anemia, hemochromatosis)	
Dietary factors	
Ascorbic acid	Phytate
Meat, fish, seafood	Iron-binding phenolic compounds
Certain organic acids	Calcium

Deficiency symptoms

The progression from adequate iron status to iron-deficiency anemia develops in three overlapping stages. The first stage consists of depletion of storage iron, which is characterized by a decrease in serum ferritin which, in turn, reflects the size of the iron stores in the liver, bone marrow and spleen. The second stage is a decrease in transported iron and is characterized by a decline in serum iron and an increase in the total iron-binding capacity, as transferrin has more free binding sites than in normal iron status. The third stage develops when the supply of iron is insufficient to provide for enough hemoglobin for new erythrocytes and insufficient to fulfil other physiological functions.

During the latter stage, free protoporphyrin, destined for hemoglobin, increases in plasma two- to five-fold, indicating a lack of tissue iron. The harmful consequences of iron deficiency occur mainly in conjunction with anemia. Iron-deficiency anemia is most common in infants, preschool children, adolescents and women of child-bearing age, particularly in developing countries.

The functional effects of iron-deficiency anemia result from both a reduction in circulating hemoglobin and a reduction in iron-containing enzymes and myoglobin. Both factors presumably play a role in the fatigue, restlessness and impaired work performance associated with iron-deficiency anemia. Other functional defects include disturbances in normal thermoregulation and impairment of certain key steps in the immune response. For example, there is evidence that iron-deficiency anemia is associated with lower T- and B-lymphocyte, macrophage and neutrophil function. Although the phagocytic uptake of neutrophils is usually normal, the intracellular killing mechanism is usually defective. This is thought to be owing to a defect in the generation of reactive oxygen intermediates resulting from a decrease in the iron-containing enzyme myeloperoxidase. Iron-deficiency anemia can also have an adverse effect on psychomotor and mental development in children, and mortality and morbidity of mother and infant during pregnancy.

Toxicity

The very effective regulation of iron absorption prevents overload of the tissues by iron from a normal diet, except in individuals with genetic defects, as in idiopathic hemochromatosis (see below). Excess iron via overuse of iron supplements could pose a possible health risk. The mechanism of cellular and tissue injury resulting from excess iron is not fully understood, but it is thought that free radical reactions may be involved. Normally in the body, iron is bound tightly to proteins, which ensures that iron is prevented from reacting with biomolecules. It is possible that excess iron intake permits some iron to be in a free form and this may promote the formation of free radicals. Liabilities may include increased risks for bacterial infection, neoplasia, arthropathy, cardiomyopathy and endocrine dysfunctions. However, there is still much debate as to the strength of evidence to support a relationship between dietary iron intake and cancer or cardiovascular disease.

Gastrointestinal distress does not occur from consuming a diet containing naturally occurring or fortified iron. Individuals taking iron at high levels (>45 mg/day) may encounter gastrointestinal side-effects (constipation, nausea, vomiting and diarrhea), especially when taken on an empty stomach. Based largely on the data on gastrointestinal effects following supplemental elemental iron intake in apparently healthy adults, the US Food and Nutrition Board established a tolerable UL of iron of 45 mg/day.

Genetic diseases

Primary idiopathic hemochromatosis is a hereditary disorder of iron metabolism characterized by an abnormally high iron absorption owing to a failure of the iron absorption control mechanism at the intestinal level. High deposits of iron in the liver and the heart can lead to cirrhosis, hepatocellular cancer, congestive heart failure and eventual death. Sufferers of this disorder can develop iron overload through consumption of a normal diet, but would be at much higher risk if consuming iron-fortified foods. Thus, early detection of the disease via genetic screening followed by regular blood removal has proven to be a successful treatment.

Assessing status

Several different laboratory methods must be used in combination to diagnose iron-deficiency anemia correctly. The most commonly used methods to assess iron status include

- serum ferritin
- transferrin saturation
- erythrocyte protoporphyrin
- mean corpuscular volume
- serum transferrin receptor
- hemoglobin or packed cell volume.

Iron-deficiency anemia is usually defined as a hemoglobin level below the cut-off value for age and sex plus at least two other abnormal iron status measurements. The most commonly used are probably low serum ferritin, high protoporphyrin and, more recently, high serum transferrin receptor.

Requirements and dietary sources

Daily (absorbed or physiological) iron requirements are calculated from the amount of dietary iron necessary to cover basal iron losses, menstrual losses and growth needs. They vary according to age and sex, and in relation to body weight, they are highest for the young infant. An adult man has obligatory iron losses of around 1 mg of iron/day, largely from the gastro-intestinal tract (exfoliation of epithelial cells and secretions), skin and urinary tract. Thus, to remain replete with regard to iron, an average adult man needs to absorb only 1 mg of iron from the diet on a daily basis. Similar obligatory iron losses for women amount to around 0.8 mg/day. However, adult women experience additional iron loss owing to menstruation, which raises the median daily iron requirement for absorption to 1.4 mg (this covers 90% of menstruating women; 10% will require daily absorption of at least 2.4 mg iron to compensate for their very high menstrual losses). Pregnancy creates an additional demand for iron, especially during the second and third trimesters, leading to daily requirements of 4–6 mg. Growing children and adolescents require 0.5 mg iron/day in excess of body losses to support growth. Physiological iron needs can be translated into dietary requirements by taking into account the efficiency at which iron is absorbed from the diet. Current RDA for iron (recommended by the US Food and Nutrition Board in 2001) are: infants 0.27 mg (first 6 months; this is an adequate intake value), 11 mg (7–12 months), children 7 and 10 mg (1–3 and 4–8 years, respectively), teenage boys 8 and 11 mg (9–13 and 14–18 years, respectively), adult men 8 mg (19 years and older), teenage girls 8 and 15 mg (9–13 and 14–18 years, respectively), adult women 18 and 8 mg (19–50 years and 51 years and older, respectively), pregnant women 27 mg and lactating women 10 and 9 mg (younger than 18 years and 19–50 years, respectively).

Iron is widely distributed in meat, eggs, vegetables and cereals, but the concentrations in milk, fruit and vegetables are low (Table 9.10). The iron content per se of individual foods has little meaning as iron absorption varies considerably. There are two types of food iron: nonheme iron, which is present in both plant foods and animal tissues, and heme iron, coming from the hemoglobin and myoglobin in animal products. Heme iron represents 30–70% of the total iron in lean meat and is always well absorbed. Nonheme iron from meat and vegetable foods enters a common nonheme iron pool in the gastric juice, from which the amount of iron absorbed depends to a large extent on the presence of enhancing and inhibiting substances in the meal and on the iron status of the individual.

Table 9.10 Iron content of some common foods

Food source	Description	Fe content (mg/100 g)
Liver	Raw, calf	8.0
Beef	Lean (from six different cuts)	2.1
Black (blood) sausage	Fried	20.0
Chicken	Raw, meat only	0.7
Cod, plaice, whiting	Raw	0.3–1.0
Eggs	Chicken, whole, raw	1.9
Pulses	Raw	0.6–11.1
Wheat flour	Whole flour	3.9
Wheat flour	White flour	1.5–2.0
Milk	Cow's (3.9, 1.6 and 0.1% fat)	0.05–0.06
Green leafy vegetables	Raw	0.7–2.2
Rice	Raw, white, polished	0.5
Potatoes	Raw	0.3–0.4

Data from Holland *et al.* (1995).

Micronutrient interactions

The fact that serum copper has been found to be low in some cases of iron-deficiency anemia suggests that iron status has an effect on copper metabolism. Copper deficiency impinges on iron metabolism, causing an anemia that does not respond to iron supplementation. Interactions between iron and copper seem to be owing to impaired utilization of one in the absence of the other. As mentioned above, calcium can inhibit iron absorption under certain circumstances. In aqueous solutions iron impairs zinc absorption, but this interaction does not take place when iron is added to an animal protein meal, indicating different uptake mechanisms for solutions and solid foods.

9.8 Zinc

The natural abundance of zinc in the Earth's crust is 0.02%. The principal ores of zinc are sphalerite or blende (sulfide), smithsonite (carbonate), calamine (silicate) and franklinite (zinc iron oxide). Zinc is used to form numerous alloys with other metals. Brass, nickel, silver, typewriter metal, commercial bronze, spring brass, German silver, soft solder and aluminum solder are some of the more important alloys. Large quantities of zinc are used to produce die castings, used extensively by the automotive, electrical and hardware industries. Zinc is also extensively used to galvanize other metals, such as iron to prevent corrosion. Zinc oxide is widely used in the manufacture of paints, rubber products, cosmetics, pharmaceuticals, floor coverings, plastics, printing inks, soap, storage batteries, textiles, electrical equipment and other products. Zinc sulfide is used in making luminous dials, X-ray and television screens, and fluorescent lights. The chloride and chromate are also important compounds. In biological systems zinc is virtually always in the divalent ($+2$) state. Unlike iron, zinc does not exhibit any direct redox chemistry.

Absorption, transport and tissue distribution

Zinc is ubiquitous in the body. It is the most abundant intracellular trace element, with $>95\%$ of the body zinc intracellular. An adult human contains about 2 g of zinc, of which about 60% and 30% are in skeletal muscle and bone, respectively, and 4–6% is present in skin (Table 9.11). Zinc turnover in these tissues is slow and, therefore, the zinc in these tissues is not accessible at times of deprivation. Because zinc is essential for the synthesis of lean tissue, it is while this is occurring that it may become a limiting nutrient. Although some zinc may be available in short-term zinc deprivation from a mobile hepatic pool, it is generally assumed that the body has no specific zinc reserve and is dependent on a regular supply of the element.

With essential roles in many fundamental cellular processes (see below), it is not surprising that whole-body zinc content is tightly controlled. Zinc in foods is absorbed via a carrier-mediated transport process, which under normal physiological conditions appears not to be saturated. Zinc is absorbed throughout the small intestine. Proximal intestinal absorption is efficient, but it has a large enteropancreatic circulation; net intestinal absorption of zinc is achieved by the distal small intestine. Zinc is transported in the plasma by albumin and α_2-macroglobulin, but only 0.1% of body zinc is found in plasma. Body zinc content is regulated by homeostatic mechanisms over a wide range of intakes by changes in fractional absorption (normally 20–40%) and urinary (0.5 mg/day) and intestinal (1–3 mg/day) excretion. For example, during periods of low zinc intake, absorption is enhanced and secretion of endogenous zinc into the gastrointestinal lumen is suppressed. In contrast, high zinc intake is associated with decreased absorption and enhanced secretion of endogenous zinc. Within cells, fluctuations in zinc content are modulated by changes in the amount of the metal associated with the storage protein metallothionein.

Table 9.11 Approximate zinc content of major organs and tissues in the adult man

Tissue	Total Zn content (g)	Percentage of body Zn (%)
Skeletal muscle	1.53	~57
Bone	0.77	29
Skin	0.16	6
Liver	0.13	5
Brain	0.04	1.5
Kidneys	0.02	0.7
Heart	0.01	0.4
Hair	<0.01	~0.1
Blood (plasma)	<0.01	~0.1

Modified from Mills (1998).

Table 9.12 Factors affecting zinc absorption

Increased absorption	Decreased absorption
Physiological factors	
Depleted zinc status	Replete zinc status
	Disease state (acrodermatitis enteropathica)
Dietary factors	
Low zinc intake	High zinc intake
Certain organic acids	Phytate
Certain amino acids	Certain metals
Human milk	

The bioavailability of dietary zinc depends on dietary enhancers and inhibitors and host-related factors (Table 9.12). Diets can be roughly classified as having a low, medium or high bioavailability, according to the content of zinc, phytate and animal protein. From a mixed animal and plant product diet, 20–30% zinc absorption can be expected. The lowest absorption, 10–15%, is seen from diets prevalent in developing countries and which are based on cereals and legumes with a high phytate content and with negligible amounts of animal protein.

Metabolic function and essentiality

Zinc has three major groups of functions in the human body: catalytic, structural and regulatory. Most biochemical roles of zinc reflect its involvement in a large number of enzymes, and over 100 different zinc metalloenzymes have been identified, including RNA nucleotide polymerase I and II, alkaline phosphatase and carbonic anhydrases. Important structural roles for zinc are in the zinc finger motif in proteins, but also in metalloenzymes [e.g. copper/zinc superoxide dismutase (Cu/Zn-SOD)]. Zinc is also required by protein kinases that participate in signal transduction processes and as a stimulator of transacting factors responsible for regulating gene expression.

Deficiency symptoms

The clinical manifestations of severe zinc deficiency in humans are growth retardation, sexual and skeletal immaturity, neuropsychiatric disturbances, dermatitis, alopecia, diarrhea, increased susceptibility to infections and loss of appetite. Many of these features, by and large, represent the dependence on zinc of tissues with a high rate of turnover. However, severe zinc deficiency in humans is rare, and more interest has been focused on marginal zinc deficiency. This is more difficult to diagnose. Furthermore, it has been a challenge to define, and the current understanding of zinc deficiency is largely based on responses to zinc supplementation. Zinc supplementation has been reported to stimulate growth and development in infants and young children, and reduce morbidity (diarrhea and respiratory infections) in children. In women, low serum zinc concentration during pregnancy was found to be a significant predictor of low birth weight, and low maternal zinc intake has been associated with an approximately two-fold increased risk of low birth weight and increased risk of preterm delivery in poor urban women.

Toxicity

Gross acute zinc toxicity has been described following the drinking of water that has been stored in galvanized containers or the use of such water for renal dialysis. Symptoms include nausea, vomiting and fever, and are apparent after acute ingestion of 2 g or more. The more subtle effects of moderately elevated intakes, not uncommon in some populations, are of greater concern, because they are not easily detected. Prolonged intakes of supraphysiological intakes of zinc (75–300 mg/day) have been associated with impaired copper utilization (producing features such as microcytic anemia and neutropenia), impaired immune responses and a decline of high-density lipoproteins, but some have argued that even short-term intakes of about 25–50 mg zinc/day may interfere with the metabolism of both iron and copper. The US Food and Nutrition Board recently reported that there was no evidence of adverse effects from intake of naturally occurring zinc in food; however, they derived a tolerable UL of 40 mg/day for adults older than 19 years, which applies to total zinc intake from food, water and supplements (including fortified foods). Data on reduced copper status in humans were used to derive this UL for zinc.

Genetic diseases

Acrodermatitis enteropathica, a rare, inborn, autosomal recessive disease, is a disorder of primary zinc malabsorption. It is characterized by alopecia; vesicular, pustular and/or eczematoid skin lesions, specifically of the mouth, face, hands, feet and groin, growth retardation, mental apathy, diarrhea and secondary malabsorption, defects in cellular and phagocytic immune function, and intercurrent infections. The disorder responds very well to zinc therapy.

Assessing status

Measurement of zinc in plasma or activities of zinc metalloenzymes in blood are frequently used to measure zinc status. They are not ideal indices, however, as they are relatively resistant to changes in dietary zinc and, moreover, metabolic conditions unrelated to zinc status cause them to decline. The development of zinc deficiency is different from that of many other nutrients because a functional reserve or store of zinc does not seem to be available when zinc intake is inadequate. Tissue zinc is conserved by reduction or cessation of growth in growing organisms or by decreased excretion in nongrowing organisms. Depending on the degree of deficiency, zinc homeostasis can be re-established by adjusting growth and excretion or, with a more severe deficiency, further metabolic changes occur, resulting in a negative zinc balance and loss of tissue zinc.

Requirements and dietary sources

The US RDA for zinc was based primarily on data derived from metabolic balance studies. Such studies are technically difficult to perform and it is uncertain whether information from these studies reflects true requirements. Recently, a different approach, using the factorial method, was proposed for estimates of zinc requirements and future RDA. Factorial calculations to estimate zinc requirements require knowledge of obligatory losses, tissue composition, and needs for growth and tissue repair. Current RDA for zinc (recommended by the US Food and Nutrition Board in 2001) are: infants 2 mg [first 6 months; this is an adequate intake (AI) value], 3 mg (7–12 months), children 3 and 5 mg (1–3 and 4–8 years, respectively), teenage boys 8 and 11 mg (9–13 and 14–18 years, respectively), adult men 11 mg (19 years and more), teenage girls 8 and 9 mg (9–13 and 14–18 years, respectively), adult women 8 mg (19 years and older), pregnant women 13 and 11 mg (younger than 18 years and 19–50 years, respectively) and lactating women 14 and 12 mg (younger than 18 years and 19–50 years, respectively).

The bioavailability of zinc in different foods varies widely, from 5 to 50%. Meat, seafood (in particular oysters) and liver are good sources of bioavailable zinc (Table 9.13). It has been estimated that approximately 70% of dietary zinc in the US diet is provided by animal products. In meat products, the zinc content to some extent follows the color of the meat, so that the highest content, approximately 50 mg/kg, is found in lean red meat, at least twice that in chicken. However, in many parts of the world, most of the zinc is provided by cereals. In cereals, most of the zinc is found in the outer fiber-rich part of the kernel, thus the degree of refinement determines the total zinc content. Whole-grain products provide 30–50 mg/kg, while a low extraction rate wheat flour contains 8–10 mg/kg. The bioavailability of zinc can be low from plant-based diets, in particular from whole-grain cereals and legumes, owing to the high content of phytic acid, a potent inhibitor of zinc absorption.

Micronutrient interactions

A decrease in copper absorption has been reported in the presence of excessive zinc. Recent data indicate that the level necessary to impair bioavailability is >40–50 mg/day; but results from balance studies indicate that it must exceed normal dietary intakes; therapeutic levels (150 mg/day) over extended periods produce symptoms of copper deficiency. As mentioned above, iron under certain circumstances impairs zinc absorption. Animal studies have suggested an interaction between calcium and zinc in phytate-rich diets, but this has not been confirmed in human studies.

9.9 Copper

Copper occurs in the environment in three oxidation states. Copper (0) metal is used widely in the building industry (e.g. water pipes, electrical wires) because of its properties of malleability, ductibility and high thermal and electrical conductivity. Brass, an alloy of copper and zinc, is used for cooking utensils and musical instruments, while bronze, an alloy of copper and tin, has been used in castings since early times. Copper-based alloys and amalgams are used in dental bridges and crowns, and copper is a constituent of intra-uterine contraceptive devices. Copper compounds are widely used in the environment as fertilizers and nutritional supplements and, because of their microbicidal properties, as fungicides, algicides, insecticides and wood preservatives. Other industrial uses include dye manufacturing, petroleum refining, water treatment and metal finishing. Copper compounds in the cuprous (1) state are easily oxidized to the more stable cupric (2) state, which is found most often in biological systems.

The most important copper ores are chalcocite (Cu_2S), chalcopyrite ($CuFeS_2$) and malachite [$CuCO_3 \cdot Cu(OH)_2$]. Copper concentrations in soil vary from 5 to 50 mg Cu/kg and in natural water from 4 to 10 µg Cu/l. Concentrations of copper in water, however, depend on acidity, softness and extent of copper pipes and municipal water supplies can contain appreciably higher concentrations. The taste threshold of copper ranges from 1 to 5 mg Cu/l, producing a slight blue–

Table 9.13 Zinc content of some common foods

Food source	Description	Zn content (mg/100 g)
Liver	Raw, calf	7.8
Beef	Lean (from six different cuts)	4.3
Lamb	Lean (from six different cuts)	4.0
Pork	Lean (from three different cuts)	2.4
Chicken	Raw, meat only	1.1
Cod, plaice, whiting	Raw	0.3–0.5
Muscles	Boiled	2.1
Oysters	Raw	90–200
Crab	Boiled	5.5
Eggs	Chicken, whole, raw	1.3
Cheese	Soft and hard varieties	0.5–5.3
Pulses	Raw	0.2–5.0
Wheat flour	Whole flour	2.9
Wheat flour	White flour	0.6–0.9
Milk	Cow's (3.9, 1.6 and 0.1% fat)	0.4
Yoghurt	Whole milk	0.5–0.7
Green leafy vegetables	Raw	0.2–0.6
Rice	Raw, white, polished	1.8
Potatoes	Raw	0.2–0.3

Data from Holland *et al.* (1995).

green color at concentrations >5 mg Cu/l. Acute copper toxicity symptoms, mainly nausea and gastrointestinal irritation, can occur at concentrations of >4 mg Cu/l.

Absorption, transport and tissue distribution

About 50–75% of dietary copper is absorbed, mostly via the intestinal mucosa, from a typical diet. The amount of dietary copper appears to be the primary factor influencing absorption, with decreases in the percentage absorption as the amount of copper ingested increases. High intakes of several nutrients can also influence copper bioavailability. These include antagonistic effects of zinc, iron, molybdenum, ascorbic acid, sucrose and fructose, although evidence for some of these is mainly from animal studies. Drugs and medication, such as penicillamine and thiomolybdates, restrict copper accumulation in the body and excessive use of antacids can inhibit copper absorption. While high intakes of sulfur amino acids can limit copper absorption, absorption of copper is promoted from high-protein diets.

Ionic copper can be released from partially digested food particles in the stomach, but immediately forms complexes with amino acids, organic acids or other chelators. Soluble complexes of these and other highly soluble species of the metal, such as the sulfate or nitrate, are readily absorbed. Regulation of absorption at low levels of copper intake is probably by a saturable active transport mechanism, while passive diffusion plays a role at high levels of copper intake. Regulation of copper absorption is also effected via metallothionein, a metal-binding protein found in the intestine and other tissues. Metallothionein-bound copper in mucosal cells will be lost when these cells are removed by intestinal flow. The major regulator of copper elimination from the body, however, is biliary excretion. Most biliary copper is not reabsorbed and is eliminated in the feces. The overall effect of these regulatory mechanisms is a tight homeostasis of body copper status. Little copper is lost from the urine, skin, nails and hair.

After absorption from the intestinal tract, ionic copper (2) is transported tightly bound to albumin and transcuprein to the liver via the portal bloodstream, with some going directly to other tissues, especially the kidney. Hepatic copper is mostly incorporated into ceruloplasmin, which is then released into the blood and delivered to other tissues. Uptake of copper by tissues can occur from various sources including ceruloplasmin, albumin, transcuprein and low molecular weight copper compounds. Chaperone proteins are then thought to bind the copper and transfer bound copper across the cell membrane to the intracellular target proteins, for example cytochrome c oxidase. The ATPase proteins may form part of the transfer process.

The body of a healthy 70 kg adult contains a little over 0.1 g of copper, with the highest concentrations found in the liver, brain, heart, bone, hair and nails. Over 25% of body copper resides in the muscle, which forms a large part of the total body tissue. Much of the copper in the body is functional. Storage of copper, however, is very important to the neonate. At birth, infant liver concentrations are some five to 10 times the adult concentration and these stores are used during early life when copper intakes from milk are low.

Metabolic functions and essentiality

Copper is a component of several enzymes, cofactors and proteins in the body. These enzymes and proteins have important functions in processes fundamental to human health (Table 9.14). These include a requirement for copper in the proper functioning of the immune, nervous and cardiovascular systems, for bone health, for iron metabolism and formation of red blood cells, and in the regulation of mitochondrial and other gene expression. In particular, copper functions as an electron transfer intermediate in redox reactions and as a cofactor in several copper-containing metalloenzymes. As well as a direct role in maintaining cuproenzyme activity, changes in copper status may have indirect effects on other enzyme systems that do not contain copper.

Deficiency symptoms

Owing to remarkable homeostatic mechanisms, clinical symptoms of copper deficiency occur in humans only under exceptional circumstances. Infants are more susceptible to overt symptoms of copper deficiency than are any other population group. Among the predisposing factors of copper deficiency are prematurity, low birth weight and malnutrition, especially when combined with feeding practices such as cow's milk or total parenteral nutrition. The most frequent symptoms of copper deficiency are anemia, neutropenia and bone fractures, while less frequent symptoms

Table 9.14 Human enzymes and proteins that contain copper

Enzyme or protein	Function
Cytochrome c oxidase	Mitochondrial enzyme involved in the electron transport chain; reduces oxygen to water and allows formation of ATP; activity is highest in the heart and also high in the brain, liver and kidney
Ceruloplasmin (ferroxidase I)	Glycoprotein with six or seven copper atoms; four copper atoms involved in oxidation/reduction reactions; role of other copper atoms not fully known; scavenges free radicals; quencher of superoxide radicals generated in the circulation; oxidizes some aromatic amines and phenols; catalyzes oxidation of ferrous iron to ferric iron; assists with iron transport from storage to sites of hemoglobin synthesis; about 60% of plasma copper bound to ceruloplasmin; primarily extracellular; activity will be low during severe copper restriction
Ferroxidase II	Catalyzes oxidation of iron; no other functions known; in human plasma is only about 5% of ferroxidase activity
Hephaestin	Membrane-bound ceruloplasmin homologue; probably a multicopper oxidase required for iron export from the intestine
Monoamine oxidase	Inactivates catecholamines; reacts with serotonin, noradrenaline, tyramine and dopamine; activity inhibited by some antidepressant medications
Diamine oxidase	Inactivates histamine and polyamines; highest activity in small intestine; also high activity in kidney and placenta
Lysyl oxidase	Acts on lysine and hydroxylysine found in immature collagen and elastin; important for integrity of skeletal and vascular tissue; use of estrogen increases activity
Dopamine β-hydroxylase	Catalyzes conversion of dopamine to noradrenaline, a neurotransmitter; contains two to eight copper atoms; important in brain and adrenal glands
Copper, zinc superoxide dismutase	Contains two copper atoms; primarily in cytosol, protects against oxidative damage by converting superoxide ion to hydrogen peroxide; erythrocyte concentrations are somewhat responsive to changes in copper intake
Extracellular superoxide dismutase	Protects against oxidative damage by scavenging superoxide ion radicals and converting them to hydrogen peroxide; small amounts in plasma; larger amounts in lungs, thyroid and uterus
Tyrosinase	Involved in melanin synthesis; deficiency of this enzyme in skin leads to albinism; catalyzes conversion of tyrosine to dopamine and oxidation of dopamine to dopaquinone; present in eye and skin and forms color in hair, skin and eyes
Metallothionein	Cysteine-rich protein that binds zinc, cadmium and copper; important for sequestering metal ions and preventing toxicity
Albumin	Binds and transports copper in plasma and interstitial fluids; about 10–15% of copper in plasma is bound to albumin
Transcuprein	Binds copper in human plasma; may transport copper
Blood clotting factors V and VIII	Role in clotting and thrombogenesis; part of structure homologous with ceruloplasmin

are hypopigmentation, impaired growth, increased incidence of infections, and abnormalities of glucose and cholesterol metabolism and of electrocardiograms. Various attempts have been made to relate these symptoms to alterations in copper metalloenzymes (see Table 9.14) and noncopper enzymes that may be copper responsive, and to identify the role of copper as an antioxidant, in carbohydrate metabolism, immune function, bone health and cardiovascular mechanisms. Notwithstanding the rarity of frank copper deficiency in human populations, some have speculated that suboptimal copper intakes over long periods may be involved in the precipitation of chronic diseases, such as cardiovascular disease and osteoporosis. The pathological significance of subtle changes, in the longer term, in those systems that respond to copper deficiency have yet to be defined for humans.

Toxicity

Acute copper toxicity in humans is rare and usually occurs from contamination of drinking water, beverages and foodstuffs from copper pipes or containers, or from accidental or deliberate ingestion of large amounts of copper salts. Symptoms include vomiting, diarrhea, hemolytic anemia, renal and liver damage, sometimes (at about 100 g or more) followed by coma and death. Clinical symptoms of chronic copper toxicity appear when the capacity for protective copper binding in the liver is exceeded. These symptoms include hepatitis, liver cirrhosis and jaundice.

Consumption of formula milks, heavily contaminated with copper after boiling or storage in brass vessels, is usually a feature of Indian childhood cirrhosis, which occurs in early weaned infants between the ages of 6 months and 5 years. Symptoms include abdominal distension, irregular fever, excessive crying and altered appetite, followed by jaundice and often death. Some believe that a genetic disorder enhances susceptibility to this toxicity syndrome, associated with excessive dietary exposure to copper and massive accumulation of liver copper.

Genetic diseases

There are several disorders that result in deficiency or toxicity from exposure to copper intakes tolerated by the general population. The most important of these are: Menkes' syndrome, an X-linked copper deficiency that is usually fatal in early childhood; Wilson's disease, an autosomal recessive disorder resulting in copper overload; and aceruloplasminemia, an autosomal recessive disorder of iron metabolism. All three disorders are characterized by low serum copper and ceruloplasmin.

Menkes' syndrome, which affects 1 in 300 000 in most populations, is caused by mutations in the gene that encodes a novel member of the family of cation-transporting p-type ATPases. The gene is expressed in extrahepatic tissues, and symptoms result from an inability to export copper from cells, particularly from intestinal cells and across the placenta. The syndrome has three forms, classic, mild and occipital horn. Among the symptoms of the classic (most severe) Menkes' syndrome are abnormal myelination with cerebellar neurodegeneration (giving progressive mental retardation), abnormal (steely, kinky) hair, hypothermia, hypopigmentation, seizures, convulsions, failure to thrive and connective tissue abnormalities resulting in deformities in the skull, long bones and ribs, and twisted, tortuous arteries. Death usually occurs in the severe forms before 3 years of age.

Wilson's disease, which affects 1 in 30 000 in most populations, is caused by numerous (over 100 recognized) mutations in the gene for a copper-transporting ATPase. The defect results in impaired biliary excretion of copper and accumulation of copper in the liver

and brain of homozygous individuals or compound heterozygotes. Abnormalities in copper homeostatis, however, may also occur in heterozygous carriers, who may make up 1–2% of the population. The age of onset is from childhood onwards and patients may present in three different ways: with hepatic symptoms (with liver cirrhosis and fatty infiltration in the latter stages), with neurological symptoms (degeneration of the basal ganglia resulting in defective movement, slurred speech, difficulty swallowing, face and muscle spasms, dystonia and poor motor control), or with psychiatric and behavioral problems (including depression and schizophrenia, loss of emotional control, temper tantrums and insomnia). Kayser–Fleischer rings (corneal copper deposits) in the eyes are generally present in neurological or psychiatric presentations. The phenotypic differences between Wilson's disease and Menkes' syndrome are probably owing to the tissue-specific expression of the ATPase genes.

If Wilson's disease is diagnosed early, copper chelation therapy, usually with D-penicillamine, can be beneficial, although neurological symptoms are often irreversible and liver disease may be advanced at the time of diagnosis. Zinc supplements limit copper absorption and subsequent accumulation, and this is the treatment of choice for maintenance therapy.

Aceruloplasminemia, which affects about 1 in 2 million individuals, is caused by mutations in the ceruloplasmin gene. Ceruloplasmin is involved in iron metabolism and, in the disease, there is an accumulation of ferrous iron within the recticuloendothelial system with pathogenesis mainly linked to the slow accumulation of iron in the brain, rather than other tissues. Symptoms include dementia, speech problems, retinal degeneration, poor muscle tone and diabetes. Early therapy with the high-affinity iron chelator desferoxamine can relieve some of the symptoms.

Disruption of copper metabolism may be involved in other neurodegenerative diseases such as the accumulation of amyloid β-protein in Alzheimer's disease and the accumulation of modified prion protein in human prion disease.

About 10% of motor neurone disease cases are familial and 20% of these are owing to autosomal dominant inheritance of mutations in the Cu/Zn-SOD (SODI) gene. It is unclear how changes in activity of this copper enzyme might be involved in the progressive muscle weakness and atrophy of motor neurone disease or in Down's syndrome, where additional Cu/Zn-SOD activity results from the *SOD1* gene being present in the extra chromosome 21.

Assessing status

It is possible to diagnose severe copper deficiency in infants from plasma or serum copper, ceruloplasmin protein and neutrophils. These measures, however, cannot be used to detect suboptimal copper status in individuals, as such measures are insensitive to small changes in copper status and there are intractable problems in interpretation. Ceruloplasmin, the major copper protein in plasma or serum, is an acute-phase reactant and is raised by cigarette smoking, oral contraceptives, estrogens, pregnancy, infections, inflammation, hematological diseases, hypertension, diabetes, cardiovascular diseases, cancer and cirrhosis, and after surgery and exercise.

Currently, there is no adequate measure of suboptimal (or supraoptimal) copper status and this is a major barrier to determining precise dietary requirements for copper and the possible role of suboptimal or supraoptimal copper status in the etiology of chronic disease. Table 9.15 gives some of the functional indices (classified as molecular, biochemical and physiological) that might be used to define suboptimal or supraoptimal status in humans. A valid functional index of copper status in humans must respond sensitively, specifically and predictably to changes in the concentration and supply of dietary copper or copper stores, be accessible for measurement and measurable, and impact directly on health. As such, indices in Table 9.15 have not been validated and many lack sensitivity and specificity. Perhaps, the best way forward is to use a combination of measures. Among the more promising are erythrocyte superoxide dismutase activity, platelet cytochrome c oxidase, plasma diamine oxidase, plasma peptidyl glycine α-amidating mono-oxygenase, urinary pyridinium cross-links of collagen (may indicate lowered activity of the cuproenzyme, lysyl oxidase) and various immunological measures.

Requirements and dietary sources

Although copper is the third most abundant trace element, after iron and zinc, in the body, precise dietary requirements for copper are still subject to conjecture because of the difficulty in assessing copper status. Current estimates suggest that the requirements for copper for the great majority of adults are below about

Table 9.15 Putative functional indices of copper status

Molecular indices
Changes in activity/concentration of Cu-metalloproteins:
    Ceruloplasmin oxidase
    Ceruloplasmin protein
    Superoxide dismutase
    Cytochrome c oxidase
    Lysyl oxidase
    Diamine oxidase
    Dopamine β-monooxgenase
    Peptidylglycine α-amidating mono-oxgenase
    Tyrosinase
    Factor V
    Factor VIII
    Transcuprein
Biochemical indices
    Pyridinium cross-links of collagen
    Various measures of oxidative stress (TBARS)
    Catecholamines
    Encephalins
    Polyamines
Physiological indices
    Immune function
    Hemostasis
    Cholesterol metabolism
    Glucose tolerance
    Blood pressure
    Arterial compliance
    Arterial plaque
    DNA damage and repair
    Bone density

1.5 mg copper/day, while most people can tolerate 3 mg copper/day or more over the long term and 8–10 mg copper/day or more in the shorter term (over several months).

Estimates of average intakes of copper are about 1.5 and 1.2 mg copper/day for men and women, respectively, on mixed diets, with higher intakes for those on vegetarian diets or those consuming water with appreciable concentrations of copper. Particularly rich food sources of copper include offal, seafood, nuts, seeds, legumes, whole-grain cereals and chocolate. Milk and dairy products are very low in copper and infants are at risk of copper deficiency if they are fed exclusively on cow's milk.

Micronutrient interactions

The major micronutrient interactions with copper are those involving zinc and iron, high intakes of which can restrict copper utilization in infants and adults. The mechanism by which zinc appears to exert on antagonistic effect on copper status is through the induction of metallothionein synthesis by zinc in mucosal cells in the intestine. Metallothionein has a particularly strong affinity for copper. Metallothionein-bound copper is not available for transport into the circulation and is eventually lost in the feces when the mucosal cells are sloughed off. Molybdenum also has a strong interaction with copper and thiomolybdates are potent systemic copper antagonists. Although both cadmium and lead can inhibit copper utilization, this inhibition only occurs at dietary intakes of these heavy metals above those normally consumed by humans. Vitamin E, selenium and manganese have metabolic interactions with copper as antioxidants, but data on beneficial interactions of these on symptoms of copper deficiency are largely confined to animal studies. Copper deficiency exerts an effect on iodine metabolism resulting in hypothyroidism, at least in animal models.

9.10 Selenium

Selenium is a nonmetallic element that has similar chemical properties to sulfur and has four natural oxidation states $(0, -2, +4, +6)$. It combines with other elements to form inorganic selenides [sodium selenide (-2) Na_2Se], selenites [sodium selenite $(+4)$ Na_2SeO_3] and selenates [sodium selenate $(+6)$ Na_2SeO_4], and with oxygen to form oxides [selenium $(+4)$ dioxide SeO_2] and oxyacids [selenic $(+6)$ acid H_2SeO_4]. Selenium replaces sulfur to form a large number of organic selenium compounds, particularly as selenocysteine, the 21st amino acid. Selenium is a component of selenoproteins, where it also occurs as selenides on the side-chains of selenocysteine at physiological pH. Selenium also displaces sulfur to form the amino acid selenomethionine. Elemental selenium is stable and has three allotropic forms, deep red crystals, red amorphous powder and the black vitreous form.

Selenium has many industrial uses in electronics, glass, ceramics, pigments, as alloys in steel, as catalysts in pharmaceutical production, in rubber vulcanization and in agriculture, as feed supplements and fertilizers. Because of its increasing use, selenium has become a potential health and environmental hazard. The primary pathway of exposure to selenium for the general population is food, followed by water (predominantly inorganic selenate and selenite) and air (mainly as elemental particulate selenium from combustion of fossil fuels and from volcanic gas).

Absorption, transport and tissue distribution

Absorption of dietary selenium takes place mainly in the small intestine, where some 50–80% is absorbed. Organic forms of selenium are more readily absorbed than inorganic forms and selenium compounds from plants are generally more bioavailable than those from animals, and particularly from fish. In general, plant foods contain a greater proportion of organic selenium compounds, especially selenomethionine, than animal foods, where selenium occurs in a variety of forms, such as sulfides and selenides, as well as selenocysteine and some selenomethionine.

The bioavailability of selenium from water (mainly inorganic selenates) and supplements is lower than from food. Overall bioavailability of selenium from the diet depends on a number of factors, including selenium status, lipid composition and metals.

Inorganic forms of selenium are passively transported across the intestinal brush border, whereas organic forms (selenomethionine and probably selenocysteine) are actively transported. On reaching the bloodstream, selenium is transported largely bound to protein (mainly very low-density β-lipoprotein with a small amount bound to albumin) for deposition in various organs. Liver and kidney are the major target organs when selenium intake is high but, at lower intakes, the selenium content of the liver is decreased. Heart and muscle tissue are other target organs, with the latter, because of its total bulk, accounting for the greatest proportion of body selenium. The total body content of selenium can vary from about 3 to 15 mg depending on dietary intakes.

In the body, dietary selenium can be bound to selenium-binding proteins but can also be directly incorporated into selenoproteins during translation at the ribosome complex using a transfer RNA specific for the amino acid selenocysteine; thus, selenocysteine can be considered as the 21st amino acid in terms of ribosome-mediated protein synthesis.

The major excretion routes of selenium are in urine (mainly as trimethylselenonium ion), in feces (via biliary pancreatic and intestinal secretions, together with unabsorbed dietary selenium) and in breath (as volatile dimethylselenide). Unlike copper, and particularly iron,

Table 9.16 Selenoproteins

Selenoprotein	Function
Glutathione peroxidases (GPx1, GPx2, GPx3, GPx4; cystolic, gastrointestinal, extracellular and phospholipid hydroperoxide, respectively)	Antioxidant enzymes: remove hydrogen peroxide, and lipid and phospholipid hydroperoxides (thereby maintaining membrane integrity, modulating eiconsanoid synthesis, modifying inflammation and likelihood of propagation of further oxidative damage to biomolecules, such as lipids, lipoproteins and DNA)
(Sperm) mitochondrial capsule selenoprotein	Form of glutathione peroxidase (GPx4): shields developing sperm cells from oxidative damage and later polymerizes into structural protein required for stability/motility of mature sperm
Iodothyronine deiodinases (three isoforms)	Production and regulation of level of active thyroid hormone, T_3, from thryoxine T_4
Thioredoxin reductases (three isoforms)	Reduction of nucleotides in DNA synthesis; regeneration of antioxidant systems; maintenance of intracellular redox state, critical for cell viability and proliferation; regulation of gene expression by redox control of binding of transcription factors to DNA
Selenophosphate synthetase, SPS2	Required for biosynthesis of selenophosphate, the precursor of selenocysteine, and therefore for selenoprotein synthesis
Selenoprotein P	Found in plasma and associated with endothelial cells; appears to protect endothelial cells against damage from peroxynitrite
Selenoprotein W	Needed for muscle function
Prostate epithelial selenoprotein (15 kDa)	Found in epithelial cells of ventral prostate; seems to have redox function (resembles GPx4), perhaps protecting secretory cells against development of carcinoma
DNA-bound spermatid selenoprotein (34 kDa)	Glutathione peroxidase-like activity; found in stomach and in nuclei of spermatoza; may protect developing sperm
18 kDa selenoprotein	Important selenoprotein, found in kidney and large number of other tissues; preserved in selenium deficiency

From Rayman (2000).

which have inefficient excretion mechanisms, selenium is rapidly excreted in the urine.

Metabolic function and essentiality

Selenocysteine is a component of at least 30 selenoproteins, some of which have important enzymic functions (Table 9.16). Selenocysteine is generally at the active site of those selenoproteins with catalytic activity, and functions as a redox center for the selenium-dependent glutathione peroxidases (cystolic, phospholipid hydroperoxide, extracellular and gastrointestinal), iodothyronine deiodinases (types I, II and III) and thioredoxin reductases. The glutathione peroxidase isozymes, which account for about 36% of total body selenium, differ in their tissue expression and map to different chromosomes.

Deficiency symptoms

Keshan disease is a cardiomyopathy that affects children and women of child-bearing age and occurs in areas of China where the soil is deficient in selenium. Despite the strong evidence for an etiological role for selenium in Keshan disease (i.e. the occurrence of the disease only in those regions of China with low selenium soils and, hence, low amounts of selenium

in the food chain, and only in those individuals with poor selenium status together with the prevention of the disease in an at-risk population by supplementation with selenium), there are certain epidemiological features of the disease that are not readily explained solely on the basis of selenium deficiency. A similar situation occurs with Kashin–Beck disease, a chronic osteoarthropathy that most commonly affects growing children and occurs in parts of Siberian Russia and in China, where it overlaps with Keshan disease. Although oral supplementation with selenium is effective in preventing the disease, it is likely that other factors, apart from selenium deficiency, are involved in the etiology of Kashin–Beck disease. There are also some selenium-responsive conditions with symptoms similar to Keshan disease that occur in patients receiving total parenteral nutrition.

One explanation for the complex etiology of selenium-responsive diseases in humans is that low selenium status may predispose to other deleterious conditions, most notably the increased incidence, virulence or disease progression of a number of viral infections. For example, in a selenium-deficient animal model, harmless coxsackie virus can become virulent and cause myocarditis, not only in the selenium-deficient host, but also when isolated and injected into selenium-replete animals. A coxsackie virus has been isolated from the blood and tissues of Keshan disease patients and the infection may be responsible for the cardiomyopathy of that disease. It has been speculated that similar events linked with other RNA viruses may explain the emergence of new strains of influenza virus in China and the postulated crossing over of the human immunodeficiency virus (HIV) to humans in the selenium-deficient population of Zaire. Many human viral pathogens (e.g. HIV, coxsackie, hepatitis and measles viruses) can synthesize viral selenoproteins and, thereby, lower the selenium available to the host. In any event, selenium deficiency is accompanied by loss of immunocompetence, with the impairment of both cell-mediated immunity and B-cell function. Covert suboptimal selenium status may be widespread in human populations, as selenium supplementation in subjects considered to be selenium replete had marked immunostimulant effects, including increased proliferation of activated T-cells. Such immunostimulant effects or the production of antitumorigenic metabolites may explain the lowering of cancer incidence after selenium supplementation in selenium-replete subjects (those who already had maximized selenoenzyme activity).

The evidence for suboptimal selenium status increasing the risk of cardiovascular disease is more fragmentary, but it has been proposed that optimizing the activity of the seleno-dependent glutathione peroxidases and, thereby, increasing antioxidant activity may be a factor. As selenium has well-recognized antioxidant and anti-inflammatory roles, other oxidative stress or inflammatory conditions (e.g. rheumatoid arthritis, ulcerative colitis, pancreatitis and asthma) may benefit from selenium supplementation. In addition, some, but certainly not all, studies have suggested beneficial (possibly antioxidant) effects of selenium on mood and reproduction in humans. The evidence, however, supporting a role for optimum selenium status preventing or ameliorating most inflammatory conditions is not strong and may be confounded by other dietary antioxidants, particularly vitamin E, compensating for low selenium status.

Toxicity

There is a narrow margin, perhaps not much more than three- or four-fold, between beneficial and harmful intakes of selenium. The dose necessary to cause chronic selenosis in humans is not well defined, but the threshold for toxicity appears to lie somewhere in the range of 850–900 mg per day. Symptoms of chronic selenium toxicity include brittle hair and nails, skin lesions with secondary infections and garlic odor on the breath, resulting from the expiration of dimethyl selenide. Toxicity depends on the chemical form of selenium, with most forms having low toxicity. Data from animal studies indicate that selenite and selenocysteine are a little more toxic than selenomethionine and much more toxic than other organic selenium compounds (dimethyl selenide, trimethyselenonium ion, selenoethers, selenobetaine). Methylation in the body is important for detoxification of the element.

Genetic diseases

Although no important genetic diseases affecting selenium status are apparent, polymorphisms in gene sequences of some selenoenzymes may determine selenium utilization and metabolic needs, and hence dietary requirements. This may explain the significant variation among individuals in the extent of the response to supplementation of selenoenzyme activities.

Assessing status

Plasma or whole blood, hair and toenail selenium concentrations can indicate changes in selenium status in humans. Plasma and serum selenium concentrations respond rapidly to changes in selenium intakes, while erythrocyte selenium is an index of longer term or chronic intake. Dietary intake data, however, are insufficient to determine selenium status in individuals because of uncertainties about bioavailability and variations in the content and form of selenium in foodstuffs. Although plasma (or preferably platelet) glutathione peroxidase activities have been used as functional indices to estimate selenium requirements, it has not been established how these measurements relate to other biochemical functions of selenium, such as thyroid metabolism, or immune function and their health sequelae. For example, at higher levels of selenium intake, glutathione peroxidase activities plateau but immunoenhancement may be evident at supplementation levels higher than those needed to optimize the selenoenzyme activity. Perhaps the best way forward is to select from a battery of functional indices, such as selenoenzyme activity, plasma thyroid hormone concentrations and immune measures, according to the function or disease under investigation.

Table 9.17 Dietary selenium intakes worldwide

Country (region)	Range (μg/day)
Australia	57–87
Canada	98–224
China (Keshan county)	3–22
China (Enshi county)	3200–6690
Greece	110–220
Mexico	10–223
New Zealand (Dunedin)	6–70
Portugal	10–100
Russia	60–80
UK	30–60
USA	62–216

After Reilly (1996).

Requirements and dietary sources

Dietary intakes of selenium vary widely with geographical spread (Table 9.17). Requirements for selenium have been estimated at intakes required to saturate plasma glutathione peroxidase activity (which corresponds to lower status and intake than that needed to saturate platelet glutathione peroxidase activity) in the vast majority (97.5%) of all individuals in a population. In the UK, the reference nutrient intake (RNI) has thus been set at 75 and 60 μg selenium/day for men and women, respectively. Blood selenium concentrations in the UK population have declined by approximately 50% over the past 30 years and current UK intakes are only about 50% of RNI. As explained previously, however, there is uncertainty as to what constitutes optimum selenium status and the intakes of selenium in various dietary regimens needed to achieve optimum status. Optimum status may not necessarily be reflected in saturated glutathione peroxidase activity.

Selenium enters the food chain through plants which, in general, reflect concentrations of the element in the soil on which the plants were grown. The absorption of selenium by plants, however, is dependent not only on soil selenium content but also on pH, microbial activity, rainfall and the chemical form of selenium. Higher plants absorb selenium preferentially as selenate and can synthesize organic selenium compounds, e.g. selenomethionine, and to a lesser extent selenocysteine. Brazil nuts contain high concentrations of selenium because of the seleniferous soils in the Andes Mountains. Selenium concentrations of cereals and staples are much lower, but the content and bioavailability of selenium in wheat usually make this a major contributor to overall selenium intakes because of the high quantities of wheat consumed as bread and other baked products. Fish, shellfish and offal (liver, kidney) are rich sources of selenium, followed by meat and eggs. Animal sources, however, have lower bioavailability of selenium than those from plant sources.

Micronutrient interactions

Selenium is an antioxidant nutrient and has important interactions with other antioxidant micronutrients, especially vitamin E (Figure 9.7). Vitamin E, as an antioxidant, can ameloriate some of the symptoms of selenium deficiencies in animals. Copper deficiency also increases oxidative stress, and the expression of glutathione peroxidase genes is decreased in the copper-deficient animal.

The metabolic interactions between selenium and other micronutrients, however, extend beyond those between selenium, vitamin E and other antioxidants. Peripheral deiodination of thyroxine (T_4), the predominant hormone secreted by the thyroid, to the more biologically active triiodothyronine (T_3) in extrathyroidal tissues is accomplished through the selenium-dependent deiodinase enzymes. Selenium deficiency, therefore, can contribute to iodine deficiency disorders, and goitre complications have been noted in up to 80% of Keshan disease casualties after autopsy. Moreover, higher serum T_4 concentrations were found in patients with subacute Keshan disease and in children with latent Keshan disease compared with respective controls. All thyroid hormone concentrations in these studies were within normal ranges, suggesting that selenium deficiency, or even suboptimal selenium status, was blocking optimum thyroid and iodine metabolism.

Excess selenium intake interferes with zinc bioavailability, decreases tissue iron stores and increases copper concentrations in heart, liver and kidney. Vitamins C and E, sulfur amino acids and sulfate, arsenic and heavy metals can decrease the toxicity of selenium. Conversely, selenium modifies the toxicity of many heavy metals. In seafoods, selenium is combined with mercury or methyl mercury and this interaction may be one of the factors that decrease the bioavailability of selenium in these foods.

9.11 Iodine

Iodine is a nonmetallic element of the halogen group with common oxidation states of −1 (iodides), +5

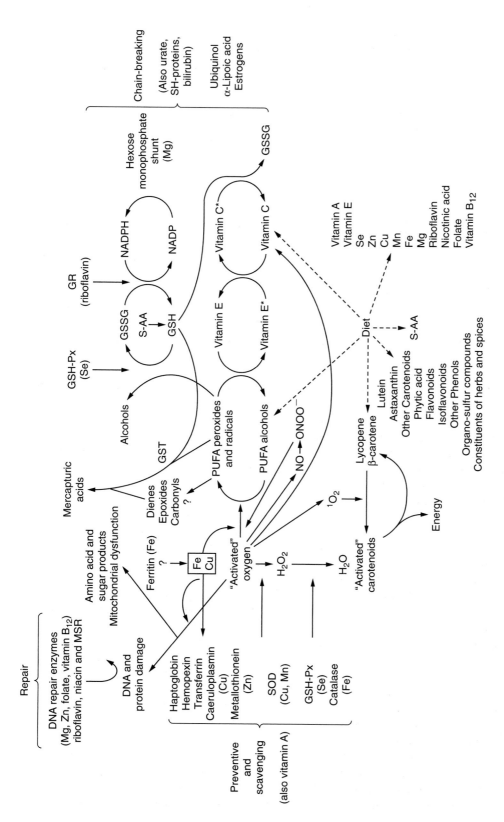

GR, glutathione reductase (EC1.6.4.2); GSH, reduced glutathione; GSH-Px glutathione peroxidase (EC1.11.1.9); GSSG, oxidized glutathione; GST, glutathione-S-transferase (EC 2.5.1.18); MSR, methionine sulfoxide reductase (EC1.8.4.5); PUFA, polyunsaturated fatty acids; S-AA, sulfur amino acids; SH-proteins, sulfydryl proteins; SOD, superoxide dismutase (EC1.15.1.1); Fe Cu , transition metal-catalyzed oxidant damage to biomolecules. ? Biological relevance.

Figure 9.7 Antioxidant defense system (from Strain and Benzie, 1999).

(iodates) and +7 (periodates), and less common states of +1 (iodine monochloride) and +3 (iodine trichloride). Elemental iodine (0) is a soft blue–black solid, which sublimes readily to form a violet gas.

The principal industrial uses of iodine are in the pharmaceutical industry, medical and sanitary uses (e.g. iodized salt, water treatment, protection from radioactive iodine and disinfectants), as catalysts (synthetic rubber, acetic acid synthesis), and in animal feeds, herbicides, dyes, inks, colorants, photographic equipment, lasers, metallurgy, conductive polymers and stabilizers (nylon). Naturally occurring iodine minerals are rare and occur usually in the form of calcium iodates. Commercial production of iodine is largely restricted to extraction from Chilean deposits of nitrates (saltpetre) and iodine in caliche (soluble salts precipitated by evaporation) and from concentrated salt brine in Japan. Iodine is the least abundant halogen in the Earth's crust, at concentrations of 0.005%. The content of iodine in soils varies and much of the original content has been leached out in areas of high rainfall, previous glaciation and soil erosion.

The concentration of iodine (as iodide and iodate) in the oceans is higher, at about 0.06 mg/l. Iodine volatilizes from the surface of the oceans and sea spray as salt particles, iodine vapor or methyl iodide vapor. Some iodine can then return to land in rainwater (0.0018–0.0085 mg iodine/l). There is a large variation of iodine content in drinking water (0.0001–0.1 mg iodine/l).

Absorption, transport and tissue distribution

Iodine, usually as an iodide or iodate compound in food and water, is rapidly absorbed in the intestine and circulates in the blood to all tissues in the body. The thyroid gland traps most (about 80%) of the ingested iodine, but salivary glands, the gastric mucosa, choroid plexus and the lactating mammary gland also concentrate the element by a similar active transport mechanism. Several sulfur-containing compounds, thiocyanate, isothiocyanate and goitrin inhibit this active transport by competing for uptake with iodide, and their goitrogenic activity can be overcome by iodine supplementation. These active goitrogens are released by plant enzymes from thioglucosides or cyanogenic glucosides found in cassava, kale, cabbage, sprouts, broccoli, kohlrabi, turnips, swedes, rapeseed and mustard. The most important of these goitrogen-containing

foods is cassava, which can be detoxified by soaking in water. Tobacco smoke also contributes thiocyanate and other antithyroid compounds to the circulation.

Metabolic functions and essentiality

Iodine is an essential constituent of the thyroid hormones, thyroxine (T_4) and triiodothyronine (T_3), which have key modifying or permissive roles in development and growth. Although T_4 is quantitatively predominant, T_3 is the more active. The mechanism of action of thyroid hormones appears to involve binding to nuclear receptors which, in turn, alter gene expression in pituitary, liver, heart, kidney and, most crucially, brain cells. Overall, thyroid hormones stimulate enzyme synthesis, oxygen consumption and basal metabolic rate and, thereby, affect heart rate, respiratory rate, mobilization and metabolism of carbohydrates, lipogenesis and a wide variety of other physiological activities. It is probable that iodine has additional roles to those of thyroid hormone activity, for example in antibiotic and anticancer activity, but these are poorly understood.

Once iodide (-1) is trapped from the circulation and actively transported to the lumen of the thyroid gland, it is oxidized to I_2 (0) and reacts with tyrosine in thyroglobulin protein to form monoiodotyrosine or diiodotyrosine. These reactions are catalyzed by thyroid peroxidase. The iodinated compounds, in turn, couple to form T_3 and T_4, which are secreted from the thyroid into the circulation.

Flavonoids, found in many plants, including pearl millet, and phenol derivatives, released into water from soil humus, inhibit thyroid peroxidase and the organification of iodide. The concentration of iodine in the thyroid gland also affects the uptake of iodide into the follicle, the ratio of T_3 to T_4 and the rate of release of these hormones into the circulation. This process is also under hormonal control by the hypothalamus of the brain which produces thyroid-releasing hormone, which then stimulates the pituitary gland to secrete thyroid-stimulating hormone (TSH) which, in turn, acts on the thyroid gland to produce more thyroid hormones.

Almost all of the thyroid hormones released from the thyroid are bound to transport proteins, mainly thyroxine-binding globulin. The longer half-life of T_4 ensures that there is a reservoir for conversion to the more active T_3 with a much shorter half-life of 1 day. The deiodination of T_4 to T_3 takes place in extrathyroidal tissues (mainly the liver). Excretion of iodine is predominantly in the urine.

Deficiency symptoms

A deficiency of iodine causes a wide spectrum of disorders from mild goitre (a larger thyroid gland than normal) to the most severe forms of endemic cretinism (congenital, severe, irreversible mental and growth retardation). Collectively, these manifestations of iodine deficiency are termed iodine deficiency disorders (IDD) and symptoms differ depending on the life stage at which iodine deficiency occurs. The most severe disorders (cretinism) arise if the fetus suffers from iodine deficiency. The clinical features of endemic cretinism are either a predominant neurological syndrome with severe to profound mental retardation including defects of hearing and speech (often deaf–mutism), squint and disorders of stance and gait of varying degrees (neurological cretinism) or predominant features of hypothyroidism and stunted growth with less severe mental retardation (myxedematous cretinism). Profound hypothyroidism is biochemically defined as high serum TSH and very low T_4 and T_3, and is accompanied by low basal metabolic rate, apathy, slow reflex relaxation time with slow movements, cold intolerance and myxedema (skin and subcutaneous tissue are thickened, because of an accumulation of mucin, and become dry and swollen). While cretinism is the severest form of IDD, varying degrees of intellectual or growth retardation are apparent when iodine deficiency occurs in the fetus, infancy or childhood and adolescence. In adulthood, the consequences of iodine deficiency are more serious in women, especially during pregnancy, than in men.

The mildest form of IDD, goitres, range from those only detectable by touch (palpation) to very large goitres that can cause breathing problems. The enlargement of the thyroid gland to produce goitre arises from stimulation of the thyroid cells by TSH and, without the ability to increase hormone production owing to iodine deficiency, the gland becomes hyperplastic.

Apart from cretinism, hypothyroidism and goitre, other features linked to IDD are decreased fertility rates, increased stillbirth and spontaneous abortion rates, and increased perinatal and infant mortality. The public health significance of iodine deficiency cannot be underestimated, with over one billion people (worldwide, but mostly in Asia and Africa) estimated to be living in iodine-deficient areas and, therefore, at risk of IDD. Estimates of those with IDD demonstrate the scale of the problem, with 200–300 million goitrous people, over 40 million affected by some degree of mental impairment and some 7 million cretins. Fortunately, these figures should decrease as public health programs using preventive interventions with iodized oil (oral or intramuscular injection) salt, bread, water or even sugar have an impact. Treatment with iodine supplementation in older children and adults can reverse many of the clinical manifestations of IDD, including mental deficiency, hypothyroidism and goitre. Although iodine deficiency is the primary cause of IDD, goitrogenic factors limiting bioavailability appear to be superimposed on the primary cause. In addition, genetic variation, immunological factors, sex, age and growth factors seem to modify expression of the conditions, producing a wide range of symptoms and severity of IDD with similar iodine intakes.

Toxicity

A wide range of iodine intakes is tolerated by most individuals, owing to the ability of the thyroid to regulate total body iodine. Over 2 mg iodine/day for long periods should be regarded as excessive or potentially harmful to most people. Such high intakes are unlikely to arise from natural foods, except for diets that are very high in seafood and/or seaweed or comprising foods contaminated with iodine. In contrast to iodine-replete individuals, those with IDD or previously exposed to iodine-deficient diets may react to sudden moderate increases in iodine intake, such as from iodized salt. Iodine-induced thyrotoxicosis (hyperthyroidism) and toxic nodular goitre may result from excess iodine exposure in these individuals. Hyperthyroidism is largely confined to those over 40 years of age and symptoms are rapid heart rate, trembling, excessive sweating, lack of sleep, and loss of weight and strength.

Individuals who are sensitive to iodine usually have mild skin symptoms, but very rarely fever, salivary gland enlargement, visual problems, skin problems and, in severe cases, cardiovascular collapse, convulsions and death may occur. The occurrence of allergic symptoms, for example to iodine medications or antiseptics, however, is rare.

Genetic diseases

Pendred's syndrome is an autosomal recessive inherited disorder with a frequency of 100 or less per 100 000. It is characterized by goitre and profound deafness in childhood and is caused by mutations in the Pendrin gene located on chromosome 7. The gene codes for pendrin, a transporter protein for chloride/iodine transport across the thyroid apical membrane. This results in defective iodination of thyroglobulin. Mutations in another gene, the sodium/iodide symporter (*NIS*) gene, occasionally cause defective iodide transport and goitre, while single nucleotide polymorphisms in the TSH receptor gene may predispose individuals to the hyperthyroidism of toxic multinodular goitre and Graves' disease.

Assessing status

The critical importance of iodine for the thyroid indicates that iodine status is assessed by thyroid function. A standard set of indicators (goitre by palpation, thyroid volume by ultrasound, median urinary iodine and whole blood TSH) is used to determine prevalence in countries with endemic deficiency. Measurement of plasma thyroid hormones (TSH, T_4 and T_3) provides useful indicators of functional iodine status in the individual. Of these, TSH is the most sensitive functional indicator of suboptimal iodine status. Concentrations of T_4 decline in more severe iodine deficiency and T_3 concentrations only in the most severe of iodine deficiencies.

Dietary intakes and requirements

Requirements in infancy and childhood range from 40 to 150 mg iodine/day. Adult requirements are estimated at 150 mg iodine/day, increasing to 175 and 200 mg/day for pregnancy and lactation.

Under normal circumstances, about 90% of iodine intake is from food, with about 10% from water. The concentration of iodine in most foods is low and, in general, reflects the iodine content of the soil, water and fertilizers used in plant and animal production. In most countries other sources, such as iodized salts or foods, are required. Seafoods and seaweed concentrate iodine from seawater and are particularly rich sources. In some populations, milk has become a major source of iodine, owing to the use of iodized salt licks and iodine-enriched cattle feed for dairy herds. Minor amounts may come from adventitious contamination from iodophor disinfectants (teat-dip). Iodine-enriched cattle feed will also increase the iodine content of meat for beef herds raised on concentrated feedstuffs. Processed foods contribute some additional iodine from food additives, such as calcium iodate used in the baking industry.

Micronutrient interactions

From a public health viewpoint, the most important metabolic interaction of iodine with other micronutrients is with selenium. Adequate selenium status is essential for thyroid hormone metabolism and, therefore, normal growth development, by ensuring sufficient T_3 supply to extrathyroidal tissues. Most T_3 is formed from T_4 by the selenium-dependent deiodinases. Iodine and selenium deficiencies overlap in various parts of the world and concurrent deficiencies of both may contribute to the etiologies of Kashin–Beck disease in Russia, China and Tibet, and myxedematous cretinism in Zaire. In addition, both nutrients are required for normal reproduction, normal gene expression, synthesis of zenobiotic and metabolizing enzymes in the liver, and normal tolerance against cold stress. It is possible that hypothyroidism associated with suboptimal selenium status may explain some of the etiology of cardiovascular disease and certain cancers.

Hypothyroidism is associated with deficiencies of other trace elements, including zinc, iron and copper, while there are close metabolic relationships at the molecular and transport levels between iodine and vitamin A. Conversely, the widespread disruption of metabolism in IDD can affect the proper utilization of a host of other nutrients.

9.12 Manganese

Manganese is widely distributed in the biosphere: it constitutes approximately 0.085% of the Earth's crust, making it the 12th most abundant element. Manganese is a component of numerous complex minerals including pyroluosite, rhodochrosite, rhodanite, braunite, pyrochite and manganite. Chemical forms of manganese in their natural deposits include oxides, sulfides, carbonates and silicates. Anthropogenic sources of manganese are predominantly from the manufacturing of steel, alloys and iron products. Manganese is also widely used as an oxidizing agent, as a component of fertilizers and fungicides, and in dry cell batteries. The permanganate is a powerful oxidizing agent and is used in quantitative analysis and medicine.

Manganese is a transition element. It can exist in 11 oxidation states from -3 to $+7$, with the most common valences being $+2$, $+4$ and $+7$. The $+2$ valence is the predominant form in biological systems, the $+4$ valence occurs in MnO_2 and the $+7$ valence is found in permanganate.

Absorption, transport and tissue distribution

The total amount of manganese in the adult human is approximately 15 mg. Up to 25% of the total body stores of manganese may be located in the skeleton and may not be readily accessible for use in metabolic pathways. Relatively high levels have been reported in liver, pancreas, intestine and bone.

Intestinal absorption of manganese occurs throughout the length of the small intestine. Mucosal uptake appears to be mediated by two types of mucosal binding, one that is saturable with a finite capacity and one that is nonsaturable. Manganese absorption, probably as Mn^{2+}, is relatively inefficient, generally less than 5%, but there is some evidence of improvement at low intakes. High levels of dietary calcium, phosphorus and phytate impair the intestinal uptake of the element but are probably of limited significance because, as yet, no well-documented case of human manganese deficiency has been reported.

Systemic homeostatic regulation of manganese is brought about primarily through hepatobiliary excretion rather than through regulation of absorption (e.g. the efficiency of manganese retention does not appear to be dose dependent within normal dietary levels). Manganese is taken up from blood by the liver and transported to extrahepatic tissues by transferrin and possibly α_2-macroglobulin and albumin. Manganese is excreted primarily in feces. Urinary excretion of manganese is low and has not been found to be sensitive to dietary manganese intake.

Metabolic function and essentiality

Manganese is required as a catalytic cofactor for mitochondrial superoxide dismutase, arginase and pyruvate carboxylase. It is also an activator of glycosyltransferases, phosphoenolpyruvate carboxylase and glutamine synthetase.

Deficiency symptoms

Signs of manganese deficiency have been demonstrated in several animal species. Symptoms include impaired growth, skeletal abnormalities, depressed reproductive function, and defects in lipid and carbohydrate metabolism. Evidence of manganese deficiency in humans is poor. It has been suggested that manganese deficiency has never been observed in non institutionalized human populations because of the abundant supply of manganese in edible plant materials compared with the relatively low requirements of mammals. There is only one report of apparent human manganese deficiency. A male subject was fed a purified diet deficient in vitamin K, which was accidentally also deficient in manganese. Feeding this diet caused weight loss, dermatitis, growth retardation of hair and nails, reddening of black hair and a decline in levels of blood lipids. Manganese deficiency may be more frequent in infants owing to the low concentration of manganese in human breast milk and varying levels in infant formulae.

Toxicity

Manganese toxicity of dietary origin has not been well documented. Toxicity has been observed only in workers exposed to high concentrations of manganese dust or fumes in air. For example, mine-workers in Chile exposed to manganese ore dust developed, possibly as a result of inhalation rather than ingestion, "manganic madness", manifested by psychosis, hallucinations and extrapyramidal damage with features of parkinsonism.

The US Food and Nutrition Board recently set the tolerable UL for manganese at 11 mg/day for adults (19 years and older). Elevated blood manganese concentrations and neurotoxicity were selected as the critical adverse effects on which to base their UL for manganese.

Assessing status

Progress in the field of manganese nutrition has been hampered because of the lack of a practical method for assessing manganese status. Blood manganese concentrations appear to reflect body manganese status of rats fed deficient or adequate amounts of manganese, but consistent changes in blood or plasma manganese have not been observed in depleted or repleted human subjects. Researchers are actively investigating whether the activities of manganese-dependent enzymes, such as manganese-SOD in blood lymphocytes and blood arginase, may be of use in detecting low manganese intake; however, there is evidence that these enzymes can be influenced by certain disease states.

Table 9.18 Dietary sources of manganese

Rich sources (>20 mg/kg)	Intermediate sources (1–5 mg/kg)	Poor sources (<1 mg/kg)
Nuts	Green leafy vegetables	Animal tissue
Whole-grain cereals	Dried fruits	Poultry
Dried legumes	Fresh fruits	Dairy products
Tea	nonleafy vegetables	Seafood

Requirements and dietary sources

Relatively high concentrations of manganese have been reported in cereals (20–30 mg/kg), brown bread (100–150 mg/kg), nuts (10–20 mg/kg), ginger (280 mg/kg) and tea (350–900 mg/kg dry tea). Concentrations of manganese in crops are dependent on soil factors such as pH, whereby increasing soil pH decreases plant uptake of manganese. Products of animal origin such as eggs, milk, fish, poultry and red meat contain low amounts of manganese (Table 9.18). Many multivitamin and mineral supplements for adults provide 2.5–5.0 mg manganese.

There is currently no RDA set for dietary manganese; instead, there is an AI value [these values were recently established by the US Food and Nutrition Board (2001)]: infants 0.003 mg (first 6 months), 0.6 mg (7–12 months), children 1.2 and 1.5 mg (1–3 and 4–8 years, respectively), teenage boys 1.9 and 2.2 mg (9–13 and 14–18 years, respectively), adult men 2.3 mg (19 years and older), teenage girls 1.6 mg (9–18 years), adult women 1.8 mg (19 years and older), pregnant women 2.0 mg and lactating women 2.6 mg. The AI was set based on median intakes reported from the US Food and Drug Administration Total Diet Study.

Micronutrient interactions

Iron–manganese interactions have been demonstrated whereby iron deficiency increased manganese absorption, and high amounts of dietary iron inhibit manganese absorption, possibly by competition for similar binding and absorption sites between nonheme iron and manganese.

9.13 Molybdenum

Molybdenum does not exist naturally in the pure metallic state but rather in association with other elements, or predominantly in solution as the molybdate anion. Insoluble molybdenum compounds include molybdenum dioxide and molybdenum disulfide. The metal has five oxidation states (2–6), of which +4 and +6 are the predominant species. Major molybdenum-containing ores are molybdenum sulfites and ferric molybdenum ores, usually produced as by-products of copper mining operations, while other molybdenum salts are by-products of uranium mining. Molybdenum is used mostly in metallurgical applications such as stainless steel and cast iron alloys, and in metal–ceramic composites. Molybdenum compounds have anticorrosive and lubricant properties and can act as chemical catalysts.

Molybdenum uptake into plants and hence into the food chain occurs mostly from alkaline or neutral soils. Water usually contains little molybdenum except near major mining operations.

Absorption, transport and tissue distribution

Molybdenum is readily absorbed (40–100%) from foods and is widely distributed in cells and in the ECF. Some accumulation can occur in liver, kidneys, bones and skin. The major excretory route of molybdenum after ingestion is the urine, with significant amounts also excreted in bile.

Metabolic functions and essentiality

Molybdenum functions as a cofactor for the iron- and flavin-containing enzymes that catalyze the hydroxylation of various substrates. The molybdenum cofactor in the enzymes aldehyde oxidase (oxidizes and detoxifies purines and pyrimidines), xanthine oxidase/hydrogenase (production of uric acid from hypoxanthine and xanthine) and sulfite oxidase (conversion of sulfite to sulfate) has molybdenum incorporated as part of the molecule.

Deficiency symptoms

Although there is a clear biochemical basis for the essentiality of molybdenum, deficiency signs in humans and animals are difficult to induce. Naturally occurring deficiency, uncomplicated by molybdenum antagonists, is not known with certainty. In animal experiments, where large amounts of the molybdenum antagonist tungsten have been fed, deficiency signs are depressed food consumption and growth, impaired reproduction and elevated copper concentrations in liver and brain.

Toxicity

A moderate (540 mg/day) intake of molybdenum has been associated with urinary copper loss in humans, and most signs of molybdenum toxicity in animals are similar or identical to those of copper deficiency. These signs include anemia, anorexia, diarrhea, joint abnormalities, osteoporosis, hair discoloration and death.

Genetic diseases

A rare unborn error of metabolism, resulting in the absence of the molybdenum pterin cofactor, may give some clue to the essentiality of molybdenum. These patients have severe neurological dysfunction, dislocated ocular lenses, mental retardation and biochemical abnormalities, including increased urinary excretion of xanthine and sulfite and decreased urinary excretion of uric acid and sulfate.

Assessing status

Determining the body status of molybdenum is difficult. Homeostatic control of molybdenum ensures that plasma levels are not elevated, except after extremely high dietary intakes. Decreased urinary concentrations of sulfite, hypoxanthine, zorithine and other sulfur metabolites, however, are generally indicative of impaired activities of the molybdoenzymes. Adult requirements for molybdenum have been estimated at about 25 mg/day. Average intakes tend to be considerably above this value. Milk, beans, bread and cereals (especially the germ) are good sources of molybdenum, while water also contributes small amounts to the total dietary intakes.

Micronutrient interactions

The major micronutrient interactions with molybdenum are those involving tungsten and copper. Molybdenum supplementation depletes body levels of the essential trace element copper, and has been used as a chelating agent for conditions such as Wilson's disease, which cause elevated concentrations of copper in the body.

9.14 Fluoride

Fluorine occurs chiefly in fluorspar and cryolite, but is widely distributed in other minerals. Fluoride is the ionic form of fluorine, a halogen and the most electronegative of the elements in the periodic table; the two terms are often used interchangeably. Fluorine and its compounds are used in producing uranium and more than 100 commercial fluorochemicals, including many well-known high-temperature plastics. Hydrofluoric acid is extensively used for etching the glass of light bulbs, etc. Fluorochlorohydrocarbons are extensively used in air conditioning and refrigeration. Fluorine is present in small but widely varying concentrations in practically all soils, water supplies, plants and animals, and is a constituent of all diets.

Absorption, transport and tissue distribution

Fluoride appears to be soluble and rapidly absorbed, and is distributed throughout the ECF in a manner similar to chloride. The concentrations of fluorine in blood, where it is bound to albumin, and tissues are small. The elimination of absorbed fluoride occurs almost exclusively via the kidneys. Fluoride is freely filtered through the glomerular capillaries and undergoes tubular reabsorption in varying degrees.

Fifty per cent of orally ingested fluoride is absorbed from the gastrointestinal tract after approximately 30 min. In the absence of high dietary concentrations of calcium and certain other cations with which fluoride may form insoluble and poorly absorbed compounds, 80% or more is typically absorbed. Body fluid and tissue fluoride concentrations are proportional to the long-term level of intake; they are not homeostatically regulated. About 99% of the body's fluoride is found in calcified tissues (bone and teeth), to which it is strongly but not irreversibly bound.

In general, the bioavailability of fluoride is high, but it can be influenced to some extent by the vehicle with which it is ingested. When a soluble compound such as sodium fluoride is ingested with water, absorption is nearly complete. If it is ingested with milk, baby formula or foods, especially those with high concentrations of calcium and certain other divalent or trivalent ions that form insoluble compounds, absorption may be reduced by 10–25%. Fluoride is absorbed passively from the stomach, but protein-bound organic fluoride is less readily absorbed.

The fractional retention (or balance) of fluoride at any age depends on the amount absorbed and the amount excreted. In healthy, young or middle-aged adults, approximately 50% of absorbed fluoride is retained by uptake in calcified tissues and 50% is excreted in urine. In young children, as much as 80% can be retained owing to the increased uptake by the developing skeleton and teeth. In later life, it is likely that the fraction excreted is greater than the fraction retained. However, this needs to be confirmed.

Metabolic function and essentiality

While there is no known metabolic role in the body for fluorine, it is known to activate certain enzymes and to inhibit others. While the status of fluorine (fluoride) as an essential nutrient has been debated, the US Food and Nutrition Board recently established a dietary reference intake for the ion that might suggest their willingness to consider fluorine to be a beneficial element for humans, if not an "essential nutrient".

The function of fluoride appears to be in the crystalline structure of bones; fluoride forms calcium fluorapatite in teeth and bone. The incorporation of fluoride in these tissues is proportional to its total intake. There is an overall acceptance of a role for fluoride in the care of teeth. The cariostatic action (reduction in the risk of dental caries) of fluoride on erupted teeth of children and adults is owing to its effect in the metabolism of bacteria in dental plaque (i.e. reduced acid production) and on the dynamics of enamel demineralization and remineralization during an acidogenic challenge. The ingestion of fluoride during the pre-eruptive development of the teeth also has a cariostatic effect because of the uptake of fluoride by enamel crystallite and formation of fluorhydroxyapatite, which is less acid soluble than hydroxyapatite. When drinking water contains 1 mg/l there is a coincidental 50% reduction in tooth decay in children. Fluoride (at relatively high intakes) also has the unique ability to stimulate new bone formation and, as such, it has been used as an experimental drug for the treatment of osteoporosis. Recent evidence has shown an especially positive clinical effect on bone when fluoride (23 mg/day) is administered in a sustained-release form rather than in forms that are quickly absorbed from the gastrointestinal tract.

Deficiency symptoms

The lack of exposure to fluoride, or the ingestion of inadequate amounts of fluoride at any age, places the individual at increased risk for dental caries. Many studies conducted before the availability of fluoride-containing dental products demonstrated that dietary fluoride exposure is beneficial, owing to its ability to inhibit the development of dental caries in both children and adults. This was particularly evident in the past when the prevalence of dental caries in communities without water fluoridation was shown to be much higher than that in communities who had their water fluoridated. Both the intercommunity transport of foods and beverages and the use of fluoridated dental products have blurred the historical difference in the prevalence of dental caries between communities with and without water fluoridation. This is referred to as a halo or diffusion effect. The overall difference in caries prevalence between fluoridated and non fluoridated area regions in the USA was reported to be 18% (data from a 1986–87 national survey), whereas the majority of earlier studies reported differences of approximately 50%. Therefore, ingestion of adequate amounts of fluoride is of importance in the control of dental caries.

Toxicity

Fluorine, like other trace elements, is toxic when consumed in excessive amounts. The primary adverse effects associated with chronic, excess fluoride intake are enamel and skeletal fluorosis. Enamel fluorosis is a dose-related effect caused by fluoride ingestion during the pre-eruptive development of the teeth. After the enamel has completed its pre-eruptive maturation, it is no longer susceptible. Inasmuch as enamel fluorosis is regarded as a cosmetic effect, it is the anterior teeth that are of most concern. The pre-eruptive maturation of the crowns of the anterior permanent teeth is finished and the risk of fluorosis is over by 8 years of age. Therefore, fluoride intake up to the age of 8 years is of most interest. Mild fluorosis (which is not readily apparent) has no effect on tooth function and may render the enamel more resistant to caries. In contrast, the moderate and severe forms of enamel fluorosis are generally characterized by esthetically objectionable changes in tooth color and surface irregularities.

Skeletal fluorosis has been regarded as having three stages. Stage 1 is characterized by occasional stiffness or pain in joints and some osteosclerosis of the pelvis and vertebrae, while the clinical signs in stages 2 and 3, which may be crippling, include dose-related calcification of ligaments, osteosclerosis, exostoses, and possibly osteoporosis of long bones, muscle wasting and neurological defects owing to hypercalcification of vertebrae. The development of skeletal fluorosis and its severity are directly related to the level and duration of exposure. Most epidemiological research has indicated that an intake of at least 10 mg/day for 10 or more years is needed to produce the clinical signs of the milder form of the condition. Crippling skeletal fluorosis is extremely rare. For example, only five cases have been confirmed in the USA since the mid-1960s.

Based largely on the data on the association of high fluoride intakes with risk of skeletal fluorosis in children (>8 years) and adults, the US Food and Nutrition Board has established a tolerable UL of fluoride of 10 mg/day for children (>8 years), adolescents and adults, as well as pregnant and lactating women.

Assessing status

A high proportion of the dietary intake of fluoride appears in urine. Urinary output in general reflects the dietary intake.

Requirements and dietary sources

Most foods have fluoride concentrations well below 0.05 mg/100 g. Exceptions to this include fluoridated water, beverages and some infant formulae that are made or reconstituted with fluoridated water, teas and some marine fish. Because of the ability of tea leaves to accumulate fluoride to concentrations exceeding 10 mg/100 g dry weight, brewed tea contains fluoride concentrations ranging from 1 to 6 mg/l depending on the amount of dry tea used, the water fluoride concentration and brewing time.

Intake from fluoridated dental products adds considerable fluoride, often approaching or exceeding intake from the diet, particularly in young children who have poor control of the swallowing reflex. The major contributors to nondietary fluoride intake are toothpastes, mouth rinses and dietary fluoride supplements.

In 1997 the US Food and Nutrition Board established AI values for fluoride: infants 0.01 mg (first 6 months), 0.5 mg (7–12 months), children and adolescents 0.7, 1.0 and 2.0 mg (1–3, 4–8 and 9–13 years, respectively), male adolescents and adults 3 and 4 mg (14–18 and 19 years and older, respectively), female adolescents and adults 3 mg (over 14 years, including pregnancy and lactation). The AI is the intake value of fluoride (from all sources) that reduces the occurrence of dental caries maximally in a group of individuals without causing unwanted side-effects. With fluoride, the data are strong on caries risk reduction but the evidence upon which to base an actual requirement is

scant, thus driving the decision to adopt an AI as the reference value.

Micronutrient interactions

The rate and extent of fluoride absorption from the gastrointestinal tract are reduced by the ingestion of foods particularly rich in calcium (such as milk or infant formulae).

9.15 Chromium

Chromium has an abundance of 0.033% in the Earth's crust. It is a transition element that can occur in a number of valence states, with 0, +2, +3 and +6 being the most common. Trivalent chromium is the most stable form in biological systems. The principal ore is chromite. Chromium is used to harden steel, to manufacture stainless steel and to form many useful alloys. It finds wide use as a catalyst. Hexavalent chromium is a strong oxidizing agent that comes primarily from industrial sources.

Absorption, transport and tissue distribution

The human body contains only a small amount of chromium, less than 6 mg. The kidney, followed by the spleen, liver lungs, heart and skeletal muscle are the tissues with the greatest chromium concentrations.

Absorbed chromium is excreted primarily in urine and only small amounts of chromium are lost in the hair, sweat and bile. Therefore, urinary chromium excretion can be used as an accurate estimation of absorbed chromium. At normal dietary chromium intakes (10–40 μg/day), chromium absorption is inversely related to dietary intake. Chromium intake is approximately 0.5% at a daily intake of 40 μg/day and increases to 2% when intake drops to 10 μg/day. The inverse relationship between chromium intake and absorption appears to be a basal control mechanism to maintain a minimal level of absorbed chromium. It is absorbed in the small intestine, primarily in the jejunum in humans. The mechanism is not well understood, but a nonsaturable passive diffusion process seems likely. Ascorbic acid promotes chromium absorption.

Chromium absorption in young and old subjects is similar, but insulin-dependent diabetic patients absorb two to four times more chromium than other apparently healthy subjects. Diabetic subjects appear to have an impaired ability to convert inorganic chromium to a usable form. Therefore, diabetic subjects require additional chromium and the body responds with increased absorption, but the absorbed chromium cannot be utilized effectively and is excreted in the urine. The chromium content of tissues of these patients is also lower.

Chromium is transported to the tissues primarily bound to transferrin, the same protein that transports iron. It has been hypothesized that iron interferes with the transport of chromium in hemochromatosis and that this may explain the high incidence of diabetes in hemochromatosis patients, and which may be induced by chromium deficiency.

Metabolic function and essentiality

Chromium in the trivalent form is an essential nutrient that functions in carbohydrate, lipid and nucleic acid metabolism. The essentiality of chromium was documented in 1977 when the diabetic signs and symptoms of a patient on total parenteral nutrition were reversed by supplemental chromium. Chromium functions primarily through its role in the regulation of insulin. Adequate dietary chromium leads to a normalization of insulin, with reductions in blood glucose concentration in subjects with elevated blood glucose levels, increases in subjects with low blood glucose levels, and no effect on subjects with near-optimal glucose tolerance. Improved insulin function is also associated with an improved lipid profile. Supplemental chromium also leads to increased insulin binding and increased insulin receptor numbers, and recent evidence suggests that chromium may be involved in the phosphorylation and dephosphorylation of the insulin receptor proteins.

Deficiency symptoms

The hallmark of marginal chromium deficiency is impaired glucose tolerance. In studies of patients whose total parenteral nutrition solutions contained no chromium or were supplemented with inadequate amounts of chromium, insulin requirements were reduced and glucose intolerance was reversed with chromium chloride supplementation. Two of these patients had weight loss that was restored with chromium supplementation. Peripheral neuropathy was seen in one of the patients and it too was reversed with chromium supplementation.

Toxicity

Trivalent chromium, the form of chromium found in foods and nutrient supplements, is one of the least toxic nutrients. The chromium often found in paints, welding fumes and other industrial settings is hexavalent and is several times more toxic than the trivalent form. Because trivalent chromium is poorly absorbed, high oral intakes would be necessary to attain toxic levels. The US Food and Nutrition Board recently concluded that there are insufficient data to establish a tolerable UL for trivalent chromium. However, because of the current widespread use of chromium supplements, more research is needed to assess the safety of high-dose chromium intake from supplements.

Assessing status

There is no accurate method for reliable detection of marginal chromium deficiency. Chromium concentrations in hair, urine, blood and tissues can be used to assess recent chromium exposure, but are not long-term measures of chromium status. The only reliable indicator of chromium status is to monitor blood levels of glucose, insulin, lipid and/or related variables before and after chromium supplementation. A response in blood glucose can often be seen in 2 weeks or less, while effects on blood lipids may take longer.

Requirements and dietary sources

Dietary chromium content of foods varies widely. Richest dietary sources of chromium are spices such as black pepper, brewer's yeast, mushrooms, prunes, raisins, nuts, asparagus, beer and wine. Refining of cereals and sugar removes most of the native chromium, but stainless-steel vessels in contact with acidic foods may contribute additional chromium.

There is currently no RDA set for dietary chromium, instead there are AI values [which were recently established by the US Food and Nutrition Board (2001)]: infants 0.2 mg (first 6 months), 5.5 mg (7–12 months), children 11 and 15 mg (1–3 and 4–8 years, respectively), teenage boys 25 and 35 mg (9–13 and 14–18 years, respectively), adult men 35 and 30 mg (19–50 years and 50 years and older, respectively), teenage girls 21 and 24 mg (9–13 and 14–18 years, respectively), adult women 25 and 20 mg (19–50 years and 51 years and older, respectively), pregnant women 29 and 30 mg (less than 18 years and 19–50 years, respectively), and lactating women 44 and 45 mg (less than 18 and 19–50 years, respectively). An AI was set based on representative dietary intake data from healthy individuals from the Third Nutrition and Health Examination Survey (NHANES III).

9.16 Other elements

In addition to the essential elements discussed in this chapter, other elements in the periodic table may emerge as being essential for human nutrition. For 15 elements, aluminum, arsenic, boron, bromine, cadmium, chromium, fluorine, germanium, lead, lithium, nickel, rubidium, silicon, tin and vanadium, specific biochemical reactions have not been defined and their suspected essentiality is based on circumstantial evidence from data emanating from animal models, from essential functions in lower forms of life or from biochemical actions consistent with a biological role or beneficial action in humans. Two elements, fluorine and lithium, have beneficial actions when ingested in high (pharmacological) amounts. Lithium is used to treat manic–depressive disorders, while fluorine is discussed in Section 9.14 because of its important beneficial actions in preventing dental caries in susceptible population groups. Some consider that the circumstantial evidence for chromium is sufficiently substantial to warrant special attention in dietary requirement recommendations, and this element is discussed in Section 9.15. The estimated or suspected requirement of all of these elements (including the essential trace elements, iodine, selenium and molybdenum) is usually less than 1 mg/day and they are defined as ultratrace elements. Cobalt is not included in the list of ultratrace elements because the only requirement for cobalt is as a constituent of preformed vitamin B_{12}.

These elements are not discussed at length in this chapter and the reader is referred to other reading material. For completeness, three tables, on absorption, transport and storage characteristics (Table 9.19), excretion, retention and possible biological roles of the ultratrace elements (Table 9.20), and human body content and food sources (Table 9.21) are included here.

9.17 Perspectives on the future

The preceding parts of this chapter have highlighted some issues in the area of minerals and trace elements for which we have an incomplete understanding. In the future, nutritional scientists, dietitians and other health care professionals will have to:

- obtain a greater understanding of the molecular and cellular processes involved in the intestinal absorption and tissue uptake of certain minerals and trace elements;
- identify functional markers of mineral and trace element status. These markers could be defined as a physiological/biochemical factor which (1) is related to function or effect of the nutrient in target tissue(s) and (2) is affected by dietary intake or stores of the nutrient (which may include markers of disease risk). Examples of such indicators or markers are those related to risk of chronic diseases, such as osteoporosis, coronary heart disease, hypertension or diabetes. However, for many nutrients there are as yet no functional indicators that respond to dietary intake and, in such cases, nutrient requirements are established using more traditional approaches, such as balance data. The lack of functional markers of mineral and trace element status is a significant disadvantage for studies relating their intake or status to health outcomes such as hypertension, cardiovascular disease, osteoporosis, diabetes and other disorders. For example, widely used biochemical indicators of essential trace element status generally lack both the sensitivity and the specificity that are required to define optimal intake at various stages of the life cycle. Recent efforts have provided a number of potential "sensors" of cellular copper, zinc and manganese status that merit further evaluation. The judicious application of methods in molecular biology (including genomics and proteomics) and noninvasive imaging techniques is likely to provide new breakthroughs and rapid advances in the nutrition and biology of trace elements;
- evaluate further the specific health risks associated with marginal deficiencies of various minerals and trace elements. There is a need to determine reliable relationships between mineral status and disease and then to demonstrate that the incidence or severity of specific diseases is reversible by repletion of mineral status. The development and validation of reliable assessment tools and functional markers of mineral status are the utmost priority for this field;

Table 9.19 Absorption, transport and storage characteristics of the ultratrace elements

Element	Major mechanism(s) for homeostasis	Means of absorption	Percentage of ingested absorbed	Transport and storage vehicles
Aluminum	Absorption	Uncertain; some evidence for passive diffusion through the paracellular pathway; also, evidence for active absorption through processes shared with active processes of calcium; probably occurs in proximal duodenum; citrate combined with aluminum enhances absorption	<1%	Transferrin carries aluminum in plasma; bone a possible storage site
Arsenic	Urinary excretion; inorganic arsenic as mostly dimethylarsinic acid and organic arsenic as mostly arsenobetaine	Inorganic arsenate becomes sequestered in or on mucosal tissue, then absorption involves a simple movement down a concentration gradient; organic arsenic absorbed mainly by simple diffusion through lipid regions of the intestinal boundary	Soluble inorganic forms, >90%; slightly soluble inorganic forms, 20–30%; inorganic forms with foods, 60–75%; methylated forms, 45–90%	Before excretion inorganic arsenic is converted into monomethylarsonic acid and dimethylarsinic acid; arsenobetaine not biotransformed; arsenocholine transformed to arsenobetaine
Boron	Urinary excretion	Ingested boron is converted into B(OH)$_3$ and absorbed in this form, probably by passive diffusion	>90%	Boron transported through the body as undissociated B(OH)$_3$; bone a possible storage site
Cadmium	Absorption	May share a common absorption mechanism with other metals (e.g. zinc) but mechanism is less efficient for cadmium	5%	Incorporated into metallothionein which probably is both a storage and transport vehicle
Germanium	Urinary excretion	Has not been conclusively determined but probably is by passive diffusion	>90%	None identified
Lead	Absorption	Uncertain; thought to be by passive diffusion in small intestine but evidence has been presented for an active transport perhaps involving the system for calcium	Adults 5–15%, children 40–50%	Bone is a repository for lead
Lithium	Urinary excretion	Passive diffusion by paracellular transport via the tight junctions and pericellular spaces	Lithium chloride highly absorbed: >90%	Bone can serve as a store for lithium
Nickel	Both absorption and urinary excretion	Uncertain; evidence for both passive diffusion (perhaps as an amino acid or other low molecular weight complex) and energy-driven transport; occurs in the small intestine	<10% with food	Transported in blood principally bound to serum albumin with small amounts bound to L-histidine and α$_2$-macroglobulin; no organ accumulates physiological amounts of nickel
Rubidium	Excretion through kidney and intestine	Resembles potassium in its pattern of absorption; rubidium and potassium thought to share a transport system	Highly absorbed	None identified
Silicon	Both absorption and urinary excretion	Mechanisms involved in intestinal absorption have not been described	Food silicon near 50%; insoluble or poorly soluble silicates ~1%	Silicon in plasma believed to exist as undisassociated monomeric silicic acid
Tin	Absorption	Mechanisms involved in intestinal absorption have not been described	~3%. Percentage increases when very low amounts are ingested	None identified; bone might be a repository
Vanadium	Absorption	Vanadate has been suggested to be absorbed through phosphate or other anion transport systems; vanadyl has been suggested to use iron transport systems; absorption occurs in the duodenum	<10%	Converted into vanadyltransferrin and vanadyl-ferritin; whether transferrin is the transport vehicle and ferritin is the storage vehicle for vanadium remains to be determined; bone is a repository for excess vanadium

Reproduced with permission from Nielsen (1999).

Table 9.20 Excretion, retention and possible biological roles of the ultratrace elements

Element	Organs of high content (typical concentration)	Major excretory route after ingestion	Molecules of biological importance	Possible biological role
Aluminum	Bone (1–12 µg/g) Lung (35 µg/g)	Urine; also significant amounts in bile	Aluminum binds to proteins, nucleotides and phospholipids; aluminum-bound transferrin apparently is a transport molecule	Enzyme activator
Arsenic	Hair (0.65 µg/g) Nails (0.35 µg/g) Skin (0.10 µg/g)	Urine	Methylation of inorganic oxyarsenic anions occurs in organisms ranging from microbial to mammalian; methylated end-products include arsenocholine, arsenobetaine, dimethylarsinic acid and methylarsonic acid; arsenite methyltransferase and monomethylarsonic acid methyltransferase use S-adenosylmethionine for the methyl donor	Metabolism of methionine, or involved in labile methyl metabolism; regulation of gene expression
Boron	Bone (1.6 µg/g) Fingernails (15 µg/g) Hair (1 µg/g) Teeth (5 µg/g)	Urine	Boron biochemistry essentially that of boric acid, which forms ester complexes with hydroxyl groups, preferably those adjacent and cis, in organic compounds; five naturally occurring boron esters (all antibiotics) synthesized by various bacteria have been characterized	Cell membrane function or stability such that it influences the response to hormone action, transmembrane signalling or transmembrane movement of regulatory cations or anions
Bromine	Hair (30 µg/g) Liver (40 µg/g) Lung (6.0 µg/g) Testis (5.0 µg/g)	Urine	Exists as Br⁻ ion in vivo, binds to proteins and amino acids	Electrolyte balance
Cadmium	Kidney (14 µg/g) Liver (4 µg/g)	Urine and gastrointestinal tract	Metallothionein, a high sulfhydryl-containing protein involved in regulating cadmium distribution	Involved in metallathionein metabolism and utilization
Germanium	Bone (9 µg/g) Liver (0.3 µg/g) Pancreas (0.2 µg/g) Testis (0.5 µg/g)	Urine	None identified	Role in immune function
Lead	Aorta (1–2 µg/g) Bone (25 µg/g) Kidney (1–2 µg/g) Liver (1–2 µg/g)	Urine; also significant amounts in bile	Plasma lead mostly bound to albumin; blood lead binds mostly to hemoglobin but some binds a low molecular weight protein in erythrocytes	Facilitates iron absorption and/or utilization

(Continued)

Table 9.20 (Continued)

Element	Organs of high content (typical concentration)	Major excretory route after ingestion	Molecules of biological importance	Possible biological role
Lithium	Adrenal gland (60 ng/g) Bone (100 ng/g) Lymph nodes (200 ng/g) Pituitary gland (135 ng/g)	Urine	None identified	Regulation of some endocrine function
Nickel	Adrenal glands (25 ng/g) Bone (33 ng/g) Kidney (10 ng/g) Thyroid (30 ng/g)	Urine as low molecular weight complexes	Binding of Ni^{2-} by various ligands including amino acids (especially histidine and cysteine), proteins (especially albumin) and a macroglobulin called nickeloplasmin important in transport and excretion; Ni^{2+} component of urease; Ni^{3+} essential for enzymic hydrogenation, desulfurization and carboxylation reactions in mostly anerobic micro-organisms	Cofactor or structural component in specific metalloenzymes; role in a metabolic pathway involving vitamin B_{12} and folic acid; role similar to potassium; neurophysiological function
Rubidium	Brain (4 µg/g) Kidney (5 µg/g) Liver (6.5 µg/g) Testis (20 µg/g)	Urine; also significant amounts excreted through intestinal tract	None identified	Role similar to potassium; neurophysiological function
Silicon	Aorta (16 µg/g) Bone (18 µg/g) Skin (4 µg/g) Tendon (12 µg/g)	Urine	Silicic acid $(SiOH_4)$ is the form believed to exist in plasma; magnesium orthosilicate is probably the form of silicon in urine. The bound form of silicon has never been rigorously identified	Structural role in some mucopolysaccharide or collagen; role in the initiation of calcification and in collagen formation
Tin	Bone (0.8 µg/g) Kidney (0.2 µg/g) Liver (0.4 µg/g)	Urine; also significant amounts in bile	Sn^{2+} is absorbed and excreted more readily than Sn^{4+}	Role in some redox reactions
Vanadium	Bone (120 ng/g) Kidney (120 ng/g) Liver (120 ng/g) Spleen (120 ng/g) Testis (200 ng/g)	Urine; also significant amounts in bile	Vanadyl (VO^{2+}), vanadate $(H_2VO_4^-$ or $VO_3^-)$ and peroxovanadyl [V-OO]; VO^{2+} complexes with proteins, especially those associated with iron (e.g. transferrin, hemoglobin)	Lower forms of life have haloperoxidases that require vanadium for activity; a similar role may exist in higher forms of life

Reproduced with permission from Nielsen (1999).
None of the suggested biological functions or roles of any of the ultratrace elements has been conclusively or unequivocally identified in higher forms of life.

Table 9.21 Human body content and deficient, typical and rich sources of intakes of ultratrace elements

Element	Apparent deficient intake (species)	Human body content	Typical human daily dietary intake	Rich sources
Aluminum	160 µg/kg (goat)	30–50 mg	2–10 mg	Baked goods prepared with chemical leavening agents (e.g. baking powder), processed cheese, grains, vegetables, herbs, tea, antacids, buffered analgesics
Arsenic	<25 µg/kg (chicks) <35 µg/kg (goat) <15 µg/kg (hamster) <30 µg/kg (rat)	1–2 mg	12–60 µg	Shellfish, fish, grain, cereal products
Boron	<0.3 mg/kg (chick) 0.25–0.35 mg/day (human) <0.3 mg/kg (rat)	10–20 mg	0.5–3.5 mg	Food and drink of plant origin, especially noncitrus fruits, leafy vegetables, nuts, pulses, legumes, wine, cider, beer
Bromine	0.8 mg/kg (goat)	200–350 mg	2–8 mg	Grain, nuts, fish
Cadmium	<5 µg/kg (goat) <4 µg/kg (rat)	5–20 mg	10–20 µg	Shellfish, grains, especially those grown on high-cadmium soils, leafy vegetables
Germanium	0.7 mg/kg (rat)	3 mg	0.4–3.4 mg	Wheat bran, vegetables, leguminous seeds
Lead	<32 µg/kg (pig) <45 µg/kg (rat)	Children less than 10 years old 2 mg, Adults 120 mg	15–100 µg	Seafood, plant foodstuffs grown under high-lead conditions
Lithium	<1.5 mg/kg (goat) <15 µg/kg (rat)	350 µg	200–600 µg	Eggs, meat, processed meat, fish, milk, milk products, potatoes, vegetables (content varies with geological origin)
Nickel	<100 µg/kg (goat) <20 µg/kg (rat)	1–2 mg	70–260 µg	Chocolate, nuts, dried beans and peas, grains
Rubidium	180 µg/kg (goat)	360 mg	1–5 mg	Coffee, black tea, fruits and vegetables (especially asparagus), poultry, fish
Silicon	<20 mg kg (chick) <4.5 mg/kg (rat)	2–3 g	20–50 mg	Unrefined grains of high fiber content, cereal products
Tin	<20 µg/kg (rat)	7–14 mg	1–40 mg	Canned foods
Vanadium	<10 µg/kg (goat)	100 µg	10–30 µg	Shellfish, mushrooms, parsley, dill, seed, black pepper, some prepared foods

Reproduced with permission from Nielsen (1999).

- define the adverse effects of acute and chronic high intakes of some minerals and trace elements. Interest in mineral fortification of foods is higher than ever before. Governments worldwide are increasingly tackling the common deficiencies of iron and iodine by adding these minerals to widely consumed staple foods such as cereal flours, sugar or soy sauce. The food industry in industrialized countries is manufacturing an increasing number of functional foods, designed to provide the consumer with protection against diseases of major public health significance, such as osteoporosis, cancer and heart disease, and fortified with minerals such as calcium, selenium, zinc, magnesium and copper. The same minerals are added to dietetic products, including infant foods, foods for pregnant and lactating women, and enteral feeds for hospital patients, all designed to cover the nutritional requirements of specific consumers. This raises the issues not only of the possible health benefits of fortification but also of possible toxicity. Therefore, there is an ever-increasing emphasis placed on upper safe levels of mineral intake and on fortification legislation;

- elucidate the impact of single nucleotide polymorphisms in the human genome on mineral and trace element dietary requirements. The key to future applications of the DNA polymorphisms will be to mine the human genome for DNA sequence information that can be used to define biovariation in nutrient absorption and use. However, before this can be accomplished, a vast amount of nutritional biology research is needed to correlate gene polymorphism with nutritional outcomes.

Further reading

Bowman B, Russel R, eds. Present Knowledge in Nutrition, 8th edn. Washington DC: ILSI Press, 2001.

Department of Health. Report on health and social subjects 41. Dietary reference values for food energy and nutrients in the UK. Committee on Medical Aspects of Food Policy. London: HMSO, 1991.

Hallberg L, Sandstrom B, Aggett PJ. In: Human Nutrition and Dietetics, 9th edn (JS Garrow, WPT James, A Ralph, eds). London: Churchill Livingstone, 1993.

Holland B, Welch AA, Unwin ID, Buss DH, Paul AA, Southgate DAT, eds. McCance & Widdowson's The Composition of Foods, 5th edn. Royal Society of Chemistry and Ministry of Agriculture, Fisheries and Food, London: HMSO, 1995

Institute of Medicine (USA). Dietary Reference Intakes for Calcium, Phosphorus, Magnesium, Vitamin D, and Fluoride. Washington DC: National Academy Press, 1997.

Mills CF, ed. Zinc in Human Biology. London: Springer-Verlag, 1989.

Nielsen F. In: Encyclopedia of Human Nutrition (MJ Sadler, JJ Strain, B Caballero, eds). London: Academic Press, 1999.

Passmore R, Eastwood MA, eds. Davidsons and Passmore Human Nutrition and Dietetics, 8th edn. London: Churchill Livingstone, 1986.

Optimal Nutrition Symposium. A series of papers. In: Proceedings of the Nutrition Society, 58: 395–512, 1999.

Rayman MP. The importance of selenium to human health. Lancet, 356: 233–241, 2000.

Reilly C. Selenium in Food and Health. London: Blackie, 1996.

Sadler MJ, Strain JJ, Caballero B, eds. Encyclopedia of Human Nutrition, Vol. 3, Parts 1–3. London: Academic Press, 1999.

Sánchez-Castillo CP, James WPT. In: Encyclopedia of Human Nutrition (MJ Sadler, JJ Strain, B Caballero, eds). London: Academic Press, 1999.

Strain JJ, Benzie IFF. In: Encyclopedia of Human Nutrition (MJ Sadler, JJ Strain, B Caballero, eds). London: Academic Press, 1999.

Website

Online Mendelian Genetics in Man (OMIM) website at the National Institute for Biotechnology Information: www.ncbi.nlm.nih.gov/Omim

10
Measuring Food Intake

Ingrid HE Rutishauser and Alison E Black

Key messages

- Measuring the food intake in free-living individuals is a complex task.
- All measurements of food intake are subject to sources of error.
- The existence of error means that it is always important to be aware of and, whenever possible, to assess the nature and magnitude of the error.

- To increase our understanding of the error associated with measurements of food intake it is also necessary to develop and use physiological and biochemical markers of food intake.
- To evaluate food intake data effectively it is important to collect sufficient additional data to allow individuals to be identified not only by age and gender, but also by body mass index, physical activity and supplement use.

10.1 Introduction

The purpose of this chapter is to describe the various ways in which one can set about the task of finding out what people eat. The task may be to find out about the national food supply, the usual intake of a group or the intake of a given individual over a specified period.

The many reasons for finding out about the food that people eat fall into three broad categories: to evaluate the adequacy and safety of the food that people eat (public health), to assist with the diagnosis and treatment of diet-related conditions (clinical), and to study the interrelationships between food intake and physiological function under controlled conditions (research). The kind and amount of food intake data required differ in each situation and may require data at the national, household or individual level.

Assessment of nutritional status

Nutritional health is maintained by a state of equilibrium in which nutrient intake is balanced by nutritional requirements. Malnutrition occurs when net nutrient intake (correcting for large fecal or urinary losses) is less than requirements. Malnutrition leads to a succession of metabolic abnormalities, physiological changes and reduced organ and tissue function, in association with a reduction in body mass. Concurrent disease states and trauma accelerate the loss of tissue and function, ultimately leading to death.

An ideal tool does not exist to measure a person's nutritional status accurately. Attempts to predict the influence of malnutrition based on single parameters fail to consider the many interacting factors between nutrition and disease state. For this reason, it is necessary to look at several parameters in order to assess a person's nutritional status.

- **a**nthropometry (discussed in detail in Chapter 2)
- **b**iochemical and hematological parameters
- **c**linical and physical assessment
- **d**ietary intake.

The rest of this chapter will concentrate on the measurement of food intake, but more detailed descriptions of the assessment of nutritional status, at the individual and population level, can be found in the Public Health Nutrition and Clinical Nutrition textbooks in this series.

Obtaining data on food intake has a number of inherent problems. A major one is that "food intake" is not a simple measure of one variable, such as weight or height, but requires data on the intake of many different food items. Another problem is that food intake data are subject to many sources of variability, since even the same individuals eat different foods, at different times, in different places and in many different combinations. The net effect of all these sources of variability is that more data are needed to generate reliable data than would be the case with a less variable measure.

A further difficulty is that we are rarely in a position to know the truth about food intake. With many biological measurements it is possible to check the results obtained against a reference method that is known to give accurate results or by means of an independent measure. For example, we can check an infant's birth weight by checking the accuracy of the weighing equipment used to measure it by means of a standard weight or, if the information was obtained by means of a questionnaire, we may be able to check the data from official records. With food intake data we rarely have an absolute source of information against which to check the data obtained.

In most circumstances we also have to rely on the individuals who eat the food to provide us with the answers to our question. For this reason one of the most important considerations, when obtaining information on food intake from individuals, is to take all possible steps to obtain their full cooperation. This may well involve much time and effort on the part of the investigator(s), but is essential for high-quality data.

It is also essential to recognize that finding out what people eat requires adequate resources. Appropriately trained personnel must be employed not only for the period of data collection but also for the time it takes to review, enter and analyze the data. It may not always be necessary to obtain detailed data on food intake in order to answer a particular question. When resources are limited it is probably more useful to collect limited data of high quality than to attempt to collect comprehensive dietary data with inadequate resources. Being able to recognize this situation is important for maximising available resources. Table 10.1 lists the different approaches to measurement of food intake that are described in this chapter.

Table 10.1 Approaches to the measurement of food intake in population groups, households and individuals

Type and nature of data	Name of method	Used for assessing differences between
Commodity-level food supply data, e.g. production, imports and exports (indirect)	Food balance sheets	Countries and regions of the world
Product-level food supply data, e.g. retail and wholesale sales data (indirect)	Food disappearance data	Country, locality and season
Household food expenditure, e.g. money spent on food (indirect)	Household expenditure surveys	Country, locality, season and type of household
Household food acquisition, e.g. amount of food entering the household (indirect)	Household budget surveys	Country, locality, season and type of household
Qualitative record of foods (but not amounts) eaten during 1 or more weeks by individuals (direct)	Menu records	Geographical, seasonal and demographic subgroups and individuals
Quantitative record of food intake, e.g. record of foods eaten during 1–7 days by individuals (direct)	Weighed records and records estimated in household measures	Geographical, seasonal and demographic subgroups and individuals
Qualitative or semiquantitative recall, usually of a specified list, of foods eaten in the previous month or year by individuals (direct)	Food frequency questionnaires	Geographical, seasonal and demographic subgroups and individuals
Quantitative recall of foods eaten on the previous day, usually obtained from individuals by interview (direct)	Single or multiple 24 h recalls	Geographical, seasonal and demographic subgroups and individuals (if multiple recalls obtained)
Quantitative recall of habitual intake in the immediate past obtained from individuals by interview (direct)	Diet history	Temporal and demographic subgroups and individuals

Finally, it is important that the interpretation and application of data derived from food intake studies take into account the limitations of the data. This clearly does not improve the quality of the data per se, but maximizes their usefulness for the purpose for which they were originally collected. Recognition of the limitations of dietary data involves more than simply stating the limitations. External comparisons to check whether the data are consistent with independent sources of information on food intake and to determine the likely direction and magnitude of any bias are an integral part of the interpretation of dietary data. Relevant sources of comparative information may include food supply and expenditure data and physiological or biochemical measures related to nutrient intake.

10.2 Indirect measurements of food intake

The essential feature of all indirect measures of food intake is that they are not derived directly from data on food intake, but indirectly from sources of information that provide data on the amount of food available for consumption (food supply data), on the volume of food traded at the wholesale or retail level (food disappearance data) or on the amount of food purchased at a household level (household budget or expenditure data).

Food supply data

Food supply data are usually produced at the national level and based on compilations of data from multiple sources. The primary sources of data are records of agricultural production, food exports and imports adjusted for changes in stocks and for agricultural and industrial use of food crops and food products. National food supply data are usually referred to as "food balance sheets" or as "apparent consumption data". A food balance sheet represents the food available for human consumption in a country, usually expressed per caput in grams or kilograms per year.

The Food and Agriculture Organization (FAO) has compiled and published food balance sheet data for most countries in the world since 1949. Regularly updated food balance sheet data are available on-line at www.fao.org for most countries for about 100 primary crop, livestock and fishery commodities and some products such as sugar, oils and fats derived from them.

The accuracy of food balance sheets and apparent consumption data depends on the reliability of the basic statistics used to derive them, i.e. population, supply, utilization and food composition data. These can vary markedly between countries not only in terms of coverage but also in terms of accuracy.

Several internal and external consistency checks are built in to the preparation of the FAO food balance sheets, but users still need to evaluate the data for themselves in the context of the purpose for which they are being used. One of the crucial factors in using the data appropriately is to understand the terminology used. Box 10.1 provides "in principle" definitions of the key terms.

Box 10.1

Production: total domestic production whether produced inside or outside the agricultural sector, i.e. includes noncommercial production and production from home gardens

Imports: all movements of the commodity into the country, e.g. commercial trade, food aid, donated quantities and estimates of unrecorded trade

Stock changes: changes in stocks occurring during the reference period at all levels between the production and retail levels, i.e. stocks held by the government, manufacturers, importers, exporters, wholesale and retail merchants and distributors. In practice, the available information often only relates to government stocks

Exports: all movements out of the country during the reference period estimated as for imports

Industrial uses: commodities used for manufacture for nonfood purposes, e.g. oils for soap

Waste: commodities lost through all stages between postharvest production and the household, i.e. waste in processing, storage and transportation, but not domestic waste. Losses occurring during the manufacture of processed products are taken into account by means of extraction/conversion rates

Food: the amounts of the commodity and any commodity derived therefrom available for human consumption during the reference period, e.g. for maize includes maize, maize meal and any other products derived from maize that are available for human consumption

Per caput supply: adjustments are made when possible to the resident population for temporary migrants, refugees and tourists. The figures represent only the average supply available for the population as a whole and not what is actually consumed by individuals. Many commodities are not consumed in the primary form in which they are reported in food balance sheets. To take this into account the protein and fat content shown against primary commodities are derived by applying appropriate food composition factors to the relevant amounts of processed foods, and not by multiplying the quantities shown in the food balance sheet by food composition factors relating to the primary commodity

In practice, the data needed to compile food balance sheets are not always available and imputations or estimates may have to be used at each stage in the calculation of per caput food and nutrient availability. Errors associated with incomplete data are by no means confined to data from nonindustrialized countries. In most industrialized countries reliable data are usually available on primary commodities, but this is not necessarily the case for the major processed products. For example, data may be available on flour but not on products such as bread and other cereal products based on flour which may have quite different nutrient characteristics. The overall impact of incomplete data will vary from country to country, but it has been suggested that in general underestimation of per caput availability of nutrients is more likely in less developed countries and overestimation in countries where most of the food supply is consumed in the form of processed products.

Food disappearance data

In some countries (e.g. Canada and the USA) data on per caput food availability are prepared from data on food available at the retail or wholesale level. Such data are derived mainly from food industry organizations and firms engaged in food production and marketing. Errors arise mainly from inappropriate conversion factors for processing, the absence of data for some processed products, and the lack of data on food obtained from noncommercial sources such as home gardens, fishing and hunting.

Commercial databases such as those produced by the AC Neilsen Company and the electronic stock-control records from individual supermarkets, from which they are compiled, have the potential for monitoring national, regional and local level trends in the food supply, at a product-specific level. Their principal disadvantage at present lies in the costs associated with processing or otherwise accessing, on a regular basis, the very large amounts of data that are involved.

FAO food balance sheets and similar sources of information are primarily useful for formulating agricultural and health policy, for monitoring changes in national food supplies over time and as a basis for forecasting food consumption patterns. They can also be used to make intercountry comparisons of food and nutrient supplies, provided that potential differences in data coverage and accuracy are taken into account.

10.3 Household food surveys

Surveys that provide information on household food supplies generally focus on household income and expenditure and are usually described as household expenditure or household budget surveys. In most countries where such surveys are conducted the primary focus is on collecting information about the amount of money spent on food over a given period. Sometimes, however, data on the quantities of food purchased are also collected but may not be processed because of the additional complexity and cost involved.

Household food expenditure data alone can provide useful information for nutritionists on food expenditure patterns of different types of households, but without quantitative information this cannot be translated into nutrient patterns.

Household budget surveys (HBS) are conducted at regular intervals in many European countries and many also collect data on food quantities as well as cost. HBS have several advantages:

- they are usually conducted at regular intervals of between 1 and 5 years
- they are conducted on representative samples of households
- the food supply information collected can be classified by sociodemographic characteristics, geographical location and season.

The large amount of nutrition-related information collected by these surveys has potential for assessing the nutritional patterns of different population groups, for identifying high-risk groups for nutrition-related conditions, for monitoring trends in food patterns over time and for developing nutrition policy. The information available from HBS, however, also needs to be considered in the context of their limitations.

- Information provided by HBS differs from country to country both in the number of food items recorded and in the type of information collected.
- Most surveys do not include expenditure information on food consumed outside the home.
- Most surveys do not collect information on domestic wastage, i.e. food given to pets, spoiled food and plate waste or food provided for guests.
- It is often difficult to estimate the nutrient content of the food available to the household because data are reported only at food group and not individual food level.

- Differences in food coding systems between countries make it difficult to compare data between countries.

Three conclusions emerge from this list. First, the data obtained from HBS are not necessarily comparable between countries. Secondly, most HBS do not collect all of the information needed to provide an accurate assessment of the total food supply available at household level. Thirdly, provided that the HBS methodology remains consistent, HBS can provide a great deal of valuable information about food patterns over time, in different sociodemographic groups and in different parts of the country, and how these relate to social, economic and technological changes in the food supply.

10.4 Direct measures of food intake

Information about food intake can be obtained in different ways. Usually it is obtained from individuals, but occasionally data may be collected at household level. For example, in societies where it is usual for members of the household to eat out of the same pot this may be the only practical approach because it does not disrupt the normal pattern of food intake. In these circumstances data on food intake is usually collected by someone external to the household who is able to weigh the food being consumed before and after preparation and also any food that is left at the end of the meal.

The procedure for measuring food and nutrient intake involves five steps (Figure 10.1):

- obtaining a report of all the foods consumed by each individual
- identifying these foods in sufficient detail to choose an appropriate item in the food tables
- quantifying the portion sizes
- measuring or estimating the frequency with which each food is eaten
- calculation of nutrient intake from food tables.

To convert the information on food intake into nutrient intake, the nutrient content of each food eaten is calculated from food tables as:

Portion size (g) $\times$ Frequency $\times$ Nutrient content per g

and summed for all foods eaten by each individual during the study period.

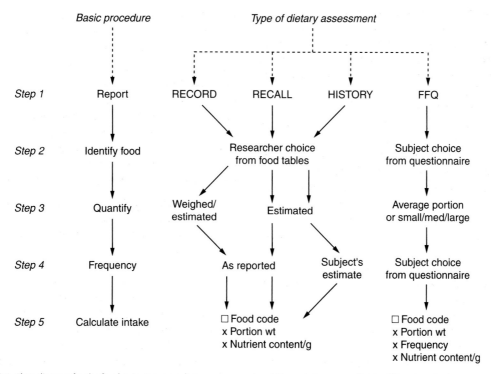

Figure 10.1 Flow diagram for the five basic steps in a dietary assessment and the variations according to different methods.

Ways of measuring food intake in individuals can be divided into two basic approaches: reports of foods actually consumed on specified days and approaches that attempt to construct typical food patterns. The first category includes weighed records, estimated records, menu records and 24 h recalls. The second includes diet histories and food frequency questionnaires. Records are usually limited to fairly short periods, usually not longer than 7 consecutive days, while recalls may relate to a single period of 24 h or occasionally 48 h. Diet histories and food frequency questionnaires relate to longer periods and their purpose is to obtain an assessment of habitual intake over the period in question and not a detailed day-to-day recall of what was eaten during that time. When records are kept portions may be either weighed or estimated in terms of standard household measures. In recalls and questionnaires quantities always have to be estimated. Dimensions, photographs of foods, food models and, sometimes, actual foods may be used to assist in this process. Each of these approaches has specific advantages and disadvantages and no single method of measuring food intake can be regarded as the ideal method for all situations.

Weighed intake recorded over a period of a week has often been taken as the reference method against which less detailed and demanding methods have been compared, but it is now recognized that this method also has limitations and that it is not only desirable but necessary to use physiological and biochemical measures to determine whether any method of measuring food intake is actually measuring what it sets out to measure.

10.5 Basic concepts

Before describing the most commonly used dietary methods it is appropriate to introduce four fundamental concepts relevant to the process of dietary assessment and evaluation. A brief definition of terms related to these concepts is given in Box 10.2. Terms are listed in the box in alphabetical order for ease of reference.

Habitual intake

The objective of virtually all dietary assessments is to obtain an estimate of the habitual or average long-term intake for the group or the individual of interest. Habitual represents what is "usual" in the long term and not

Box 10.2

Accuracy: the extent to which an estimate approximates the true value

Bias: the extent by which an estimate differs from the true value

Coefficient of variation: the standard deviation of a set of observations expressed as a percentage of their mean

Habitual intake: an estimate of the long-term average intake of an individual

Precision: the extent to which a method is repeatable. Usually expressed in terms of the coefficient of variation, i.e. the standard deviation of the results of repeated analyzes of the same parameter expressed as a percentage of their mean

Random errors: errors that are randomly distributed about the true value. Random errors increase the variability of a set observations but do not affect their mean

Repeatability: a method is repeatable or reproducible when it gives the same result on repeated measurement

Systematic errors: errors that are not randomly distributed about the true value. Systematic errors can increase or decrease the variability of a set of observations and also affect the estimate of their mean. The effect on the mean is referred to as bias

Validity: a method is valid if it measures what it is intended to measure, i.e. the true value:

- **Absolute validity or accuracy:** terms used to describe the extent to which a method measures the true value. It is not possible to determine the absolute accuracy of a dietary method by comparison with another dietary method
- **Face or content validity:** a method which gives results that are consistent with other data related to the parameter it is intended to measure
- **Relative validity:** the extent to which a test method performs in relation to a criterion or reference method, i.e. the dietary method judged to provide the "best" available measure of the true value
- **Validity at group level:** a method is valid at the group level if it provides an unbiased estimate of mean intake for the group
- **Validity at individual level:** a method is valid at the individual level if it is able to rank subjects correctly (usually evaluated in terms of the same proportion in the same quintile or tertile of the distribution compared with the "true" or more usually a "reference" value)

Variance: statistical term to describe the variation that occurs in a set of observations. It is equal to the square of the standard deviation of the individual observations:

- **Between-person variance:** the variance arising from differences between individuals
- **Within-person variance:** the variance arising from differences within individuals

simply at a specific moment in time. It is this level of intake that is relevant for maintenance of energy balance and nutrient status, and for the assessment of relationships between nutrient intake and health in the long term. Habitual intake, however, is difficult to measure because food intake varies widely from day to day and to a lesser extent from week to week and month

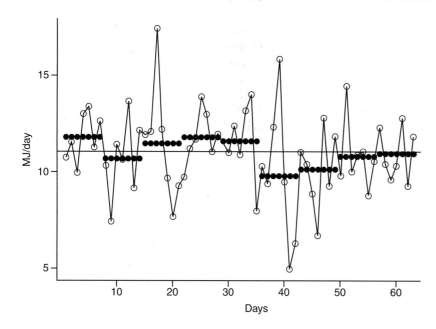

Figure 10.2 Energy intake of one individual from weighed records obtained for 1 day every sixth day over 1 year. —: overall mean; •••: weekly mean; ○: intake on individual days.

to month. Figure 10.2 illustrates the energy intake of one individual who maintained a weighed record every sixth day for 1 year. The horizontal line indicates the overall average intake over the year in MJ per day. The open circles show the intake on individual days and the solid circles the average intake over 7 day periods. It is obvious that intake on a single day does not provide a reliable estimate of habitual intake and that even average intake over 7 days can differ by as much as 20% from the overall mean.

The nature of error

There is not, and probably never will be, a method that can estimate dietary intake without error.

This means not that we should stop collecting dietary data but rather that dietary data need independent validation and that methods need to be developed to assess the error structure of dietary data sets so that it can be taken into account in analyzing and evaluating the data. Basically, there are two types of error, random error and systematic error.

Random error increases the variance of the estimates obtained and consequently reduces their precision (see below). The effects of random error can be reduced by increasing the number of observations. Day-to-day variation in food intake in individuals is one example of

a random error that can be reduced by increasing the number of days of observation (Figure 10.2).

In contrast, the effects of systematic error cannot be reduced by increasing the number of observations. Systematic error arises from errors that are non randomly distributed in the group or in the data from a given individual. For example, inappropriate nutrient data for some food items will not affect the food intake data for all individuals in the same way. Systematic error leads to bias in the estimates of intake obtained.

Precision/repeatability

In the laboratory the precision of a method is given by the coefficient of variation of repeated determinations on the same sample made under the same conditions (see Box 10.2). In the context of dietary studies we determine whether the same method gives the same answer when repeated in the same individuals, and the terms repeatability and reproducibility are commonly used to describe the precision of a method. It is important to note that it is possible for a method to have high precision (good repeatability) yet not to provide an accurate (valid) estimate of intake.

Accuracy/validity

An accurate method is one that measures what the method intends to measure, that is, the "truth".

In the context of dietary studies the truth represents the actual intake over the period of the study. For example, a valid diet record is a complete and accurate record of all the food and drink consumed over the period of the record. To be a valid record of habitual intake it also needs to reflect what would have been eaten and drunk had the individual not been keeping a record. If the process of recording influenced what was eaten then the record is not a valid record of habitual intake, although it may be a true record of actual intake over the period. Similarly, a valid 24 h recall is a complete and accurate account of all food and drink consumed during the specified period.

Determining the validity of a dietary technique has been impossible in the absence of external markers of intake, except for the 24 h recall or for individual meals.

10.6 Options for measuring intake on specified days

Menu records

Menu records are the simplest way of recording information on food intake. They only require the participant to write down descriptions of the food and drink eaten at each meal and snack throughout the day for the specified days without quantifying the portions. A menu record is useful when information on food patterns rather than intake is required over a longer period or when subjects have difficulty in providing quantitative information. For example, elderly people may have difficulty in reading the divisions on household scales or in measuring out food portions. To derive information on nutrient intake from menu records investigators also need to obtain information on portion sizes of commonly eaten foods. The method works well when the diet is relatively consistent, does not contain a great variety of foods and has been adapted for use in nonliterate communities. The method can also be used to distinguish differences in the frequency of use of specific foods over time, to determine whether quantitative short-term intake records are likely to be representative of habitual intake and as a way of assessing compliance with special diets.

Weighed records

Weighed records require the subject, or the investigator, to weigh each item of food or drink at the time it is consumed and to write down a description of this item and its weight in a booklet specially designed for this purpose. Weighed records are usually kept for 3, 4, 5 or 7 consecutive days. To obtain accurate information it is necessary to use trained investigators to collect the data or to demonstrate the procedure and to provide clear instructions to the subjects on how food should be weighed. Weighing can be carried out in two different ways:

- the ingredients used in the preparation of each meal, as well as the cooked amounts obtained and consumed, are weighed together with any food waste
- all food and beverage items are weighed, in the form in which they are consumed, immediately before they are eaten, and any previously weighed food that is not consumed is also weighed.

The first approach is sometimes referred to as the precise weighing technique and is usually carried out by trained fieldworkers rather than the subjects themselves. It is most appropriate when the food composition tables available contain few data on cooked and mixed dishes or when subjects are not able to weigh the food themselves. It should be noted, however, that the precise weighing technique does not allow for nutrient losses in cooking. To take these into account information on cooking losses for the most commonly used cooking methods must also be available.

The second procedure, which is more widely used, involves weighing all food eaten in the form in which it is consumed. It is sometimes referred to as the weighed inventory method. Using this method the nutrient content of the diet can be determined either by chemical analysis of duplicate portions of individual foods or aliquots of the total food consumed or from tables of food composition. Scales used for weighing food need to be robust and able to weigh up to 2 kg with a precision of at least ±5 g and preferably ±2 g. Record books need to be easy to use and of a convenient size. They should contain basic guidelines for weighing and an example page illustrating the level of detail required.

Metabolic studies carried out to determine absorption and retention of specific nutrients from measurements of intake and excretion are a specialized application of the weighed food intake record. In metabolic studies all foods consumed by the subjects are usually either preweighed or weighed by the investigators at the time of consumption. The foods consumed are usually also analyzed for the nutrient constituents of interest or prepared from previously analyzed ingredients.

Estimated records

This method of recording food intake is essentially similar to weighed records except that the amounts of food and beverages consumed are assessed by volume rather than by weight, that is, they are described in terms of cups, teaspoons, or other commonly used household measures, dimensions or units. Photographs or models may be used to assist quantification. These descriptive terms have then to be converted to weights by the investigator, using appropriate conversion data when available, or by obtaining the necessary information when not. For example, the investigator can determine the volume of the measures commonly used in a given household and then convert these to weights by weighing food portions of appropriate size or using information about the density (g/ml) of different kinds of foods. A record book for this kind of study is similar to that for a weighed record study. In some situations a precoded record form that lists the commonly eaten foods in terms of typical portion sizes may be appropriate, but an open record form is generally preferred. Since there is no need for weighing scales to be provided the record forms can be distributed by mail rather than by interviewers. This is convenient if a large number of subjects located over a large geographical area is involved. In this situation the follow-up interview, after completion of the record, could be conducted by telephone.

Weighed records are favored in countries where kitchen scales are a common household item and quantities in recipes are given by weight, for example the UK. Estimated records are favored in countries where it is customary for recipe books to give quantities by standard spoons and cups, for example the USA and Canada. The dietary literature frequently uses the phrase "diet record" without specifying how portions were quantified. In these instances, estimated records are most likely to have been used.

Recalled intake

Information on dietary intake over a specified period can also be obtained by asking individuals to recollect the types and amounts of food they have eaten. This approach therefore does not influence the type of food actually consumed in the way that a food record may do. However, it is open to misrepresentation of the dietary pattern, with subjects reporting a "good" dietary pattern in order to project a good self-image. Response rates in short-term recall studies tend to range from 65% to 95% and depend largely on how, under what conditions and from whom the information is obtained. A recall may consist of a face-to-face or telephone interview or of a self-completed questionnaire.

The 24 h recall is probably the most widely used method of obtaining information on food intake from individuals. It is often used in national surveys because it has a relatively high response rate and can provide the detailed information required by regulatory authorities for representative samples of different population subgroups.

The 24 h recall is an attempt to reconstruct quantitatively the amount of food consumed either in the previous 24 h or on the previous day. This period is considered to provide the most reliable recall of information. With longer periods memory becomes an increasing limitation. Incomplete recalls are more likely with self-completed records unless these records are subsequently checked with the subject by the investigator. Traditionally, the food intake has been reviewed chronologically. Problems encountered in estimating the amounts of foods consumed are similar to those encountered with estimated records. Recalls conducted by means of a face-to-face interview often use aids such as photographs and food models to help the subject to describe how much food was eaten. In telephone recalls subjects may be provided with pictures or other two-dimensional aids to help them with the task of describing the amounts consumed. There is, however, very little information on how effective these aids are. For this type of study a standardized interview protocol, which is based on a thorough knowledge of local food habits and commonly used foods, is essential when more than one interviewer is involved.

Recently, the multiple-pass 24 h recall has been described. First, the subjects provide a list of all foods eaten on the previous day using any recall strategy they desire, not necessarily chronological. Interviewers then obtain a more detailed list by probing for additions to foods such as cream in coffee and giving respondents an opportunity to recall food items that were initially forgotten. In a third pass the interviewer reviews the list of foods to stimulate reports of more foods and eating occasions. This approach is thought to provide better cues for subjects' cognitive processes than chronological cues.

Of the methods so far described weighed records should contain the least error as they report all food consumed on specified days with weighed portions. Estimating the size of portions increases error and if menu records are quantified with average portions, then the error at the individual level is further increased. If food that has already been eaten has to be recalled then poor memory can introduce an additional source of error. All methods that report intake on specified days are also subject, in individuals, to the error associated with day-to-day variation in intake, but this error can be reduced by increasing the number of days studied.

10.7 Options for measuring intake over the longer term

Diet history

The principal objective of the diet history is to obtain information on the habitual intake of an individual. As first proposed by Burke in the 1940s, the method had several components:

- an interview to obtain usual diet
- a cross-check of this information by food group
- a 3 day record of food consumed in household measures.

The 3 day record component is now seldom used as regular component of a diet history. Its purpose originally was as a way of checking the data obtained from the diet-history interview. A diet history is usually obtained by an experienced nutritionist by means of an open interview followed by some kind of cross-check using a standard list of commonly consumed foods. The interview usually begins with a review of the food that was eaten in a specific time-frame (e.g. yesterday) or on a typical day, and then moves on to explore the variations in food intake that occur for each meal over a given period. Information on the usual size of food portions is obtained with the aid of food models or photographs in the same way as for a 24 h recall. The time-frame for a diet history can range from the previous month to the previous year.

In practical terms it is easier for subjects to reconstruct the immediate past, but the past year is often used to capture seasonal variation. Whatever the time-frame used it is important for it to be clearly specified.

In the literature the term "diet history" is sometimes used loosely to describe any form of diet recall, including the 24 h recall and self-administered food frequency questionnaires, as well as interviewer-administered recalls of habitual or longer term intake. This broader use can be confusing and is best avoided. The dependence of the diet history on both subject and interviewer skills may make the results obtained less comparable between individuals than those obtained from other methods, and for this reason it is often considered more appropriate to categorize diet-history data (e.g. as high, medium, low) rather than to treat them as intakes expressed in terms of absolute units per day.

The diet history is favored in Scandinavia and the Netherlands, where a structured interview may be used. The structured interview is more standardized but may miss elements specific to the individual or bore the subjects with irrelevant questions. The open-ended interview allows for tailoring to the individual, but risks missing important items.

Food frequency questionnaires

The food frequency questionnaire provides the subject with a list of foods and a selection of options for how often each food is consumed. Typical options might be:

- daily
- 3–4 times per week
- 1–2 times per week
- 1–2 times per month
- occasionally
- never.

Subjects are required to indicate the best option for frequency of consumption for each of the foods on the list by marking the appropriate option column. The list may contain only a few food items or it may contain up to 200 items. The length of the list in part depends on the focus of interest. If the purpose of the questionnaire is to obtain an estimate of calcium intake the list may be restricted to foods that are major sources of calcium in the diet. If the questionnaire also aims to provide information on total energy intake it needs to include both a wider range and a longer list of foods.

Food frequency questionnaires are usually designed to be self-administered. This is because such questionnaires have been developed as a practical and cost-effective way of collecting dietary data from a large number of individuals (often several thousands) in

Please completely fill one oval in every line. Please MARK LIKE THIS: ○ ● ○ ○	N E V E R	1 time	2 times	3 or more times	1 time	2 times	3 to 4 times	5 to 6 times	Less than once	1 to 3 times
		per month			per week				per day	
Flavoured milk drink (cocoa, Milo™ etc.)	○	○	○	○	○	○	○	○	○	○
Nuts	○	○	○	○	○	○	○	○	○	○
Peanut butter or peanut paste	○	○	○	○	○	○	○	○	○	○
Corn chips, potato crisps, Twisties™ etc.	○	○	○	○	○	○	○	○	○	○
Jam, marmalade, honey or syrups	○	○	○	○	○	○	○	○	○	○
Vegemite™, Marmite™ or Promite™	○	○	○	○	○	○	○	○	○	○
Dairy products, Meats and Fish										
Cheese	○	○	○	○	○	○	○	○	○	○
Ice-cream	○	○	○	○	○	○	○	○	○	○
Yoghurt	○	○	○	○	○	○	○	○	○	○
Beef	○	○	○	○	○	○	○	○	○	○
Veal	○	○	○	○	○	○	○	○	○	○
Chicken	○	○	○	○	○	○	○	○	○	○
Lamb	○	○	○	○	○	○	○	○	○	○
Pork	○	○	○	○	○	○	○	○	○	○
Bacon	○	○	○	○	○	○	○	○	○	○

Figure 10.3 Typical layout of a food frequency questionnaire suitable for optical scanning. (Reproduced with permission of Anti Cancer Council of Victoria, Melbourne, Australia.)

etiological and analytical studies of the relationships between diet and disease. When appropriately designed, such questionnaires can also be optically scanned, which saves time on data entry and checking procedures (Figure 10.3). Food frequency questionnaires are not suitable for small-scale studies as the random errors are large and precision at the individual level is limited.

Most food frequency questionnaires obtain information only on the frequency of consumption of a food over a given period and not on the context in which the foods were eaten, that is, on meal patterns. Meal-based food frequency questionnaires have also been used on the basis that it may be easier for subjects to provide the information in the context of meals. The information on meal patterns obtained from such questionnaires is, however, more limited than that which can be obtained from a dietary history. Additional questions, if included, can provide some information on cooking methods.

Some food frequency questionnaires also attempt to quantify the frequency information by obtaining data on portion size. Information on the quantity of each food consumed may be obtained by asking subjects to indicate on the questionnaire whether their usual portions are small, medium or large relative to those eaten by others, by asking subjects to describe their usual portion size in terms of a standard portion size described on the questionnaire or by reference to a picture atlas of food portions.

Food frequency questionnaires are mainly used in studies that are designed to look for associations between food intake and disease, particularly when specific foods rather than the level of consumption of a nutrient are thought to be the important factor. A detailed discussion of the design and evaluation of food frequency methods for use in epidemiological studies is given by Willett.

10.8 Sources of error in dietary studies

The major sources of error in dietary studies have been reviewed in detail by Bingham (1987). Four possible sources of error occur to some degree with all dietary methods, but can be minimized by careful study design and execution:

- sampling bias
- response bias
- inappropriate coding of foods
- use of food composition tables in place of chemical analysis.

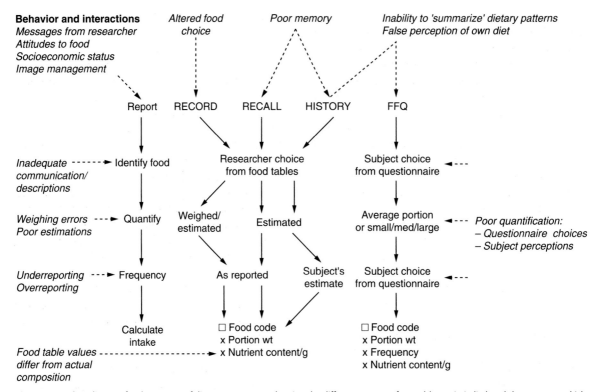

Figure 10.4 Flow diagram for the process of dietary assessment showing the different sources of error (shown in italics) and the stages at which they operate in different dietary methods. FFQ: food frequency questionnaire.

In contrast, the errors that are associated with specific methods are generally much more dependent on the nature of the method and the abilities of the subjects, and therefore less easy to control. Errors of this type include:

- estimation of portion size
- recall or memory error
- day-to-day variation in intake
- effect of survey method on food intake.

Figure 10.4 illustrates the points in the dietary assessment process at which different kinds of error operate.

Sampling bias

Sampling bias arises when the sample studied is not truly representative of the population of interest. The importance of minimizing sampling bias depends on the purpose of the dietary study. Except in methodological studies, volunteers are not generally appropriate subjects because frequently the objective is to study a representative sample of a particular group to be able to extrapolate the results to the population group from

which the sample was drawn. For this purpose it is clearly important that as many as possible of the sample group originally selected participate in the study.

The proportion of the sample that agrees to participate in the study can vary considerably even with the same method. It depends not only on the group being studied but also on the circumstances of the study. In general, response rates tend to be greater in studies that use methods such as the 24 h recall (which make fewer demands on subjects) and lower in studies such as 7 day weighed records (which require much more co-operation, effort and time from the subjects). It is always important to try to maximize response rates, for example by increasing subject motivation, providing specific assistance if required and by allowing subjects as much flexibility as possible in participation within the context of the study objectives.

Response bias

Response bias arises when subjects provide incomplete or inappropriate responses. The extent of this problem is not easy to assess, but can be investigated by making measurements that are independent of dietary intake, both during and after dietary study periods. Measurements suitable for this purpose will be discussed further in the context of validity. Response bias can probably best be minimized by providing the subjects with clear and well-presented instructions, as well as adequate support and appropriate incentives. Such incentives may include relevant dietary feedback where this is appropriate, monetary or other rewards.

In dietary studies that involve more than one interviewer, the training of interviewers and the use of standard procedures for interviewing is one way of reducing unnecessary random variation (error) that might otherwise arise because different interviewers conduct interviews in different ways. The use of standard procedures, however, can also introduce systematic error, for example if one interviewer is assigned to interview all subjects in areas of low socioeconomic status and another to interview all subjects in areas of high socioeconomic status. It is important to recognize also that standard interview procedures do not necessarily "standardize" subject response. To date, relatively little work has focused on the subject response aspect of dietary assessment.

> Since all dietary methods engage the cognitive processes of respondents, an appreciation of the properties of human cognition and its limitations is fundamental to improving the accuracy of dietary assessments.

Some of the important issues in this area that are relevant to improving the quality of dietary data include identification of:

- factors that improve communication between subject and investigator
- the most effective cues for recall over different periods
- factors that influence retention of dietary information over time
- the ways in which individuals conceptualize foods and food quantities.

Coding

Coding errors arise when the food that has been consumed is not described in sufficient detail to enable unambiguous allocation, by the investigator, to a food category in a food composition table or database. Making it easy for subjects to describe foods with the level of detail required is therefore an important consideration in study design. This is increasingly difficult, particularly in industrialized countries where the food supply now consists of thousands of different manufactured foods, the names of which are often no longer a good guide to their nutrient content.

Coding errors are also likely to arise when more than one person is involved in coding and there is no agreed procedure and/or comprehensive coding manual. Coding errors arising exclusively from inadequate description of foods have resulted in coefficients of variation ranging from 3% to 17% for different nutrients. Note that a standard procedure for coding foods, while minimizing differences between coders (random error), can also introduce bias if the coding decisions that are made are not based on up-to-date knowledge of the local food supply and food preparation methods. Gross errors associated with weights of foods can be checked, before analysis, by means of computer routines that identify values outside a prescribed range.

Use of food composition tables

Most dietary studies use food composition tables or databases rather than chemical analysis to derive the nutrient content of the foods consumed. Chapter 2 describes in detail the way in which data on food composition are derived and compiled. The purpose of this section is simply to review briefly the kinds of error that can arise as a consequence of using food composition tables to calculate nutrient intake, compared with chemical analysis of the diet, and which can lead to both random and systematic errors.

Systematic error can result from:

- the way in which results are calculated or expressed
- the analytical method used
- the processing and preparation methods in common use.

Food composition tables for different countries often use different ways of expressing results and different analytical methods. The ways in which food items are processed or prepared are also likely to differ and for these reasons different sources will not necessarily provide comparable data for the same foods. Systematic differences, which may not necessarily be errors (e.g. when foods are prepared differently in different countries), often only become evident when different food composition tables are used to evaluate the same diets.

Random error arises from the fact that most foods vary in their composition as a result of changes in composition associated with the conditions of production, processing, storage preparation and consumption. The random error associated with the use of food composition databases generally decreases as the size of the sample group increases. This may not be true, however, in institutional settings where everyone is likely to be consuming food from the same source.

To compare calculated and analyzed data without the complication of other sources of error it is necessary that the diets to be analyzed (a duplicate of what has been eaten) are collected at the same time as the diet record. At group level it has been observed that mean intakes calculated from the food tables are generally within approximately 10% of the mean analyzed value for energy and macronutrients, but not for micronutrients. However, a large proportion of individuals have values that fall outside this range.

In general, calculated and analyzed values for nutrients agree more closely:

- for groups than for individuals
- for macronutrients than for micronutrients
- when data for locally analyzed foods are used.

Estimation of portion size

Estimation of portion size has long been recognized as an important source of error in dietary studies (Young et al., 1953) with coefficients of variation of the differences between estimates and weights of food portions regularly reported to be around 50% for foods and 20% for nutrients (Bingham and Nelson, 1991). However, despite the fact that individuals are known to vary widely in their ability to estimate portion size, relatively few studies have attempted to quantify the size of this error or to "calibrate" their subjects in this respect. The influence of some factors on the determination of portion size is summarized in Box 10.3.

Experimental studies of cognitive aspects of portion size estimation suggest that: "individuals appear to have fragile memories about the size of portions they have seen and tend to be insensitive to the definitions of portion size provided on food-frequency questionnaires". Given this state of affairs it would seem prudent to avoid the need for individuals to estimate portion size whenever this is possible.

Box 10.3

Food characteristics:
- no consistent associations observed with type of food, although foods of indeterminate shape are more often associated with larger and liquid foods with smaller errors
- large portion sizes appear to be more difficult to estimate accurately than small portion sizes

Visual aids:
- household measures may be associated with considerable errors
- food models produce more reliable results than household measures, but because only one size is usually available they may "bias" subjects to report portion sizes similar to those shown
- graduated food models and two-dimensional pictures may be as helpful as three-dimensional models for estimating portion size
- the range of reference portion sizes available may influence the estimates
- the use of multiple photographs results in more accurate estimates

Subjects:
- subjects of all ages have been reported to have difficulty with portion size estimates
- women have sometimes, but not invariably, been reported to be better able to estimate portion size than men, but this may simply reflect the fact that they tend to handle food more often than men

---

Recall errors

Factors that have been studied in relation to the accuracy of dietary recall include food consumption patterns, weight status, gender and age. Many other characteristics, such as intelligence, mood, attention and salience of the information, however, have also been demonstrated to influence performance tests of general recall, but not studied in the context of dietary recall.

Short-term memory

Like the ability to estimate portion size, the ability to remember what was eaten varies with the individual. Studies that have compared the abilities of different groups to remember what they have eaten conclude that women are generally better than men and that younger adults are better than older adults. In short-term recalls of intake (e.g. 24 h recalls) individuals more often tend to omit an item or items that they have consumed than to include ones that they have not consumed. For this reason, 24 h recall studies often provide estimates of food intake that are lower than food records obtained over the same period. The size of the error incurred by the omission of one or more food items clearly depends on what is omitted and not only on the proportion of food omitted. For example, the effect, on 24 h energy intake, of omitting a cup of black coffee, a glass of milk or a bar of chocolate is quite different.

The omission of food items in 24 h recall studies can be reduced by appropriate probing by the interviewer in relation to meals, between-meal snacks and other activities on the previous day, but even when subjects have previously weighed their food the average energy intake may still be underestimated by as much as 20%.

Long-term memory

The diet history and most food frequency questionnaires set out to measure the habitual intake of an individual over a period of weeks or months. Individuals are not asked to recall their food intake on specific days, but to construct a picture of their "usual" food consumption pattern over a specified reference period. To provide reliable information individuals thus need to be able to remember the range of foods that they usually consume, to judge the frequency of consumption on a long-term basis and to be able to estimate correctly the average amount that is usually consumed. These are complex cognitive tasks.

As in the case of 24 h recalls, no attempt is usually made to assess how well individuals are able to perform these various tasks. From the limited amount of data available from comparative studies between diet histories and long-term diet records, it appears that the two methods do not give concordant results in individuals. Food frequency questionnaires are subject to the same difficulties, and have the added problem that estimates of portion size are based on standard measures or made in the absence of visual aids such as food models or photographs.

When subjects are asked to report their intake over a period of weeks they rely largely on generic knowledge of their diet and tend to report items that they are likely to have eaten or items that they routinely eat, rather than items that they specifically remember having eaten during the reference period. This tendency increases with the time interval between the recall and the reference period. The accuracy of frequency estimates also deteriorates with time. While individuals appear to report more frequently eaten foods with greater frequency than less frequently eaten foods, there are differences between individuals in the way that they report the same frequency of consumption. Ranking of individuals on the basis of the usual frequency of intake is thus likely to lead to misclassification unless the extent of the differences between

individuals is known and can be taken into account. It is difficult to see how such misclassification can be reduced unless it is possible to classify individuals, in some way, in terms of their ability to provide reliable information on habitual long-term intake.

10.9 Day-to-day variation in intake

We have already seen that individuals vary considerably in their intake of nutrients from day to day (Figure 10.2). In addition, the magnitude of day-to-day variation differs between nutrients. The implication of the first observation is that short-term intake data (e.g. 24 h recall data) are unlikely to provide a reliable estimate of habitual intake for most individuals. The implication of the second observation is that the length of time for which dietary data need to be collected, in order to estimate habitual intake with any given level of confidence, varies with the nutrient of interest.

Table 10.2 expresses the impact of this variation in terms of the number of days of dietary information needed to classify 80% of individuals into the correct third of the distribution. It is clear from the table that not only 24 h recalls but also 7 day records are likely to be inadequate to classify 80% of individuals correctly into the appropriate third of the distribution for most micronutrients. This is an important reason, although

Table 10.2 Number of days of records required to enable 80% of men to be assigned into their correct third of the intake distribution

Nutrient	British civil servants	Random sample of British men	Random sample of Swedish men
Energy	7	5	7
Protein	6	5	7
Fat	9	9	7
Carbohydrate	4	3	3
Sugar	2	2	–
Dietary fiber	6	10	–
P : S ratio	11	–	–
Cholesterol	18	–	–
Alcohol	4	–	14
Vitamin C	–	6	14
Thiamin	–	6	15
Riboflavin	–	10	–
Calcium	–	4	5
Iron	–	12	9

P : S ratio: ratio of polyunsaturated to saturated fatty acids in the diet.
Source: Bingham and Nelson (1991).

not the only reason, why short-term records are only rarely used for epidemiological studies, in preference to food frequency questionnaires, despite the loss of detail and precision inevitably associated with the use of the latter.

Effect on usual diet

Recall methods clearly cannot change what has already been eaten, but what has been eaten can be misreported either consciously or unconsciously. When individuals are asked to keep records, however, they may also alter their normal habits as a consequence of the recording process. One obvious reason for doing so would be to simplify the process of recording. Other reasons may include a desire to eat less in order to lose weight or to be seen to conform with dietary recommendations. If this is what happens in practice, then what is measured in short-term dietary records may be actual intake or desired intake, but not normal intake.

> Many studies have now demonstrated that there is a tendency, in most population subgroups, for short-term dietary records to provide estimates of energy intake that are on average around 16% lower than would be expected on the basis of measured and/or estimated levels of energy expenditure.

These studies will be discussed further in the section on precision and validity. The fact that for some groups measurements of energy intake and energy expenditure agree quite closely indicates that it is possible to achieve recording without a concomitant change in diet when there is full co-operation from subjects, and highlights the importance of efforts to achieve such co-operation.

10.10 Choosing a dietary method

It is not possible to decide which dietary method to use until the purpose of the study has been clearly defined, since this will govern the kind of information and the length of time for which it needs to be collected from each individual. Often, the purpose of the study also determines the level of precision that is required to meet the study objectives and therefore the sample size. These two considerations are the most important ones in determining the method to be used, because both the method and the size of the sample have implications

for the human and financial resources needed for the study.

Purpose of the study

When dietary data are collected to describe the diet of a group for comparison with that of another group or groups, it is possible to use either a short-term method such as a 24 h recall or record, or a longer term method such as food records obtained over several days, a diet history or a questionnaire about habitual intake. The final choice will depend on factors such as the importance of a representative study sample, the resources available and the level of precision required. Usually the most efficient approach is to measure the diet of as many individuals as possible for one day.

However, if the purpose of the dietary study is to determine the proportion of individuals in the group who are at risk of dietary inadequacy or excess, relative to some standard of reference, then a single day of information on each individual is no longer adequate because it is necessary to have a reliable estimate of the distribution of habitual intake in the group. As Figure 10.2 shows, a single day of intake is generally not a reliable measure of an individual's habitual intake.

To determine the distribution of habitual food intake in a group, at least 2 days (preferably not consecutive) of information from each individual or a representative subsample of individuals from the group of interest are needed. If several days of intake are available they can be used to derive a mean intake for each individual and from this the distribution of average intakes for the group. Alternatively, statistical techniques can be used to adjust 1 day intake data, for the day-to-day variation that occurs in individuals, to provide a better estimate of the underlying distribution of habitual intake for the group than is given by the 1 day data. While the use of appropriate statistical techniques can improve estimates of the proportion of individuals at risk of deficiency by adjusting for within-person variation, they do not enable at-risk individuals to be identified.

When the purpose of the study is to assess the diet of specific individuals it is necessary to obtain dietary information over at least a week and preferably longer. This is best done by obtaining either multiple 24 h recalls or 24 h food records over an extended period. The minimum number of days needed to obtain an estimate of nutrient intake with a specified level of confidence differs for different nutrients. Information on energy intake, which tends to show less day-to-day variation than other nutrients, can be obtained over a shorter period (days) than information on a nutrient for which day-to-day intake is much more variable, such as vitamin A (weeks).

Precision

In studies of groups, precision is primarily a function of sample size, while in studies of individuals it is a function of the number of days of information available. Precision increases with sample size and with the number of days for which information is collected, but so does the cost of the study. Precision therefore needs to be defined in relation to the purpose of the study.

Usually, what is required of the nutritionist is to be able to provide the statistician with an estimate of the level of difference that it is important to be able to detect (in nutritional, not statistical terms) and an estimate of the variance or standard deviation for the measurement(s) in question. For example, when looking for differences in energy intake between two groups, would a difference of 500 kJ or 1500 kJ be regarded as biologically significant?

Since the variance of a dietary measurement depends not only on the real variation within or between subjects but also on the error of the measurement, the precision of a dietary estimate can be improved not only by increasing sample size but also by reducing measurement error.

Resources

It is inevitable that the resources available, both financial and human, also influence the choice of method. They should not, however, be the primary consideration. The method used should be determined by the question to be answered. If the method or methods needed to answer the question are beyond the resources available it is better either to abandon the study or to redefine the question than to collect inadequate data.

Repeatability and validity

This section looks at ways in which it is possible to assess the repeatability and validity of dietary methods.

Repeatability

Assessing the repeatability of a laboratory method is relatively straightforward because, with care, it is possible to reproduce both what is measured and the conditions of measurement. This is almost always impossible in the case of a dietary intake measurement. Individuals do not eat exactly the same quantities or the same foods on different days or weeks.

All measures of repeatability obtained by applying the same method to the same individuals on more than one occasion include not only measurement error but also real day-to-day or week-to-week variability in intake.

While at first sight it might appear easier to measure the repeatability of recall methods such as the 24 h recall and diet histories, this process also introduces additional sources of variation since the interviews have to be conducted at different times and possibly by different interviewers. Measures of repeatability for all dietary methods will thus tend to give an overestimate of the extent of measurement error because they will always include an element of variation due to real differences in what is being measured and in the conditions under which it is being measured.

Usually, the repeatability of a dietary method is determined by repeating the same method on the same individuals on two separate occasions, that is, by a test–retest study. The interval between tests depends on the time-frame of the dietary method being assessed, but should generally be short enough to avoid the effects of seasonal or other changes in food habits and long enough to avoid the possibility of the first interview or recording period influencing the second one.

The difference between the results obtained on the two occasions can be expressed in a number of different ways. Table 10.3, which was compiled from data reported in the literature, shows various measures of repeatability for energy intake obtained with different dietary methods repeated after an interval of time.

The different measures of repeatability provide different information. The correlation coefficient is widely quoted but is not a good measure of repeatability since a good correlation may be obtained even if one set of measurements has been systematically biased and has a different mean from the other set. The mean difference is not a good measure of repeatability in individuals since it depends primarily on whether the differences are random or systematic. Measures that reflect the differences between repeated measurements within individuals are to be preferred. The coefficient of variation of the differences within individuals and the coefficient of repeatability (which is simply twice the standard deviation of the differences and represents

Table 10.3 Measures of repeatability for energy intake obtained for a 3 day food record, a dietary history and a food-frequency questionnaire (FFQ)

Measure of repeatability	3 day food record	Dietary history	FFQ
Mean difference (kJ/day)	156	105	954
Mean difference (% of overall mean intake)	1.6	1.1	12.5
Coefficient of variation of the differences within individuals (%)	16.5	18.6	28.5
Coefficient of repeatability (kJ)	±3266	±1819	±4294
Correlation coefficient	–	0.86[a]	0.70[a]
Individuals classified in the same quartile or tertile* on both occasions (%)	56	–	60*

[a]Intraclass correlation.

the 95% confidence limits of agreement) give much better measures of their magnitude. They are also more readily interpreted in practical terms than either a correlation coefficient or the percentage of individuals classified in the same quintile, quartile or tertile. If the standard deviation of the difference within individuals is of the order of 20–30% of mean intake, one is unlikely to describe the method as precise or repeatable even if the mean difference at group level is only 1%.

Validity

Demonstrating that a dietary method measures what it is intended to measure is even more difficult than demonstrating that a method is repeatable, because in effect it "requires that the truth be known".

This is almost always impossible unless it is possible to observe, surreptitiously, what is consumed over short periods such as 24 h or at most a few days. Observation is usually only feasible in institutional settings or in situations specially set up to allow unobtrusive observation of what people eat.

For methods that are designed to obtain information on habitual longer term intake, such as the diet history or food frequency questionnaires, unobtrusive observation is impossible. This is a problem that has been faced by all investigators of dietary assessment methods and until relatively recently was usually "solved" by assessing one dietary method in relation to another dietary method, usually a 7 day weighed dietary record, which was considered as the best available or criterion measure. Comparison with another

dietary method provides at best only a relative form of validity and at worst information that is unrelated to validity but reflects either real differences or similar errors between the methods. For example, comparison of data from a single 24 h recall or a diet history with data from a 7 day weighed record for the same individuals does not compare the same information because the time periods are not concurrent. However, because of the lack of a suitable external standard against which true validity could be judged before the 1980s it was usually assumed that most dietary intake data, and weighed records in particular, provided valid data. Usually, a method was judged acceptable if the mean intake, as measured by both methods, did not differ significantly and if correlations for nutrient intake in individuals exceeded 0.5. The magnitude of the coefficient of variation of the differences within individuals was generally ignored.

Table 10.4 shows data from three studies that provide additional information on agreement. All three studies compared data from a food frequency questionnaire with multiple days of food intake records. When different methods are compared the mean differences tend to be higher (there is greater bias) than those found in repeatability studies. However, the range of values obtained for other measures of agreement is generally similar to that obtained in repeatability studies. Agreement at the individual level is also not high, with coefficients of variation for differences in individuals ranging from 17 to 33% in these studies and less than 50% of subjects classified in the same quintile of intake. Note that even good agreement between two dietary methods does not necessarily indicate validity, but may merely indicate similar errors.

Table 10.4 Measures of relative validity for energy intake obtained from a food-frequency questionnaire (FFQ) compared with multiple days of records in three different studies

Measure of validity	7 days of weighed records	12 days of weighed records	15 days of records in household measures
Mean difference (kJ/day) (FFQ – record)	800	926	351
Mean difference (% of overall mean intake)	6	11	4
Coefficient of variation of the differences within individuals (%)	32.7	26.6	16.9
Coefficient of repeatability (kJ)	±8248	±4542	±2950
Correlation coefficient	–	0.69	0.71
Individuals classified in the same quintile or tertile* on both occasions (%)	43*	42	44

10.11 Biological measures to validate energy and nutrient intake

It is now clearly recognized that to assess the validity of any dietary method, including weighed records, it is necessary to compare the dietary data with one or more objective measures that reflect but are independent of food intake. At the group level such measures include food supply or food expenditure data, and at the individual level biochemical or physiological measures that reflect energy and nutrient intake. The latter are often referred to as biological or biochemical markers and include energy expenditure, urinary breakdown products of protein, sodium and potassium, plasma levels of vitamins, tissue levels of minerals and the fatty acid composition of subcutaneous adipose tissue.

> **Biological marker** – any biochemical index in an easily accessible biological sample that in health gives a predictive response to a given dietary component (Bingham, 1987).

The three most widely used measures to assess the validity of dietary intake data are: urinary nitrogen to validate protein intake, energy expenditure as measured by the doubly labeled water (DLW) method to validate energy intake in weight-stable individuals, and the ratio of energy intake to basal metabolic rate to identify "plausible" records of food intake.

Urinary nitrogen

One of the first to suggest an external measure as a means of validating dietary intake data was Isaakson, who proposed urinary nitrogen as an independent measure of protein intake according to the equation:

Reported protein intake (g)
$$= (24\,h\ \text{urinary N} + 2) \times 6.25\ (g)$$

Like the 24 h recall, a single 24 h urine collection does not necessarily reflect what is "usual". However, it appears that urinary nitrogen excretion is less variable from day to day than dietary protein intake, and that while 16 days of food intake are needed to assess habitual protein intake only eight 24 h urine collections are needed to assess nitrogen excretion with the same level of confidence.

Although fewer 24 h urine collections may be needed they are, in general, no more acceptable to subjects than 24 h food records and also require access to laboratory facilities. Nevertheless, they can provide a practical independent assessment, not only of protein but also of potassium and sodium intake.

Very few validation studies have attempted to evaluate how well the different methods rank individuals. It has been observed that the correlation between urinary nitrogen and dietary nitrogen measured by diet records was better (0.65 and 0.79) than between urinary nitrogen and dietary nitrogen measured by food frequency questionnaires (0.15 and 0.24).

Doubly labeled water method

The DLW technique allows the measurement of energy expenditure in free-living subjects over several days with minimal inconvenience to the subject and with a high level of accuracy and precision. Under controlled conditions the DLW method gives a small overestimate of 2–3% compared with whole body calorimetry, and under field conditions bias is not expected to exceed 5%.

The DLW method requires that the subject drinks a small measured dose of water enriched with naturally occurring stable isotopes of deuterium and ^{18}O. The two isotopes disperse throughout the body, and are metabolized and then gradually lost from the body. Since the deuterium labels the body water pool and the ^{18}O both the water and the bicarbonate pools, the difference between the disappearance rates of deuterium and ^{18}O can be used to calculate carbon dioxide production. The level of both isotopes is determined, using mass spectrometry, in a small sample of urine collected each day for between 5 and 28 days. Energy expenditure is calculated from carbon dioxide production using calorimetric equations. Further details of the DLW technique and the main factors influencing its accuracy and precision are provided in Chapter 3.

Using the DLW technique several investigators have compared self-reported dietary energy intake with energy expenditure based on the equation:

$$\text{Energy expenditure (EE)} = \text{Energy intake (EI)} \pm \text{Change in the body energy store}$$

Differences between measured energy intake and expenditure varied from -44% to $+28\%$ depending on the population subgroup studied. This finding confirms the need to include one or more independent measures of validity in all dietary studies to ascertain the level applicable to the particular group under study, since it is not readily predicted on the basis of gender, age or body mass index (BMI).

The main advantage of the DLW method is that it makes minimal demands on the subjects and does not in any way interfere with their normal daily activities and therefore their habitual level of energy expenditure. Its main disadvantage is that the cost of the DLW required for each estimate is exceedingly high and the method also requires access to sophisticated laboratory equipment for mass spectrometric analysis. It is, therefore, not available for use on a routine basis for the validation of dietary intake data.

Ratio of energy intake to basal metabolic rate

Because of the limitations of the DLW method, another approach that is used compares the energy intake (EI) reported from published studies with the presumed requirements for energy expenditure, both intake and expenditure being expressed as multiples of the basal metabolic rate (BMR). The relevant equation is:

$$\text{EI} : \text{BMR} = \text{EE} : \text{BMR (PAL)}$$

where PAL is the physical activity level. To determine whether reported energy intake is a "plausible" measure of actual diet during the measurement period (i.e. represents either the habitual diet or is a low/high energy intake obtained simply by chance) an equation was developed by Goldberg and colleagues to calculate the 95% confidence limits of agreement between EI : BMR and PAL. This equation allowed for variation in EI, BMR and PAL and also for the length of the dietary assessment period and study sample size.

For a group, if mean reported EI : BMR is below the lower 95% confidence limit (cut-off) for the given study period and sample size, then there is definitely bias to the underestimation of energy intake.

However, the identification of individual underreporters is much more difficult, since reported EI can deviate quite markedly from energy expenditure (EE) before it falls outside the limitations of the methods. Figures 10.5 and 10.6 illustrate the limitations of both techniques. Figure 10.5 shows the energy intake and DLW EE of 264 women. The solid lines indicate EI : EE of 0.76 and 1.24. These are the 95% confidence limits of agreement between EI and EE, allowing for day-to-day variation in food intake and within-subject variation on repeat DLW measurements. Only women with EI : EE above 1.24 can be confidently identified as overreporters, and those below 0.76 as underreporters. In Figure 10.6, the same data are expressed as EI : BMR and EE : BMR, and each subject is represented by the same symbol as in Figure 10.5. The line at EI : BMR = 1.05 indicates the Goldberg cut-off for $n = 1$ and PAL $= 1.55$ which has been widely used to identify low energy reporters (LER). These data demonstrate that only about 50% of underreporters (as defined by EI : EE < 0.76) are identified as LER. The second line at EI : BMR of 1.35 is the Goldberg cut-off for $n = 1$ and PAL $= 1.95$. This cut-off identifies more of the underreporters, but also includes some of the acceptable reporters. To improve on identification of underreporters it is necessary to have information on physical activity to enable subjects to be classified into different levels of activity and to calculate cut-offs appropriate for each activity level.

The ability to be able to separate the food and nutrient intake data of those with and without plausible energy intakes is a very important step forward in the evaluation of dietary intake data and is discussed further in the next section on dietary evaluation.

Figure 10.5 Reported energy intake (EI) against energy expenditure measured by doubly-labeled water (DLW) (EE) in 264 women aged 18–90 years. The solid lines represent the 95% confidence limits of the expected agreement between EI and EE (±24%). UR: underreporters; AR: acceptable reporters; OR: overreporters. (After Black, 2000b, reproduced with permission.)

Figure 10.6 Energy intake: estimated basal metabolic rate (EI : BMR$_{est}$) against physical activity level [PAL; energy expenditure: measured BMR (EE : BMR$_{meas}$)]. Subjects are designated as acceptable reporters (AR), overreporters (OR) or underreporters (UR) by the direct comparison of EI : EE. The horizontal lines indicate the lower Goldberg cut-off for PAL = 1.55 and 1.95, 7 day records and $n = 1$. (After Black, 2000b, reproduced with permission.)

10.12 Characteristics of low energy reporters

A number of studies have examined the characteristics of LER. Associations between low energy reporting and a constellation of factors including high body weight, high BMI, obesity, dieting and awareness of body image were found in every study that looked at these measures. Associations with other sociodemographic factors of the type normally included in nutrition studies, such as gender, age, education, socioeconomic status and smoking, were inconsistent.

10.13 Evaluation of food intake data

Recognizing the impact of underreporting

As indicated in Section 10.10, dietary studies are often conducted to be able to compare food and nutrient intake between different groups in the population, to determine the proportion of individuals at risk of dietary inadequacy or excess, or to determine the habitual intake of individuals.

In each case it is important first to assess the validity of the data. For most investigators the use of the Goldberg cut-offs is currently the most practical option to indicate whether, and to what extent, the results are likely to be biased. However, to use the Goldberg cut-offs effectively dietary studies need to include:

- measurements of weight and height, to be able to estimate BMR from equations
- questions on activity level to provide guidance on suitable PAL for evaluation of both mean and individual data.

While the characteristics of "true" underreporters (as opposed to LER identified by a single EI : BMR cut-off) remain to be confirmed, the associations consistently observed between high BMI, weight consciousness and low energy reporting suggest that, in addition, questions on self-perception of body shape, dieting and dietary restraint may also help in identifying true underreporters.

It cannot be overemphasized that it is always important to examine all dietary intake data critically because false conclusions generate false hypotheses that may take years to be disproved.

A classic case was the *luxus konsumption* hypothesis, namely that lean individuals are energy prodigal and obese individuals energy efficient. This hypothesis was generated by studies apparently showing that obese persons did not consume more energy than their lean controls. Subsequently, DLW studies demonstrated beyond doubt that obese persons recruited for studies of obesity grossly underreported their food intake.

Allowing for the effects of underreporting

At the time of writing (in the year 2000), techniques for identifying individuals who underreport their food intake, and for handling biased dietary data, are in their infancy. However, the following suggestions serve to promote critical examination of data and wariness in drawing conclusions.

If the proportion of individuals who report implausibly low intakes of energy differs between population subgroups of interest, then any comparisons between them that do not take this into account will be biased. One way to draw attention to the possibility of bias between groups is to report not only the mean or median energy intake of the groups being compared but also the EI : BMR ratio. If differences are evident then the groups should be compared both with and without LER included. One problem that arises is that by subdividing the groups the sample size is reduced and imprecision increased, so that a difference of biological significance may be missed, not because it does not exist, but because the sample size is too small to detect it statistically.

When dietary inadequacy or excess is the question of interest it is again important to consider LER separately. Energy intake is highly correlated with the intake of many nutrients and, consequently, intake of nutrients is also likely to be underestimated in underreporters and more likely to indicate inadequacy relative to recommendations for nutrient intake. An alternative approach is to compare nutrient intake per unit energy for both groups. If this differs between LER and the rest of the population it provides evidence that the reporting of food intake is also likely to be selective. The nutrients for which significant differences are observed can also provide clues as to the types of food likely to be involved.

Studies that have examined macronutrient intake between subjects above and below a given value of EI : BMR have generally found that the percentage of energy derived from protein was higher and that from fat lower in LER than in non-LER. Results for carbohydrate have been more variable, but when separated into starch and sugars, energy from starch tended to be higher and energy from sugars lower in LER. Nutrient density also tends to be higher for most nutrients in LER than in non-LER, providing further indication of differences in food patterns between the two groups.

Table 10.5 illustrates these general trends with data from the 1995 Australian National Nutrition Survey.

Table 10.5 Nutrient intakes in low energy reporting (LER) and non-LER adults in the 1995 Australian National Nutrition Survey

Nutrient	LER (n = 1291)	Non-LER (n = 9451)	Total (n = 10 851)
Energy (MJ)	4.62	10.19	9.24
Protein (g/MJ)	11.0	9.8	9.9
Fat (g/MJ)	8.1	9.0	9.0
Starch (g/MJ)	15.9	14.9	15.0
Sugars (g/MJ)	12.9	12.4	12.4
Vitamin (µg/MJ)	159	122	127
Riboflavin (mg/MJ)	0.26	0.22	0.23
Folate (µg/MJ)	37	28	29
Vitamin C (mg/MJ)	19	13	13
Calcium (mg/MJ)	106	90	92
Iron (mg/MJ)	1.8	1.5	1.5

Data used with permission from the Australian Bureau of Statistics (abs.gov.au) (ABS, 1998).

Twelve per cent of men and 21% of women in this survey were identified as LER. The median energy intake in non-LER was approximately 6% higher in men and 10% higher in women than for all men and women, and vitamin and mineral intake approximately 5–10% higher in non-LER men and 6–15% higher in non-LER women. Differences of this order of magnitude are important in the context of the assessment of dietary adequacy.

Relatively few studies have reported on differences in foods eaten, but there appears to be a general tendency for LER to report more foods such as meat, fish, vegetables, salads and fruit, and fewer cakes, biscuits, sugar, confectionery and fats.

10.14 Assessment of dietary adequacy

Methods for evaluating dietary adequacy are described in Chapter 7. This section simply draws attention to the limitations of these methods.

The first limitation is that the evaluation of nutrient intake can only provide an estimate of the risk of nutrient inadequacy for a population or an individual. None of the methods can identify the specific individuals who have a nutrient deficiency. Individuals with a nutrient deficiency or excess can only be identified on the basis of biochemical or clinical measures of nutritional status.

The second limitation is that all estimates of dietary adequacy/inadequacy obtained by comparison with reference values for nutrient requirements depend on how the estimate is derived (see Chapter 7).

However, irrespective of the approach that is used to assess dietary adequacy, unless the extent of under-reporting is known and taken into account, the proportion of individuals at risk of inadequacy will be overestimated. While it may become possible to distinguish more reliably in population-based studies valid from invalid reports of dietary intake, this still does not enable population-based estimates of inadequacy to be made unless those who provide valid intakes are also representative of the population as a whole. All the evidence available to date suggests that this is highly unlikely.

When the principal objective of a dietary survey is to identify the proportion of the population who may have inadequate intakes of energy and nutrients, it is essential that the dietary intake information is interpreted in the light of appropriate biological measures of nutritional status.

Assessing food intake

Nutritionists usually analyze dietary intake data by converting the information on food intake into nutrient intake using relevant food composition databases. This approach simplifies the process of analysis and enables the resulting data to be compared with energy and nutrient requirements (see Chapter 7). Describing food intake in terms of foods rather than nutrients presents two practical difficulties that do not exist when food intake is analyzed in terms of nutrients. First, the variety of foods consumed is much greater than the range of nutrients for which food composition data are available. Secondly, while essentially all individuals in a group contribute to nutrient intake data, not all individuals contribute food data for all foods, that is, not all individuals are "consumers".

There are, however, several uses for which information on food intake is more relevant or for which information on food intake is needed in conjunction with data on nutrient intake. For example, food regulatory authorities and agencies concerned with food safety and nutritional surveillance require data on the availability and intake of foods in addition to information on nutrient intake. Similarly, nutritional epidemiologists are also interested in the relationship of different foods and dietary patterns with specific health outcomes. The use of dietary data in the context of epidemiological studies is covered in the textbook on Public Health Nutrition.

To describe dietary intake data in terms of foods rather than nutrients it is necessary to reduce the data to manageable proportions by grouping foods into appropriate categories. While this can be done in different ways, for example in terms of composition, biological origin or cultural use, the process is relatively straightforward within a given culture or country. It is more difficult, however, to develop a classification that can be used consistently across different countries or food cultures. National food classification systems tend to differ not only because the type and range of foods differs but also because the same foods are used in different ways. For the purpose of comparing food intake patterns between countries or regions it is, therefore, necessary to develop a food classification or coding system that allows food data from individual regions or countries to be assigned in a consistent way.

The United Nations University Food and Nutrition Program for an International Network of Food Data Systems (INFOODS) was developed for the purpose of supporting work on the classification and naming conventions for individual foods and food groups (see Chapter 2).

Indirect information on food consumption, such as that provided by FAO food balance sheets and by data from household budget and similar surveys, is usually presented in terms of foods or food groups, but may also be converted to nutrients to provide information on the nutrient contribution of individual foods or groups of foods.

Tracking changes in the food sources of nutrients and nonnutrients is particularly important in the context of technological developments in food production and manufacture that result in the addition of nutrients to foods, in the development of foods for specific functional purposes and in the genetic modification of foods. A specific example of the need for individual food, rather than nutrient, intake data is provided by exposure assessments to dietary nonnutrients such as food additives, pesticide residues and other possible food contaminants.

Food safety assessments

Safety assessments for food additives are expressed in terms of the acceptable daily intake (ADI) estimated on the basis of lifetime exposure. While it is clearly not possible to collect food consumption data over the lifetimes of individuals, it is important that the dietary data used for the purpose of estimating acceptable levels of intake over a lifetime reflect, as far as is possible, the habitual level of intake of the foods being assessed.

For the purpose of food safety assessments only the intake of "consumers" is of interest. It follows, therefore, that the dietary data need to be adequate to obtain both an accurate estimate of the proportion of the population who are consumers and of the average habitual intake of consumers. Because the frequency of consumption varies between foods (some foods are eaten by most people on most days, but many other foods are eaten less frequently), the duration of the dietary recording period influences both the estimate of the proportion of consumers and the average intake of consumers. One-day intake data will inevitably underestimate the true number of consumers for most foods and overestimate the average habitual intake of those consumers, because not all foods are eaten every day. However, it appears that 75% or more of household menu items are normally consumed within a 14 day period and that a 14 day diary provides a good estimate of the habitual intake of most foods by consumers.

Most studies of the food intake of individuals, however, do not last for 14 days because of the increased cost and nonresponse associated with such a long study period. For the purpose of food safety assessment an approach that combines a 3 day food intake record with a food frequency questionnaire has the potential to give estimates for the intake of consumers that are comparable with those obtained from 14 day records.

10.15 Perspectives on the future

It is unlikely that either the measurement or the evaluation of food intake will become less complex in future. If anything, the reverse is likely to be true given the increasing diversity in the food supply and the increasing recognition of the need to be able to assess accurately not only the intake of foods and nutrients but also the intake of nonnutrient constituents of foods and dietary supplements. While the existence of errors in association with measurements of food intake is now widely appreciated, much work still remains to be done in this area.

Other aspects of food intake measurement that also require further development in the immediate future are likely to include the following.

As all direct methods of food intake measurement involve interaction between investigators and individuals and our understanding of the cognitive aspects of these interactions is still limited, more work is needed to improve the communications aspect of dietary assessment.

As the food supply becomes more complex individuals will no longer be able to describe the foods they have eaten in adequate detail unless technological developments such as the use of barcodes and similar systems of food identification become an integral part of dietary assessment.

As the number of food constituents of interest, in relation to health, increases it is important that appropriate physiological and biochemical markers are also developed for these constituents, as well as for the nutrient constituents of foods.

Finally, since food intake data serve no useful purpose unless they can be appropriately evaluated it is essential that dietary studies include sufficient ancillary information to allow this to occur. This means routinely collecting information not only on age, gender, body size and physiological status, but also on key aspects of lifestyle such as physical activity and the consumption of nonfood items such as supplements (both nutrient and nonnutrient) and drugs (both social and medicinal).

Further reading

Australian Bureau of Statisics. Australian National Nutrition Survey. ABS, 1998.

Bingham SA. The dietary assessment of individuals; methods, accuracy, new techniques and recommendations. Nutr Abstr Rev (Series A) 1987; 57: 705–742.

Bingham SA, Nelson M. Assessment of food consumption and nutrient intake. In: Design Concepts in Nutritional Epidemiology (BM Margetts, M Nelson, eds), p. 153. Oxford: Oxford University Press, 1991.

Black AE. Critical evaluation of energy intake using the Goldberg cut-off for EI : BMR. A practical guide to its calculation, use and limitations. Int J Obes 2000a; 24: 1119–1130.

Black AE. The sensitivity and specificity of the Goldberg cut-off for EI : BMR for identifying dietary reports of poor validity. Eur J Clin Nutr 2000b; 54: 395–404.

Gibson RS. Principles of Nutritional Assessment, p. 21. Oxford: Oxford University Press, 1990.

Willett W. 5. Food-frequency methods. In: Nutritional Epidemiology, 2nd edn (W Willett, ed.), p. 74. New York: Monographs in Epidemiology and Biostatistics, Oxford University Press, 1998.

Young CM, Chalmers FW, Church HN, Murphy GC, Tucker RE. Subjects' estimation of food intake and calculated nutritive value of the diet. JADA 1953; 29:1216–1220.

11
Food Composition

Clive E West and Hettie C Schönfeldt

Key messages

- Reliable good-quality food composition data of foods for human consumption are critical resources for a variety of applications.
- These data are required for a spectrum of users ranging from international, to national, regional, household and individual levels.
- In general, data obtained on food intake by individuals, or groups of individuals, are converted to the consumption of nutrients and interpreted to nutritional requirements and health guidelines.
- The determination of the consumption of nutrients can be achieved either by analyzing the foods con-

sumed directly (by far the most accurate, but also the most costly method) or by using food composition tables.
- The food described in the food composition table should be recognizably similar to that being consumed by the individual or group.
- Factors such as sampling, variability and analytical methods involved must be considered when developing such tables.
- Inadequacies of food composition tables can be minimized by calculating nutrient losses and gains during food processing and preparation. Future composition tables may examine bioavailability and the glycemic index.

11.1 Introduction

Although the amount, quality and availability of food composition data vary among countries and regions, in general most developing countries do not have adequate and reliable data. This is despite the fact that the components of specific foods have been published for over 150 years. Over time food composition data have assumed more scientific, academic and political importance owing to their utility. Refer to Table 11.1 for practical examples of the uses of food composition data. It was only in 1961 that a regional food composition table was developed and published for Latin America, followed by a food composition table for Africa (1968), the Near East (1970) and Asia (1972). The data in these tables were based on a very limited number of samples, a limited number of nutrients and, in today's terms, unacceptable analytical methodologies. However, these tables are still being used today as there are no more up-to-date tables readily available.

Worldwide there are currently over 150 food composition tables or nutrient databases, which are their electronic/magnetic equivalent, in use, excluding most of the tables that exist in the USA, as most are based on the data from the United States Department of Agriculture (USDA). A comprehensive list of the food composition tables available can be obtained from the Food and Agricultural Organization of the United Nations (FAO) homepage on the world wide web (http://www.fao.org/infoods/fdtables).

There is still a continued need to carry out food analyses as the number of foods consumed all over the world, especially unique foods, is probably still several times greater than the number for which analytical data exist. Food analyses are also needed under the following circumstances:

- when the data in the tables are based on a single or very limited number of samples
- when the content of a nutrient or other food component is not available in an existing food table

Table 11.1 Examples of the uses of food composition data

Level	Examples
International	Role of food in the provision of nutrients and/or the estimation of adequacy of the dietary intake of population groups
	Investigation of relationships between diet, health and nutritional status, e.g. epidemiologists correlate patterns of disease with dietary components
	Evaluation of nutrition education programs
	Nutrition intervention and food fortification programs such as in food assistance programs; foods are distributed or enriched to address the specific nutritional needs of populations, e.g. iodine or vitamin A
	In food trade nutritional labeling
National	Monitoring at governmental level, the availability of foods produced and estimating the individual intake for specific dietary requirements, e.g. protein and energy
	Food balance sheet data are used to provide data on food available nationally for the whole population and are useful in monitoring trends in food consumption over time
	Researchers work to improve the food supply by selecting or developing new strains or cultivars, improving cultivation, harvesting, preservation and preparation
	Estimation of adequacy of the dietary intake of groups within populations
	Investigation of relationships between diet, health and nutritional status
	Evaluation of nutrition education programs
	Food and nutrition training
	Nutrition intervention and food fortification programs
	Food and nutrition regulation and food safety
	Nutrition labeling
Regional (influenced by meal patterns and food preferences)	Institutions such as hospitals, schools, dormitories and troops/armies (ration scale) formulate nutritionally balanced diets to the individuals in their care
	Food industries regulate the quality of their foods by routinely analyzing the components in their products
	Food industries change and improve their products to appeal to new customers by improving nutrient content or sensory appeal through the change in ingredients
	Product development
Household	Household food surveys provide data on household food consumption
	Household budget surveys
	Household food economics
Individual	Dietary intake of the individual is assessed to understand present health and to monitor changes in dietary intake
	Impact of interpretation of choice and preference via data composition
	Individual energy expenditure is the only true measurement of energy need, e.g. in the management of a sportsman's diet or in obesity
	Personal dietary needs and goals with associated likes and dislikes can be assessed on an individual basis
	Individual nutritional balance studies
	Therapeutic or restricting diets with specific nutrient contents, e.g. management of diabetes and hypertension, can only be described on an individual basis
	Individual shoppers scan the ingredient list and nutrient content on the labels of packaged foods

- when there is no information available on which foods are important sources of a nutrient or another food component of interest
- when there is no information on the loss or gain of nutrients in foods during preparation by the methods being used by the population under investigation
- when it is necessary to check the comparability of the various food composition tables being used in a multicenter study
- when the method available to determine a particular nutrient is considerably improved

- to keep up with the proliferation of foods and processing techniques.

11.2 Foods

Food composition tables normally consist of a list of selected foods with data on the content of selected nutrients in each food. For a food composition table to be of value in estimating nutrient content, a significant portion of the foods consumed by the group or individual being studied, as well as the nutrients of interest, should be present in the table. To a large extent this relationship is critical in determining the quality of the information obtained by using the tables, assuming that the data in the tables are of a desirable quality.

Criteria for inclusion in tables

The identification of potential contributions of foods to the diet of the population group being studied is arguably the first step in identifying and selecting which foods should and should not be included in the production of a database. However, common sense dictates that it is unreasonable to expect that all foods consumed by all individuals at all times be included in a specific food composition table at any one time. Therefore, most tables aim to include all foods that form a major part of the food supply and that are major contributors to the diet in the forms most commonly obtained or consumed, and as many as possible of the less frequently consumed foods. For instance, in the USA the number of foods contributing to quartiles of critical nutrient intakes was identified as the following: 50 foods contribute to 25% of food intake, 200 foods to 50%, 660 to 75% and 3604 to approximately 100%.

Databases can be compiled directly, where the compiler initiates sampling and analyses to obtain the data, or indirectly by drawing on the following sources of data, in order of preference:

- original analytical values
- imputed values derived from analytical values from a similar food, e.g. values for "boiled" used for "steamed"
- calculated values derived from recipes, calculated from the ingredients and corrected for preparation factors
- borrowed values (refers to using data originally generated or gathered by someone else) from other tables and databases.

Today, database compilers normally draw on a combination of the direct and indirect methods.

Description of foods

The food described in the food composition table should be recognizably similar to that being consumed by the individual or group. The precise description of foods is a difficult task and much is required to ensure that foods are described adequately. Recently, it has become clear that the introductory material (description and explanation) in a printed table may be almost as important as the data values. By using several words to describe a food, called an extended or multifaceted description, the chance of misinterpreting the data is reduced. As internationalization of food composition data continues, linguistic aspects of defining foods, with one definition meaning different things in different cultures and even from place to place within countries, is highlighted. For instance, sorbet or sherbet is made by beating whisked egg whites into the partly frozen mixture such as in apple sorbet and lemon sorbet. However, the term sorbet is preferred to sherbet, since the latter can also refer to a flavored sweet sparkling powder or drink, or a drink of sweet diluted fruit juice. The name tortilla is also applied to a variety of foods in Latin America. Using scientific names for food items is not necessarily a solution, since the relationship between common name and scientific name is neither consistent nor universally unique, for example the German tables group pears and apples in the same genus, while the British and US tables separate them.

Many structured food description systems have been proposed. For example, the International Food Data System Project (INFOODS) Nomenclature and Terminology Committee has developed guidelines for describing foods. INFOODS is a comprehensive effort, begun within the United Nations University Food and Nutrition Program to improve data on the nutrient composition of food from all parts of the world. The Food and Drug Administration (FDA) of the USA has developed an international framework for food description, based on the principle of a faceted thesaurus, where each food indexed is described by a set of standard terms grouped in facets characteristic of the nutritional and/or hygienic quality of a food. Examples are the biological origin, the methods of cooking and conservation, and technological treatments. It is an automated method for describing, capturing and retrieving data about food, adapted to computerized national and international food composition and consumption databanks, and is therefore language independent. In Table 11.2 an example of the application of LanguaL is presented. More information can be obtained from the LanguaL (Langua aLimentaria or "language of food") homepage on the world wide web (http://food.ethz/LanguaL). Since 1996, the European LanguaL Technical Committee has administered this thesaurus.

Classification of foods

Most food composition tables are organized according to the classification of foods into food groups, with

Table 11.2 Example of the international use of LanguaL

Facet	Code	English term	French term	Danish term	Hungarian term
Product type	A178	Bread	Pain	Brød	Kenyér
Food source	B1418	Hard wheat	Blé de force (*Triticum aestivum*)	Hård hvede (*Triticum aestivum*)	Kemény búza (*Triticum aestivum*)
Part of plant or animal	C208	Seed or kernel, skin removed, germ removed (endosperm)	Graine ou grain sans enveloppe et sans germe	Frø eller kerne, skaldele (pericarp/caryopse) fjernet, kim fjernet (endosperm)	Szénhidrát vagy hasonló vegyület
Physical state, shape or form	E105	Whole, shape achieved by forming, thickness 1.5–7 cm	Entier façonné épais de 1,5 à 7 cm	Hel, facon dannet ved formning, tykkelse 1.5–7 cm	Egész, formázott, 1.5–7 cm közötti vastagság
Extent of heat treatment	F14	Fully heat treated	Transformation thermique complète	Fuldt varmebehandlet	Teljesen hőkezelt
Cooking method	G5	Baked or roasted	Cuit au four	Bagt eller ovnstegt	Sütött vagy piritott
Treatment applied	H256	Carbohydrate fermented	Fermenté au niveau des glucides	Kulhydratfermenteret	Szénhidrátos fermentált
Preservation method	J3	No preservation method used	Sans traitement de conservation	Igen konservering	Tartósitási eljárást nem alkalmaztak
Packing medium	K3	No packing medium used	Sans milieu de conditionnement	Intet pakningsmedium anvendt	Csomagoló eszközt nem alkalmaztak
Consumer group/dietary use/label claim	P24	Human food, no age specification	Alimentation humaine courante	Levnedamiddel uden aldersspecifikation	Emberi fogyasztásra szánt élelmiszer, kormeghatározás nélkül

food items listed alphabetically within each food group, for example the fruit group starts with apples and ends with tangerines. A simple coding system could supplement the alphabetically listed foods (used in the British tables), but it presents a problem when a new food is introduced and all the codes have to change. Although food groups of different countries and organizations are never completely identical, they are usually recognizably similar. However, problems normally arise with the description of cooked mixed dishes where a dish can be equally well described by one or more food group. In some tables, particularly those for educational purposes, there are subgroups based on the content of specific nutrients such as high-fat and low-fat dairy products. Table 11.3 provides an example of major food groups that is used by the FAO for their food balance sheets and regional food composition tables.

Another example of food coding and descriptor system is the Eurocode 2 food coding system that was originally developed within the European Food-Linked Agro-Industrial Research (FLAIR) Eurofoods-Enfant Project to serve as a standard instrument for nutritional

Table 11.3 Major food groups that are utilized by the Food and Agricultural Organization

Cereals and grain products
Starchy roots, tubers and fruits
Grain legumes and legume products
Nuts and seeds
Vegetables and vegetable products
Fruits
Sugars and syrups
Meat, poultry and insects
Eggs
Fish and shellfish
Milk and milk products
Oils and fats
Beverages
Miscellaneous

surveys in Europe and to serve the need for food intake comparisons. Representatives from 27 countries have agreed on the food coding system, which involves grouping foods together on the basis of their similarities. In the Eurocode 2, there are 13 main food groups (Table 11.4) with subgroups within some groups based on species for animal foods and variety for plant foods,

Table 11.4 Major food groups that are utilized by the EUROCODE

1 Milk and milk products
2 Eggs and egg products
3 Meat and meat products
4 Fish, molluscs, reptiles, crustaceans and their products
5 Oils, fats and their products
6 Grains and grain products
7 Pulses, seeds, kernels, nuts and their products
8 Vegetables and vegetable products
9 Fruits and fruit products
10 Sugar, sugar products, chocolate products and confectionery
11 Beverages (nonmilk)
12 Miscellaneous, soups, sauces, snacks and products
13 Products for special nutritional use

plus data on methods of food preparation. Each main food group of Eurocode 2 is divided into first, the general policies and listing of the classification and, secondly, the documentation of individual categories. The classification section starts with policy statements for the main group, including the types of food item that are covered and those that are excluded, general points of policy and revisions. The second part of the classification section is a listing of the classification. The scientific names of the food, similar products or examples of the food have been included where possible. Links are provided where more detailed documentation is available. The categories section provides specific documentation for individual categories (at each level within the main group) in the same order as the classification listing, so that related items are grouped together for convenient review. The latest information on Eurocode 2 can be obtained on the world wide web (http://www.vfdz.dk/eurocode).

Sampling of foods for inclusion in tables

Food sampling concerns the selection of the individual units of foods, food products or bulk foodstuffs from the food supply or source, whether it be the marketplace, manufacturing outlet, field or the homes of the members of the study population. Sampling also concerns the selection of the representative aliquot from the individual unit or homogenized mixture in the laboratory just before analysis. The objectives for sampling will, in the large part, determine the type and nature of the sampling plan. One of the major objectives of food sampling is to provide representative mean values for individual components in foods. The sampling process is described in detail in Table 11.5.

Food sampling is a critical step in any food composition program. For any research project, personnel and financial resources are always limited. The selection, procurement, shipping and storage of sample units require a significant portion of available resources. Therefore, sampling must follow a specific and detailed statement of the objectives and procedures to ensure that the selection of units is sufficient in number and weight and representative of the foods of interest. Pilot studies, conducted by the investigator(s) or published in the scientific literature, can be used as the basis of sampling decisions for the current study.

Variability in foods: regional and other differences

Foods are biological materials and, as such, have a naturally variable composition. Even processed foods produced under highly controlled circumstances show some variability. Therefore, a database must be able to predict the composition of a single sample of food within the limits defined by its natural variability. Variability may be contributed by one or more of the following factors: brand or cultivars, season, climate, geographical location (e.g. soil type), fertilizer treatment, method of husbandry, harvesting, preservation state, stage of maturity, enrichment/fortification standards, preparation methods, food color, variation in recipes and formulations, distribution and marketing practices, and other factors. For critical components variability may affect the sufficiency, deficiency or excess of the intake of a given component. Estimates of variability must be based on sampling and analyses specifically planned to yield such data. The intended use of the data should determine the specificity and level of precision for the estimates.

For instance, it was found that the nutrient composition of whole milk in South Africa differed among the five localities investigated and between winter and summer, with the fat-soluble vitamins showing the greatest variation of all the nutrients. Vitamin A is commonly regarded as one of the micronutrients that are deficient in most developing countries and specifically in black schoolchildren in South Africa. Considering the results of the nutrient composition of whole milk, a recommendation was made to the health authorities to fortify summer milk with retinol in the South African school-feeding intervention program, where milk is served as a mid-morning snack to five million primary school children.

Table 11.5 Sampling process of foods for food composition data

1 *Prioritizing foods for inclusion*
May be based on:
- type
- frequency and
- amount of specific foods or products consumed
- quality and quantity of existing data
- appropriateness of prior analytical methods or
- perceived benefit/risk of particular foods as sources of components of interest

May be affected by:
- changes in the forms of foods or
- levels of components, including reformulation or fortification

Levels of available resources will impact on the process of setting priorities

2 *Defining prioritized foods*
Within the context of the objective, define the specific characteristics of the food that may contribute to the variability of the estimate:
- uncooked or raw foodstuffs versus cooked forms of the food
- composition of prepared or multicomponent foods (i.e. mixed dishes)
- individual brands or cultivars or generic value

3 *Definition of sampling unit*
Collection of units (packages, bunches, or items) representative of the total population of food units:
- sample units must be taken from the available types and forms of the food for which the composition estimates are being determined. Production, consumption or sales statistics may be used. The population of items may be supplied to or distributed through an entire nation or region or be only typical of a particular subpopulation (e.g. ethnic group or tribe)
- select sample units from all the various types of food and geographical or manufacturing locations of food consumed by the population of interest. The units may be selected according to the relative importance (e.g. frequency of consumption) for given types
- sample units that are collected can be analyzed as individual units or may be combined together or composited and analyzed. The analysis of composite samples reduces the costs associated with the analysis of individual samples, but information about the variability of the component in that food will be lost

4 *Definition of sampling size*
Amount of material required:
- objective of analyses
- analyses of individual samples or composite samples of the food
- number of components to be measured; determine the number and weight of aliquots needed as required by the chemical methods
- policy for saving reserve or archive aliquots

5 *Protocol for sample collection*
Foods should be typical of the usual preparation and consumption practices

Correct units of foods should be selected

Protocols should be tested for the adequacy of food storage and transportation facilities, sample unit documentation and labeling, and packaging and short-term preservation requirements

Policies for the substitution of units should be in place in the event of unavailable sample units

Sampling among ethnic or native populations may impose additional restrictions owing to cultural or religious customs

Samples should be clearly coded for identification. Documentation should start from the planning stage, throughout purchasing, transporting, preparation and the combining of samples, to analyses including storage condition, use of reference samples, recording of data obtained (duplicate or triplicate values), as well as manipulation of the data, e.g. expression of the data on a wet (as eaten) basis, as opposed to the content of a freeze-dried sample. Correction factors applied or calculations (e.g. N × Jones factor = protein) should be recorded for each foodstuff analyzed

Documentation and handling of sample units should be under the careful control of the principal co-ordinator and all laboratory personnel should be informed before the start of the project of the reasons for handling the samples in a specific manner. The samples should preferably be marked with three-digit random codes for analysts to ensure that analyses are unbiased. Values should only be decoded as results become available, by the principal investigator. This will improve the reliability of the results if performed on a double-blind basis

11.3 Nutrients, nonnutrients and energy

Analytical methods

Judgement should be made on the availability of suitable methods of analyses for nutrients and whether the resources, laboratory equipment and experience are adequate before deciding which nutrients should be included in a nutrient database. If the methods available are not well developed, one should reconsider the importance of the nutrient and whether it justifies using limited resources, in most instances and countries,

to develop the method and train the staff accordingly. It will not be cost-effective to analyze food for a particular nutrient, however high in priority, if methods yield conflicting values. This implies that, as new or improved methods for measuring a nutrient emerge, foods that are important in the food supply and are known or suspected to be a good source of that nutrient should be analyzed or reanalyzed. Food regulation sometimes limits the choice of methods.

The choice of method selected should be that which most closely reflects the nutritive value of the foodstuff analyzed. A basic understanding of the chemistry of the nutrients, the nature of the food substrate (the way in which the nutrient is distributed and held in the food matrix) to be analyzed, the effect of processing and preparation on both the food matrix and the nutrient, and the expected range of concentration of the nutrient determine the choice of method. An understanding of the role of the nutrient in the diet of individuals or populations is also a prerequisite.

The basic principle is that the method used should provide information that is nutritionally appropriate. For instance, traditionally, carbohydrate was estimated by difference, that is, by directly measuring the percentage of protein (from the nitrogen content), fat, ash and water, and deducting these from 100 to give the percentage of carbohydrate. This method is inadequate for all nutritional purposes because it combines in one value all of the different carbohydrate species: sugars, oligosaccharides and polysaccharides (starch and non-starch), together with all of the errors in the other determinations, as the physiological effects of all of the components are quite different. Therefore, the sum of the individually analyzed carbohydrates is widely recommended today.

In studying the relationship between particular foods and health or disease, the biological action of related nutrients may be crucial information for particular uses of food composition data. For example, a study on the role of vitamin A and carotenoids in lung cancer requires more information than the vitamin A activity expressed in retinol equivalents. At the very least, vitamin A and provitamin A activity are required separately. Information on provitamin A could be divided into the various provitamin A carotenoids, and it may also be desirable to have information on other carotenoids present. This is also true for the vitamers of other vitamins, including vitamin B_6 (pyridoxal, pyridoxal phosphate and pyridoxamine), folic acid (with a side-chain with one, three or seven glutamic acid residues), vitamin D (D_2 or D_3), vitamin E (various tocopherols and tocotrienols) and vitamin K (with various numbers of saturated and unsaturated isoprene units in the side-chain).

Criteria for inclusion in tables

As the number of nutrients is reasonably infinite, it is to some extent easier to choose and prioritize food items. Core nutrients for a nutritional database include the major proximate constituents, those that are essential and for which there are recommended

intakes. The inclusion of micronutrients, especially trace elements, fatty acid profiles, amino acid composition and the various forms of vitamins is normally limited by the resources available. Many databases give limited coverage of the carbohydrates and carotenoids in foods, but methods are available and this limitation will probably disappear in the future.

Nutrients to be included in the food composition table will depend on the proposed use of the table. For instance, when assessing nutrient intake, two types of nutrient can often be distinguished: those nutrients that are found in small quantities in a large number of foods, such as iron and most of the B vitamins, and those that are found in large quantities in a small number of foods, such as cholesterol and vitamin A. The FAO limits the inclusion of nutrients in the table for group feeding schemes to 11 nutrients per 100 g edible portion. The nutrients that have been selected as the most important for developing countries are energy, protein, fat, calcium, iron, vitamin A, thiamine, riboflavin, niacin, folate and vitamin C.

Complete coverage of all nutrients in a single food database is unlikely, as priorities are set according to the importance of a food in the provision of a nutrient, resulting normally in analyses of proximates and major nutrients. However, with the growing interest in the role of biologically active compounds, residues and toxicants in food there is increased pressure to include these in special-purpose food composition tables. Phytochemicals or phytoprotectants, often used in functional foods, are bioactive compounds found in food that may have benefits to human health. A provisional database for food flavonoid composition has recently been developed and will be maintained by the United States Department of Agriculture on its National Nutrient Databank website. A European network established to compile and evaluate data on natural food plant toxicants, the EU AIR Concerted Action NETTOX, has identified 31 major compound classes called the NETTOX – list of toxicant classes with 307 major food plants listed in Europe. They are proposing a relational database consisting of 23 data tables linked to the international coding system (LanguaL). For a food composition database to include all these substances will imply that there may be an overemphasis on "nonnutrients". In general, levels of pesticides, residues, toxicants and additives in food, except those that contribute to energy and nutrients, are not reported in food composition tables.

Modes of expression

An increasing amount of attention is being paid to how data are presented in food composition tables. Interchange and compatibility of food composition databases are only possible if the data are uniformly expressed. To overcome ambiguities in the naming of nutrients and also to allow for the transfer of data among food composition tables, INFOODS has developed a system for identifying food components, referred to as tags. The term "tag" refers to the significant part of a generic identifier. Generic identifiers are predefined word-like strings of characters used to distinguish one element type from another. An example of a tagname and its definition is presented in Table 11.6. The latest information on this system is available on the world wide web via the INFOODS home page (http://www.fao.org/infoods). As already mentioned, LanguaL is a multilingual system that provides a standardized language for describing food products using faceted classification. Each food is described by a set of standard, controlled terms chosen from facets characteristic of the nutritional and/or hygienic quality of a food, for example the biological origin, method of cooking and conservation, and technological treatments.

Other problems related to the method of expression of nutrients may arise from the long-standing convention of using protein values derived by applying a factor to measured total nitrogen values and from the calculation of energy values using energy conversion factors. Calculation of total carbohydrate content by difference as opposed to the sum of the individual carbohydrates is no longer the norm. The bases of expression in databases are the most commonly unit (such as g) per 100 g edible portion. In some instances unit per 100 g dry mass is presented, or unit per 100 ml. However, some tables list nutrient content per serving size or household measure, either as purchased or as prepared.

Quality of data

Both the quality of the sampling protocol in providing a representative sample for analysis (description of the sampling process, place and time of sampling, number of samples, origin of samples and state of sample when purchased) and the application of appropriate analytical methods controlled by a suitable quality-assurance program determine the quality of the data in the nutrient database. An example of a quality-assurance program is an expert system developed to evaluate the quality of the analytical data according to a four-point rating scale for factors such as analytical method, analytical quality control, number of samples, sample handling and sampling plan. Confidence codes for component values for specific foods can then be assigned in databases. For example, a "0" is assigned when information is not adequate to permit evaluation of data for use in food composition databases, or when certain procedures or practices are inappropriate, and a "3" is assigned when procedures are well documented and appropriately applied.

With cooked foods, the cooking procedures such as the internal end-point temperature of meat and recipe should be known. Some data in food composition tables are based on the analyses of pooled samples and this may influence the value of the data obtained. In addition, information on the treatment of samples before analysis, such as the removal of inedible material, and details of the portion taken for analysis should be documented.

At present, the quality of data in most nutritional databases is considerably superior to the quality of

Table 11.6 Example of an INFOODS tagname and its definition for a food component

<ENERC>

Energy, total metabolizable; calculated from the energy-producing food components

Unit: kJ. The value for <ENERC> may be expressed in kilocalories instead of the default unit of kilojoules. However, if expressed in kilocalories, kcal must be explicitly stated with the secondary tagname <Unit>

Note: It would be confusing and would imply additional information that does not exist if two <ENERC> values, i.e. one expressed in kilocalories and the other expressed in kilojoules, were included for a single food item when one value has simply been calculated from the other using the conversion equation: 1 kcal = 4184 kJ. Consequently, one or the other should be used, but not both

Synonyms: kilojoules; kilocalories; calories; food energy

Comments: In addition to a value for the quantity of total metabolizable energy, <ENERC> includes a description or listing of the conversion factors used to calculate this energy value from the proximate quantities. The conversion factors may be described by a keyword, or the conversion factors may be listed using secondary tagnames within <ENERC>. (More than one <ENERC> tagname may exist for a single food item if the values were calculated from the proximate components using different conversion factors.)

food intake data and this is the major limitation in using nutritional databases to assess nutrient intakes.

11.4 Information required on sources of data in tables

It is important to have information on the source of the data in a food composition table to be able to check its appropriateness for the study and to confirm its authenticity. The four major categories of sources of data are:

- primary publications, e.g. peer-reviewed articles in scientific literature
- secondary publications, e.g. reviews or published compilations with compositional data
- unpublished reports ranging from analytical records to documents prepared with limited circulation, e.g. confidential reports for clients or internal use within a company
- unpublished analytical data that can either be specifically commissioned analyses for the generation of nutrient data or analytical data that were not particularly generated for the purpose of generating food composition data.

Data in food composition tables may be original analytical values, imputed, calculated or borrowed. Original analytical values are those taken from published literature or unpublished laboratory reports. Unpublished reports may include original calculated values, such as protein values derived by multiplying the nitrogen content by the required factor, energy values using energy conversion factors for some constituents of food and "logical" values, such as the content of cholesterol in vegetable products, which can be assumed to be zero. Imputed values are estimates derived from analytical values for a similar food or another form of the same food. This category includes those data derived by difference, such as moisture and, in some cases, carbohydrate and values for chloride calculated from the sodium content. Calculated values are those derived from recipes by calculation from the nutrient content of the ingredients corrected by the application of preparation factors. Such factors take into account losses or gain in weight of the food or of specific nutrients during preparation of the food. Borrowed values are those derived from other tables or databases without referring to the original source. When a value for the content of a specific nutrient in

Table 11.7 Proportion of various types of data in food composition tables

Types of data	McCance and Widdowson tables, UK (developed country)	South African food composition table (developing country)
Analyses	70%	41% in 1999 (improved from 18% in 1991)
	10%	49%
Calculated	15%	10%
Estimated	5%	–

a food is not included, there is a "–" or "0" value and, when a table has no values for a particular nutrient, the value is regarded as being "not included".

The proportion of the various types of data differs between tables and for different nutrients (Table 11.7). Details on food tables can be obtained on the world wide web (http://www.fao.org/infoods). In other tables, such as those in the Netherlands, where sources of the data are given in the references, information on how the data have been obtained can also be obtained. However, this is not the case for all tables of food composition.

11.5 Overcoming the inadequacies of food composition tables

Nutrient losses and gains during food processing and preparation

The content of nutrients per unit mass of food changes when foods are prepared, and such losses and gains can be classified in two ways. The first is related to yield, when the primary ingredients at the precooking stage are compared with the prepared food at the cooking stage and also with the food as consumed at the postcooking stage. The second is related to changes in the amount of specific nutrients when foods are prepared. Although original analytical data will be the most desirable for foods at all stages of preparation, they are seldom available.

As food composition data are frequently lacking for cooked foods, estimates based on the use of factors for calculating the nutrient content of prepared foods from raw ingredients are made. Thus, the nutrient composition of a prepared or cooked food is calculated from the analytical data of uncooked food by applying suitable nutrient retention and yield factors. To obtain the nutrient content per 100 g cooked food, the nutrient content per 100 g of raw food is multiplied by the percentage retained after cooking, and this is divided by the percentage retained after cooking, divided by the percentage yield of the cooked product:

Nutrient content of cooked food

$$= \frac{\text{Nutrient content of raw food} \times \text{Retention factor}}{\text{Yield of cooked food}}$$

The retention factor accounts for the loss of solids from foods that occurs during preparation and cooking. The resulting values quantify the nutrient content retained in a food after nutrient losses due to heating or other food preparations.

The following example using only the yield factor to predict the nutrient content of the cooked food. The USDA Nutrient Database for Standard Reference, Release 12, lists the yield from cooked carrots as 92%. Selected nutrient values for 100 g raw carrots are: 1.03 g protein, 27 mg calcium and 9.3 mg ascorbic acid. Using the yield factor the composition of 100 g cooked carrots is calculated as: 1.03 g/0.92 = 1.12 g protein, 27 mg/0.92 = 31 mg calcium and 9.3 mg/0.92 = 10.1 mg ascorbic acid. This compares favorably to the determined values for carrots of 1.09 g protein and 29 mg calcium, but less so for ascorbic acid at a value of 2.3 mg, probably because it is heat sensitive; therefore, applying the retention factor for ascorbic acid would have resulted in a more accurate prediction.

This example uses both the yield and retention factors to predict the nutrient content of the cooked food. In the USDA Nutrient Database for Standard Reference, Release 12, the folacin content of 100 g of raw onions is 19.9 μg, with a yield of 95% for cooked onions and a retention factor (for root vegetables) of folacin of 70%. The folacin content of 100 g cooked onions is calculated as: 19.9 μg × 0.07/ 0.95 = 14.7 μg. This compares with the determined value of 12.7 μg.

Missing values in food composition tables

In general, original analytical data provide information of the highest quality for inclusion in a food composition table or nutrient database. However, it is seldom possible to construct a food composition table with only such data. A plan of action should be developed by the compilers of the database to deal with missing food items and values for particular nutrients. Very often, values of a biologically similar food are used. For composite or mixed dishes the composition of the dish is estimated by calculation from a standard recipe and applying appropriate nutrient retention factors and, in some cases, adjusting for changes in moisture content due to cooking loss or gain in the different cooking procedures. If a food item forms an important part of the population's diet and analysis is not possible, existing food composition databases should be searched to see whether data on the same or a similar food item could be borrowed. If a value for a nutrient is missing a similar approach can be followed, as it is more desirable to have a slightly incorrect estimated value of lower quality than no value at all. A value of "–" or "0" assigned to missing nutrient values may lead to underestimation of nutrient intakes, especially when there are no values for a nutrient in those foods that make a significant contribution to the supply of that nutrient in the diet, resulting in incorrect conclusions being drawn.

Bioavailability and glycemic index

Nutrient composition information in food composition tables indicates the amount of nutrients as analyzed in that specific food sample and does not give an indication of the absorption or bioavailability of the nutrient from that food item. However, when dietary reference intakes such as recommended dietary allowances (RDA) are drawn up, the recommendation makes provision for the amount of ingested nutrient that may not be absorbed. The concept of bioavailability has developed from observations that measurements of the amount of a nutrient consumed do not necessarily provide a good index of the amount of a nutrient that can be utilized by the body. The bioavailability of a nutrient can be defined as the proportion of that nutrient ingested from a particular food that can be absorbed and is available for utilization by the body for normal metabolic functions. This is not simply the proportion of a nutrient absorbed, and cannot be equated with solubility or diffusibility in *in vitro*-simulated physiological systems. Bioavailability is not a property of a food or of a diet per se, but is the result of the interaction between the nutrient in question, other components of the diet and the individual consuming the diet. Owing to the many factors influencing bioavailability, tables of food composition cannot give a single value for a nutrient's bioavailability. Most research until now has centered upon inorganic constituents, particularly iron, but the concept is applicable to virtually all nutrients. Iron incorporated into heme is more readily absorbed than iron in the nonheme form, and these two forms of iron are sometimes listed separately in food composition tables. Yet, such information does not take into account, for example, the effect of ascorbic acid (vitamin C) and organic acids (citric, malic, tartaric and lactic acid) on nonheme iron absorption. Iron absorption is also increased in a state of iron deficiency. In the coming years, it can be expected that much more work will be carried out on bioavailability than in the past, because of its key role in relating functional nutritional status to nutrient intake.

Future research will probably also focus more on the measurement of the bioavailability of food constituents. Several vitamins and minerals, such as calcium, iron, zinc and a number of B vitamins, are already being studied, with limited attention to carotenoid bioavailability. Inhibitors of absorption, and the effects of processing and storage on the foodstuffs must be determined. As bioavailability is also influenced to a large extent by the meal in which a food constituent is consumed, this means that more information will be needed not only on daily food consumption but also on intake of other constituents at individual meals.

There is an increasing demand from users of food composition tables for information on the glycemic index (GI) of food, which is used as a tool in the selection of food in the management of diabetes, as opposed to the previous system of carbohydrate exchange. The GI is a food-specific measure of the relative tendency of carbohydrate in food to induce postprandial glycemia. The body's response to a 50 g carbohydrate dose induced by either glucose or white bread is taken as the reference and assigned a value of a 100. Responses to all other foods are rated in comparison and listed in tabular format. New data sets with complementary values, based on the GI and available carbohydrate content of food, are being proposed, of which one is a measure of the relative glycemic response to a given mass of whole food and the other is the mass of a food responsible for a given glycemic response.

Both bioavailability and GI are food indices that are influenced not only by the characteristics of the food, but also by the response of the individual to the food (i.e. absorption, metabolism and excretion of the metabolites). For example, quantitative analysis of carotenoids alone could lead to a misinterpretation of vitamin A value. Therefore, the bioavailability of test foods in a single mixture may be investigated using the digestive system of nutrient-depleted rats (i.e. measuring retinol accumulation factor as a measure of total carotenoid bioavailability), or in humans using the relative dose–response test. Advances in analytical chemistry such as improvements in analytical methods, information science, computer hardware and software will assist in filling these gaps in special-purpose databases in the future.

How to calculate a recipe not included in the table

If the composition of a composite or mixed dish is not known, it can be estimated by calculation from a standard recipe and applying appropriate nutrient retention factors and, in some cases, adjusting for changes in moisture content due to cooking loss or gain during cooking. The following guideline are suggested.

- Identify the ingredients of the recipe from the most appropriate foods available in the food composition table.
- Quantify the ingredients in mass (g).
- Calculate the nutrient values for the specific amount of each ingredient.
- Add up the nutrient values of the individual ingredients.
- Calculate the nutrient composition for 100 g of the recipe.
- Apply suitable retention factors to the mineral and vitamin nutrient values if the recipe food is cooked. Note that if individual ingredients were in a cooked form this step is not necessary.
- Compare the moisture content of the calculated recipe with a similar cooked composite dish. If the moisture content differs by more than 1%, adjust the moisture content of the recipe food. All of the nutrients of the recipe food must be adjusted (concentrated or diluted) according to either the decrease or increase in moisture content.
- Assign to a suitable food group and list.

This is only an estimation of the make-up of a composite or mixed dish of unknown composition. Refer to Table 11.8 for an example of the calculation of the composition of a dish from a recipe. However, if this dish is a very important part of the diet of an individual or group and the information is crucial in assessing the adequacy of the diet, analysis should be considered.

Table 11.8 Calculation of the composition of a dish from a recipe

Recipe for scrambled eggs with onions
2 large eggs
⅛ cup whole milk
⅛ teaspoon salt
¼ cup chopped raw onions
2 teaspoons oil
Add milk and salt to eggs and beat with a fork. Fry onions in the oil. Pour egg mixture into frying pan with the onions, and stir mixture with a fork while cooking until it solidifies. Makes one serving.

Calculation of nutrient content of scrambled eggs from nutrient values for raw ingredients
Step 1: Add nutrient levels for the specified quantities of ingredients
  The nutrients in the raw eggs, whole milk, salt, raw onions and oil are added together
Step 2: Readjust quantities of those nutrients in the raw ingredients that are lost during cooking due to evaporation or heat

Nutrient loss on cooking	Eggs	Milk	Onions
Thiamin (%)	15	10	15
Riboflavin (%)	5		
Niacin (%)	5		
Ascorbic acid (%)		25	20
Folacin (%)			30

Step 3: Determine weight of the recipe before cooking
  1 large egg = 57 g; 57 g × 2 eggs = 114 g; refuse factor to calculate weight without shell of 11%;
  114 g × 0.89 = 101.46 g
  1 cup whole milk = 244 g × ⅙ = 40.66 g
  1 teaspoon salt = 5.5 g × ⅛ = 0.69 g
  1 cup chopped raw onions = 170 g × 0.25 = 42.5 g
  1 teaspoon oil = 4.53 g × 2 = 9.06 g
  Total weight = 194.37 g
Step 4: Determine weight of recipe after cooking
  Weight loss during cooking due to evaporation is estimated to be 8%
  Weight of recipe after cooking = 194.37 g × 0.92 = 179 g
Step 5: Determine the nutrient levels of the recipe per 100 g and per serving
  Divide the nutrient levels by 1.79 to determine the nutrient content of 100 g scrambled eggs
  The calculated nutrient levels represent the nutrient content of one serving

Accurate estimation of portion size

Food composition tables are mainly used in nutritional epidemiology to estimate the composition of foods consumed by individuals. All subjects have difficulties in estimating the exact portion sizes of food consumed. This issue is further complicated by the difference between the weight of a product as purchased and that of the actual item consumed (e.g. in meat after cooking there is at least a 25% cooking loss, without bone and with or without visible fat). Standardized portion sizes for individual foods within countries may help, but a set of standard food models (small, medium and large) for use in dietary assessment may be of more value.

11.6 Description of food composition tables and how to retrieve data

A food composition table is easier to use if the format allows easy access to the data available. Advances in information technology have led to more and more food composition tables being available in electronic form, progressively replacing the printed format. Printed food composition tables, although limited by physical proportions such as the size of both the written text and the printed table, continue to be popular in developing and underdeveloped countries. The printed word is seen as authoritative and only a limited level of literacy or knowledge on nutrition is necessary to be able to access the data. Electronic data and access to them are more limited in remote areas in these countries, and a higher level of computer literacy and equipment is necessary, which is generally seen as a luxury and not a necessity.

However, electronic databases have many advantages over printed tables, including virtually unlimited capacity to store information, rapid access to individual data items, and easy sorting and manipulation of data for use in a wide range of calculations. However, the ease of accessing data in an electronic or a computerized database is dependent on the database access software and not only on the way in which data are stored. The development of relational databases has led to the opening up of possibilities to link different databases in regions and countries with each other. This has led to the identification of new challenges such as food identification, compatibility of data, data interchange and data quality.

11.7 Converting foods to nutrients

Entering data

Before the computer age, the conversion of food consumption into nutrient intake had to be done manually, which was a laborious and time-consuming task. Later, much of the work, especially for larger surveys, was done on mainframe computers, and has since passed on to microcomputers, because of their ready accessibility and ease of use. Data on food and nutrient intakes were often subsequently transferred to a mainframe computer, where they were combined with other survey data for further analysis. Today, there is little that cannot be done on a microcomputer, including data manipulation such as sorting and calculations.

Before proceeding to calculate nutrient intake from data on food consumption, it is necessary to ensure that mistakes that have crept into the data set during acquiring, coding, merging, transcription and storage are reduced to an acceptable level. Regardless of the method used for the collection of data on food consumption, consideration should be given to how the data will be entered into the computer. Suitable forms should be designed for the collection of data. These can be on paper or in a personal computer-based program that can save time and eliminate errors associated with the transcription of data from paper to the computer. The use of carefully prepared forms, with information to guide those collecting the data, can reduce the chance of error during the collection of data and, if a separate process, during entry into the computer. The collection and entry of data are subject to human and computer error; therefore, procedures must be developed to ensure that the quality of data is as high as possible. Editing and error-checking routines should be incorporated in the data-entry process and subsets of data entered into the computer should be compared with the original written records. Where mistakes are found, the extent of the error should be determined, because it could involve data for the previous (or next) subject or day, or those previously (or subsequently) entered by the operator involved. In addition to such checks, frequency distributions of all amounts of food and food codes should be carried out.

Converting data in food intake to nutrient intake

A crucial aspect of food composition research is the transmission of information from those working in food composition and analysis to those working in food monitoring, scientists trying to improve the food supply, workers in epidemiological, training and nutrition programs, and regulators. Yet there is little discussion in the scientific literature of the issues relating directly to the compilation of food composition databases, which are the primary means of transmission of food composition data to most professionals in the field. If good

Table 11.9 Comparison of two international systems

Criteria	LanguaL	INFOODS
Language independence	Good	Poor
Culture independence	Good	Poor
Compiler friendliness	Very poor	Very good
Ease of maintenance	Very poor	Very good
Usefulness in food composition tables	Very poor	Very good
Usefulness in software	Very poor	Very good
Ability to document visually	Poor	Poor
Usefulness in food trade	Potentially good	Neutral
Usefulness in nutrition	Good	Good
Usefulness in toxiciology	Good	Neutral

food statistics are available in a country, as well as access to food intake and food composition databases, estimates of a higher quality can be made regarding the nutrient intake of the individual or population as a whole. However, few data on food composition exist for the 790 million people in developing countries who are chronically undernourished and where malnutrition in the form of deficiencies of iron, iodine and vitamin A is rife.

11.8 Perspectives on the future

No universal food database system has been developed that fulfils all of the needs of compilers and users of food databases, despite the fact that it would represent the primary scientific resource from which all other nutritional studies flow. Two international systems are compared in Table 11.9. It is clear that neither system is adequate alone. However, recent international collaboration has considerably improved the development and compatibility of food composition data. It is essential for the development of nutritional sciences that this resource be maintained and improved to serve at both national and international levels.

Further reading

Greenfield H, Southgate DAT. Food Composition Data. Production. Management and Use. London: Elsevier Applied Science, 1992.
Gry S, Holden J. Sampling strategies to assure representative values in food composition data. Food Nutr Agric 1994; 12: 12–20.
Klensin JC. INFOODS Food Composition Data Interchange Handbook. Tokyo: United Nations University Press, 1992.

Rand WM, Pennington JAT, Murphy SP, Klensin JC. Compiling Data for Food Composition Data Bases. Tokyo: United Nations University Press, 1991.

Southgate DAT. Food composition tables and nutritional databases. In: Human Nutrition and Dietetics, 10th edn (JS Garrow, WPT James, A Ralph, eds), pp. 303–310. Edinburgh: Churchill Livingstone, 2000.

Truswell AS, Bateson DJ. Madafiglio KC *et al.* (1991) INFOODS guidelines for describing foods: a systematic approach to describing foods to facilitate international exchange of food composition data. J Food Comp Anal 1991; 4: 18–38.

Websites

Eurocode2: http://www.vfd2.dk/eurocode/

Food and Agricultural Organization of the United Nations: http://www.fao.org/

INFOODS: United Nations University of International Food Data Systems Project: http://www.fao.org/infoods

LanguaL: http://food.ethz.ch/LanguaL

Nutrient Data Laboratory Food Composition Data: http://www.nal.usda.gov/fnic/foodcomp/

United Nations University: http://www.unu.edu/

12
Food Policy and Regulatory Issues

Barbara O Schneeman and John R Lupien

Key messages

- A national food policy encompasses the various programs, policies and regulations that ensure a safe, wholesome and nutritious food supply for a population.
- In developing a comprehensive food policy, several components of the policy need to be considered, including the creation of a regulatory framework that ensures the quality and safety of the food supply, as well as the appropriate use of food-based approaches to promote health and prevent disease in the population.
- A food policy should be used by regions of the world to ensure that their population has a food supply that is adequate to meet the needs of the population and to address the special needs of target populations that may be vulnerable to nutritional stress.
- An effective food policy can enable countries or regions to plan for crises, conflicts or natural disasters that may affect the availability of food for the population.

12.1 Introduction

The complex nature of food policy shown in Figure 12.1 is by no means an exhaustive illustration. From the point of view of food and nutrition, it is to the health dimension of food policy that we must turn. This health dimension has two major elements, food safety (chemical and microbiological) and nutrition. However, nutritionists and food scientists must maintain links with the totality of food policy since it is that totality which determines quality and adequacy of the food supply.

Given the complex nature of food policy, its development requires a multidisciplinary approach that encompasses the food system from production through consumption. Table 12.1 illustrates the various disciplines that affect the development of a food policy in relation to the objectives outlined above. The two critical starting points are with nutrition and with agricultural production and trade. The food supply, whether obtained through production or through trade, must meet the nutritional needs of the population, including any special requirements for groups such as pregnant and lactating mothers, children and those at risk for certain diseases. Consequently, planners must understand

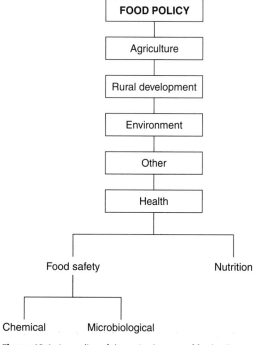

Figure 12.1 An outline of the main elements of food policy.

Table 12.1 Types of data gathered in monitoring surveys

Food availability and security	Food choices	Nutrient status
Crop production	Disappearance data	Food composition tables
Exports and imports	Consumption surveys	Anthropometrics
Food balance sheets	Diet and nutrition knowledge	Biochemical measures
Household economics Socioeconomic factors Participation in food assistance programs	Food expenditures	Clinical measures

nutrient needs in accordance with the population demographics. However, to achieve this understanding integration of concepts from economics, public health, food science and technology, education, behavioral sciences and environmental sciences, with a knowledge of nutrition and agricultural production and trade is needed.

Freedom from hunger is viewed as a basic human right. However, as the sciences of nutrition and food safety have advanced, we have come to realize that adequate nutrition and the quality and safety of our food supply are not only critical for basic human dignity, but also essential for productivity, health and the quality of life. Economists view a healthy population as a prerequisite to sustaining increases in productivity in a region. In this context a safe food supply that lowers risk of food-borne illness and a nutritious food supply that meets nutrient requirements in conjunction with lifestyle factors that promote health must work together. While each of the disciplines outlined in Table 12.1 has a unique responsibility for its part of the food policy, opportunities for interaction and working together must exist for a policy to be of greatest benefit for the health and well-being of the population. In a sense, each of these disciplines provides essential input into the overall policies that are relevant to meet the needs of a particular population but is not sufficient by itself for an effective policy.

The overall goals of a national food policy are to ensure that food production, food purchase, import and export, food processing and marketing are adequate to meet national, local, household and individual food and nutritional needs. The UN World Food Summit, convened at the Food and Agriculture

Organization of the United Nations (FAO) Rome headquarters in 1996, stated in the Plan of Action adopted by the 176 countries attending, that "food security exists when all people, at all times, have physical and economic access to sufficient, safe and nutritious food to meet their dietary needs and food preferences for an active and healthy life". While other definitions of food security have also been devised, the meaning is clear: nations must take action to ensure that all people have access to adequate amounts of good-quality and safe foods throughout the year. This requires the participation of many different disciplines, as outlined below.

12.2 Food and nutrition monitoring

A food policy is effectively a vision of the optimal and attainable goals of food security, food safety and nutrition. By definition, this requires the gathering of data against which optimal and attainable goals are compared. Where the observed performance falls short of these goals, programs to attain the full vision of the food policy are enacted. Table 12.1 lists some of the types of data gathered in nutrition monitoring and categorizes them in terms of the types of information provided.

Information on food and nutrient intake and access to food can be used for several purposes relevant to maintaining public health. The data can be used to track nutritional deficiency diseases, the level of food security, risk of excessive intakes, issues related to food safety and problems specific to vulnerable groups such as children or the elderly. Although household surveys of food and nutrient intake are useful to gather basic monitoring information, additional detail is needed to use monitoring data to provide insight into the linkages among dietary patterns, economic status, risk of exposure to food-borne illness, the level of food insecurity, and risk of nutrient deficiencies or noncommunicable diseases. Data on agricultural production and trade may provide information on the adequacy of the food supply to meet the energy and nutrient needs of the population, as well as gaps in the ability of the food supply to meet critical needs, but individual intakes and variability in intake among sectors of the population are needed to understand the potential for diet-related diseases in the population. Linking food monitoring data to public health monitoring is needed to determine the diet–food relationships to any of the major public health problems within a population. In some regions of the world food insecurity may be measured by inadequacy of food availability at the household level; however, in more developed areas a deficiency of foods may not be the primary indicator of food insecurity. Rather, the inability to have assured access to safe food in socially acceptable ways is more indicative of this problem, which requires a different set of monitoring data than just examining food availability and intake. The challenge for policy makers is often to realize that several approaches to monitoring are needed to develop sound food and nutrition policy and to use the data available in an appropriate manner.

Evaluating food availability and security is dependent on understanding the production of food as well as the amount of food obtained through trade. Some consideration should be given to understanding local and household food production as well as large-scale production that enters the commodity markets and/or is purchased by food processors. FAO has used food balance sheets as a means to understand the ability of regions to meet the food energy needs of various populations and identify regions at risk for food inadequacy (http://apps.fao.org/). Relying on production figures and food disappearance can overestimate food availability in a region. Non-human food uses of commodities, waste and spoilage all decrease the actual amount of food consumed by humans. A bias toward overestimations of food availability can result in an underestimate of problems with micronutrients (vitamins and minerals) while exaggerating problems due to intake of macronutrients such as fat and sugar, and total energy intake. To understand fully the level of food security, it is not sufficient simply to know what food is available but also to understand household economics and related socioeconomic factors, to understand the level of access to safe food in socially acceptable ways as well as food availability at the household level. Food choices are measures of the foods actually consumed by the population and are most accurately obtained through household or individual consumption surveys. Surveys of food consumption can underestimate actual food intake because of underreporting. Underreporting can result in inaccurate estimates of micronutrient intake or excess intake of macronutrients and energy.

Knowledge of food choices by the population are essential to develop intervention strategies that encourage changes in behavior as well as to predict the effects of modifying the food supply. However, the information is most useful if food choices can be understood in relation to population demographics such as age, gender, ethnicity and socioeconomic status. Additional information can be obtained on the factors that influence food choice by surveying diet and nutrition knowledge and information on food expenditure. Nutritional status can be estimated by determining the nutrient profile of the foods actually consumed. The nutrient profile of foods consumed can be compared with standards for recommended nutrient intake to estimate potential gaps that may lead to health problems. Chapter 7 discusses the development of dietary reference standards. To be useful in food policy, these standards should include estimations of the biological requirement, variability in the required intake of a nutrient and an estimation of upper levels of safe intake (Food and Nutrition Board, 1999). This information will allow policy makers to understand whether the nutrient intake of a population is barely adequate to meet minimal requirements, includes a safety factor to account for variability or has the potential to be excessive. In addition to standards for evaluating the adequacy of the food supply, information on nutritional status from anthropometric, biochemical and clinical data is extremely valuable. For example, iron intake and/or iron content of the food supply may provide an indication of whether the population is at risk for iron-deficiency anemia; however, measures of hemoglobin, hematocrit and/or ferritin levels will provide insight into the actual incidence of anemia that may be related to inadequate iron intakes. Having both dietary and clinical assessment data also allows public health workers to consider other environmental or lifestyle factors that are influencing the risk of diet-related disease. For example, a population that has relatively high calcium intake but high risk of osteoporosis may need to consider other dietary or lifestyle factors that contribute to bone density than simply calcium intake alone.

12.3 Food policy and food production

A wide range of legislation, including basic laws and accompanying regulations, plays an important part in ensuring that countries and individuals have continued access to adequate amounts of good-quality and safe food. Basic agricultural legislation which assists food producers through fundamental and applied research, extension advice and education, subsidies and other forms of financial support is extremely important in the overall maintenance of an adequate food supply, at the local, national and global levels. Policies and legislation in this area can also cause some distortion in food production and marketing. Price supports, subsidies and export incentives are often directed to food groups which, while important to overall food supplies, cause excess production of certain grains, meat and dairy products, while other food groups important to a balanced diet such as fruit and vegetables receive little or no attention or support. By and large across the globe, the process of farming and fishing is tightly regulated for social, rural developmental, environmental, economic, health and many other reasons. All of those involved in the food supply must take heed of these regulatory aspects. From the point of view of nutritionists, a primary interest must be how the totality of food production can be altered to improve the balance of nutrients available to the population. Consider the issues that must be addressed in this regard, taking as an example a desire to increase the supply of fruit and vegetables to the consumer.

- A first step would be to look at the available data gathered in a food supply monitoring system to determine the differential in the supply of fruit and vegetables if a target of five servings of fruits and vegetables per day is to be achieved by 75% of the population over a 7 year period.
- A second issue might be to examine the trade implications. For example, the climate of some countries does not allow for many fruits to be grown and thus increasing fruit intake will necessitate increased imports. In some countries a mix of an increased domestic supply and increased imports may be needed.
- A third issue might be to look at the availability of land to grow more of the foods in question and to look at this availability in the context of the suitability of the soil and of the local climate.
- A fourth issue is to consider which crops might be displaced by increased production of fruit and vegetables or some other target crops.
- Finally, when all the realistic issues have been addressed, the question remains of how to persuade farmers to grow these crops and how to persuade consumers to buy them. Price support and subsidies are an option, as discussed later in this chapter.

12.4 Regulatory aspects of food safety

Low-quality foods that are partially spoiled, adulterated, damaged by insects, rodents or birds, mislabeled, or otherwise unacceptable from a basic quality point of view can cheat consumers, cause unnecessary food losses, and harm the reputation of food producers or of an entire food sector or country. Similarly, unsafe foods that present either acute or possible chronic health risks can harm consumers, cause tremendous food losses, and damage or destroy the reputation and economic base of countries or food producers, processors and marketers.

Laws and regulations designed to control the quality and safety of food have existed for over 2000 years. It should be pointed out at the start of this discussion that there are many problems related to food quality and safety that cannot be easily detected by consumers buying food in the marketplace. Because of concerns about hidden adulteration of basic foods in ancient times and the Middle Ages, authorities enacted laws governing the sale of basic grains, beverages and spices, all of which were subject to weight or volume abuses, and adulteration with foreign substances, water or other diluents that could cheat consumers. The Industrial Revolution in the latter part of the eighteenth century brought about concerns about the sanitary conditions of new and larger food processing plants, and led to new food laws in several countries designed to add sanitary requirements and health protection to existing antiadulteration laws.

During the twentieth century food law and regulations became progressively more comprehensive to control existing or newly discovered food quality and safety problems as the methods of producing, processing, packaging and marketing of foods became more complex, and food distribution systems became global. The advent and increasing use of food additives and pesticides in the production and processing of most foods, veterinary drugs in animal production, or contaminants such as heavy metals, industrial chemicals or mycotoxins in many foods, along with pathogenic microorganisms, have required new and more sophisticated systems of food laws, regulations and means to ensure that their requirements are met. Work on ensuring the quality and safety of foods has also taken on both national and international dimensions, and the realization that there can never be a "zero risk" with any food has led to additional emphasis on risk analysis of various food problems so that consumers can receive adequate protection from the many risk factors of quality or safety that can occur in the food supply.

In recent years the process of risk analysis has been split into three components. The first is risk assessment, where a team of scientists (toxicologists, chemists, microbiologists, geneticists, medical and veterinary doctors, biologists, etc.) review data from *in vitro* studies and multispecies and multigeneration animal studies before approval for use in the human or animal food supply. Such studies may also be accompanied by data on humans. The purpose of risk assessment is to establish the risk to people of a given food chemical, and to evaluate the acceptability of that risk. It is of paramount importance to understand that the process of toxicological risk assessment is to find a level of intake up to which a lifetime's exposure will not have any adverse effects. This is done by examining the myriad of data generated in the necessary animal studies to search for a statistically significant adverse effect. Whatever the effect, the minimum exposure level at which these adverse effects do not occur (no observable adverse effect level or NOAEL) is sought. It is then divided by 10 to allow for an animal to human extrapolation and by a further 10 for safety reasons. This figure is known as the acceptable daily intake (ADI). It is not a toxicological threshold but rather a level of lifetime exposure, at or below which no adverse effects are anticipated.

The second component is risk management, implying adequate trained industry and government personnel to ensure that levels set by the risk assessment process are not exceeded, and to help to identify new areas of concern where risk assessment may be needed.

The third component is risk communication, implying adequate sharing of information among scientists, and between the scientific community in industry and government with consumers, legislators and other policy makers, and media so that the general public is assured that risk factors are being adequately controlled. Effective risk communication is extremely important to alert and/or reassure consumers when adverse events occur such as the Chernobyl accident with subsequent radionuclide contamination of foods, bovine spongiform encephalopathy (BSE or "mad cow disease"), or dioxin contamination of animal feed and animal products. Advice and information in such instances should be science based and clear, so that consumers and the general media will be properly informed.

Ensuring the quality and safety of foods and food ingredients requires concerted and co-operative efforts by government authorities, food producers, processors, marketers, consumers and academia. Food problems receive high priority in media reporting, and cause concern among consumers and legislators. Increasingly strict controls over food additives, residues of pesticide and veterinary drug residues in foods, pathogenic microorganisms and packaging materials have all been seen to be necessary, and newer technologies such as genetically modified foods have led to additional concerns. Control of such problems and concerns should be based on sound scientific evidence and judgement, and this requires a strong commitment by both the food industry and government to have adequate human and scientific resources to evaluate and monitor current or new problems, and to explain to and assure consumers, legislators and other policy makers that the quality and safety of the food supply are fully acceptable. Many countries are finding this task difficult, particularly since the dynamics of politics often causes imbalances within food control systems so that overemphasis on one area of problems leads to neglect of other problems. For example, emphasis on food safety in several countries has led to the neglect of food quality problems, with consequent increased food losses, increased amounts of adulterated or mislabeled foods on the markets, and a proliferation on food products that are of questionable value.

To develop effective national food quality and safety control systems it is first necessary to have a basic food law. The FAO cooperated with the World Health Organization (WHO) and the United Nations Environment Program (UNEP) to prepare a model food law that is simple but comprehensive, and gives to the responsible government ministries the power to prepare and publish adequate regulations that can control the many food problems that may occur. The same food law sets basic definitions, enforcement mechanisms, co-ordination systems and penalties for noncompliance. The FAO model food law was based on a study of the essential elements of food laws in many countries, and is patterned after the Canadian food and drugs act which was in force in the 1970s, because of its clarity and simplicity. The concept in such a law is to leave the details to regulations that can be published, and altered if necessary, by government ministries without the need for additional laws to be amended or added. The FAO model food law has been enacted by several developing countries and has been found to be a fully adequate vehicle for ensuring the quality and safety of domestic food supplies, and foods for export to developed and developing countries. At the same

Table 12.2 Structure of the FAO/WHO model food law (www.fao.org/es/ESN/foodlaw.pdf)

Part I: Preliminary
  1. Short title and commencement
  2. Interpretation

Part II: General provisions
  3. Prohibition against sale of poisonous, unwholesome or adulterated food
  4. Deception
  5. Standard of foods
  6. Prohibition against sale of food not of the nature, substance or quality demanded
  7. Sale and preparation of food under insanitary conditions

Part III: Legal procedures
  8. Importation
  9. Warranty
  10. Defences

Part IV: Regulations relating to food standards, food safety and other matters
  11. Regulations

Part V: Administration and enforcement
  12. Food Standards Board
  13. Powers of authorized officers
  14. Appointment and duties of authorized officers for official laboratories
  15. Other authorized officers
  16. Power of Minister to obtain particulars of certain food ingredients

Part VI: Legal procedures
  17. Power of court to order license to be canceled and articles to be disposed of
  18. Prosecution
  19. Penalties
  20. Certificates of analysis and presumptions
  21. Saving of other written laws

time, many developed countries have taken an opposite approach, with the growth of basic food laws with hundreds of pages of detailed texts, accompanied by thousands of pages of virtually impenetrable regulations, leading to confusion, unnecessary litigation and consumer confusion. The main elements of the FAO/WHO model food law are given in Table 12.2.

Compliance with food quality and safety legislation requires a food industry that is familiar with the requirements of the laws and regulations, and has in place the quality- and safety-control systems needed to ensure adequate levels of control. Government must have adequate levels of properly trained and equipped food control administrators, inspection and laboratory personnel, and scientists to perform premarketing approval processes for substances such as food additives, pesticides and veterinary drugs and their residues in foods, and risk analyses of these substances and of pathogenic microorganisms, mycotoxins, heavy metals, and industrial contaminants such as dioxins and polychlorinated biphenyls (PCBs). Relationships between food control officials and the legal community must also be emphasized, since many food problems can be quite technical and difficult for lay people, including judges, to understand. All groups should have trained personnel to inform the public regularly of ongoing food quality-and safety-control programs to provide reassurance that food supplies are of good quality and safe.

Since food production and processing has become progressively more complex, concentrated and worldwide in nature since the 1960s, there is an increased need for all involved in the production, storage, processing and marketing of foods, food ingredients, of other food-related substances such as packaging, agricultural and food industry chemicals to have fully functional quality-control systems in place, which include food safety components where needed. Each entity involved in the food chain needs to know the quality, safety and appropriate use of all inputs used in the production or processing of foods, and keep adequate records to show that these systems are working properly. Government activities to monitor compliance with food legislation need to be equally comprehensive so that properly trained inspectors can inspect food entities for compliance, and chemists, microbiologists and technicians in adequately equipped laboratories can carry out analyses of food samples for compliance with legislation. Systems of this type, when adequate, can also carry out the risk management and risk communication functions mentioned previously.

Food labeling has become an important part of the overall marketing of food. While many foodstuffs are still purchased in a raw or semiprocessed form for further processing and preparation in the home or food catering establishment, a progressively larger percentage of foods in many countries is now sold in packaged form. Informative labeling that provides the purchaser with reliable information is necessary. Packaged foods should have labels that bear, as a minimum, the name of the product, an accurate ingredients statement, the name and address of the manufacturer or distributor, and a statement of net weight or volume.

In many countries there are mandatory or voluntary systems for nutritional labeling, which can be an important adjunct to overall nutrition education programs, but when viewed in isolation may lead to as much confusion as clarity in the minds of average consumers. Labels are also important with regard to possible allergenic substances, and can enable individuals with allergies or other adverse reactions from certain ingredients to avoid foods that may cause problems. In recent years the food label in some countries has also become a vehicle for certain health and nutritional claims, despite a general prohibition on false and misleading claims on food labels. Many countries continue to disallow such claims because of their possible misleading nature, even when they are based on some level of current scientific information.

Since the 1930s the provision of an adequate food supply in each country has become more international. Virtually no country is fully self-sufficient in all aspects of its food supply, ingredients or ancillary materials. Imports of some foods and exports of other cash crops and surpluses are a feature of many national economies, and a mainstay of the economy of many developing countries. The increasing trade in foods since the 1930s led to international work on food requirements immediately following World War II. FAO was created in 1945, following the 1943 United Nations Hot Springs Conference on Food and Agriculture, which emphasized in its final declaration the need for agreed international food standards for foods that were regularly traded between countries.

In the 1950s FAO began working with the WHO in the expert evaluation of food additives, and established the Joint FAO/WHO Expert Committee of Food Additives (JECFA). In the early 1960s a similar Joint FAO/WHO Meeting on Pesticide Residues (JMPR) was set up to provide FAO and WHO with recommendations from panels of independent experts on the use of pesticides in agricultural, and safe levels of residues in foods. JECFA, over the years, has provided similar advice on food additives, and has added to its work evaluation of veterinary drug residues in foods, mycotoxins, heavy metals and industrial chemical contaminants in food. FAO also saw the need for the preparation of agreed international standards, recommendations, codes of practice and guidelines for foods in international commerce, and with the WHO set up the Joint FAO/WHO Food Standards Program in 1962. The secretariat of this program, which is located at FAO headquarters in Rome, Italy, serves as the secretariat to the Codex Alimentarius Commission (CAC).

CAC activities started in 1962 with about 40 nations as member countries. In 2001 there were 165 CAC member countries, and CAC work has grown with the growing membership. At the outset the CAC concentrated on individual standards for various foods, and over 200 such standards have been produced. The standards for individual food products, often called "vertical standards", include basic compositional information, lists of approved additives, pesticide residues, labeling, hygiene components and other related information. Work on such vertical standards has been reduced in recent years, while work on codes of practice, guidelines and recommendations that apply to many different food and food processes, often called "horizontal" standards, is underway to produce or update food hygiene codes, general standards for food additives, labeling, limits for pesticide residues, and guidelines or codes for biotechnology, animal feedstuffs, import and export inspection and certification, and general principles involving risk analysis and related topics. The participation of developing countries in Codex work has grown dramatically and world food trade has grown to about $500 billion per year.

Meeting CAC standards, recommendations and guidelines has become extremely important since the completion of the 1986–1994 GATT Uruguay Round of Multilateral Trade Negotiations and the creation of the World Trade Organization (WTO) on 1 January 1995. Two of the Uruguay Round Agreements, the Agreement of Sanitary and Phytosanitary Measures (SPS) and the Agreement on Technical Barriers to Trade (TBT), give explicit or implicit recognition to the work of the CAC as the benchmark standards for foods in international trade. Both the SPS and TBT Agreements call on WTO member countries to seek harmonization or equivalence of national regulations and regulatory procedures based on CAC work, and recognize that foods which meet CAC standards, recommendations and guidelines should be able to be traded freely in international commerce. The WTO also provides a regulatory mechanism for countries that feel they have been discriminated against by arbitrary rules of other countries to appeal for WTO review and adjudication. The work of the CAC has been cited in several such appeals, and has been upheld as representing standards and recommendations that are based on sound science and appropriate levels of risk protection.

The importance of CAC work is thus obvious to all countries, and continued collaboration between the CAC and the WTO will continue to reinforce the need for all countries to make vigorous efforts to meet CAC requirements in their growing international food trade and national food control and consumer protection programs.

12.5 Nutritional aspects of food policy

The use of food policy to guide food choice indicates that a government has a level of understanding of dietary patterns that are consistent with health in the population, the gap between the recommended pattern and current consumption, as well as public health issues for the population that are related to diet. These optimal patterns are dietary guidelines or dietary reference values and can be expressed in many ways: as nutrients or as foods and in quantitative or qualitative terms. Where the policy analysis sees a gap between the optimal prevailing values, then several choices are available in terms of food policy strategy.

Supply-driven versus demand-driven policies

Demand-driven options to alter population nutrient intake involve the familiar public health nutrition promotion strategies. These are largely based on information that is communicated to the consumer using methods as diverse as label information and claims, media campaigns and work-based programs. If the consumer can be persuaded to "demand" an altered food supply, then the food supply must be enabled or obliged to meet these demands.

Supply-driven options try to manipulate the balance of foods produced by managing agricultural policy to make the production of certain foods more attractive to the primary producer. Equally, it can involve leaving the food supply as it is but manipulating price so that consumers will find the consumption of specific foods more attractive or less attractive as the strategy dictates.

It would be wrong to think that the choice is always one or the other, that is demand or supply driven. Often, both strategies are involved and indeed no matter how exhaustive supply-driven policies are pursued, unless consumers can be persuaded to go along with the strategy through demand-driven approaches, no progress will be made.

Options to change the food supply versus changing the property of foods

Another strategy is to leave the pattern of food selection alone but to change the properties of foods consumed. In many parts of the world dairy products are the main sources of saturated fatty acids, which raise blood cholesterol levels and increase the risk for cardiovascular disease. Processors can change this property of milk by making low or non-fat products available in the marketplace, and people can continue to consume the other nutrients in milk while lowering their intake of saturated fatty acids. These types of change are dependent on changes in demand and are thus allied to demand-driven food supply. However, there are instances where the nutritional properties of food are altered through mandatory fortification of specific foods with specific nutrients. Examples are given in Table 12.3. This is an example of supply-driven food policy combined with a policy to alter the property of the target food through mandatory fortification. Since it is mandatory, all who consume the fortified food are exposed to the target nutrient, with their right to choose limited by the regulatory authority. Sometimes the target population is everybody and sometimes it is a specific group. Thus, whereas fortifying salt with iodine will help to tackle goitre across the whole population, fortifying chapatti flour with vitamin D has been used to tackle rickets among Asian immigrants to Europe.

Altering the nutritional or functional properties of foods to improve health will become an increasingly important part of food policy. While processing technology has been the traditional approach for this type of modification, plant breeders and biotechnologists have demonstrated that genetic approaches will continue to make inroads into altering the nutritional composition of foods. These new technologies will widen the options and challenges open to those charged with implementing food and nutrition policy.

Table 12.3 Examples of nutrients used in fortification programs to prevent specific diet-related conditions

Fortified nutrient	Target condition
Folic acid	Neural tube defects
Vitamin D	Rickets
Iron	Anemia
Vitamin A	Xerophthalmia
Iodine	Goitre

Irrespective of the strategy involved, with the exception of mandatory fortification, consumers must be directed to specific food choices. The UN agencies, FAO and WHO, recognized the needs for an analytical guide to reaching optimal food choices or "food-based dietary guidelines", and these are outlined in the next section. This detailed analysis on the basis for guiding food choice was presented by FAO/WHO in their consultation of the preparation and use of food-based dietary guidelines (FAO/WHO, 1998). Figure 12.2, which is reprinted from that report, outlines the integration of information on public health issues, nutrient

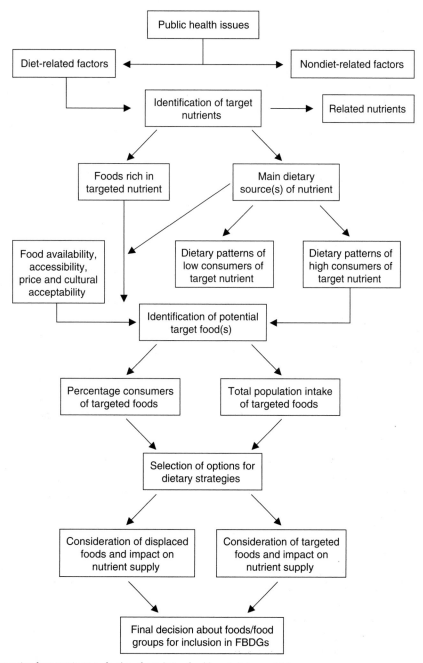

Figure 12.2 Reorientation from nutrients to foods in formulating food based dietary guidelines.

composition of foods, monitoring data on food and nutrient intakes into recommendations about food-based dietary guidelines and the development of messages to communicate to the public and to health professionals.

Figure 12.2 is organized into five stages based on the boxes in the center of the diagram. The beginning stage is to identify the major public health problems within a population and decide the degree to which these problems are due to dietary factors. If the major public health problems do not have a relationship to diet then other means must be used to address these problems. A population may not be open to messages on diet and health if other issues are more pressing for their survival. Nonetheless, most populations in the world today will have several public health issues that are related to diet and nutrition, whether due to over-nutrition or to undernutrition. The identification of these issues allows the identification of target nutrients related to the public health problem. It is important to note that there may be a tendency to rely on nutrient monitoring data to identify issues for nutritional intervention. Under these circumstances a policy maker may focus on the gap between recommended nutrient intakes and actual consumption by the population and focus on addressing that gap. Focusing on these gaps may not address the key public health issues; to develop relevant food and nutrition policy it is more constructive to begin with the public health issues and identify those that have a diet–nutrient relationship. If gaps are observed between recommended intakes and actual consumption, it is important to consider whether the public health monitoring system can identify potential problems associated with the nutrient in question. Once target nutrients have been identified, these must be translated into potential target foods. Two strategies are useful: one to identify those foods that are relatively high in the targeted nutrient and the other to identify the primary dietary sources of the nutrient. Both categories of foods can become targets for changing the nutrient intake of the population, depending on the availability, cost and acceptability of the foods. Further analysis of food choices by the population will determine the most viable options for food-based strategies. The final stage of this process is to focus on food-based dietary guidelines to address the public health issues identified at the beginning of the process, but it is important to consider the broader implications of the food-based strategies to

ensure that new problems are not created in the process. A key part of this process is to integrate food-based dietary guidelines into a sustainable food policy for a region. Hence, the process of identifying foods can help to guide agricultural and trade policy to ensure that the products are available to the targeted population. Likewise, it is important to identify those foods that can be made available to a population in a sustainable manner.

The implementation of food policy can also incorporate the use of food assistance programs for a region. Food assistance should be targeted to reduce the degree of food insecurity in a region. Depending on the resources available, strategies may include subsidies for feeding programs that target vulnerable populations, such as feeding programs at schools, for pregnant women or for the elderly. In addition, governments, through the support of foreign partners or the World Food Program (http://www. wfp. org), can provide foods for distribution that have been unavailable, often because of conflicts or natural disasters. In some cases governments may make resources available through vouchers for purchase of foods in the marketplace. (For examples of these types of program see http://www.fns.usda.gov/fns/) Distribution of vitamin or mineral supplements has been used in certain populations to address micronutrient deficiency problems. However, this is a therapeutic approach to a specific nutrient deficiency and should not be considered as food assistance. Food assistance requires a food-based approach to address nutritional problems within a population.

12.6 Research on food, nutrition and health

Research is an important part of developing relevant policy. The research efforts may focus on devising better tools to monitor the nutritional status of populations, especially those who are at risk, on developing better analytical skills to determine the composition of the food supply, including the various factors involved with safety and quality of foods, on new knowledge to determine the essential role of nutrients and intake levels associated with health, on approaches to improve the quality and safety of the food supply, and on behavioral approaches that will motivate choices that lower the risk of disease. Research is ongoing to identify the association between food components and the prevention of disease. If we simply look at the 100 years encompassed in the twentieth century, the dynamic nature of this research effort is evident. As you read the chapters on nutrient metabolism, keep in mind the evolving nature of our understanding of nutrient function and the need to link that new knowledge to the development of policy. During the first half of the twentieth century the essential role of vitamins and minerals in the prevention of deficiency diseases was understood. In the latter half of the century this research evolved to understand the functions of nutrients at the cellular and molecular levels (Centers for Disease Control, 1999). In the process of understanding the metabolic function of nutrients we have begun to understand new roles for nutrients. For example, it has been known since the 1940s that folic acid is required to prevent macrocytic anemia. In recent years an association has been discovered between low folate intake and the risk of neural tube defects, heart disease and certain types of cancer. This association between folates and disease risk raises additional research questions on the need for new methodology to measure accurately the folate content of foods and monitor intake in the population, and to define the relationship between folate metabolism and disease. However, advancing our understanding of folates and disease prevention has resulted in new policies of fortification of the food supply.

Research that helps to improve the quality and safety of the diet is important and valuable. However, this information will be most useful if we understand how to motivate consumers to take actions that will lower their risk for disease. Simply knowing the benefits of a dietary pattern or safe food handling is not sufficient if social or economic factors prevent consumers from acting on their knowledge. Research to understand these issues from a consumer's perspective is a necessary complement to using policy effectively for behavioral change.

12.7 International work on food policy

From the above discussion, it can be seen that food policy is usually a national responsibility. However, many countries look to international organizations for guidance and assistance in formulating and implementing national policies for food production and nutritional improvement. FAO and WHO, as the two main UN specialized agencies in food and health, have prime importance in this area, as shown by the 1992 International Conference on Nutrition and the 1996 World

Food Summit, in addition to the CAC and expert committee work on food quality, safety and nutrition. The publications and assistance given by FAO and WHO to their member countries are in constant demand and highly valued by all member countries, both developing and developed.

Other international organizations are also actively involved in certain aspects of nutrition. The United Nations Children's Fund (UNICEF), with its mandate to improve conditions for infants and children, has active programs to improve breast-feeding and prevent low birth-weight babies, in co-operation with the WHO. The United Nations Educational, Scientific and Cultural Organization (UNESCO) has active programs to promote nutrition education in schools at all levels, and the United Nations University is active in promoting nutrition policy considerations in university activities around the world. The World Bank and regional international banks also have nutrition improvement activities built into many of their projects in developing countries, as does the United Nations Development Program. Food aid in emergency situations, and in some development activities, is provided by the UN World Food Program and by the UN High Commission for Refugees. The International Food Policy Research Organization also carries out economic-based nutritional studies in developing countries and makes recommendations to countries on the basis of these studies.

The WTO plays a crucial role in the area of food production and marketing policy, subsidies and related support to agriculture, and in resolving food quality and safety disputes between countries.

12.8 Perspectives on the future

Food policy will be most effective when it is constantly updated to reflect changing circumstances and new knowledge. Such updating requires a commitment to core principles in the food policy and the ability to use new information to develop new strategies. The overriding principle should be the use of food and nutrition policy to improve the health of the population. It is difficult to find a region of the world that has consistently used an integrated approach to food policy in this manner. For example, an analysis by the Economic Research Service of the United States Department of Agriculture illustrates that significant gaps exist between the recommended intakes of various food groups and the production capacity of these foods (ERS, 1999). So, while agricultural policies have ensured that the USA has an abundant, low-cost food supply available, it has not adjusted agricultural production policies to reflect the recommendations made in the Dietary Guidelines for Americans. Some regions of the world have placed more emphasis on expanding crops for export than on diversifying production for local nutrition needs.

New technologies for producing and processing food are constantly emerging. Clear criteria are needed to evaluate the nutritional impact of these new technologies, especially for those technologies that have a stated goal of improving nutritional status. Some of the questions that need to be asked concern the replacement of foods in the diet, stability of nutrients under normal processing and handling conditions, bioavailability of the nutrients and interaction with other food components. In developing new technologies to improve nutritional status it is also important to understand the factors that contribute to inadequate nutrition. For example, one strategy for improving nutritional status is to improve the diversity of food crops available for consumption. At subsistence levels of agriculture, grains are frequently a staple crop and provide significant amounts of energy. However, grains are lacking in many nutrients and need to be complemented with other foods. Most populations that subsist primarily on grain experience a number of nutritional deficiencies.

Food systems that can diversify beyond subsistence farming and include fruits, vegetables, legumes and animal products result in improved nutritional status. As a consequence, biotechnology approaches to increase the content of two or three nutrients in a crop such as rice may have less impact on overall nutritional status than using the technology to adapt new crops to regions that depend primarily on rice. Likewise, using new technologies to extend shelf-life, prevent storage losses, improve taste and reduce the cooking time of foods such as dry beans may make valuable contributions to improving nutritional status by allowing a more diversified diet.

Further reading

Bloom DE, Canning D. The health and wealth of nations. Science 2000; 287: 1207–1209.

Centers for Disease Control. Achievements in public health, 1900–1999: safer and healthier foods. MMWR Weekly 1999; 48: 905–913.

Cordian L. Cereal grains: humanity's double-edged sword. World Rev Nutr Diet 1999; 84: 19–73.

Economic Research Service. Moving Toward the Food Guide Pyramid: Implications for U.S. Agriculture. Washington, DC: United States Department of Agriculture, Agric Econ Report 779, 1999.

Food and Agricultural Organization and World Health Organization. Preparation of Use of Food-based Dietary Guidelines. Geneva: WHO Technical Report Series 880.

Food and Nutrition Board. Institute of Medicine. Dietary Reference Intakes: A Risk Assessment Model for Establishing Upper Intake Levels for Nutrients. Washington, DC: National Academy Press, 1999.

13
Nutrition Research Methodology

J Alfredo Martínez and Miguel A Martínez González

Key messages

- This chapter identifies critical aspects and factors involved in nutritionally orientated investigations as well as the measurement qualities concerning research procedures.
- It describes how to select methods and techniques as well as animal models to assess nutrient utilization and functions.

- It defines indicators and markers of dietary intake and metabolism in human studies.
- It helps to choose methods to investigate the causal relationships between diet and disease.

13.1 Introduction

Research is a meticulous process to discover new or collate old facts by the scientific study of a subject or through a critical investigation. In this context, nutrition research involves advances in knowledge concerning not only nutrient functions and the short- or long-term influences of food and nutrient consumption on health, but also studies on food composition, dietary intake, and food and nutrient utilization by the organism.

The design of any investigation involves the selection of the research topic accompanied by the formulation of both hypotheses and the aims, the preparation of a research protocol with appropriate and detailed methods and, eventually, the execution of the study under controlled conditions and the analysis of the findings leading to a further hypothesis. These stages of a typical research program are commonly followed by the interpretation of the results and subsequent theory formulation. Other important aspects concerning the study design are the selection of statistical analyses as well as the definition of the ethical commitments.

This chapter begins with a review of some of the important issues in statistical analysis and experimental

design. The ensuing sections look at *in vitro* techniques, animal models and finally human studies. The primary purpose is to provide a primer in nutrition research methods early in a student's career to allow a more critical review of the many studies that, from time to time, a student will need to consider in the course of their study.

13.2 Statistical analysis and experimental design

In all areas of research, statistical analysis of results and data plays a pivotal role. This section is intended to give students some of the very basic concepts of statistics as it relates to research methodology.

Validity

Validity describes the degree to which the inference drawn from a study is warranted when account is taken of the study methods, the representativeness of the study sample and the nature of its source population. Validity can be divided into internal validity and external validity. Internal validity refers to the subjects actually sampled. External validity refers to the extension of the findings from the sample, to a target population.

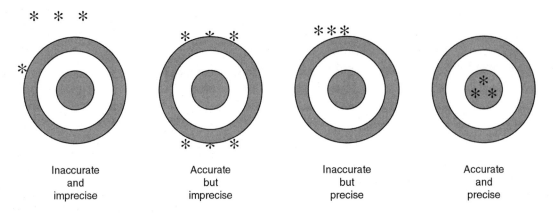

Inaccurate and imprecise   Accurate but imprecise   Inaccurate but precise   Accurate and precise

Figure 13.1 Accuracy and precision.

Accuracy

Accuracy is a term used to describe the extent to which a measurement is close to the true value, and it is commonly estimated as the difference between the reported result and the actual value (Figure 13.1).

Reliability

Reliability or reproducibility refers to the consistency or repeatability of a measure.

Precision

Precision is described as the quality of being sharply defined or stated; thus, sometimes precision is indicated by the number of significant digits in the measurement.

In a more restricted statistical sense, precision refers to the reduction in random error. It can be improved either by increasing the size of a study or by using a design with higher efficiency. For example, a better balance in the allocation of exposed and unexposed subjects, or a closer matching in a case–control study usually obtains a higher precision without increasing the size of the study.

Sensitivity and specificity

Measures of sensitivity and specificity relate to the validity of a value. Sensitivity is the proportion of subjects with the condition who are correctly classified as having the condition. Specificity is the proportion of persons without the condition who are correctly classified as being free of the condition by the test or criteria. Sensitivity reflects the proportion of affected individuals who test positive, while specificity refers to the proportion of nonaffected individuals who test negative (Table 13.1).

Table 13.1 Estimation of sensitivity and specificity

	True condition or outcome present	True condition or outcome absent
Test +	A	B
Test −	C	D

$$\text{Sensitivity} = \frac{A}{A+C} \qquad \text{Specificity} = \frac{D}{B+D}$$

Data description

Statistics may have either a descriptive or an inferential role in nutrition research. Descriptive statistical methods are a powerful tool to summarize large amounts of data. These descriptive purposes are served either by calculating statistical indices, such as the mean, median and standard deviation, or by using graphical procedures, such as histograms, box plots and scatter plots. Some errors in the data collection are most easily detected graphically with the histogram plot or with the box-plot chart (box-and-whisker plot). These two graphs are useful for describing the distribution of a quantitative variable. Nominal variables, such as gender, and ordinal variables, such as educational level, can be presented simply tabulated as proportions within categories or ranks. Continuous variables, such as age and weight, are customarily presented by summary statistics describing the frequency distribution. These summary statistics include measures of central tendency (mean, median) and measures of spread (variance, standard deviation, coefficient of variation). The standard deviation describes the "spread" or variation around the sample mean.

Hypothesis testing

The first step in hypothesis testing is formulating a hypothesis called the null hypothesis. This null hypothesis can often be stated as the negation of the research hypothesis that the investigator is looking for. For example, if we are interested in showing that, in the European adult population, a lower amount and intensity of physical activity during leisure time has contributed to a higher prevalence of overweight and obesity, the research hypothesis might be that there is a difference between sedentary and active adults with respect to their body mass index (BMI). The negation of this research hypothesis is called the null hypothesis. This null hypothesis simply maintains that the difference in BMI between sedentary and active individuals is zero. In a second step, we calculate the probability that the result could have been obtained if the null hypothesis were true in the population from which the sample has been extracted. This probability is usually called the p-value. Its maximum value is 1 and the minimum is 0. The p-value is a conditional probability:

$$p\text{-Value} = \text{Prob}(\text{differences} \geq \text{differences found} \mid \text{null hypothesis (H}_0) \text{ were true})$$

where the vertical bar (|) means "conditional to". In a more concise mathematical expression:

$$p\text{-Value} = \text{Prob}(\text{Difference} \geq \text{Data} \mid \text{H}_0)$$

The above condition is that the null hypothesis was true in the population that gave origin to the sample. The p-value by no means expresses the probability that the null hypothesis is true. This is a frequent and unfortunate mistake in the interpretation of p-values.

An example of hypothesis testing is shown in Box 13.1. Hypothesis testing helps in deciding whether or not the null hypothesis can be rejected. A low p-value indicates that the data are not likely to be compatible with the null hypothesis. A large p-value indicates that the data are compatible with the null hypothesis.

Many authors accept that a p-value lower than 0.05 provides enough evidence to reject the null hypothesis. The use of such a cut-off for p leads to treating the analysis as a decision-making process. Two possible errors can be made when making such a decision (Table 13.2).

A type I error consists of rejecting the null hypothesis, when the null hypothesis is in fact true. Conversely, a type II error occurs if the null hypothesis is accepted when the null hypothesis is in fact not true. The

---

Box 13.1 Example of hypothesis testing

Among a representative sample of 7097 European men, the authors found that each 10 unit increase in the leisure-time physical activity was associated with $-0.074 \, \text{kg/m}^2$ in BMI. Physical activity was measured in units of MET-hours/week (1 MET-hour is the energy expenditure during 1 resting hour).

What is the probability of finding, in such a sample, a BMI $0.074 \, \text{kg/m}^2$ lower (or still lower) for those whose energy expenditure is 10 MET-hours higher, if the actual difference in the whole European population were 0? This probability is the p-value; the smaller it is, the stronger is the evidence to reject the null hypothesis.

In this example, the p-value was 0.001, i.e. chance would explain a finding like this, or even more extreme, in only 1 out of 1000 replications of the study. The conclusion is that we reject the null hypothesis (population difference in BMI = 0) and (provisionally) accept the hypothesis that states that lower physical activity during leisure time is associated to a higher BMI. We call this the alternative hypothesis (Martínez-González et al., 1999).

Table 13.2 Right and wrong decisions in hypothesis testing

Decision	Truth (Population)	
	Null hypothesis	Alternative hypothesis
Null hypothesis	Right decision (probability = $1 - \alpha$)	Type II error (probability = β)
Alternative hypothesis	Type I error (probability = α)	Right decision (power = $1 - \beta$)

probabilities of type I and type II errors are called alpha (α) and beta (β), respectively.

Power calculations

The power of a study is the probability of obtaining a statistically significant result when a true effect of a specified size exists. The power of a study is not a single value, but a range of values, depending on the assumption about the size of the effect. The plot of power against size of effect is called a power curve. The calculations of sample size are based in the principles of hypothesis testing. Thus, the power of a study to detect an effect of a specified size is the complementary of beta ($1 - \beta$). The smaller a study is, the lower is its power. Calculation of the optimum sample size is often viewed as a rather difficult task, but it is an important issue because a reasonable certainty that the study will be large enough to provide a precise answer is needed before starting the process of data collection (see Box 13.2).

Box 13.2 Example of sample size calculation

Let us suppose that we want to compare the proportion of subjects who develop a given outcome depending on whether they have been assigned to diet A or diet B. We expect that 5% of subjects in the group assigned to diet A and 25% of those assigned to diet B will develop the outcome of interest. We are willing to accept a type I error with a 5% probability and a type II error with a 10% probability. A simplified equation* for sample size (n) calculation would be:

$$n = \frac{(z_{\alpha/2} + z_\beta)^2 \, (p_A q_A + p_B p_B)}{(p_A - p_B)^2}$$

$$= \frac{(1.96 + 1.28)^2 [(0.05 \times 0.95) + (0.25 \times 0.75)]}{(0.05 - 0.25)^2}$$

$$= 62$$

where $z_{\alpha/2}$ and z_β are the values of the normal distribution corresponding to alpha 0.05 ($z_{\alpha/2} = 1.96$) and beta 0.10 ($z_\beta = 1.28$), p_A and p_B are the expected proportions, and q_A and q_B are the complementary values of the proportions ($q = 1 - p$). Therefore, in this example:

$$z_{\alpha/2 \,=\, 0.05 \text{ (two tailed)}} = 1.96$$
$$z_{\beta \,=\, 0.10 \text{ (one tailed)}} = 1.28$$
$$p_A = 0.05 \,(q_1 = 0.95)$$
$$p_B = 0.25 \,(q_2 = 0.75)$$

These values are substituted in the equation and thus the required sample size for each group is obtained (62). Therefore, we shall need 124 participants, 62 in each group.

*When the outcome is a quantitative variable, sample means ($\bar{x}_A$ and $\bar{x}_B$) replace proportions in the denominator, while the product terms $p_A q_A$ and $p_B q_B$ are replaced by the respective variances (s^2) of the two groups in the numerator:

$$n = \frac{\left(z_{\alpha/2} + z_\beta\right)^2 \times \left[s_A^2 + s_B^2\right]}{\left(\bar{X}_A - \bar{X}_B\right)^2}$$

The necessary sample size for a study can be estimated taking into account at least three inputs:

- the expected proportion in each group and, consequently, the expected magnitude of the true effect.
- the beta error (or alternatively, the power) that is required
- the alpha error.

The p-value has been the subject of much criticism because a p-value of 0.05 has been frequently and arbitrarily misused to distinguish a true effect from lack of effect. Until the 1970s most applications of statistics in nutrition and nutritional epidemiology focused on classical significance testing, involving a decision on whether or not chance could explain the observed association. But more important than the simple decision is the estimation of the magnitude of the association. This estimation includes an assessment about the range of credible values for the association. This is more meaningfully presented as a confidence interval, which expresses, with a certain degree of confidence, usually 95%, the range from the smallest to the largest value that is plausible for the true population value, assuming that only random variation has created discrepancies between the true value in the population and the value observed in the sample of analyzed data.

Options for statistical approaches to data analysis

Different statistical procedures are used for describing or analyzing data in nutritional epidemiology (Table 13.3). The criteria for selecting the appropriate procedure are based on the nature of the variable considered as the outcome or dependent variable. Three main types of dependent variable can be considered: quantitative (normal), qualitative (very often dichotomous) and survival or time-to-event variables.

Within bivariate comparisons, some modalities deserve further insights (Table 13.4).

The validity of most standard tests depends on the assumptions that:

- the data are from a normal distribution
- the variability within groups (if these are compared) is similar.

Tests of this type are termed parametric and are to some degree sensitive to violations of these assumptions. Alternatively, nonparametric or distribution-free tests, which do not depend on the normal distribution, can be used. Nonparametric tests are also useful for data collected as ordinal variables because they are based on ranking the values. Relative to their parametric counterparts, nonparametric tests have the advantage of ease, but the disadvantage of less statistical power if a normal distribution should be assumed. Another additional disadvantage is that they do not permit confidence intervals for the difference between means to be estimated.

A common problem in nutrition literature is multiple significance testing. Some methods to consider in these instances are analysis of variance together with multiple-comparison methods specially designed to make several pairwise comparisons, such as the least significant difference method, the Bonferroni and

Table 13.3 Common statistical methods used in nutritional epidemiology

Dependent variable ("outcome")	Univariate description	Bivariate comparisons	Multivariable analysis
Quantitative (normal)	Mean, standard deviation	t-Tests (two groups) Analysis of variance (more than two groups) Regression and correlation (two quantitative variables)	Multiple regression
Qualitative (dichotomous)	Proportion, odds	Chi-squared Fisher's exact test Cross-tables Odds ratio Relative risk	Multiple logistic regression
Survival	Kaplan–Meier (product-limit) estimates and plots	Log-rank test (Mantel–Haenszel)	Proportional hazards model (Cox regression)

Table 13.4 Common statistical methods for comparison of means

	Two samples		More than two samples	
	Parametric	Nonparametric	Parametric	Nonparametric
Independent samples Paired or related samples	Student's t-test Paired t-test	Mann–Whitney U-test Wilcoxon test	Analysis of variance Analysis of variance for repeated measurements, general linear models	Kruskal–Wallis test Friedman's test

Scheffé procedures, and the Duncan test. Analysis of variance can be also used for replicate measurements of a continuous variable.

Correlation is the statistical method to use when studying the association between two continuous variables. The degree of association is ordinarily measured by Pearson's correlation coefficient. This calculation leads to a quantity that can take any value from -1 to $+1$. The correlation coefficient is positive if higher values of one variable are related to higher values of the other and it is negative when one variable tends to

be lower while the other tends to be higher. The correlation coefficient is a measure of the scatter of the points when the two variables are plotted. The greater the spread of the points, the lower the correlation coefficient. Correlation involves an estimate of the symmetry between the two quantitative variables and does not attempt to describe their relationship. The nonparametric counterpart of Pearson's correlation coefficient is the Spearman rank correlation. It is the only nonparametric method that allows confidence intervals to be estimated.

To describe the relationship between two continuous variables, the mathematical model most often used is the straight line. This simplest model is known as simple linear regression analysis. Regression analysis is commonly used not only to quantify the association between two variables, but also to make predictions based on the linear relationship. Nowadays, nutritional epidemiologists frequently use the statistical methods of multivariable analysis (Table 13.3). These methods usually provide a more accurate view of the relationship between dietary and nondietary exposures and the occurrence of a disease or other outcome, while adjusting simultaneously for many variables and smoothing out the irregularities that very small subgroups can introduce into alternative adjustment procedures such as stratified analysis.

Most multivariate methods are based on the concept of simple linear regression. An explanation of the variation in a quantitative dependent variable (outcome) by several independent variables (exposures or predictors) is the basis of a multiple regression model. However, in many studies the dependent variable or outcome is quite often dichotomous (diseased/nondiseased) instead of quantitative and can also be explained by several independent factors (dietary and nondietary exposures). In this case, the statistical multivariate method that must be applied is multiple logistic regression. In follow-up studies, the time to the occurrence of disease is also taken into account. More weight can be given to earlier cases than to later cases. The multivariate method most appropriate in this setting is the proportional hazards model (Cox regression) using a time-to-event variable as the outcome (Table 13.3).

13.3 In vitro studies

Scientific research involves studies across a reductionist spectrum. As studies become more reductionist, more and more confounding factors are stripped away. In vitro studies represent part of the reductionist approach in nutrition research. The range of techniques used is large.

- Chemical analysis studies provide data on nutrient and nonnutrient content of foods.
- Digestibility techniques, in which a substrate is exposed to enzymes capable of digesting the substrate, help to refine the gross chemical analytical data to predict nutritional potential.

- Intact organs such as the liver of experimental animals can be used in studies such as perfused organ studies. In such studies, the investigator can control the composition of material entering an isolated organ and examine the output. Sections of organs can also be used, such as the everted gut sac technique. A small section of the intestine is turned inside out and placed in a solution containing some test material. Uptake of the test material into the gut can be readily measured.
- Another approach is the construction of mechanical models that mimic an organ, which in nutrition research is usually the gut. Many of these models very successfully predict what is observed in vivo but have the obvious advantages such as cost and, most of all, flexibility in altering the experimental conditions with great precision.

The application of molecular biology techniques to tissue and cell culture systems has provided researchers with powerful strategies to evaluate and establish metabolic pathways and regulatory roles of nutrient and nonnutrient components of food. Thus, Northern, Southern and Western blotting techniques to quantitate specific RNA, DNA and proteins in tissues in response to nutrients are common tools in the nutrition laboratory. The influence of some nutrients or nutritional conditions on ribosomal dynamics as well as on cell hyperplasia or hypertrophy processes has been estimated through RNA, DNA or protein/DNA values, respectively.

Furthermore, molecular biological approaches have allowed numerous in vitro discoveries that have aided our understanding of the genetic basis of nutrient functions and metabolic states in vivo. The polymerase chain reaction (PCR) can be used for DNA and/or messenger RNA (mRNA) amplification to determine the genetic background and/or gene expression in very small cellular samples. Transfection studies allow the insertion of DNA into cells to examine nutrient function. Thus, cell lines that usually lack the expression of a particular gene can be transfected with DNA containing the gene promoter, as well as all or part of the transfected gene of interest, to study the interactions of various nutrients with the expression of a particular gene. Conversely, knockout cell lines allow us to investigate the consequences of losing a specific gene. In either case, nutrient function at the cell level and the cell–gene level may be studied and provide definitive results. Gene regulation by nutrients has been assessed in different isolated cells and tissues using appropriate indicators and markers of gene expression RNA levels.

13.4 Animal models in nutrition research

Whole animal systems have been used in measuring the utilization, function and fate of nutrients. Thus, a part of our knowledge regarding nutrition concepts stems from animal experiments, which are often extrapolated to humans and referred to as animal models. There are many reasons for choosing an animal study over a human study. We can and do subject animals to experimental conditions that we would ethically not be allowed to apply to humans. For example, to study the manner in which a nutrient influences the scale and histopathology of atherosclerosis, animal studies are needed. Just as studies with humans are governed by the rules of ethics committees, so too are studies with animals. These rules involve the regulation of facilities, accommodation and animal care, competence, alternatives to animal experimentation, anesthesia and euthanasia procedures, registration, supply of animals and the involvement of an ethical committee.

In general, the use of animals as models for human nutrition research can be examined from three aspects:

- the animal model
- the experimental diet and its delivery
- the experimental techniques available.

The animal model

Many species have been used in the study of nutrition. Many are pure-bred strains such as the Wistar rat, the Charles River mouse or the New Zealand white rabbit. Some animal models have been specially selected to exhibit particular traits, making them very useful models for research. The Wattanable rabbit has defective low-density lipoprotein (LDL) receptor function, making this animal model very useful for studying the role of diet in influencing LDL receptor-mediated arterial disease. The ob/ob mouse develops gross obesity because of an alteration in a genetic profile. In recent times there has been a rise in the use of transgenic animal models which have been produced through advanced molecular genetic techniques. In such models, specific genes can be inserted or deleted to fulfil specific functions. For example, the peroxisomal proliferating activating receptor-alpha (PPAR-α) is not expressed in

one knockout mouse model, giving rise to fat accumulation. Another example of a transgenic mouse presents an overexpression of the Cu/Zn-superoxide dismutase enzyme.

The experimental diet and its delivery

The nature of the diet and its mode of delivery are centrally important in understanding the role of animal models in human nutrition issues. There are several types of diets offered to laboratory animals.

Commercially available diets made to internationally accepted nutritional norms are often referred to as chow diets or laboratory chow. For the vast majority of laboratory animals in studies where nutrient intake is not the central area of interest, such chow diets are used. However, when nutrition is the area of research, special diets will almost always have to be formulated. The type of diet that needs to be formulated will depend on the nature of the research question.

Terms such as semipurified, purified and chemically defined diets are often used but frequently it is difficult to know exactly which type of term fits different formulations. The least refined experimental diet uses ingredients such as barley, soyabean and wheat. An example is given in Table 13.5, taken from a study of rapeseed glucosinolates on the iodine status of piglets.

The purpose of the study was to assess the effects of glucosinolate derived from ground rapeseed. A direct comparison between the ground rapeseed and the

Table 13.5 An example of less refined experimental diets to test the effects of rapeseed-derived glucosinolate

	Control (g/kg)	Rapeseed oil (g/kg)	Ground rapeseed (g/kg)
Soyabean meal[a]	220	240	195
Rapeseed oil	5	40	–
Ground rapeseed	–	–	100
Barley	755	700	685
Mineral/vitamin	20	20	20
Total	1000	1000	1000
Energy (MJ/kg)[b]	12.6	13.3	13.0
Protein (g/kg)	183	177	182
Fat (g/kg)	29	56	58
Glucosinolate (mmol/kg)	0	0	1.9

[a] Solvent-extracted soyabean meal.
[b] Metabolizable energy.
From Schone et al. (2001). Reproduced with permission.

control is not possible because the ground rapeseed contains twice as much fat as the controls. Thus, the rapeseed oil diet is included because it contains no glucosinolate, but the same amount of fat as the control diet. The ingredients used in these diets, in general, contain several nutrients. Thus, the main ingredient, barley, contains protein, carbohydrate and fat as well as fiber and micronutrients. That can create problems when there is a need to examine the effects of specific nutrients, such as fatty acids. The fatty acids naturally present in barley cannot be ignored. In the case of the rapeseed oil diet in Table 13.5, 40 g of the 56 g of fat per kilogram of diet comes from the rapeseed oil, but 16 g (or 28.6%) comes from barley lipid.

To deal with this, more refined diets are used. An example of such a diet is given in Table 13.6. In this instance, the authors were examining how different dietary fats influence blood cholesterol in normal mice and in transgenic mice not expressing the gene for the protein cholesteryl ester transfer protein (CETP), which is a key protein in lipid metabolism. In this instance, the ingredients are almost all pure. Thus, casein is pure protein and nothing else. Similarly, sucrose is pure carbohydrate and cellulose is pure fiber. The diets differ only in the source of fat. The high-fat diet obviously has more fat and thus more energy per kilogram of diet. It is thus critically important to note that as the energy density goes up, most other things must also go up to ensure a common concentration, not on a weight-for-weight basis but on a weight-for-energy basis. A simple illustration is the level of the mineral mix used: 2.5 g/100 g in the control diet, 3.2 g/100 g in the low-fat diet and 4.2 g/100 g in the high-fat diet. But when considered on a weight-for-energy basis, all five diets contain 2.0 g/MJ. The only changes are in fat and in maize starch, which always vary in opposite directions.

Variations in diet composition are often the key for the design of nutrition experiments. In this context, different feeding regimens can be applied to laboratory animals depending on scientific criteria. In *ad libitum* feeding the animals have free access to food; in controlled feeding animals are offered a limited amount of food (restricted feeding) or receive as much food as can be fed to them (forced feeding). A specific form of restricted feeding is pair feeding, which involves the measurement of food consumed by some animals to match or equalize the intake of a test group on the following day. There are many reasons why pair feeding

Table 13.6 An example of more refined experimental diets to examine the cholesterolemic effects of fats in transgenic CETP mice

	Control diet		Low-fat diet		High-fat diet	
	(g/100 g)	(g/MJ)	(g/100 g)	(g/MJ)	(g/100 g)	(g/MJ)
Casein	20	12	19	12	24	12
L-Cystine	0.03	0.18	0.28	0.18	0.36	0.18
Maize starch	40	24	48	31	13	6
Dextrinized starch	13	8	12	8	16	8
Sucrose	10	6	9	6	12	6
Cellulose	5	3	5	3	6	3
Soyabean oil	7	4	0	0	0	0
Safflower oil	0	0	2	1.2	2.4	1.2
Experimental oil[a]	0	0	0	0	22	11
Mineral mix	3.5	2.1	3.3	2.1	4.2	2.1
Vitamin mix	1	0.6	0.9	0.6	1.2	0.6
% Energy						
Total fat	16.9		5.7		48.6	
Sugar	10.1		10.9		10.5	
Starch	54.1		22.3		22.1	
Protein	20.2		20.9		20.7	
MJ/kg	16.7		15.9		20.1	

[a] Three different experimental oils were used (butter, safflower, high oleic safflower) for three different high-fat diets varying in types of fatty acids.
From Chang and Snook (2001). Reproduced with permission.

is critically important. An experiment may seek to examine how a new protein source, rich in some nutrient of interest, influences some aspect of metabolism. Let us consider a compound in the protein source that may reduce blood LDL cholesterol. A control diet is constructed based on casein. In the experimental diets, this casein is replaced on an isonitrogenous basis with the test protein source. Otherwise the diets are identical. After several weeks of *ad libitum* feeding a blood sample is taken and the results show that blood cholesterol rose with the experimental diet. Then the researcher begins to look at other data and observes that growth rates in the control rats were far higher than in the experimental group because the latter had a much lower food intake. Quite simply, the new protein source was unpalatable. The experiment will now have to be carried out as a pair-fed study. The food intake of rats given the experimental diet will be measured each day. On the following day the control rats will be rationed to that amount. Food intakes and probably growth rates are identical. Only the protein source differs. Now the researcher can truly reach conclusions as to the effect of the new protein source on LDL cholesterol metabolism. The intake or supply of nutrients may be administered orally, intravenously, intraperitoneally or by means of some specific tools (gavage, stereotaxis, etc.).

13.5 Human studies

In human nutrition, man is the ultimate court in which hypotheses are both generated and tested. Nutritional epidemiology, through its observational studies, demonstrates possible links between diet, physical activity and disease. It is not the only way in which such possible links are generated but it is a critically important one in modern nutrition. Experimental human nutrition takes the hypothesis and through several experiments tries to understand the nature of the link between nutrients and the metabolic basis of the disease. Once there is a reasonable body of evidence that particular nutritional conditions are related to the risk of disease, experimental nutritional epidemiology examines how population-level intervention actually influences the incidence of disease (see Section 13.6). In effect, experimental human nutrition and experimental nutrition epidemiology both involve hypothesis testing. However, the former is more often intended to understand

mechanisms and generally involves small numbers. The latter, in contrast, uses very large numbers to examine the public health impact of a nutrition intervention which, under the controlled conditions of the laboratory, showed promise.

Human nutrition experimentation

The use of experimental animals for human nutrition research offers many possible solutions to experimental problems. However, the definitive experiments, where possible, should be carried out in humans. Studies involving humans are more difficult to conduct for two major reasons. First, humans vary enormously compared with laboratory animals. They vary genetically and they also vary greatly in their lifestyle, background diet, health, physical activity, literacy and many other ways. Secondly, it is far more difficult to manipulate human diets since we do not eat purified or semi-purified diets.

Experimental diets in human nutrition intervention studies

In the 1950s, an epidemiological study across seven countries presented data to suggest that the main determinant of plasma cholesterol was the balance of saturated, monounsaturated and polyunsaturated fatty acids (MUFA and PUFA). To test this hypothesis, a series of studies was carried out on human volunteers using "formula diets". Dried skimmed milk powder, the test oil and water were blended to form a test milk with specific fatty acid compositions. The volunteers lived almost exclusively on these formulae. Although this type of study is simple to conduct, it does not represent the true conditions under which normal humans live. At the other end of the spectrum of options for manipulating human diets is that of issuing advice that the subjects verify by way of a food record. It is difficult to prove that subjects actually ate what they say they have eaten. Sometimes, adherence to dietary advice can be ascertained using tissue samples (blood, saliva, hair, fat) and biomarkers. For example, adherence to advice to increase oily fish intake can be monitored using platelet phospholipid fatty acids.

In between these two extremes of formula feeds and dietary advice lies an array of options in which convenience is generally negatively correlated with scientific exactitude. In the case of minerals and vitamins, it is possible simply to give out pills for the volunteers to take and measure compliance by counting unconsumed pills and perhaps using biomarkers. When it comes to macronutrients this is not generally possible. Whereas asking someone to take a mineral supplement should not alter their eating habits, asking someone to consume a litre of milk a day or a bowl of rice bran per day will alter other aspects of the diets of the volunteers. It will not then be possible to attribute definitively an event to the intervention (1 litre/day of milk or 1 bowl/day of rice bran). The event could have been caused by possible displacement of some other foods by the intervention. The only option in human intervention experiments is to prepare foods for volunteers to eat, which differ only in the test nutrient. If the objective is to examine the effect of MUFA relative to saturated fatty acids (SFA) on blood lipids, then fat-containing foods can be prepared that are identical except for the source of fat. The more foods and dishes that can be prepared in this way, the more successful the experiment will be.

The final dilemma is where the test foods will be consumed. A volunteer may share the test foods, which are almost always supplied free of charge, with friends or family. To be sure of consumption, volunteers may be asked to consume the test meal in some supervised space, usually a metabolic suite. This, however, is a very costly option.

Study designs in human nutrition

As the researcher designs the options for altering the intake of nutrient under investigation, so too the design of the study requires careful thought. The metabolic effect of the nutrient in question may be influenced by age, gender and other variables, such as high levels of alcohol intake or physical activity, smoking, health status, prescribed drug use and family history. On an experiment-by-experiment basis, the researcher must decide which attributes will exclude a volunteer (exclusion criteria). The volunteers recruited can now be assigned to the various treatments. When the numbers are small, randomly assigning subjects to the treatments may lead to imbalances that could confound conclusions. For example, if one has 45 volunteers for three treatments, it could be that the 15 assigned to treatment A include the five heaviest subjects and the five lightest subjects. Another treatment may be predominantly one gender. In such instances, a minimization scheme can be used. Minimization is a technique in which individuals are allocated to treatment groups, ensuring a balance by minimizing

the differences between groups in the distribution of important characteristics (age, weight, physical activity). To apply minimization, during the recruitment process, the investigators must keep an ongoing analysis of differences between groups in the major variables that may affect the result and allocate new individuals to the group that leads to a more balanced distribution of these characteristics. Another option is stratified randomization in which strata are identified and subjects are randomly allocated within each stratum. While stratification and minimization are potentially very useful, it is impractical to stratify individuals for many variables at the same time or to try to minimize every conceivable variable that may affect the result. To a considerable extent, the need to balance groups becomes less important when all subjects are rotated through all treatments (cross-over designs). For this to happen, the number of experimental periods must equal the number of treatments. For any given period, all treatments must be represented. An important factor to consider in this type of design is whether or not a washout period is needed between treatments, and its duration.

Consider the situation above if the study was to examine the effect of fish oil (treatment A) versus olive oil (treatment B) on lymphocyte function. If it is deemed necessary that 20 days are needed to alter the membrane phospholipids of lymphocytes, then it is likely that 30 days will be needed to return to baseline. If it is necessary that each treatment should commence at baseline, then a washout period, where volunteers resume their normal routine, is needed.

A final consideration is the occasion when it is not possible to balance all confounding factors. Take as an example a study to examine the effect of supplemental calcium on bone mineral density in premenopausal women. The treatment group will receive a supplement of 1000 mg of calcium as a tablet and the control will receive a placebo tablet. What factors might one wish to balance in such a study? Among the possibilities are age, parity, use of oral contraceptives, intake of coffee, smoking and physical activity. To balance these factors adequately is impossible. However, if they are recorded, then, when the data are being evaluated on a statistical basis, they can be included to ascertain their effect on the measured outcome, bone mineral density. To accomplish this aim, multivariate methods such as multiple regression or logistic regression should be used (see Section 13.2).

13.6 Epidemiological designs

Epidemiology is a health-related science dealing with the distribution and determinants of health and illness in populations. Nutritional epidemiology integrates the knowledge derived from nutrition research, to examine diet–disease relationships at the level of free-living populations. Nutritional epidemiology provides scientific evidence to understand the role of nutrition in the cause and prevention of disease.

The comparison and choice of different epidemiological study designs depends on exposure measures, outcome measures, costs and expected length of follow-up. The selection of a study method is often influenced by pragmatic issues such as feasibility, as well as by ethical questions.

Epidemiological studies can be divided into two broad categories (Figure 13.2): experimental and non-experimental (observational) studies. Observational studies can be further divided into descriptive and analytical studies. In a wide sense, an experiment is a set of observations, conducted under controlled circumstances, in which the scientist manipulates the conditions to ascertain the effect of such manipulation on the observations.

Experimental studies in nutritional epidemiology

It is necessary to consider that in biological experimentation, it is not possible for the scientist to control completely all of the relevant circumstances, and the manipulation will consist of increasing at most the degree of variation in the factor that the scientist is investigating. The ideal will be to obtain two almost identical sets of circumstances where all factors are the same. If a strong variation is then introduced in only one of these factors, all of the observed differences between the two sets that occurred thereafter would be causally attributed to the single factor that the investigator had manipulated.

Experimental epidemiological designs are those in which the investigator assigns the exposure to each subject. In these studies, the treatment (or exposure) is assigned with the aim of attaining maximum comparability between treated and untreated groups regarding all other characteristics of the subjects apart from the treatment or exposure of interest. In epidemiological research, the best way to achieve identical sets of circumstances is to assign subjects randomly to expo-

sure (treatment) or control groups. This process is called randomization. All randomized studies are experimental designs.

Exposure, from an epidemiological point of view, describes lifestyle or environmental factors that may be relevant to health. Outcome is another generic term used to describe the health-related events or variables that are being studied in relation to the effect of an exposure. In nutritional epidemiology, the primary exposure of interest is dietary intake, whereas outcome measures usually involve disease occurrence or nutritional status indicators (anthropometry, clinical signs of disease/health status, biological or physiological measures or dietary habits).

It is also possible to design experimental studies assigning whole population groups to different exposures. These studies are called community trials. For example, if a whole town is assigned to receive an educational program about healthy eating and another neighboring town is assigned to control (no educational program), this would be a community trial when randomization is used, it is termed "cluster-randomization". However, when the number of randomized units is scarce, even though each unit may be large, there would be no guarantee that the groups to be compared would be identical. Conversely, if the randomization has been done on an individual basis and the whole sample is large enough, a random scheme will usually accomplish its objective of distributing the participants in groups that are essentially homogeneous in all measured and unmeasured factors. This balance makes groups directly comparable and ensures the validity of causal inferences extracted from a randomized design (individual randomization).

In general, experimental studies with individual randomization provide the strongest evidence for the effect of an exposure on an outcome. Experimental studies are the inferentially strongest designs to demonstrate causality, but they may raise substantial ethical problems because the scheme of random assignment is used to help not the subject, but the experiment. Subjects are exposed only to meet the needs of the protocol of the study and not the individual needs of the participant. Therefore, randomized experiments with humans can only be conducted under strict ethical conditions (see Boxes 13.3 and 13.4). It is not permissible to carry out experimental studies where the exposure is potentially harmful. Therefore, under these conditions, nonexperimental (observational) study designs must be applied. The design options in nutritional epidemiology must take into account the setting, uses, advantages and limitations (Table 13.7).

Experimental epidemiology

Experimental epidemiologists try to conduct controlled studies and in these studies is the investigator who assigns the exposure. Human studies, however, unlike animal studies, involve aspects that the investigator cannot control. This is particularly so when they are carried out on a free-living population. Two study designs dominate this area of epidemiology: randomized controlled trials and cross-over studies. In these studies, subjects are randomly assigned to either an exposed or a nonexposed group, commonly referred to as the treatment and the placebo group. The placebo is a substance that is indistinguishable from the treatment and enables both subjects and investigators to be blinded to the treatment. Changes in indicators of health or disease status are compared between the two groups at the end of the experiment to identify the effect of the exposure.

Cross-over designs in epidemiology operate on the same principles as the repeated-measures designs common to basic science research. All study subjects receive the treatment and the placebo for equal periods, with a washout period in between, and the order of treatment or placebo administration is selected at random for each study subject. Cross-over designs are appropriate only for studies of treatments that have no lasting effects, a feature that limits their utility in nutritional epidemiology.

In general, experimental epidemiological study designs are well suited to the identification of causal relationships between specific exposures and indicators of health or disease status. Application of these methods is limited, however, by the difficulty in controlling exposures and by the enormous expense associated with population-based intervention trials aimed at modifying risk or chronic diseases. It is perhaps more feasible to apply experimental study designs to contrast the effects of pharmacological doses of specific nutrients or food components the exposures of which can

---

Box 13.3 Sample ethics form for completion prior to research

The proposal respects the fundamental ethical principles including human rights and will deal only with individuals adequately informed and willing to participate. Also, all research data partners will obtain national authorization from an ethical committee or equivalent body before any intervention with subjects. The study does not involve any genetic manipulation.

- Requested specifications:
  - Human embryos or fetus — No   Yes
  - Use of human embryonic or fetal tissue — No   Yes
  - Use of other human tissue — No   Yes
  - Research on persons — No   Yes
  - If yes, further specify if it involves:
    - children — No   Yes
    - persons unable to consent — No   Yes
    - pregnant women — No   Yes
    - healthy volunteers — No   Yes
  - Use of nonhuman primates — No   Yes
  - Use of transgenic animals — No   Yes
  - Use of other animals — No   Yes
  - Genetic modification of animals — No   Yes
  - Genetic modification of plants — No   Yes
- Other specifications:
  - The regulations, concerning human and medical research, will be respected with precise reference to the recommendations of the Helsinki (1964), Tokyo (1975), Venice (1983) and Hong Kong (1989) committees, as well as other EU regulations RD 561/1993, 65/65 CEE, 75/318 CEE, Directive 91/507 and 89/843 EN-C (ISBN 92-825-9612-2).

Box 13.4 Sample of an informed consent form

This form will cover the following aspects:

I .... (name)

I have read the volunteer's information

I have felt free to make questions concerning the study

I have received enough information

I have talked to the following personnel responsible (names ...)

I understand that my participation is on a voluntary basis

I understand that I can withdraw from the study:

1. If I wish
2. Without further explanations

Therefore, I freely confirm my availability to be involved in the trial

Date
Signature

In addition, all the partners agree with the following statement

In implementing the proposed research I shall adhere most strictly to all national and international ethical and safety provisions applicable in the countries where the research is carried out.

I shall conform in particular to the relevant safety regulations concerning the deliberate release into the environment of genetically modified organisms.

Table 13.7 Design options in nutritional epidemiology

Design	Setting	Uses	Advantages	Limitations
Clinical trial	Secondary prevention (diseased participants)	Treatment–outcome association	Strongest evidence for causality Highest internal validity Very low potential for bias	Low external validity Ethical problems High cost
Field trial	Primary prevention (healthy participants)	Exposure–onset of disease association	Strong evidence for causality High internal validity Low potential for bias	Very large sample and long follow-up Low external validity Can assess only single-nutrient effects Highest costs
Community trial	Group randomization (towns, work-sites, schools)	Evaluation of community interventions or educational activities	If multiple and small groups are randomized, it has the advantages of an experimental design	Low internal validity if the number of randomized units is low
Quasi-experiment	Intervention study (not randomized)	Evaluation of community interventions or educational activities	High feasibility More applicable Investigator controls exposure	Difficulties in finding comparable groups High potential for bias Underlying trends may alter results
Cohort	Participants are initially classified as exposed or nonexposed and followed up in time to monitor the incidence of the outcome	The most powerful observational tool in nutritional epidemiology to study diet–health associations	Very low potential for bias Ability to study rare exposures, complex dietary patterns and multiple outcomes of a single exposure Allows direct estimation of risks and rates Minimal ethical problems	Large sample and very long follow-up No ability to study rare outcomes Bias by low follow-up (attrition) Requires collaborative participants High costs
Case–control	Exposure is compared between subjects with and without the outcome	Practical analytical tool in nutritional epidemiology to study diet–health associations	Ability to study rare outcomes Ability to study multiple potential causes of a single outcome No problems with losses to follow-up Minimal ethical problems Low cost	Potential for biased recall of exposure and biased participation of controls Inability to study rare exposures and multiple outcomes of a single exposure Inability to estimate risks and rates
Cross-sectional	Past exposure and outcome are simultaneously assessed in a representative sample of the population	Estimation of the prevalence of a disease or an exposure Population assessment in health planning Monitoring trends if it is periodically repeated	Highest external validity Relatively low costs Minimal ethical problems A wide spectrum of information about diet and health can be collected	Difficult to assess the temporal sequence: very low ability for causal inference Potential for biased participation and response bias

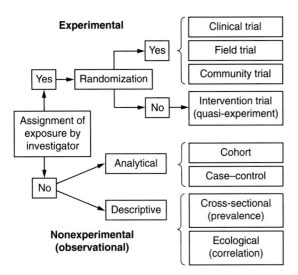

Figure 13.2 Classification of epidemiological designs.

be more easily controlled. This approach has been increasingly selected from the 1990s to assess the effects of specific micronutrients (β-carotene, α-tocopherol, folic acid, and other minerals and vitamins) using large-scale randomized trials.

Experimental studies keep the highest internal validity among epidemiological designs and therefore provide the most compelling evidence for supporting a cause–effect relationship. However, they may lack generalization (i.e. they may have low external validity) and their applicability to free-living populations may be poor insofar as the dietary intake patterns do not correspond to isolated nutrients but to the combination of more complex food items. Moreover, the induction time needed to appraise the effect of a postulated cause may last longer than the observation period of a randomized trial, thus precluding the ability of the trial to ascertain the causal relationship.

Quasi-experimental studies are those in which the assignment of exposure is controlled by the investigator, but subjects are not randomly allocated. They are sometimes called intervention trials (Figure 13.2). When only one micronutrient is compared with a placebo, the study is called a single trial, whereas multiple or factorial trials involve designs where several micronutrients are compared with a placebo. In a 2 × 2 factorial design, two treatments are evaluated simultaneously by forming four groups (treatment A, treatment B, both treatments and placebo).

Some randomized trials are referred to as primary prevention trials and others as secondary prevention trials. Primary prevention trials are those conducted among healthy individuals with the aim of preventing the onset of disease. For example, in the Alpha-Tocopherol, Beta Carotene Cancer Prevention Study (ATBC trial, 1994) almost 30 000 healthy men were randomly assigned to receive either α-tocopherol, β-carotene, both or placebo to prevent the onset of lung cancer, in a 2 × 2 factorial design. All participants were free of this disease at the start of the study and they were followed up for several years to assess the incidence of lung cancer. This is an example of a primary prevention trial. Primary prevention trials are also called field trials.

Secondary prevention trials are conducted among patients who already suffer from a particular disease and they are randomly assigned to treatment or placebo groups to prevent adverse outcomes. For example, to study the benefits of a Mediterranean-style diet, in the Lyon Diet Heart Study, patients were randomized to two different dietary patterns after suffering a myocardial infarction (de Lorgeril *et al.*, 1999). The outcome was not the onset of disease but the incidence of reinfarction or cardiac death during the follow-up period.

Nonexperimental (observational) studies

When experiments are not feasible or are unethical, other nonexperimental designs are used. In experimental investigations, exposures are assigned to subjects by the investigator, whereas in nonexperimental (observational) studies the investigator has no control over the exposure, because the participants freely assign themselves or not to the exposure. In nonexperimental studies the investigator may take advantage of "natural experiments", where exposure only appears in some defined groups. An example of this would be an "experiment" where dietary intake is culturally determined, such as in Indonesia, where the rice consumed is white rather than brown, and beriberi is common as a result of vitamin B_1 deficiency.

Nonexperimental (observational) designs can be further classified into four main subtypes:

- cross-sectional studies
- case–control studies
- cohort studies
- ecological studies.

Among observational studies, the main differences between study designs relate to the time when exposure and outcome are measured.

Cross-sectional (prevalence) studies

Cross-sectional or prevalence studies measure both exposure and outcome in the present and at the same point in time. Cross-sectional surveys provide a snapshot of descriptive epidemiological data on nutrition, identifying nutritional needs in the population and forming a basis for health promotion and disease prevention programs at a single point in time. Several countries conduct regular cross-sectional surveys on representative samples of their populations focusing on dietary habits and frequencies of illness. Dietary factors can then be correlated with prevalence of illness, which may be helpful for national nutrition policy.

Case–control studies

In case–control studies, outcome is measured in the present and past exposure is ascertained. An example would be where the dietary and lifestyle patterns of patients with a disease (cases) are compared with those of age- and gender-matched people (controls).

Subjects are identified and recruited on the basis of the presence or absence of the disease or the health outcome variable of interest. Ideally, the controls are randomly selected from the same study base as the cases, and identical inclusion and exclusion criteria are applied to each group. The presence of specific dietary exposures or other factors of etiological interest in subjects is generally established using interviews, questionnaires or medical record reviews. Within the general framework for case–control studies, there are several options for study design and control selection.

For example, controls may be matched with cases at an individual level on the basis of age, gender or other variables believed to affect disease risk. Matching eliminates variability between cases and controls with respect to the matching variables and thus leads to a higher efficiency in the analysis. Nevertheless, matching does not control for the confounding effects of these risk factors on the observed relationship. Case–control studies are by far the most logistically feasible of the analytical study designs in epidemiology, but their application to questions of interest to nutritionists is limited by the particular nature of diet–disease relationships.

The insight to be gained from a comparison of dietary exposures between cases and controls is limited by the possibility that the dietary patterns of subjects have changed since the time when diet was most important to the disease initiation process. Retrospective case–control studies attempt to overcome this limita-

tion by measuring past diet using food frequency or diet history methods. One concern is that recall of past diet by cases may be influenced by their present disease status. For example, patients who have had a heart attack may attach an unfair level of importance to their intake of specific foods, based on misinformation.

A primary factor in choosing between a case–control design and a cohort design is whether the exposure or the outcome is rare. If the outcome is rare, case–control studies are preferable, because a cohort would need a very large sample to have sufficient subjects with different levels of exposure. If the exposure is rare, cohort studies are preferable.

Cohort studies

In cohort studies exposure is evaluated in the present and outcome ascertained in the future.

Cohort studies are most commonly longitudinal or prospective, with subjects being followed forward in time over some predefined period to assess disease onset. They may also be retrospective (historical cohorts), with groups identified on the basis of exposure sometime in the past and then followed from that time to the present to establish presence or absence of the outcome. The feasibility of retrospective cohorts depends on the availability of good-quality data from pre-existing files. The research costs associated with cohort study designs mean that such studies are less common than other approaches. Nevertheless, a substantial effort to develop large cohort studies in nutritional epidemiology has been made since the early 1980s. Cohort studies can assess multiple outcomes, whereas case–control studies are restricted to assessing one outcome, but may be able to assess many different exposures. If an absolute measure of the effect of the exposure on the outcome is required, the only design that is appropriate is a cohort study, as case–control studies cannot be used to estimate incidence.

For example, to ascertain the relationship between olive oil consumption and coronary heart disease, a case–control study would compare the previous consumption of olive oil between cases of myocardial infarction and healthy controls. A cohort study would start with a roster of healthy individuals whose baseline diet would be recorded. They would then be followed up over several years to compare the occurrence of new cases of myocardial infarction between those consuming different levels of olive oil as recorded when they were healthy at baseline.

Ecological design

Epidemiological studies can be classified according to whether measurements of exposure and outcome are made on populations or individuals. Observational investigations in which the unit of observation and analysis is not the individual but a whole community or population are called ecological studies. In ecological studies, measures of exposure routinely collected and aggregated at the household, local, district, regional, national or international level are compared with outcome measures aggregated at the same level. An example of an ecological study would be plotting the mortality rates for colon cancer in several countries against the average intakes of saturated fat in these same countries and calculating the correlation between the two variables.

Studies considering the individual (instead of the population) as the unit of observation are always preferable because in an individually based study it is possible to relate exposure and outcome measures more directly, preventing many flaws that are likely to invalidate the findings of ecological studies. One of these flaws is known as the "ecological fallacy" and it is the bias resulting because an association observed between variables on an aggregated level does not necessarily represent the association that exists at an individual level. A major advantage of individually based studies over aggregated studies is that they allow the direct estimation of the risk of disease in relation to exposure.

Ecological studies measure diet less accurately because they use the average population intake as the exposure value for all individuals in the groups that are compared, leading to a high potential for biased ascertainment of diet–disease associations. Ecological studies, also termed correlation studies, may compare indicators of diet and health or disease within a single population over time to look for secular trends, or to compare the disease incidence rates and dietary intake patterns of migrant groups with those of comparable populations in the original and new country. Ecological comparisons have been important in hypothesizing diet and disease associations. Nevertheless, they are not able to establish causal relationships.

Epidemiological outcomes

Epidemiological outcomes must be clearly defined at the outset of a study. For example, a study of diet and cardiovascular disease (CVD) may specify that the outcome (CVD) is verified by specific clinical tests such as cardiac enzyme level or electrocardiographic changes. Taking the word of the patient or the doctor is not sufficient. Two main measures of the frequency for an outcome are used in epidemiology: prevalence and incidence.

Prevalence

The prevalence of an outcome is the proportion of subjects in a population who have that outcome at a given point in time. The numerator of prevalence is the number of existing cases and the denominator is the whole population:

$$\text{Prevalence} = \frac{\text{Existing cases}}{\text{Total population}}$$

Incidence

The incidence of an outcome is the proportion of new cases that occur in a population during a period of observation. The numerator of incidence is the number of new cases developing during the follow-up period, while the denominator is the total population at risk at the beginning of the follow-up time:

$$\text{Incidence} = \frac{\text{New cases}}{\text{Population initially at risk}}$$

When calculated in this fashion, incidence is a proportion. However, incidence can also be expressed as a rate (velocity or density), when the time during which each person is observed (i.e. person-time of observation) is included in the denominator. Then it is called incidence rate or incidence density and it is expressed as the number of new cases per person-time of observation.

Other epidemiological methods

Epidemiological studies have been also conducted to assess consumer attitudes to and beliefs about food, nutrition, physical patterns and health to provide policy makers, researchers and the food industry with data to promote health messages concerning the relation between food or nutrient intake and chronic diseases. These surveys seek information about influences on food choice, health determinants, criteria about perceptions of healthy eating, regular sources of nutritional information, expected benefits and barriers to healthy diet implementation, in order to identify consumers' knowledge, attitudes and beliefs concerning food and health interactions and to promote more focused nutrition education messages.

Meta-analysis and pooled analysis

The role of meta-analysis for systematically combining the results of published randomized trials has become routine, but its place in observational epidemiology has been controversial despite widespread use in social sciences. Some have argued that the combining of data from randomized trials is appropriate because statistical power is increased without concern for validity since the comparison groups have been randomized, but that in observational epidemiology the issue of validity is determined largely by confounding and bias rather than limitations of statistical power. Thus, the greater statistical precision obtained by the combination of data may be misleading because the findings may still be invalid. An alternative to combining published epidemiological data is to pool and analyze the primary data from all available studies on a topic that meets specified criteria. Ideally, this should involve the active collaboration of the original investigators, who are fully familiar with the data and its limitations. This kind of study conducted with a combination of the original data from several studies, is the basis of pooled analysis or pooling projects. In a pooled analysis, the range of dietary factors that can be addressed may be considerably greater than in the separate analyses because any one study will have few subjects in the extremes of intake and, sometimes, the studies will vary in distribution of dietary factors. The advantages of pooled analyses in nutritional epidemiology are so substantial that they are becoming common practice for important issues, such as alcoholic intake and breast cancer, body size and breast cancer, or alcohol beverages and coronary heart disease.

Analysis of epidemiological data requires careful consideration of the criteria for acceptable data quality, but also of the presentation of categorized or continuous independent variables and the application of empirical scores. The study of subgroup analysis and interactions and error correction are other issues of interest. Other limitations are the requirement of sample to be considered as representative, compliance, inaccuracies of information in retrospective studies and confounding effects by factors that are simultaneously associated with both the exposure and the outcome.

13.7 Perspectives on the future

Future nutrition research will develop new methods for studying those processes whereby cells, tissues and the whole body obtain and utilize substances contained in the diet to maintain their structure and function in a healthy manner. Particular emphasis will be paid to molecular and cellular based strategies devised to understand better the genetic basis of nutritional outcomes.

It can also be anticipated that many ongoing large cohort studies with tens of thousands of participants will provide valuable information on the role of nutrition in disease prevention, and also on nutritional management of a large number of diseases by dietary means, and gene–nutrient and gene–environment interactions. Moreover, pooling of data from several cohort studies may provide a very powerful tool to assess the benefits of a healthy diet. An increasing interest in a dietary pattern approach instead of a single nutrient approach will be seen in nutritional epidemiology in the forthcoming decades.

Nutritional epidemiology will also adopt a wider, multidisciplinary approach, with more studies concerning the impact of factors affecting social determinants of eating patterns, food supplies and nutrient utilization on health, to facilitate the decisions of policy makers, food industry managers, investigators and consumers.

Further reading

Alpha-Tocopherol, Beta Carotene Cancer Prevention Study Group. The effect of vitamin E and beta carotene on the incidence of lung cancer and other cancers in male smokers. N Engl J Med 1994; 330: 1029–1035.

Altman DG. Practical Statistics for Medical Research. London: Chapman & Hall, ITP, 1996.

Armitage P, Colton T. Encyclopaedia of Biostatistics. New York: Wiley and Sons, 1998.

Breslow NE. Statistics. Epidemiol Rev 2000; 22: 126–130.

Chang CK, Snook JT. The cholesterolaemic effects of dietary fats in cholesteryl ester transfer protein transgenic mice. Br J Nutr 2001; 85: 643–648.

Fernandez J, Martínez E, Prado M et al. Risk of non-fatal myocardial infection negatively associated with olive oil consumption: a case-control study in Spain. Int J Edemiol 2002; 31: 474–480.

Kumanyika SK. Epidemiology of what to eat in the 21st century. Epidemiol Rev 2000; 22: 87–94.

Leedy PD. Practical Research: Planning and Designs, Vol. 2. New York: Macmillan, 1980.

de Lorgeril M, Salen P, Martin JL et al. Mediterranean diet, traditional risk factors, and the rate of cardiovascular complications after myocardial infarction: final report of the Lyon Diet Heart Study. Circulation 1999; 99: 779–785.

Martínez-González MA, Martínez JA, Hu FB et al. Physical inactivity, sedentary lifestyle and obesity in the European Union. Int J Obes 1999; 23: 1192–1201.

Schone F, Leiterer M, Hartung H, Jahreis G, Tischendorf F. Rapeseed glucosinolates and iodine in sows affect the milk iodine concentration and the iodine status of piglets. Br J Nutr 2001; 85: 659–670.

14

Food Safety: A Public Health Issue of Growing Importance

Alan Reilly, Christina Tlustos, Wayne Anderson, Lisa O'Connor, Barbara Foley and Patrick Wall

---

Key messages

After reading this chapter the student should have an understanding of:

- the reasons for increased concern about the safety of food
- chronic effects of food-borne illness
- vulnerable groups
- economic consequences of food-borne illness

- emerging food-borne pathogens
- types and sources of bacterial contamination in foods
- bacteria
- food-borne viruses
- parasites
- transmissible spongiform encephalopathies and food
- chemical contamination and food
- possible control and prevention strategies
- food safety control programs.

14.1 Introduction

In recent years the reported incidence of food-borne diseases has continued to increase worldwide, with a number of extremely serious outbreaks occurring on virtually every continent. A major crisis of consumer confidence in the safety of food was triggered in 1996 when a possible link was discovered between the animal disease bovine spongiform encephalopathy (BSE) and the human disease new variant Creutzfeldt–Jacob disease (vCJD). In 1999, consumer confidence in the safety of the food supply was again brought into doubt when it was discovered that dioxin-contaminated feed had been fed to animals and that there was a possibility that toxic foods of animal origin were on sale around the world. Other scares relating to chemical residues and the emergence of antibiotic-resistant bacteria in the food chain have resulted in food safety becoming both a major public health concern and a political issue relating to global food trade.

International bodies, such as the World Health Organization (WHO) and the Food and Agricultural Organization of the United Nations (FAO), have worked since the 1960s on the development of food standards that aim to protect the health of consumers

and facilitate international trade of foods and animal feeding stuffs. This work is carried out by the Codex Alimentarius Commission (CAC), an intergovernmental body managed by FAO and WHO. Food safety standards developed by the CAC serve as the baseline for harmonization of global food standards, codes of practice, guidelines and recommendations. Harmonization of standards and recognition that different national food safety controls are equivalent are enshrined in the international agreements of the World Trade Organization (WTO). At national level, governments are evaluating their food safety controls and reviewing food safety legislation to ensure the best possible levels of consumer protection.

Globally, hundreds of millions of people are affected by illnesses caused by contaminated food. The toll in terms of human life and suffering is enormous, particularly among infants and young children, the elderly and other vulnerable groups. Food-borne diarrhea remains one of the most common illnesses of children, and one of the major causes of infant and childhood mortality in nonindustrialized countries. Although major in-roads have been made in decreasing infant mortality worldwide, WHO believes that children under five still suffer an estimated 1.5 billion annual

---

episodes of diarrhea which result in more than three million premature deaths. The implications of food-borne illness are extremely serious, particularly for poorer communities in nonindustrialized countries. The long-term consequences of repeated bouts of diarrhea are malnutrition and increased vulnerability to a wide range of diseases. Many infants do not survive under these circumstances and those who do can suffer from stunted physical and mental development. The importance of food-borne illness is often overlooked and the economic consequences are not fully appreciated at national level. In a nutritional context, food-borne illness is often associated with malnutrition due to increased nutrient losses through vomiting and diarrhea, loss of appetite and nutritional inadequacy, and increased nutritional requirements through elevated basal metabolic rate and elevated nitrogen losses. In recent times food safety issues are perceived by the public and governments alike as posing a greater potential risk to consumer health than nutritional aspects of the diet. To convey positive public health nutritional messages, nutritionists must understand the scientific basis of "food scares" that affect attitudes to food, nutrition and health. This chapter aims to highlight reasons for increased concern about the safety of food, the types and sources of biological and chemical contaminants in foods, and possible control and prevention strategies.

14.2 Factors contributing to food safety concerns

The increased incidence of food-borne diseases is due to a number of factors, that including changes that are taking place in food production on the farm, new systems of food processing, longer distribution chains, and new food preparation and storage methods. Changing lifestyles around the world are leading to a far greater reliance on convenience foods that are prepared outside the home. The food chain has become longer and more complex, and opportunities for the contamination of food have increased. International trade in foods has expanded dramatically over recent decades as a result of the globalization of world markets. Today, FAO estimates that over 500 million tonnes of food move in international trade, valued around US$400–500 billion annually. Globalization of food trade presents a major challenge to food safety control

authorities, in that food can become contaminated in the country where it is produced and can cause outbreaks of food-borne illness in another.

It is not unusual for an average meal to contain foods from many countries that have been produced and processed under different standards of food safety, increasing the risk of food-borne disease. Many large supermarkets in industrialized countries now carry up to 70 000 or more different food products that can contain ingredients from different continents. The intensification of food production and the consolidation of multinational food industries present opportunities for food-borne pathogens to infect large numbers of consumers. Many countries at different stages of development are experiencing rapid changes in their health and social environments. Government policies are focusing on decreasing public sector spending, resulting in poor surveillance of food-borne disease and an underestimation of the problem in many countries. In the poorer nonindustrialized countries other factors that contribute to an unsafe food supply are expanding urbanization, the increased dependence on stored foods, and insufficient access to safe water and essential facilities for safe food preparation.

Millions of travelers cross international borders every year, and the number is increasing. According to the World Tourism Organization, over 657 million people made international visits in 1999, at a value of US$455 billion. Many countries are investing heavily in developing their tourism industries. However, such investment is jeopardized whenever tourists return home with symptoms of diarrhea and vomiting caused by contaminated foods. It is estimated that, depending on the area visited, about 20–50% of travelers run the risk of contracting diarrhea. The growing popularity of "off-track" tourism in tropical regions can expose travelers to unexpected sources of food-borne parasites.

Chronic effects of food-borne illness

Food-borne diseases can be classified as either infections or intoxications. Food-borne infections are caused when viable micro-organisms are ingested and these can then multiply in the human body. Intoxications are caused when microbial or naturally occurring toxins are consumed in contaminated foods. Illnesses that relate to the consumption of foods that are contaminated with chemical toxins or micro-organisms are collectively referred to as food poisoning.

The health consequences of food-borne illness are varied and will depend on such factors as a person's age and state of health, the virulence of the pathogenic species, the type of disease and an individual's susceptibility. Symptoms are often mild and self-limiting in healthy individuals and people recover within a few days from acute health effects. Acute symptoms include diarrhea, stomach pain and cramps, vomiting, fever and jaundice. With the emergence of some newly recognized pathogens the health consequences of food-borne illness can be serious or even life-threatening. There is growing evidence that micro-organisms or their products are either directly or indirectly associated with long-term health effects. A number of chronic sequelae may result from food-borne infections, including reactive arthritis and rheumatoid syndromes, endocarditis, Reiter's syndrome, Guillain–Barré syndrome, renal disease, cardiac and neurological disorders, and nutritional and other malabsorptive disorders. It is generally accepted that chronic, secondary after-effect illnesses may occur in 2–3% of cases of food-borne infections and that the long-term consequences to human health may be greater than the acute disease.

The secondary chronic complications are not always linked epidemiologically to a food-borne illness because these data are not routinely collected and the symptoms are difficult to link temporally to a specific incident. Some cases, however, have been reported; for instance, in one outbreak, about 2% of patients developed reactive arthritis as a result of salmonellosis associated with drinking contaminated milk. It is estimated that up to 10% of patients with hemorrhagic colitis can go on to develop the hemolytic uremic syndrome (HUS), a life-threatening complication of *Escherichia coli* O157:H7 infection that is characterized by acute renal failure, hemolytic anemia and thrombocytopenia. *Listeria monocytogenes* is a bacterial pathogen causing serious human illness such as perinatal infections, septicemia and meningitis affecting mainly vulnerable groups.

Vulnerable groups

Some food-borne infections can be very serious in vulnerable groups such as the elderly, infants, young children, pregnant women, and malnourished, immunocompromised individuals. By the year 2025 more than 1000 million of the global population will be over 60 years old and more than two-thirds will live in developing countries. Aging is the regression of physiological functions with advancing years which predisposes the elderly to increased risk from food-borne, as well as other diseases. Many factors associated with the aging process influence the susceptibility of this group to food-borne infections and intoxications. For instance, aging is associated with a decline in gastric secretions, which may be one of the factors that makes the elderly more vulnerable to food-borne disease. The acid environment of the stomach is a major barrier to the entry of food-borne pathogens and a reduction in gastric acidity can increase the susceptibility to infection. There is an age-related decline in the body's immune function that renders the elderly more susceptible to infection. Where the diet of elderly people is poor or where such populations are malnourished and nutritionally deficient, immune responses to food-borne infections are adversely affected.

Loss of or reduced sensory abilities are associated with growing old, for instance the reduced ability to see, smell and taste foods. Reduced vision and mental facilities can lead to difficulties in choosing foods and comprehending specialized instructions on labels, such as cooking time, temperature requirements and expiry dates. Impaired vision may also lead to increased risk of cross-contamination during food preparation and reduced levels of hygiene in the kitchen environment. Loss of smell and taste can result in the inability to recognize that foods have spoiled and to the consumption of unsafe foods.

In addition to the elderly, the proportion of the population susceptible to food-borne infections is increasing. The number of immunocompromised individuals is also increasing, owing to human immunodeficiency virus (HIV) infection, malignancy and immunosuppressive treatments. In nonindustrialized countries, political unrest, war and famine lead to increased malnutrition and can expose poorer populations to increased risks of food-borne diseases.

Listeria monocytogenes mainly affects vulnerable groups such as immunocompromised individuals, pregnant women, neonates and the elderly. Although listeriosis occurs infrequently, at an annual incidence rate of 2–10 cases per million, the fatality rate is high, usually in the range of 20–30%. *Toxoplasma gondii*, a parasitic infection associated with eating raw or undercooked meat, can cause serious problems in pregnant women leading to death of the fetus or damage to the nervous system that may lead to blindness in later life.

The long-term health effects of food-borne trematode infections, which are common in south-east Asia, are liver and lung damage, and in severe cases death may occur.

With the increase in the number of immunocompromised individuals in the population, particularly patients with the acquired immunodeficiency syndrome (AIDS), many pathogens of an opportunistic nature, for instance *Cryptosporidium parvum* and *T. gondii*, have emerged as a health threat to this subset of the population. Infection due to *Vibrio vulnificus, which* is associated with eating raw oysters harvested from warm coastal environments, may be fatal in susceptible individuals. Results from a study in the USA showed the case–fatality rate for patients with pre-existing liver disease to be 63% and for those without liver disease 23%.

Economic consequences of food-borne illness

As well as morbidity and mortality associated with food-borne diseases, there are direct economic costs to society in treating sick people. There are also economic losses due to food being rejected in export markets and loss of consumer confidence in brand names on the domestic market. Consumer confidence in foods can be lost at a moment's notice, for instance an outbreak of food-borne illness associated with *E. coli* O157:H7 in 1996 in Japan caused a major loss in consumer confidence in products of animal origin, with a 56% reduction in the sales of beef and a 42% reduction in the sales of fish. Each year in the USA, food-borne diseases cost billions of dollars. Government sources in the USA estimate the cost of human illnesses of seven food-borne pathogens to be between US$5.6 and 9.4 billion annually. The cost of salmonellosis in England and Wales in 1992 was estimated at between US$560 and 800 million. Over 70% of costs were directly associated with treatment and investigation of cases, and costs to the economy of sickness related to absence from work. Estimates made in 1999 showed that food-borne diseases annually cause approximately 76 million illnesses, 325 000 hospitalizations and 5000 deaths in the USA. The BSE crisis in Britain is predicted to cost over US$5.5 billion. These costs are associated with the loss of export sales, compensating farmers, paying slaughterhouses, and research and control measures. The dioxin crisis in Belgium in 1999 saw the fall of the national government and economic costs in excess of US$2 billion to the Belgium economy. During the cholera outbreak in 1991, Peru lost over US$700 million due to rejection of fish and fishery product exports. Over a 3-month period following the start of this cholera epidemic, US$70 million was lost owing to the closure of food service establishments and a decrease in tourism.

The true estimates of food-borne disease and the likely economic costs are unknown. In industrialized countries only a small proportion of cases of food-borne diseases comes to the notice of health services and even fewer are investigated. Very few non industrialized countries have established food-borne disease reporting systems, and in those that have, only a small fraction of cases is reported. The incidence of food-borne disease is likely to be far higher than in industrialized countries because of such factors as poor nutritional status, inadequate sanitation, low standards of hygiene and the reduced likelihood of immediate medical attention. There are many hidden costs associated with food-borne illnesses. Tourists will shun regions with a high incidence of food-borne illness, as will multinational firms choosing the location of foreign investment. Repeated bouts of diarrhea damage children's mental and physical development and play havoc with their schooling.

Increase in numbers of virulent microbes: emerging food-borne pathogens

During the twentieth century improvements in sewage treatment, milk pasteurization and water disinfection all led to the control of food-borne and water-borne diseases such as typhoid and tuberculosis. However, in the last two decades new food-borne pathogens have emerged. The reasons are complex but can be attributed to current intensive food production systems and the globalization of the food supply. Food-borne organisms such as *E. coli* O157, *Campylobacter jejuni* and *Salmonella enteritidis* phage type 4 were virtually unknown in the 1970s, but have come to prominence as virulent pathogens associated with foods of animal origin. *Cyclospora cayetanensis* emerged as a food-borne pathogen in 1995 when it was associated with outbreaks of illness traced to imported raspberries in the USA. *Cryptosporidium parvum* emerged as a pathogen of worldwide significance during the 1990s and has been linked to contaminated drinking water and to a range of foods including salads, unpasteurized milk and apple juice. Some known pathogens such as *L. monocytogenes* have only recently been shown to be predominantly food borne and have increased in importance with the expansion of the cold chain for food distribution. *Listeria monocytogenes* is a psychrophile (cold loving) and grows at low temperatures (2–8°C) in coleslaw, pâté and soft cheeses. Many of these emerging pathogens have common characteristics in that most have an animal reservoir and they do not usually cause serious illness in the animal host.

During the 1980s and 1990s, antibiotic-resistant food-borne pathogens emerged that are associated with the inappropriate use of antibiotics in animal husbandry. For example, *Salmonella typhimurium* DT 104 routinely shows resistance to five different antibiotics. Strains of *Salmonella* and *Campylobacter* are showing resistance to fluroquinolines since these compounds were introduced for use in animals.

In recent years a range of new food vectors has been implicated in the spread of these emerging pathogens. For instance, the internal contents of an egg were always presumed to be safe to eat raw and uncooked eggs have been traditionally used in many different food products. This situation has changed with the emergence of *S. enteritidis* infection in egg-laying flocks, resulting in contamination in shell eggs and a major increase in food-borne illness worldwide associated with uncooked eggs. Outbreaks of *Salmonella* poisoning have also been associated with raw lettuce and beansprouts. *Escherichia coli* O157 has been implicated in illness due to the consumption of radish sprouts, lettuce and unpasteurized apple juice. Recent studies have shown that it is possible for pathogens such as *Salmonella* and *E. coli* O157 to enter the vascular system of beansprouts during the sprouting process, when the pathogens are present in the water used for seed germination. Similarly, these pathogens have been shown to enter the vascular system of lettuce leaves when they are present in the water used in the preparation of ready-to-eat salad packs.

In summary, factors contributing to food safety concerns include:

- chronic effects of food-borne illness
- vulnerable groups
- economic consequences of food-borne illness
- increase in numbers of virulent microbes.

The major cause of food-borne diseases is the consumption of microbiologically contaminated foods. There are many types of food-borne pathogens, including bacteria, viruses and parasites.

14.3 Food-borne bacteria

Bacteria can cause food poisoning by:

- production of harmful toxins in the food. This occurs when organisms such as *Clostridium botulinum* and *Staphylococcus aureus* grow in foods;
- direct infection of the intestinal tract, e.g. when *Campylobacter* or *Salmonella* species are ingested in contaminated foods. Some bacteria in this group also form toxins in the intestine following infection, e.g. *Clostridium perfringens* and verocytotoxin-producing *Escherichia coli* (VTEC).

Characteristics of food-borne bacterial intoxication and infections are summarized in Tables 14.1 and 14.2, respectively. The following is a summary of some of the key features of these bacteria.

Clostridium botulinum

Clostridium botulinum produces a neurotoxin that is one of the most poisonous substances known to man. Food-borne botulism occurs when food becomes contaminated with spores from the environment, which are not destroyed by initial cooking or processing. If the food provides a suitable environment for growth the spores will germinate, leading to toxin production. The toxin is heat sensitive and so a further heat treatment of the food would prevent illness. Botulism can be prevented by using food preservation methods that are designed to inhibit the growth of *C. botulinum*. For example, low acid (pH > 4.4) canned foods are heat treated to 121°C for 3 min (known as the "botulism cook") or equivalent.

Staphylococcus aureus

By contrast to other forms of food poisoning, food handlers play a major role in the transmission of this organism. *Staphylococcus aureus* is carried in the nose and throat of approximately 40% of healthy individuals and as such can be easily transferred to food via the hands. Most foods that have been associated with *S. aureus* poisoning have been ready-to-eat, often precooked foods that have been contaminated by poor handling practices and stored at incorrect temperatures. *Staphylococcus aureus* must grow to levels of $>10^5$ cells/g before producing the heat-stable staphylococcal toxin. This type of food poisoning can be minimized by the use of good personal hygiene and handling practices to prevent the contamination of ready-to-eat foods.

Table 14.1 Characteristics of food-borne bacterial intoxications

Food-borne bacteria	Onset of illness	(a) Symptoms (b) Infectious dose	Duration of illness	Temperature (°C) Min.	Temperature (°C) Opt.	Min. pH[a]	Min. A_w[a]	Forms spores	Heat resistance	(a) Gram stain (b) Aerobic/anaerobic	(a) Source (b) Associated foods[b]
Clostridium botulinum Group I (proteolytic)	12–36 h, but may be as long as 8 days	(a) Blurred and/or double vision, dryness of the mouth followed by difficulties in swallowing and finally breathing. Vomiting and mild diarrhea may occur in the early stages (b) 0.005–0.5 µg toxin	Variable (from days to months)	10	30–40	4.6	0.94	Yes	Toxin: destroyed by 5 min at 85°C Spores: $D_{100} = 25$ min	(a) Gram positive (b) Obligate anaerobe	(a) Soil, sediment, intestinal tract of fish and mammals (b) Canned foods, smoked and salted fish, honey
Group II (nonproteolytic)				3.3	25–37	5.0	0.97		Spores: $D_{100} < 0.1$ min		
Staphylococcus aureus	1–6 h	(a) Nausea, vomiting, abdominal pain and diarrhea (b) <1.0 µg toxin (>10^5 cells needed to produce toxin)	1–2 days	7	35–37	4.5	0.83	No	Toxin: heat resistant (i.e. able to withstand boiling for up to 30 min)	(a) Gram positive (b) Facultative anaerobe	(a) Exposed skin lesions, nose, throat and hands (b) Generally foods of animal origin that have been physically handled and have not received a subsequent bactericidal treatment
Bacillus cereus Emetic	1–5 h	(a) Nausea and vomiting (b) >10^5 cells (12–32 µg toxin/kg)	6–24 h	10	30–35	4.3	0.95	Yes	Toxin: extremely heat resistant (i.e. can withstand 121°C for 90 min) Spores: $D_{121} = 0.03$–2.35 min	(a) Gram positive (b) Facultative anaerobe	(a) Soil, dust and vegetation (b) Cooked rice, cereals and cereal-based products, herbs and spices

[a] Under otherwise optimal conditions; limits will vary according to strain, temperature, type of acid (in the case of pH), solute (in the case of A_w) and other factors.
[b] Not an exhaustive list.
Min.: minimum; Opt.: optimal; A_w: water activity.

Table 14.2 Characteristics of food-borne bacterial infections

Food-borne bacteria	Onset of illness	(a) Symptoms (b) Infectious dose	Duration of illness	Temperature (°C) Min.	Temperature (°C) Opt.	Min. pH[a]	Min. A_w^a	Heat resistance	(a) Gram stain (b) Aerobic/ anaerobic	(a) Source (b) Associated foods[b]
Bacillus cereus Diarrheal	8–16 h	(a) Abdominal pain and diarrhea (b) >10^5 cells	12–24 h	10	30–35	4.3	0.95	HS but can form heat-resistant spores: (D_{121} = 0.03–2.35 min)	(a) Gram positive (b) Facultative anaerobe	(a) Soil and dust (b) Meat, milk, vegetables, fish and soups
Clostridium perfringens	12–18 h (can be 8–22 h)	(a) Diarrhea and severe abdominal pain (b) >10^6 cells	24 h	15	43–45	5.0	0.95	HS, but forms heat-resistant spores (D_{95} = 1.3–2.8 min)	(a) Gram positive (b) Obligate anaerobe	(a) Soil and animal feces (b) Meat, poultry, gravy, dried and precooked foods
Campylobacter	2–5 days	(a) Moderate to severe diarrhea. Severe abdominal pain and sometimes bloody diarrhea. Vomiting is rare. Complications are uncommon but include bacteremia, reactive arthritis and Guillain–Barré syndrome (GBS) (b) <500 cells	1–7 days	32	42–43	4.9	0.98	HS	(a) Gram negative (b) Fastidious microaerophile	(a) Chickens, birds, cattle, flies and water (b) Undercooked chicken, raw milk, beef, pork, lamb, shellfish and water
VTEC *Escherichia coli*	1–6 days	(a) Diarrhea and severe abdominal cramps, bloody diarrhea, hemorrhagic colitis (HC), approx. 5% (mostly children) develop hemolytic uremic syndrome (HUS) (b) 10–100	4–6 days (if HUS does not develop)	7	37	4.5	0.97	HS	(a) Gram negative (b) Facultative anaerobe	(a) Cattle, sheep, pigs, deer (b) Undercooked beef burgers, raw milk, radish sprouts
Listeria monocytogenes	3 days to 10 weeks	(a) Flu-like symptoms, meningitis and/or septicemia. While pregnant women may experience a mild flu-like illness, infection which may result in miscarriage, stillbirth or birth of a severely ill infant (b) Unknown	Days to weeks	0	30–37	4.3	0.92	HS	(a) Gram positive (b) Facultative anaerobe	(a) Soil, improperly made silage (b) Fresh soft cheeses, raw milk, deli meats, pâté and hot dogs, raw vegetables, ice cream and seafood

Organism	Incubation period	Symptoms and infective dose	Duration	Min. temp (°C)	Opt. temp (°C)	Min. pH	Min. A_w	Heat	Characteristics	Sources[b]
Salmonella	Usually 12–36 h but may be 6–72 h	(a) Fever, abdominal pain, diarrhea, nausea and sometimes vomiting. It can be fatal in the very young and old and those with weakened immune systems due to illness (b) ~10^6 cells; however, under certain conditions and with certain certain foods (e.g. chocolate or cheese where the high fat content and low water activity appears to protect the organisms from stomach acidity), small numbers (<100 cells) are sufficient to cause illness in the very young and the elderly	2–5 days	7	35–37	4.0	0.93	HS	(a) Gram negative (b) Facultative anaerobe	(a) Water, soil, animal feces, raw poultry, raw meats and raw seafood (b) Raw meats, poultry, eggs, raw milk and other dairy products, raw fruits and vegetables (e.g. alfalfa sprouts and melons)
Vibrio cholera serogroup non-O1	1–3 days	(a) Diarrhea, abdominal cramps, fever, some vomiting and nausea (b) >10^6 cells	Diarrhea lasts 6–7 days	10	37	5.0	0.97	HS	(a) Gram negative (b) Facultative anaerobe	(a) Coastal waters, raw oysters (b) Shellfish
Vibrio parahaemolyticus	12–24 h	(a) Diarrhea, abdominal cramps, nausea, vomiting, headache, fever, chills (b) >10^6 cells	<7 days	5	37	4.8	0.94	HS	(a) Gram negative (b) Facultative anaerobe	(a) Coastal and estuarine waters, raw shellfish (b) Fish and raw shellfish
Vibrio vulnificans	16 h	(a) Wound infections, gastroenteritis, primarily septicemia (b) Unknown in healthy individuals but in predisposed <100 cells	Days to weeks	8	37	5	0.96	HS	(a) Gram negative (b) Facultative anaerobe	(a) Coastal waters, sediment, plankton, shellfish (b) Oysters, clams, crabs
Yersinia enterocolitica	3–7 days	(a) Diarrhea abdominal pain and fever. Intestinal pain, especially in young adults, may be confused with appendicitis (b) Unknown	1–3 weeks	−1.3	25–37	4.1	0.96	HS	(a) Gram negative (b) Facultative anaerobe	(a) Wide range of animals (e.g. pigs, dogs, cats) and water (b) Undercooked pork, raw milk and water

[a] Under otherwise optimal conditions; limits will vary according to strain, temperature, type of acid (in the case of pH), solute (in the case of A_w) and other factors.

[b] Not an exhaustive list.

HS: Heat-sensitive cells destroyed by typical cooking temperatures; Min.: minimum; Opt.: optimal; A_w: water activity; VTEC: verocytotoxin-producing *E. coli*.

A notable feature of this organism is its ability to grow in salty environments.

Bacillus cereus

Bacillus cereus is ubiquitous in the environment and is found on virtually all agricultural commodities. Most incidents of food-borne illness associated with this organism have been in cereal products or foods containing cereals or spices. The vegetative cells are inactivated at normal cooking temperatures; however, their spores are quite heat resistant. *Bacillus cereus* produces several toxins, only two of which are responsible for food poisoning: an emetic toxin and a diarrheal enterotoxin. The emetic toxin is produced in food when vegetative cells sporulate. Rice dishes have been most often implicated because rice, particularly in mass catering, is often precooked, cooled, stored and reheated before consumption. Spores if present may survive the initial cooking, and if the rice is left in warm conditions (i.e. either not cooled to <5°C within a few hours and/or not kept at <5°C before thorough reheating) *B. cereus* can form the heat-stable emetic toxin which will survive reheating. The diarrheal enterotoxin is produced when spores germinate in the gastrointestinal tract after consumption of contaminated food.

Clostridium perfringens

Clostridium perfringens causes a much less severe but more common food poisoning than *C. botulinum*. Illness results from the consumption of food containing high numbers of cells ($>10^6$/g) followed by enterotoxin production in the intestine. When contaminated food (typically meat) is cooked, the heat drives off the dissolved oxygen and induces sporulation. As cooling occurs the spores germinate and the vegetative cells continue to multiply, unless the food is cooled rapidly and kept refrigerated. *Clostridium perfringens* produces at least 11 separate toxins in addition to the enterotoxin primarily responsible for symptoms. At its optimum temperature, *C. perfringens* has one of the fastest rates of growth of any bacterium.

Escherichia coli

Escherichia coli is part of the normal flora of the intestinal tract of humans and warm-blooded animals. Its presence in food or water is generally an indication of fecal contamination. Many strains are harmless; however, some cause gastroenteritis or more serious forms of illness. Pathogenic strains are grouped as follows:

- enteroaggregative (EAggEC)
- enteropathogenic (EPEC)
- enteroinvasive (EIEC)
- enterotoxigenic (ETEC)
- verocytotoxin-producing *E. coli* (VTEC), also called shiga-toxin-producing *E. coli* (STEC). Enterohemorrhagic *E. coli* (EHEC), which causes HUS, is a subset of VTEC.

In nonindustrialized countries, diarrhea caused by pathogenic *E. coli* is a major cause of morbidity and mortality. In industrialized countries, where hygiene standards are generally higher, little diarrheal illness has been associated with *E. coli* other than traveler's diarrhea in which ETEC strains play a role. VTEC, however, is of considerable concern in the developed world, due to the severity of the illness. The organism is not particularly heat resistant and is easily killed by cooking, but the low infective dose means that foods must be cooked thoroughly and be protected after cooking from cross-contamination with raw foods. Foods of bovine origin, such as undercooked beef burgers or unpasteurized milk, have been implicated in a number of VTEC outbreaks.

Campylobacter

Campylobacter jejuni is the most common cause of bacterial food poisoning in many industrialized countries. These are fragile organisms that require microaerophilic conditions for growth and do not survive or multiply very well on foods. However, the low infectious dose means that a small level of contamination may result in illness. Compared with other food-borne bacteria with low infective doses, relatively few outbreaks have been identified. Undercooked poultry and other meats, unpasteurized milk and water are considered to be the principal sources of food-borne campylobacteriosis. *Campylobacter* species are especially common in birds, but have also been isolated from a wide range of animals. Wild birds are considered to be an important reservoir of infection for domestic and food animals.

Salmonella

Salmonella species can be split into more than 2000 serotypes according to the Kauffman–White surface antigens scheme. A small number of serotypes accounts for most of the infections, with *S. typhimurium* and *S. enteritidis* predominating. *Salmonella typhi* and *S. paratyphi* are responsible for the so-called enteric fevers (typhoid and paratyphoid, respectively), which are primarily water-borne. *Salmonella* is the second most commonly reported bacterial cause of gastroenteritis after *Campylobacter*. Undercooked (or improperly heat treated) food from infected food animals is most commonly implicated. Egg-associated salmonellosis is an important public health problem in the USA and Europe. It is caused by *S. enteritidis* that infects the ovaries of apparently healthy hens, which then lay contaminated eggs. If the eggs are eaten raw or undercooked, salmonellosis may result.

Listeria monocytogenes

Listeria monocytogenes causes serious human illness such as perinatal infections, septicemia and meningitis. In pregnant women it can cause a flu-like illness, which can result in miscarriage, stillbirth or birth of a severely ill infant. More recently, it has been recognized that *L. monocytogenes* can cause mild gastrointestinal symptoms. Listeriosis is a comparatively rare but very serious human illness with a case–fatality ratio of around 20%. Highly susceptible individuals include pregnant women, neonates, elderly people and immunocompromised individuals. *Listeria monocytogenes* is ubiquitous in the environment and so can be transferred to foods from a wide variety of sources. Foods associated with transmission are characteristically highly processed, have extended shelf-lives at refrigeration temperatures, are capable of supporting the growth of *L. monocytogenes* and are consumed without further cooking. *Listeria monocytogenes* is psychrotrophic, i.e. potentially capable of growing, albeit slowly, at refrigeration temperatures as low as 0°C.

Vibrio species

Vibrio species are indigenous marine halophilic (salt loving) or halotolerant organisms that are commonly isolated from estuarine and coastal environments. They are particularly prevalent in warm tropical waters and can be isolated in temperate zones during warm summer months. Three species of *Vibrio* that dominate as food-borne pathogens are *Vibrio parahaemolyticus*, *V. cholerae* and *V. vulnificus*. *Vibrio cholerae* non-O1 is related to *V. cholerae* O1 (the organism that causes Asi-

atic or epidemic cholera), but causes a disease reported to be less severe than cholera. Consumption of raw, improperly cooked or cooked but recontaminated shellfish may lead to gastroenteritis. It has been generally believed that water was the main vehicle for transmission; however, an increasing number of cases has been associated with food. *Vibrio parahaemolyticus* can be considered to be the leading cause of seafood-borne bacterial gastroenteritis. It is frequently isolated from fish both from marine and brackish-water environments. *Vibrio vulnificus* is considered to be one of the most invasive and rapidly lethal of human pathogens. Infection starts with a gastrointestinal illness and rapidly progresses to a septicemic condition. It is most frequently associated with the consumption of raw oysters. Human infections from this organism are rare and the populations most at risk are those with underlying illnesses or those who are immunocompromised.

Yersinia enterocolitica

Yersinia enterocolitica is psychrotrophic and is known to be quite resistant to freezing, surviving in frozen foods for extended periods. The organism is present in a wide range of animals, especially pigs. It is also found in the environment, including water, but most of these environmental strains are not pathogenic. Humans are another source of *Y. enterocolitica* and a food handler has been implicated in at least one outbreak in the USA. Milk and pork have been implicated in outbreaks, especially in countries where the pork is eaten raw. The incidence of yersiniosis is unknown, but it is often reported in the cooler regions of Europe and North America. Symptoms can vary, with diarrhea and abdominal pain being the most common. Intestinal pain can sometimes be so severe as to be confused with appendicitis.

14.4 Food-borne viruses

It is only in recent years that the role of viruses as etiological agents of food-borne illness have emerged. A recent Centers for Disease Control (CDC) report from the USA in 2000, on surveillance of food-borne disease outbreaks from 1993 to 1997, revealed that viruses accounted for 6% of all food-borne outbreaks and 8% of cases. Hepatitis A accounted for the majority of these, followed by Norwalk-like virus (NLV). In addition, hepatitis A is the only notifiable food-borne viral disease in many countries, so it is highly likely that the incidence of food-borne illness attributed to viruses is grossly underestimated. These failures in attributing viral illness to food have mainly been due to the diagnostic difficulties in detecting viruses in an implicated food and underreporting owing to the mild nature of illness.

Food-borne viruses are generally enteric, being transmitted by the fecal–oral route. However, transmission by person-to-person contact and via contaminated water is common, as with other enteric viruses. Hepatitis A and NLV are more commonly transmitted via foods than other food-borne viruses. The most important food-borne viruses are: hepatitis A, NLV, astrovirus and rotavirus. These will now be discussed individually in more detail.

Hepatitis A virus

Hepatitis A is one of the more severe food-borne diseases. The illness results from immune destruction of infected liver cells, and a few weeks of debility are common (Table 14.3).

Infections are more likely to be asymptomatic or mild in young children than in adolescents or adults. The virus can be shed in feces for up to 14 days before the onset of illness. It is therefore possible for an infected food handler with poor personal hygiene (hand-washing, in particular) to contaminate food

during this period. The virus may be shed in the feces for 1–2 weeks after onset of symptoms.

Food becomes contaminated with this virus via infected persons or via fecally contaminated water, as is usual with shellfish. Examples of other foods implicated in hepatitis A outbreaks are oysters, raw mussels and drinking water, bakery products and caviar. Hepatitis A has been shown to be more heat resistant than most enteric viruses and is also quite resistant to drying. The virus is susceptible to chlorination treatment, however, and water-borne hepatitis A outbreaks have been linked to untreated water.

Norwalk-like viruses

Norwalk virus was the first gastroenteritis virus reported to be food borne. This group of viruses has recently been classified as members of the calicivirus family. The term "small round structured viruses" (SRSV) was originally applied to these agents owing to their appearance under the electron microscope. NLV are difficult to detect, especially from foods.

Exposure is by contact with infected individuals or fecally contaminated water or other materials. Shellfish (bivalve molluscs) have been the predominant food vehicle. Shellfish beds may frequently become contaminated with human feces from sewage discharge. Aerosolization of vomitus-containing virus particles

Table 14.3 Characteristics of the illnesses caused by hepatitis A and Norwalk-like virus

Hepatitis A (Picornavirus)	Norwalk-like virus (Calicivirus)
Properties	
Particles are featureless spheres 28 nm in diameter, single-stranded RNA coated with protein	Particles are spheres 25–35 nm in diameter, single-stranded RNA coated with protein that has characteristic supped surface depressions
Infection	
Infection via intestine to liver, incubation period 15–20 days (mean 28 days)	Infection of intestinal lining, incubation 24–48 h
Illness	
Illness from immune destruction of infected liver cells: fever, malaise, anorexia, nausea, abdominal discomfort, often followed by jaundice; severity tends to increase with age: ranges from inapparent infection to weeks of debility, occasionally with permanent sequelae	Nausea, vomiting, diarrhea, etc., lasting for 24–48 h
Shedding	
Shedding of virus peaks during the second half of the incubation period (10–14 days), usually ends by 7 days after onset of jaundice	During illness (in vomitus and feces), possibly 7 days after onset
Diagnosis	
Diagnosis is based on detection of IgM class antibody hepatitis A virus in the patient's blood serum (kits available)	Detection of virus in stool ELISA or PCR or of antibody against the virus in patient's blood serum; no standard methods, reagents not readily available for most agents
Immunity	
Immunity is durable (possibly lifelong) after infection	Apparently transient

ELISA: enzyme-linked immunosorbent assay; PCR: polymerase chain reaction.

has been proposed as another mode of transmission of the virus and may also be a source of food contamination. Sensitive detection assays have now revealed that shedding of the virus in feces may continue for up to a week after the illness subsides.

Other viruses transmitted via foods

There are many other groups of enteric and gastroenteritis-causing viruses, but these are reported to be associated with foods either infrequently or not at all.

Astroviruses

Under the electron microscope, astroviruses appear as small, round viruses that have surface projections resembling a five- or six-pointed star (Greek *astron*, "star"). The illness differs from the NLV in that the incubation period is longer (3–4 days), the duration of illness is longer (often lasting for 7–14 days) and vomiting is less common, with diarrhea being the predominant symptom. In addition, the very young (<1 year) appear to be the most susceptible group, whereas NLV affect all age groups. Many astrovirus outbreaks have been reported to occur in crèches, schools, hospital wards and nursing homes, but in many cases there was no well-defined mode of transmission. One large food-borne outbreak has been reported. In Osaka, Japan, in 1991, a large outbreak of acute gastroenteritis occurred, affecting 4700 teachers and pupils from 14 schools in the city. The source was linked to contaminated food from a common supplier.

Rotaviruses

Serogroup A rotaviruses are the single most important cause of infantile gastroenteritis worldwide, affecting an estimated 130 million infants and causing 873 000 deaths every year. The rotavirus genome consists of 11 segments of double-stranded RNA surrounded by a double-shelled viral capsid. When examined by electron microscopy, the double-shelled particles resemble a wheel-like structure morphologically (Latin *rota*, "wheel"). The incubation period of the illness is 1–3 days, and illness is characterized by fever, vomiting and diarrhea. Although the majority of rotavirus infections involve infants, outbreaks of food-borne and waterborne disease affecting all age groups have been reported, albeit infrequently.

Other viruses

Picornaviruses other than hepatitis A can also be transmitted by the food-borne route. Polioviruses are transmitted by food but virulent strains of this agent are now extremely rare. Coxsackie virus and echovirus (also members of the picornavirus family) have been associated with food-borne outbreaks, but data are limited. Hepatitis E has been linked to a number of water-borne outbreaks but there has been no association with food. One food-borne outbreak of parvovirus was reported, linked to consumption of cockles.

14.5 Food-borne parasites

Food-borne parasitic diseases are a major public health problem affecting millions of people, predominantly in nonindustrialized countries. The incidence of parasitic disease associated with the consumption of foods of animal origin has declined in industrialized countries in recent years, where improvements in animal husbandry and meat inspection have led to considerable safety and quality gains. The situation in nonindustrialized countries is very different, in that these diseases are associated with poor standards of sanitation and hygiene, low educational standards and extreme poverty.

Parasites are organisms that live off other living organisms, known as hosts. They may be transmitted from animals to humans, from humans to humans, or from humans to animals. Food-borne parasitic disease occurs when the infective stages of parasites are eaten in raw or partially cooked protein foods, or in raw vegetables and fruits that are inadequately washed before consumption. These organisms then live and reproduce within the tissues and organs of infected human and animal hosts, and are often excreted in feces. The parasites involved in food-borne disease usually have complex life cycles involving one or two intermediate hosts (Figure 14.1). The food-borne parasites known to cause disease in humans are broadly classified as helminths (multicellular worms) and protozoa (single-celled microscopic organisms). These include the major helminthic groups of trematodes, nematodes and cestodes, and some of the emerging protozoan pathogens, such as cryptosporidia and cyclospora. The illnesses they can cause range from mild discomfort to debilitating illness and possibly death.

These infections occur endemically in some 20 countries, where it is estimated that over 40 million people worldwide, mainly in eastern and southern Asia, are affected. Of major concern are the fish-borne trematode infections. The trematode species concerned all have similar life cycles involving two intermediate hosts. The

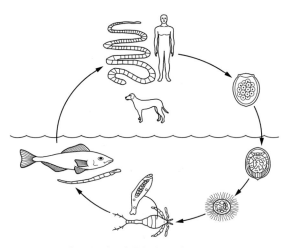

Figure 14.1 Life cycle of *Diphyllobothrium latum*.

definitive host is man and other mammals. Food-borne infection takes place through the consumption of raw, undercooked or otherwise underprocessed freshwater fish or crustaceans containing the infective stages (metacercariae) of these parasites. Table 14.4 summarizes the distribution, the principal reservoirs and freshwater fish or crustaceans involved in the transmission of these parasites in the food chain. The most important parasites with respect to the numbers of people affected are species of the genera *Clonorchis*, *Opisthorchis* and *Paragonimus*. The diseases caused by food-borne trematodes include cholangiocarcinoma, gallstones, severe liver disease and gastrointestinal problems.

Nematodes

The food-borne roundworms of primary importance in humans belong to the phylum Nematoda and are known as nematodes. Undercooked or raw fishery products and pork meat are the usual foods involved.

Where fishery products are the food vector, the definitive hosts of roundworms causing disease in humans are piscivorous marine mammals such as seals. Marine invertebrates and fish are the two intermediate hosts and humans are infected when they consume raw or minimally processed products. Fish are the secondary hosts and are infected when they consume the invertebrate primary host or fish that are already infected. There are many species of nematodes and a very large number of species of fish, worldwide, that are known to act as intermediate hosts. The most common species of nematode causing disease in humans is *Anisakis simplex*, sometimes referred to as the herringworm. The

other species involved in anisakiasis in North America, Europe and Japan is *Pseudoterranova decipiens* (the codworm or sealworm).

Nematodes are commonly present in fish caught in the wild, most frequently in the liver and belly cavity, but can also occur in the flesh. Anisakiasis is an uncommon disease because the parasite is killed by heating (55°C for 1 min), and by freezing (−20°C for 24 h). There is a risk of illness from fishery products consumed raw, for example sushi, or after only mild processing, such as salting at low concentrations or smoking. Many countries now require that fish used for these mildly processed products be frozen before processing or before sale.

Trichinella spiralis is the cause of trichinosis in humans. This most commonly results from the consumption of contaminated raw or undercooked pork or pork products. Isolated cases have been reported from the consumption of bear meat and ground beef in the USA. The incidence of trichinosis can be controlled by avoiding feeding infected waste foods to pigs or by fully cooking pig swill. Freezing pork products (−15°C for 20 days) or thorough cooking (78°C at the thermal center) before human consumption will destroy trichina larvae.

Cestodes

Cestodes are tapeworms and the species of major concern associated with consumption of fish is the fish tapeworm, *Diphyllobothrium latum*. Humans are one of the definitive hosts, along with other fish-eating mammals. Freshwater copepods and fish are the intermediate hosts. The plerocercoid is present in the flesh of the fish and infects humans following the consumption of raw or minimally processed fish. The recorded epidemiology of *D. latum* shows it to be prevalent in many countries worldwide. The incidence is relatively high in Scandinavia and the Baltic region of Europe. Diphyllobothriasis in humans can be prevented by cooking or freezing fish before consumption. Infections with tapeworms are also associated with eating undercooked or raw pork and beef.

Taenia saginata (the beef tapeworm) and *Taenia solium* (the pork tapeworm) are unique among parasites in that they have no vascular, respiratory or digestive systems. Humans are their definitive hosts and they rely solely on the human body for all of their nourishment. Infections can be prevented by sanitary disposal and treatment of human waste and by thorough cooking and freezing of contaminated pork and beef.

Table 14.4 Food-borne trematode infections

Parasite	Distribution	Principal reservoirs (other than humans)	Food involved in transmission to humans	Disease
Liver flukes				
Clonorchis sinensis	Widespread in China, including Taiwan and Hong Kong, Macao, Japan, Korea and Vietnam. Migrants to many other countries found to be infected; cases in Hawaii attributed to consumption of fish imported from China	Dogs, cats and many other species of fish-eating mammals	Many species (c. 110) of freshwater fish, mainly Cyprinidae, e.g. carp, roach and dace, most important being *Pseudorasbora parva*. Metacercariae in fish muscles	The liver flukes, *Opisthorchis viverrini*, *O. felineus* and *Clonorchis sinensis*, are biologically similar, food-borne trematodes that chronically infect the bile ducts and, more rarely, the pancreatic duct and gallbladder of humans and other mammals
Opisthorchis felineus	Commonwealth of Independent States (CIS), eastern and central Europe	Cats, dogs and other mammals that eat fish or fish waste	Freshwater fish of family Cyprinidae, e.g. whitefish, carp and tench (*Tinca tinca*). Metacercariae in muscle and subcutaneous tissue	
Opisthorchis viverrini	Laos and north-eastern Thailand (Mekong River basin)	Dogs, cats, fishing cats (*Felis viverrina*) and other mammals that feed on fish and fish waste	Some 10 species of freshwater fish including *Puntius orphoides* and *Hampala dispar*. Metacercariae in fish muscles	
Faciola hepatica	Europe, the Middle East, the Far East, Africa, Australia, USA	Sheep, cattle		Inflammation of the bile ducts which causes thickening of the lining and eventually leads to fibrosis
Intestinal flukes				
Heterophyes heterophyes	Mediterranean basin, especially Egypt and eastern Asia	Dogs, cats, jackals, foxes, pelicans, hawks and black kite	Brackish water and freshwater fish, especially mullet (*Mugil spp.*), *Tilapia* and others. In Japan, species of fish genera *Acanthogobius* and *Glossogobius* also involved. Metacercariae in muscle and skin	The parasite can irritate the lining of the small intestine, resulting in diarrhea and abdominal pain. In some instances the lining of the small intestine breaks down, and the eggs produced by the parasite enter the bloodstream. Once in the bloodstream the eggs can be carried to other organs where they can cause significant pathology, especially in the liver, heart and brain

(Continued)

Table 14.4 (Continued)

Parasite	Distribution	Principal reservoirs (other than humans)	Food involved in transmission to humans	Disease
Metagonimus yokogawai and related species	Eastern and southern Asia	Dogs, cats, pigs and fish-eating birds	Freshwater fish, e.g. sweetfish (*Plecoglossus altivelis*), dace (*Tribolodon hakonensis*), trout and whitebait. Metacercariae in gills, fin or tail	Similar to *Heterophyes heterophyes*
Nanophyetus spp.	Eastern Siberia (mountain tributaries of Amur River) and parts of Sakhalin peninsula, north-western USA	Dogs, cats, rats (?) and badgers	Salmonid and other fish. Metacercariae in muscles, fins and kidneys	Nanophyetiasis Diarrhea, usually accompanied by increased numbers of circulating eosinophils, abdominal discomfort and nausea. Sometimes asymptomatic
Spelotrema brevicaeca	Philippines	Sea birds	Crustaceans, amphipods, isopods and brachyures	
Haplorchis spp.	Eastern and southern Asia	Cats, dogs and fish-eating birds	Fish, frogs and toads. Metacercariae in muscle	
Fasciolopsis buski	Oriental countries	Pigs	Uncooked contaminated water plants such as water cress	Most infections are light and asymptomatic. Heavy infections show symptoms of diarrhea, abdominal pain, fever, ascites, anasarca and intestinal obstruction
Lung fluke				
Paragonimus westermani and related species in Asia, Africa and the Americas	Siberia, west Africa (Nigeria, Cameroon), the Americas (Ecuador to USA), Japan, Korea, Thailand, Laos, China	Domestic and wild carnivora that feed on crustaceans	Freshwater and brackish water crabs (*Eriocheir, Potamon, Parathelphusa*), crayfish and shrimps. Metacercariae in muscles, gills, liver (hepatopancreas) and cardia region. Wild boar meat suspected as a source of infection	Paragonimiasis

Based on Abdussalam *et al.* (1995). Data reproduced with permission from Elsevier Science.

Table 14.5 Food-borne protozoa

Occurrence	Transmission	Definite host	Incubation	Infective dose	Pathogenesis
Giardia intestinalis Worldwide	Food-borne, water-borne, person–person	Humans, domestic and wild animals	3–25 days	Low (~10 cysts)	Chronic diarrhea, malabsorption, weight loss
Entamoeba histolytica Worldwide	Food-borne, water-borne, person–person (food handlers)	Humans	2–4 weeks	Very low (~1 cyst)	Amebiasis, abdominal pain, fever, diarrhea, ulceration of the colon (severe cases)
Toxoplasma gondii Worldwide	Food-borne (raw or inadequately cooked infected meat), water-borne, fecal–oral (infected cats)	Humans, cats, several mammals	5–23 days	~1–30 cysts	Mostly asymptomatic. In severe cases: hepatitis, pneumonia, blindness, severe neurological disorders. Can also be transmitted transplacentally resulting in a spontaneous abortion, a stillborn or mental/physical retardation
Cyclospora cayetanensis Worldwide	Food-borne, water-borne,	Humans	Several days to weeks	Not known, probably very low	Often asymptomatic. Abdominal cramps, vomiting, weight loss, diarrhea
Cryptosporidium parvum Worldwide	Food-borne, water-borne, animal–person, fecal–oral	Humans, domestic and wild animals	It is not usually possible to define accurately the incubation period, but in most cases symptoms appear within 3 days to a week or occasionally longer	Very low (~1 cyst)	Often asymptomatic. Abdominal cramps, vomiting, weight loss, diarrhea

Protozoa

The protozoal human parasites are unicellular organisms that colonize the intestinal epithelium and form cysts. These are excreted and may survive for long periods in the environment. There are five genera of concern in foods: *Giardia*, *Entamoeba*, *Toxoplasma*, *Cyclospora* and *Cryptosporidium*.

Table 14.5 summarizes the distribution, principal reservoirs and route of transmission of these parasites in the food chain.

14.6 Transmissible spongiform encephalopathies and food

Transmissible spongiform encephalopathies (TSE) are fatal degenerative brain diseases which include BSE in cattle, scrapie in sheep and kuru, CJD and new variant CJD (vCJD) in humans. They are characterized by the appearance in the brain of vacuoles – clear holes that give the brain a sponge-like appearance – from which the conditions derive their name.

Several theories have been proposed to explain the nature of the agents that cause TSE. Prusiner was awarded the Nobel Prize in 1997 for the prion theory, which postulates that the agent is a proteinaceous infectious particle (PrP) that is capable of replication without the need of an agent-specific nucleic acid. The disease-associated prion (PrP^{Sc}) has been shown to have a different helical shape to normal cellular prion protein (PrP^C) found on neuronal cells and some other cells, for example lymphoid cells. However, while it is widely acknowledged that PrP^{Sc} is very closely associated with the causative agent, there is a reluctance by some to accept PrP^{Sc} as the sole agent responsible for transmission. Another hypothesis suggests the agent is an unconventional virus, while a third suggests that it is a virion that has similar properties to a virus but uses host proteins to coat its nucleic acid.

Bovine spongiform encephalopathy

BSE, sometimes referred to as "mad cow disease", was first identified in the UK in 1986. The disease is fatal to cattle within weeks to months of its onset. The incubation period is between 2 and 10 years. Affected animals may display changes in temperament, such as nervousness or aggression, abnormal posture, lack of coordination and difficulty in standing; decreased milk production or loss of body weight despite continued appetite. Most cattle with BSE show a gradual development of symptoms over a period of several weeks or even months, although some can deteriorate very rapidly. While the original source of the agent responsible for BSE remains unknown, currently the most plausible explanation is that a novel TSE appeared in the UK cattle population in the 1970s and subsequently spread through contaminated meat and bone meal fed to cattle.

The International Office for Epizootic Diseases (OIE) reports cases on its website (www.oie.int).

Creutzfeldt–Jakob disease and new variant CJD

CJD is a fatal disease of humans, first described in the 1920s and found worldwide. CJD is predominantly a sporadic disease, but about 14% of cases are familial (inherited) and associated with genetic mutations. Less than 1% are iatrogenic (i.e. accidentally transmitted from person to person as a result of medical or surgical procedures). Classically, sporadic CJD occurs in those over 65 years of age and presents as a rapidly progressive dementia with myoclonus (shock-like contractions of isolated muscles), usually fatal within 6 months. Surveillance of CJD, a human neurological disease, was reinstituted in the UK in 1990 to evaluate any changes in the pattern of the disease that might be attributable to BSE. The overall incidence of CJD rose in the UK in the 1990s, although a portion of this increase was due to improved ascertainment of CJD in the elderly as a result of the reinstitution of surveillance.

New variant CJD, also referred to as variant CJD (vCJD), is a newly recognized disease in humans, which was first diagnosed in the UK in the mid-1990s. In contrast to the traditional forms of CJD, vCJD has affected younger patients (average age 29 years) and has a longer duration of illness (approximately 14 months). Early in the illness, patients usually experience behavioral changes, which most commonly take the form of depression or, less often, a schizophrenia-like disorder. Neurological signs such as unsteadiness, difficulty walking and involuntary movements develop as the illness progresses and, by the time of death, patients become completely immobile and mute.

The link between BSE and vCJD

A geographical association exists, whereby the majority of BSE cases occurred in the UK and the majority of vCJD cases were also reported there. The emergence of BSE preceded vCJD, indicating a temporal association. Studies of stored human brain tissue internationally have not identified the histopathological changes characteristic of vCJD before the current BSE epidemic. Incubation period and pathological lesion studies in mice and molecular typing studies demonstrate that vCJD is similar to BSE but different from other TSE. It is now widely accepted that vCJD was transmitted to humans through the consumption of contaminated food.

Estimates of future prevalence of vCJD vary widely as too little is known about the disease, especially regarding the incubation period between exposure to the infective agent and the emergence of symptoms.

14.7 Chemicals affecting food safety

Chemicals may be present in food owing to their natural occurrence in soil (e.g. cadmium, lead) or from fungal contamination (e.g. aflatoxins, ochratoxin), from algal contamination (e.g. ASP, DSP, AZP, PSP), from industrial or other pollution (e.g. lead, mercury, PCB, dioxins), from agricultural and veterinary practices (e.g. pesticides, fertilizers, veterinary drugs) or from food processing and packaging techniques (e.g. PAH, 3-MCPD, BADGE) (see Box 14.1).

Toxicological assessment of these substances is largely carried out on an international basis by expert groups such as the Joint Expert Committee on Food Additives and Contaminants (JECFA) or Joint Meeting on Pesticide Residues (JMPR), both jointly organized by the WHO and FAO. These expert groups advise on acceptable or tolerable levels of intake of these substances.

Acceptable and tolerable levels of intake

The acceptable daily intake (ADI) level of a chemical is the daily intake which, during a lifetime, would pose no appreciable risk to the consumer, on the basis of all facts known at the time. It is expressed in mg/kg of body weight (see Box 14.2).

The tolerable weekly intake (TWI) represents permissible human weekly exposure to those contaminants unavoidably associated with the consumption of otherwise wholesome and nutritious foods. The term

Box 14.1   Principal groups of chemicals affecting food safety

Box 14.2   Levels of intake of a chemical

No observed effect level (NOEL)	Greatest concentration or amount of an agent, found by study or observation, that causes no detectable, usually adverse, alteration of morphology, functional capacity, growth, development, or lifespan of the target
↓ /Safety factor	Uncertainty factor for extrapolating animal data to humans
↓ /Safety factor	Human interspecies variation
↓ Acceptable daily intake (ADI)	Daily intake that, during a lifetime, would pose no appreciable risk to the consumer, on the basis of all facts known at the time. It is expressed in mg/kg of body weight

tolerable signifies permissibility rather than acceptability for the intake of contaminants that have no necessary function in food, in contrast to those of permitted pesticides or food additives. For cumulative toxicants, such as lead, cadmium and mercury, the tolerable intakes are expressed on a weekly basis to allow for daily variations in intake levels, the real concern being long-term exposure to the contaminant.

For potent carcinogens, such as certain mycotoxins, safe levels cannot be set. JECFA addressed this issue in 1978 and introduced the concept of an "irreducible level", which it defined as "that concentration of a substance which cannot be eliminated from a food without involving the discarding of that food altogether, severely compromising the ultimate availability of major food supplies" (FAO/WHO, 1978).

The maximum tolerable daily intake (MTDI) has been established for food contaminants that are not known to accumulate in the body, such as tin, arsenic and styrene. The value assigned to the PMTDI represents permissible human exposure as a result of the natural occurrence of the substance in food and drinking water.

Setting the acceptable daily intake

JECFA generally sets the ADI of a substance on the basis of the highest no-observed-effect level in animal studies. In calculating the ADI, a "safety factor" is applied to the no-observed-effect level to provide a conservative margin of safety on account of the inherent uncertainties in extrapolating animal toxicity data to potential effects in humans and for variation within the human species. JECFA traditionally uses a safety factor of 100 (10 × 10) in setting ADI values based on long-term animal studies. It is intended to provide an adequate margin of safety for the consumer by assuming that the human being is 10 times more sensitive than the test animal and that the difference in sensitivity within the human population is in a 10-fold range. However, different safety factors apply depending on the substance and test species in question.

Maximum levels for food commodities

These levels are calculated taking the above-mentioned levels into consideration. Depending on the substance, different principles apply. Residues such as pesticides and residues of veterinary drugs in foodstuffs are limited by setting a maximum residue limit (MRL). Additives are regulated by setting maximum limits or by applying the "quantum satis" principle (the least amount required to exert the desired technological function).

For contaminants maximum levels/limits are established for those foods that provide a significant contribution to the total dietary exposure. However, as a general principle the levels in all foods should always be kept as low as reasonably achievable (the ALARA principle).

In Europe, additives, pesticides, veterinary residues and a wide range of contaminants are regulated by EU legislation in the form of directives or regulations that are transposed into national legislation by each member state.

Pesticide residues

Pesticides are chemicals or biological products used to control harmful or undesired organisms and plants, or to regulate the growth of plants as crop protection agents. They are classified into the groups shown in Box 14.3.

Most pesticides are toxic substances that are highly selective, especially those developed since the early 1980s, and only have an effect on those pests or plants to which they are applied. Unlike other environmental contaminants, pesticides are applied under controlled conditions that should conform to "good agricultural practice" (GAP). This defines the effective use of pesticides, up to the maximum allowable dose, applied in a manner that ensures the smallest amount of residue in the foodstuff.

Pesticides can also be toxic to humans since certain biochemical pathways are relatively conserved across species, as are some enzymes and hormones. In the context of food safety, exposure to pesticides is classified as acute or chronic. An acute intoxication usually has an immediate effect on the body, whereas a chronic effect may reveal itself over the lifespan. The severity depends on the dose and the toxicity of the pesticide compound or breakdown product. Toxic effects that have been identified include enzyme inhibition, endocrine disruption and carcinogenic action, depending on the compound in question.

In Europe the control of pesticides is based on Council Directive no. 91/414/EEC. Under this regulation, pesticides must be evaluated for safety based on dossiers prepared by their manufacturers. If a pesticide is accepted it is placed on a positive list with an MRL assigned to it.

In the case of a limited number of highly toxic pesticides, for which the ADI is necessarily based on acute toxicity rather than chronic toxicity, the level of exposure is considered in relation to the acute reference dose (ARfD). ARfD values are measures of the maximum level of intake at one meal, or consumption over a day. This is the maximum intake level, which is judged to result in no adverse toxicological effect following such exposure. The ARfD value includes a safety factor to ensure that the elderly, infants and

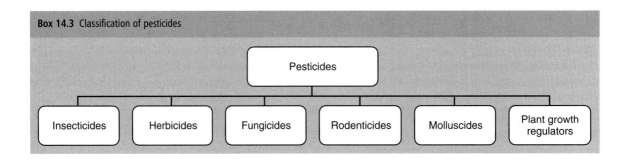

Box 14.3 Classification of pesticides

Pesticides

Insecticides | Herbicides | Fungicides | Rodenticides | Molluscides | Plant growth regulators children, and those under stress due to illness, are protected.

Veterinary drug residues

Veterinary drugs include antibacterial compounds, hormones and nonsteroidal anti-inflammatory preparations. As animal husbandry practices have intensified over the past few decades, antibacterial substances have been increasingly used as growth promoters to increase feed conversion efficiency, and for prophylaxis and therapy to prevent outbreaks and treat disease. Similarly, hormones are administered to increase growth rate and meat yield. Table 14.6 shows the main types of antibacterial and hormonal compounds.

Veterinary drugs are metabolized in the animal and are excreted in the urine and feces over time as the detoxification process continues. Hence, residue traces of drugs or their metabolites can be found in major organs, muscles and body fluids. In general, antibacterial drugs are found in greatest concentration in the kidney, lesser concentrations in the liver and lowest concentrations in the muscle tissue, whereas hormones tend to concentrate in the liver.

The excessive use of antibacterial compounds in animal husbandry has raised concerns about the development of resistant bacteria and the effect that this may have on the usefulness of antibiotics in human medicine. There have also been concerns about the risk of allergic reactions in humans to antibacterial residues in food of animal origin. The use of hormones has raised issues surrounding the effects of hormone residues in foods of animal origin on human metabolism.

Environmental and industrial contaminants

These contaminants are of environmental origin or are by-products of industrial processes.

Polyhalogenated hydrocarbons (PHH) are a category of environmental contaminants that includes

Table 14.6 Main types of veterinary drugs

Antibacterial compounds	Hormones
Aminoglycosides	β-Agonists
β-Lactams	Resorcylic lactones
Fluoroquinolones	Steroids
Macrolides	Stilbenes
Sulfonamides	Thyrostat
Tetracyclines	
Quinolones	

toxophene, dioxins and polychlorinated biphenyls (PCB). Certain polyhalogenated hydrocarbons are manufactured for use in plastics, paints, transformers and herbicides, although their use is now either banned or severely restricted. In most industrialized nations the compounds have become ubiquitous in the environment. Hence, contamination of the food chain is inevitable and it has been estimated that in Western industrialized countries 90% of human exposure is through ingestion of contaminated foods such as fish and milk.

Foods that are rich sources of fats and oils tend to accumulate PHH because the compounds are lipophilic and bioaccumulate in lipid-rich tissues and fluids. Oily fish from areas such as the Baltic Sea, where levels of PHH in the water are high, may contain elevated levels of these contaminants. Similarly, cows that graze on polluted pasture can accumulate unacceptable concentrations of PHH in their milk. A recent incident in Belgium introduced PCB and dioxins into the food chain via contaminated animal feed resulting from the accidental incorporation of industrial oil into the feed ration. The biological half-life of PHH can range from a matter of months to 20 years in human adipose tissue. Hence, they are persistent and accumulate in the body. Exposure to PHH can result in a variety of toxic effects that can be carcinogenic, including dermal toxicity, immunotoxicity, reproductive effects and endocrine disruption.

Metals, metalloids and their compounds have long been associated with food poisoning, and lead and mercury are probably the best documented hazards. Metals are released into the environment as a result of natural geological action and also as a result of man-made pollution from industrial processes.

Metals have an affinity for biological tissue and organic compounds, and hence they are often easily absorbed into the body and can often accumulate in organs and fat deposits. Table 14.7 shows some of the main metals linked with food-borne toxicity

Lead toxicity has many symptoms, but the main issue relates to its effects on the nervous system of children. Here, lead interferes with the transmission of nervous signals around the body. This can manifest itself in a reduced intelligence quotient (IQ) and coordination problems. In adults, exposure to lead can result in hypertension and other blood effects such as anemia. Cadmium is most often accumulated from occupational exposure or smoking and is known to affect the

Table 14.7 Metals in the foodchain

Metal	Main food sources
Lead	Shellfish, finfish, kidney, liver
Cadmium	Shellfish, kidney, cereals, vegetables
Mercury	Finfish
Arsenic	Meat, vegetables, seafood

respiratory system. However, food exposure tends to be at a low level over longer periods. In this regard, cadmium bioaccumulates in the kidney and can cause renal damage. Mercury and its compounds also bioaccumulate in the body, where they are most frequently associated with neural effects and renal damage. Arsenic is most often an occupational hazard, but it can also be ingested with food and is responsible for acute and chronic poisoning. The toxicity of arsenic depends on its oxidation state and the type of complex that it forms with organic molecules in the body. Chronic effects include gastroenteritis, nephritis and liver damage. Arsenic is also considered to be a carcinogen. Other metals are also known contaminants and their toxic effects are diverse. Although this is not an exhaustive list, these metals include aluminum, copper, tin, zinc and chromium.

Process contaminants

These types of contaminant occur during the processing and production of foods, and include polyaromatic hydrocarbons (PAH), chloropropanols and nitrosamines.

PAH are a group of over 100 different chemicals that are formed during certain technological processes and are common environmental contaminants. They are formed during incomplete combustion of coal and oil. They are also formed during barbecuing or grilling meat. Human exposure usually results from air pollution and from cigarette smoke. Foods most likely to be contaminated by PAH are grilled or charred meats. PAH are toxins that have been documented by the WHO as genotoxic, immunotoxic and carcinogenic. Long-term exposure to foods containing PAH can lead to serious health risks. In a recent Europe-wide incident, PAH were found in Pomace olive oil, which resulted in a major product recall.

Chloropropanols include known genotoxic animal carcinogens such as 3-monochloropropane-1,2-diol (3-MCPD) and 1,3-dichloropropan-2-ol (1,3-DCP). 3-MCPD is a by-product in soy sauce and in hydrolyzed

vegetable protein produced through acid hydrolysis. It can also be present as a contaminant in some food additives, and in epichlorhydrin/amine copolymers, used as flocculants or coagulant aids in water treatment, and may be present in drinking water (Opinion of the European Scientific Committee on Food, adopted on 30 May 2001).

Microbial toxins

Food poisoning can occur as a result of the ingestion of food containing preformed toxins that originate from bacterial growth, fungal growth or algal growth. In the case of bacteria the toxin is absorbed into the bloodstream via the intestine and therefore illness results from intoxication rather than infection. In the case of fungi, several species are involved in the production of toxic substances during growth on foodstuffs. These toxins are known as mycotoxins. Algal toxins are usually associated with seafood, most notably molluscan shellfish.

Bacterial toxins

Three bacteria are most commonly associated with preformed toxin production: *C. botulinum*, *S. aureus* and *B. cereus*.

Fungal toxins (mycotoxins)

Mycotoxins are secondary metabolites of moulds that can induce acute and chronic symptoms, such as carcinogenic, mutagenic and estrogenic effects in humans and animals. Acute toxicity due to mycotoxins is associated with liver and kidney damage. Chronic toxicity resulting from the exposure of low levels of mycotoxins in the human diet is a major food safety concern. In nonindustrialized countries mycotoxins have been reported to be responsible for increased morbidity and mortality in children owing to suppression of their immune systems and greater susceptibility to disease.

The principal fungi that are associated with mycotoxin production are the genera *Aspergillus*, *Penicillium* and *Fusarium*. *Aspergillus* and *Penicillium* are sometimes referred to as storage fungi as they can grow at low water activity levels and are associated with the post-harvest spoilage of stored food commodities such as cereals, nuts and spices. *Fusarium* species are plant pathogens and can infect plants in the field and produce mycotoxins preharvest. Table 14.8 provides an overview of the most important mycotoxins.

Table 14.8 Mycotoxins in the food supply

Mycotoxin	Producing fungi	Main foods affected	Toxicity
Aflatoxins	*Aspergillus flavus* and *A. parasiticus*	Nuts, cereals, dried fruit, herbs and spices, milk (aflatoxin M1)	Carcinogenic, hepatotoxic
Ochratoxin A	*Aspergillus ochraceus, Penicillium verrucosum* and other *Aspergillus* and *Penicillium* spp.	Coffee, dried fruit, cereals, beans, pulses, wine, beer, grape juice; kidney, liver and blood from animals fed with contaminated feed	Nephrotoxic, immunotoxic
Patulin	*Aspergillus clavatus*, also several species of *Penicillium, Aspergillus* and *Byssochlamys*	Fruits and grains, predominantly apples and apple products	Cytotoxic
Trichothecenes (nivalenol, deoxynivalenol, T2-toxin, etc.)	*Fusarium* spp.	Wheat, maize, barley, oats, rye, malt, beer, bread	Dermotoxic, enterotoxic, hemotoxic, immunotoxic
Fumonisins	*Fusarium* spp.	Cereals, mainly corn	Carcinogenic, cytotoxic, hepatotoxic
Sterigmatocystin	*Aspergillus versicolor, A. nidulans* and other *Aspergillus* spp.	Cereals, green coffee, herbs and spices, raw meat products	Hepatotoxic and nephrotoxic, carcinogenic
Citrinin	*Penicillium* spp., *Aspergillus* spp.	Cereals	Nephrotoxic
Zearalenone	*Fusarium graminearum*	Maize, barley, oats, wheat, rice, sorghum, bread	Estrogenic effects, feed refusal, vomiting
Moniliformin	*Fusarium* spp.	Cereals, maize	Nephrotoxic, causes necrosis of the heart muscle

Seafood toxins

Fish and fishery products are nutritious foods and are desirable components of a healthy diet. Food-borne illnesses resulting from the consumption of seafood are associated with both finfish and molluscan shellfish. The major risk of acute illness is associated with the consumption of raw shellfish, particularly bivalve molluscs. Molluscan shellfish are filter feeders and continually pump water through their gills, where particulate matter is removed and ingested. Consequently, any toxin associated with the phytoplankton ingested can rapidly accumulate and hence become concentrated in the bivalve mollusc. The consumption of these toxic shellfish by humans can cause illness, with symptoms ranging from mild diarrhea and vomiting to memory loss, paralysis and death. Toxins associated with phytoplankton are known as phyco-toxins. These toxins have been responsible for incidents of wide-scale death of sea-life and are increasingly responsible for human intoxication.

Various seafood poisoning syndromes are associated with toxic marine algae and these include paralytic shellfish poisoning (PSP), amnesic shellfish poisoning (ASP), diarrhetic shellfish poisoning (DSP), neurotoxic shellfish poisoning (NSP) and azaspiracid shellfish poisoning (AZP). There are also different types of food poisoning associated with finfish and these include ciguatera poisoning, scombroid or histamine poisoning and puffer fish poisoning. Consumption of raw molluscan shellfish poses well-known risks of food poisoning, but intoxication from finfish is not so well known. Most of the algal toxins associated with seafood poisoning are heat stable and are not inactivated by cooking. It is also not possible visually to distinguish toxic from nontoxic fish. Many countries rely on biotoxin monitoring programs to protect public health and close harvesting areas when toxin algal blooms or toxic shellfish are detected. In nonindustrialized countries, particularly in rural areas, monitoring for harmful algal blooms does not routinely occur and deaths due to red-tide toxins commonly occur. Table 14.9 provides an overview of the most important types of fish poisoning.

Naturally occurring plant toxins

Certain plants contain naturally occurring compounds that are toxic to humans or that reduce the bioavailability of nutrients in foods. Examples of naturally occurring toxins are listed in Table 14.10. Some species of mushroom also contain toxic compounds, for instance agaritine. Some cereal-based diets have restricted bioavailability of nutrients as a result of the presence of antinutritional factors such as phytate and tannins or polyphenols.

Table 14.9 Types of fish poisoning

Poisoning	Implicated foods	Associated toxin	Symptoms	Occurrence
Paralytic shellfish poisoning (PSP)	Mussels, oysters, clams or scallops that have fed on toxigenic dinoflagellates (*Gonyaulax* spp.)	Saxitoxins	Neurotoxic; symptoms include numbness, tingling and burning of the lips, staggering, drowsiness and in severe cases respiratory paralysis	Worldwide
Amnesic shellfish poisoning (ASP)	Mussels and clams that have recently fed on a marine diatom *Nitzchia pungens*, viscera of crabs and anchovies		Vomiting, cramps, diarrhea, disorientation and difficulty in breathing	USA, Canada and Europe
Diarrhetic shellfish poisoning (DSP)	Toxic mussels, clams and scallops that have fed on marine dinoflagellates (*Dinophysis* spp.)	Okadaic acid and associated toxins	Abdominal pain, nausea, vomiting and severe diarrhea	Europe, Japan, Chile, New Zealand and Canada
Neurotoxic shellfish poisoning (NSP)	Shellfish that have fed on the dinoflagellate *Gymnodinidum breve*	Brevitoxins	Nausea, diarrhea, tingling and burning of the lips, tongue and throat	
Azaspiracid shellfish poisoning (AZP)	Mussels, oysters, clams, scallops and razor fish	Azaspiracid	Nausea, vomiting, severe diarrhea and stomach cramps	Ireland, suspected cases in Norway, the Netherlands, Scotland and Japan
Ciguatera fish poisoning (CFP)	Flesh of toxic reef fish from tropical areas feeding on dinoflagellates (*Gambierdiscus toxicus*) and their toxins. Common species are amberjack, barracuda, moray eel, groupers, trevally, Spanish mackerel and snapper	Ciguatera	Gastrointestinal (diarrhea, vomiting, abdominal pain, nausea); neurological (paresthesia of the extremities, circumoral paresthesia, temperature reversal, ataxia, arthralgia, malign headache, severe pruritus, vertigo and stiffness, convulsions, delirium, hallucinations, photophobia, transient blindness, salivation, perspiration, watery eyes, metallic taste in mouth, blurred vision, hiccups, exacerbation of acne, dysuria); cardiovascular (dyspnea, bradycardia, hypotension, tachycardia)	Tropical reef waters, particularly in the island states of the South Pacific
Scombroid or histamine poisoning	Consumption of scombroid and scombroid-like marine fish species that have not been chilled immediately after capture. Commonly involved are members of the Scombridae family, e.g. tuna and mackerel, and a few nonscombrid relatives, e.g. bluefish, dolphin fish and amberjack	Scombroid or histamine. Production is due to the action of histidine decarboxylase that is produced by species of the Enterobacteraceae, mainly *Morganella* and *Klebsiella* spp.	Initial symptoms are that of an allergic response with facial flushing and sweating, burning–peppery taste sensations around the mouth and throat, dizziness, nausea and headache. A facial rash can develop as well as mild diarrhea and abdominal cramps. Severe cases may blur vision and cause respiratory stress and swelling of the tongue. Symptoms usually last for approximately 4–6 h and rarely exceed 1–2 days	Worldwide
Puffer fish poisoning (PFP)	Consumption of fish species belonging to the Tetraodontidea family, particularly those species caught in waters of the Indo-Pacific Ocean regions	Tetrodotoxin	Symptoms of PFP are similar to PSP as the actions of both toxins are similar. Mild poisoning results in tingling and numbness of the lips, tongue and fingers, and in severe cases death by asphyxiation due to respiratory paralysis	Most frequent in Japan, where puffer fish (called fugu in Japan) are eaten as a delicacy, Indo-Pacific Ocean region

Food processing methods have evolved that reduce human exposure to both natural toxins and antinutritional compounds. For instance, cassava is a staple food of over 500 million people worldwide. Certain bitter varieties of cassava contain high levels of linamarin, a cyanogenic glycoside. The consumption of these varieties has been associated with health defects such as goitre and paralysis of the legs. Traditional processing of cassava in Africa that involves grating, soaking roots in water and lactic acid fermentation completely removes the cyanide.

Adequate cooking of legume seeds such as kidney beans and disposal of the cooking water will remove the natural toxins present in these food products.

Antinutritional factors are those components of plants that interfere with metabolic processes and can lead to deficiencies of key nutrients in the diet. These are generally classified as enzyme inhibitors and mineral binding agents. Enzyme inhibitors are polypeptides and proteins that inhibit the activities of digestive enzymes, and most are thermolabile and are reduced by cooking. For example, trypsin inhibitors may cause poor protein digestion and a shortage of sulfur-containing amino acids in the diet. Lectins are proteins that occur in beans that alter the absorption of nutrients in the intestinal wall. Cooking beans will inactivate lectins. Tannins (polyphenols) occur in cereals, specifically in the seed coat. These form complexes with proteins and inhibition of digestive enzymes. Phytate is a natural component in plants and on digestion forms insoluble complexes with metal ions in the body. The result is reduced bioavailability of essential minerals such as iron. In addition, a range of natural plant toxins can cause allergic reactions in humans, but there is a general lack of knowledge about their properties and modes of action.

Food additives

Food additives are added to foods for a specific technological purpose during manufacture or storage and become an integral part of that foodstuff. Additives can be natural or synthetic and are usually categorized by their function (Table 14.11). For example, preservatives prevent the growth of bacteria, gelling agents maintain the structure of some foods during storage and emulsifiers maintain the stability of fat structures. Without additives it would not be possible to manufacture many of the foods available today, especially convenience foods and low-fat foods.

Safety considerations involving additives have centered on allergic reactions and food intolerances. Additives have also been blamed for inducing hyperactivity in children. Studies have been conducted into allergies and they often find that the actual prevalence rate is much lower than the perceived prevalence rate.

At the international level, additives are controlled by means of safety evaluation and the development of a positive list. To ensure transparency and choice, all additives that are used in prepackaged food should be labeled with their function and their name or approval number (E-number). However, there are some exemptions, specifically applying to additives that are in a foodstuff as a result of carry-over from an ingredient.

Table 14.10 Naturally occurring plant toxins

Compound	Food species	Common name
Glycosides:		
Linamarin	*Manihot escaleatum*	Cassava
Dhurrin	*Sorghum* spp.	Sorghum
Prunasin	*Prunus* spp.	Cherries
Glycoalkaloids:		
Solanin	*Solanium tuberosiem*	Potatoes
Pyrrolizidine alkaloids:		
Acetyllycopsaimine	*Symphytum* spp.	Comfrey
Senecionine	*Senccio jacobata*	Ragwort
Glucosinolates:		
Sinigrin	*Brassica* spp.	Cabbage
		Broccoli
		Brussels sprouts

Table 14.11 Categories of food additives according to function

Acid	Flour treatment agent
Acidity regulator[a]	Gelling agent
Anticaking agent	Glazing agent[c]
Antifoaming agent	Humectant
Antioxidant	Modified starch
Bulking agent	Preservative
Color	Propellant gas and
Emulsifier	packaging gas
Emulsifying salt	Raising agent
Enzyme[b]	Sequestrant[d]
Firming agent	Stabilizer[e]
Flavoring	Sweetener
Flavor enhancer	Thickener

[a] These can act as two-way acidity regulators.
[b] Only those used as additives.
[c] These substances include lubricants intended for the final consumer.
[d] Inclusion of these terms in this list is without prejudice to any future decision or mention thereof in the labeling of foodstuffs.
[e] This category also comprises foam stabilizers.
Source: European Union Directive 89/107/EEC. © European Communities, 1995–2002.

14.8 Food safety control programs

Each nation has a responsibility to ensure that its citizens enjoy a safe and wholesome food supply. The challenges facing national food safety control authorities have expanded in recent times and many countries are struggling to manage their food regulatory systems effectively. Increasingly our diets are becoming more complex, involving a wide range of foods and food ingredients, and diverse and changing eating arrangements. Hence, food safety authorities responsible for consumer protection must deal with an increasing range of complex issues. For instance, some of the major food scares that have plagued the EU in recent years, such as BSE and dioxin in animal feeds, have resulted in consumer confidence in regulatory agencies being damaged. These agencies were perceived to have taken decisions on economic grounds to protect the interests of the food sector rather than protecting consumer health. Many countries are now separating the role of food safety and consumer protection from the role of support and developing agri-food businesses and farming, to ensure that there is no conflict of interest.

Managing the food chain so that the public has access to a safe diet requires an effective food safety program that sets the strategic direction for food control activities. The goal of a food safety program is to safeguard the quality and safety of the total food supply, leading to a reduction in the incidence of food-borne disease, and improvements in nutrition and quality of life. The organization and enforcement food safety controls will vary from country to country, reflecting differing stages of development, nature of food safety problems and administrative arrangements. Food laws and regulations are developed and administered by a range of national agencies, including central government departments and regional and local authorities.

To ensure consumer protection, each nation requires a food safety program that identifies food safety needs, and establishes an integrated food control infrastructure that links food legislation and regulations with food inspection and surveillance initiatives, and education programs. This is best achieved by establishing a national food safety control agency that has responsibility for all sectors of the food chain, from farms to the point of sale to consumers. Many countries have gone down the road of establishing food safety authorities with the aim of coordinating the work of all government agencies that are involved in food legislation enforcement. In Europe, national food agencies are in place in Denmark, France, Germany, Ireland, the Netherlands, Sweden and the UK. Similar agencies have been established in Canada, Australia and New Zealand. Progress towards establishing single food agencies is slow in nonindustrialized countries, where food safety controls tend to focus only on foods for export. Controls for foods moving in domestic trade tend to be neglected. In addition, food legislation is enforced in isolation by separate government departments, such as agriculture and fisheries, and the role of the health sector in consumer protection from unsafe foods is minimal.

A national food safety authority would assist in overcoming the problems of overlaps and duplication of functions that sometimes exist between the food control services from different ministries. The roles of a national food safety agency include:

- developing more effective and coherent national food safety policy
- preparation and harmonization of food legislation
- coordination of food surveillance, collection and analysis of data, identifying and monitoring trends in food-borne diseases, and developing a code of practice for the control and prevention of food-borne illness
- coordinating food analysis and food laboratory networks
- coordinating food inspection and the introduction of food safety management systems based on the principles of the hazard analysis critical control point (HACCP) system
- conducting risk assessment and implementing risk management and risk communication strategies
- coordinating food research and training in food safety.

Modern food control programs also take into consideration the role of the food producers and food processors in managing the safety of their products. The various sectors of food production, processing and distribution possess knowledge about the safety and shelf-life of their products and have an important role in assisting regulators in achieving national food safety goals. One of the most effective ways for the food sector to protect the health of consumers is to base their food safety management programs on the principles of the HACCP system.

HACCP is a structured systemic approach to achieving food safety, which involves identifying potential hazards and measures for their control. The HACCP system marks a departure from the traditional end-point analysis of food. Instead of trying to detect microbial contamination in the finished product, the aim of this food safety management system is to minimize contamination by focusing on control procedures at critical points in the production process. The system was developed in the 1960s as a collaborative project between the Pillsbury Company, NASA (National Aeronautics and Space Administration) and the US Army Research Laboratory, designed to produce safe food for astronauts. While HACCP was originally developed to ensure microbiological safety of foodstuffs, it has since been broadened to include chemical and physical hazards in foods. In 1993 the CAC endorsed the HACCP system. European food hygiene law requires that food business operators identify any step in their activities that is critical to ensuring food safety and ensure that adequate safety procedures are identified, implemented, maintained and reviewed on the basis of the principles used to develop the system of HACCP.

The HACCP system consists of seven basic principles.

- Conduct a hazard analysis. List all potential hazards associated with each step and describe the preventive measures.
- Determine the critical control points (CCP) in the process.
- Establish critical limit(s) for each CCP.
- Establish monitoring programs to ensure control of the CCP.
- Establish corrective action to be taken when monitoring indicates that a CCP is not under control.
- Establish verification procedures to demonstrate the effectiveness of the HACCP system.
- Establish documentation concerning all procedures and records appropriate to these principles and their application.

14.9 Perspectives on the future

As our society changes, so do the bacteria involved in food-borne disease. Changes in food production systems and the globalization of the food supply, as well as changes in the food we are eating, and where this food is prepared, expose us to an ever-changing spectrum of contamination. The global nature of our food supply poses greater risks to consumer health from the mass production and distribution of foods and increased risk for food contamination. New food development has led to changing vectors for the spread of disease. Inappropriate use of antibiotics in animal husbandry can lead to the emergence of antibiotic-resistant food-borne pathogens such as *Salmonella typhimurium* DT 104.

Food safety and nutrition are inextricably linked because food-borne infections are one of the most important underlying factors of malnutrition, especially in poorer countries. Repeated episodes of food-borne infections can, over a period of time, lead to malnutrition, with serious health consequences. A safe food supply is essential for proper nutrition, basic health and well-being.

Maintaining a safe food supply is not difficult; however, it requires attention to detail at all stages of the food chain from agricultural inputs through farms, processing, the distribution network to retailers and catering outlets to consumers. There can be no gaps in the continuum from farm to fork if consumer protection is to be optimum. To ensure consumer protection, food standards have to be based on sound science and the principles of risk analysis. At the national level, food safety controls must be well coordinated and based on proportionate food legislation. The food industry must also recognize its primary responsibility for producing safe food and for ensuring that foods placed on the market meet the highest standards of food safety and hygiene. A multisectoral effort on the part of regulatory authorities, food industries and consumers alike is required to prevent food-borne diseases.

Further reading

Abdussalam M, Käferstein FK, Mott K. Food safety measures for the control of food borne trematode infections. Food Control 1995; 6: 71–79.

FAO/WHO. Evaluation of certain food additives and contaminants. 22nd Report of the Joint FAO/WHO Expert Committee on Food Additives. WHO Technical Report Series No. 631. Geneva: WHO, 1978: 14–15.

15
Food and Nutrition: The Global Challenge

Prakash Shetty

Key messages

- This chapter deals with the incidence of malnutrition through the life cycle, from intrauterine growth retardation to undernutrition in the older adult.
- It discusses "hidden hunger", which is the global problem of micronutrient deficiency, in particular iron, iodine and vitamin A deficiency.

- The emerging burden of obesity and the role of nutrition in the development of chronic disease are examined.
- Current major global challenges in food and nutrition are discussed.

15.1 Introduction

Fluctuations in disease rates depend on several environmental factors, which include food and nutrition. Nutrition is now recognized as a major determinant of a wide range of diseases of public health importance worldwide. In the developing world, numerous deficiency diseases continue to persist, especially in the rural areas, as a result of essential nutrient deficiencies in the daily diet. These now coexist with the increasing presence of diet-related chronic diseases in adults hitherto seen only in industrialized and developed countries.

Changes in the patterns of disease and the causes of premature death within a population have little to do with advances in medicine and therapeutics. Changes in health depend largely on environmental changes, including improvements in social and economic conditions, changes in agriculture and food systems and in the availability of and access to food, the implementation of immunization programs, and improvements in women's social and educational status within the society. These changes are, in turn, influenced by economic growth and changes in the sociocultural milieu of societies, political will and legislative influences, global trade, which affects agricultural practices

and the industrial sector, and the impact of globalization, which influences individual lifestyles. Most of these environmental influences that affect food and nutrition operate through changes in the provision of and access to adequate and safe food, namely hygienic and nutritious food, the availability of uncontaminated and safe drinking water, clean housing, sanitary surroundings and lack of exposure to environmental toxins. Economic development is thus normally accompanied by improvements in the quantity, quality and safety of a nation's food supply and an individual or a household's access to the same.

These quantitative and qualitative changes in our food patterns, which accompany such dramatic changes in life expectancy, often also result in the problems of diet-related noncommunicable diseases, but these problems are not inevitable. The diet-related chronic diseases occur typically in middle and later adult life and can undermine the gains in life expectancy. These diseases of developed societies are traditionally regarded as manifestations of excess intake and self-indulgence in an "affluent" society. In practice, some of these chronic diseases may be associated with relatively deficient intakes of some nutrients and are compounded by dramatic lifestyle changes. Thus, a "balanced" diet and an appropriate lifestyle are essential ingredients that need to be kept in mind when considering the disease patterns of adult life.

Food and nutrition are now regarded as being of fundamental importance in public health in both developed and developing societies. Nutritional issues are often seen in industrialized and developed societies as those relating to inadequate food or due to deficiency diseases that were conquered in the early part of the twentieth century, while continuing to persist in the poor, developing countries. Now, however, food and nutrition along with lifestyle changes are recognized as the principal environmental components affecting a wide range of diseases of public health importance throughout the world. These diseases reflect the cumulative impact of several pathophysiological processes developing over a lifetime. These interactions within a society are often seen as reflecting individual genetic susceptibility, but the different disease patterns of groups living on different diets are manifestly a societal reflection of the impact of dietary factors.

The display of nutrient–gene interactions is evident in:

- obesity
- alcoholism
- cardiovascular disease
- noninsulin-dependent diabetes mellitus
- many gastrointestinal disorders
- neural tube defects
- most prevalent cancers.

As clinical studies and molecular epidemiology unravel the basis for genetic susceptibility to these disorders and as gene inducers or repressors are identified, they prove to be of dietary or environmental origin. Societal characteristics that determine human behavior and economic well-being, as well as climate, tradition and culture, all affect food patterns and dietary practices. These are the features that need to be recognized as being causal determinants rather than simply the epidemiological aspects of nutrient–disease relationships. This chapter seeks to take a global view of food and nutrition in public health terms, and so nutritional deficiency disorders as well as other diet-related diseases of public health importance will be considered. This is particularly important because deficiency diseases are widespread in several parts of the world and yet coexist in the same country with chronic adult diseases usually found in affluent, developed societies.

Vitamin deficiencies continue to manifest, and the threat of food insecurity and dietary inadequacy resulting in malnutrition rapidly emerges following natural disasters and during conflict situations.

15.2 Malnutrition through the life cycle

Malnutrition in the community, particularly in developing societies, is a global challenge. Poor nutrition starts *in utero* and extends throughout the life cycle: from birth into infancy and childhood, through adolescence into adulthood and on to the elderly. It encompasses the critical periods of growth, development and maturation, both physical and mental, the active reproductive and economically productive phases of an individual's life, and the twilight years of old age and senescence. Malnutrition due to inadequacy and lack of access to food compounded by other environmental constraints and insults thus affects all individuals in a community, although some groups such as infants, pregnant and lactating mothers and the elderly may be considered as being more vulnerable than others.

Low birth weight and intrauterine growth retardation

The most significant precursor to malnutrition in infancy and childhood is intrauterine growth retardation (IUGR), which results in low birth weight (LBW). LBW is indicated when the birth weight of a full-term baby ($>$37 weeks gestational age) is $<$2500 g. IUGR is a serious public health problem in developing countries, since 23.8% of births (i.e. 30 million out of 126 million births per year) have LBW, compared with 2% in developed countries. Among developing countries, southern Asia, that is the Indian subcontinent, has the highest incidence of LBW. One of the major determinants of IUGR in developing countries is maternal undernutrition characterized by low pre-pregnancy body weights, short maternal stature and inadequate or low gestational weight gain. Maternal anemia, infections, particularly malaria, and smoking are important additional risk factors. LBW due to IUGR is a serious public health problem as it poses an increased risk of morbidity and mortality in the infant and susceptibility to severe malnutrition in childhood, along with poor cognitive, mental and physical development. There is now compelling evidence that it also increases the risk of chronic disease in adulthood, thus increasing the health burden of societies. The high prevalence of stunting among children in southern Asia may be related to the high incidence of LBW in these regions which, in turn, perpetuates the intergenerational cycle of malnutrition, poverty and disease and contributes to the costs of unachieved human and socioeconomic developmental potential of nation states.

Childhood malnutrition

Clinical protein–energy malnutrition in children

The clinical conditions of childhood malnutrition are widely recognized as kwashiorkor, marasmus and the mixed condition of marasmic kwashiorkor. These severe forms of malnutrition are, however, the tip of an iceberg of widespread mild and moderate childhood undernutrition within the community. The dominance of the three forms varies from country to country and this seems to reflect the breast-feeding and weaning practices and staple foods of the area, as well as the impact of recurrent infections. It is also determined by the manner in which the body responds to the various environmental insults.

Kwashiorkor presents with a variety of clinical features that include edematous appearance with a moon face, a scaling, crazy-paving pigmentation and ulceration of the skin with sparse, thin, discolored hair. Children with kwashiorkor are morose and lethargic, and have a large liver and often reasonable amounts of trunkal and limb fat, which obscures an atrophied muscle mass. The condition is associated with high mortality, and is often precipitated or accompanied by recurrent infections and growth failure. It can occur in epidemic form once a measles outbreak affects a society living on a low-protein staple diet, for example of cassava, yam, plantain or banana, but an additional feature may be the exposure to toxins in food such as aflatoxin. An important factor is the impact of iron overload from the ready absorption of bacterial iron, leading to marked free radical damage in a liver that is limited in dietary free radical scavengers, such as glutathione and vitamins E and C. Not only can the measles infection induce diarrhea with protein loss, but further protein can be lost as amino acids are used up in antibody production and other inflammatory responses.

The child with marasmus is a wizened, shrivelled, growth-retarded and skeletal child who is often alert and with normal but shrivelled skin. Absence of edema in the presence of severe muscle wasting is characteristic of marasmus. Thus, the marasmic child is very thin and wasted, with no subcutaneous fat and wasted muscles. Mortality rates in marasmus are lower than seen in kwashiorkor.

When a child presents with wasting of muscles and fat characteristic of marasmus along with edema as in kwashiorkor, the child has a severe form of protein–energy malnutrition called marasmic kwashiorkor. Marasmic kwashiorkor may occur if a marasmic and sick child is overfed early with too high a sodium intake, which may cause the child to become edematous.

Diarrheal disease is an important contributor to severe childhood malnutrition that is often perceived only as a nutritional disorder. There are millions of children with chronic diarrhea who fail to respond completely to the usual treatment for acute gastroenteritis. The residual problem is essentially nutritional in origin. A vicious cycle is established whereby an intestinal infection in a young child leads to anorexia, intestinal damage with malabsorption and secretory diarrhea, which then does not remit because the poor nutritional state of the child sustains the immunological deficits and this impairs the recovery of the intestine. These malnourished children with diarrhea typically have pronounced potassium depletion and are very sensitive to sodium retention.

Children, particularly in Africa and Asia, fail to thrive once they have succumbed to an infectious disease and they then languish, responding poorly to therapy and failing to grow even when presented with adequate amounts of food. New treatment schemes are now being developed based on the recognition that intestinal bacterial overgrowth is common and that for recovery to take place it is necessary to provide the full complement of minerals and vitamins. Once the child has re-equilibrated its fluid and electrolyte balance, the need is not only for the full supply of minerals and vitamins but also for adequate amounts of easily consumable and palatable energy-dense feeds. This is often best met by adding vegetable oil, which is energy dense, to the diet. The manufacture of energy-dense foods for rehabilitating malnourished children in underdeveloped countries is hampered by their tendency to oxidise, but locally produced food and oils can make an extremely valuable contribution to increasing the energy density of the diet. Shifting strategies of rehabilitation by coping with malnourished children at home rather than in rehabilitation centers clearly show the cost–benefit advantages of home care to both mother and child.

Childhood malnutrition in the community

Undernutrition in infancy and childhood is character-ized by growth failure, resulting in a body weight and height that are less than ideal for the child's age. Hence, in infants and children under 5 years of age, assessment of growth has been the single most important measure-ment that best defines their nutritional status. Disturb-ances in nutrition and health as a result of inadequacy of food intake or severe and repeated infections, or a combination of both operating very often as a vicious spiral, invariably affect the growth of a child.

These adverse conditions are closely linked to the general standard of living and the population's ability to meet its basic needs for:

- nutritious food
- safe water
- good housing
- acceptable levels of environmental sanitation
- ready and easy access to health care.

Anthropometric indices are used as the main cri-teria for assessing the adequacy of growth and hence optimal nutritional status in infancy and childhood. Assessment of the nutritional status of the child by the use of nutritional anthropometric indicators of growth has thus been used not only to provide information on the nutritional and health status of children, but also as an indirect measure of the quality of life of the entire community or population, and thereby an indicator of the nutritional status and adequacy of food of all mem-bers of that community.

Measurements of height and weight are used as indi-cators of the nutritional status of a child. Classification of malnutrition in infancy and childhood based on height, weight and age thus continues to be the back-bone of nutritional assessment methods for both popu-lation and individual assessments. The presence of undernutrition in children is assessed using these three anthropometric parameters (weight for age, height for age and weight for height) and by comparing them with internationally accepted reference standards, such as the National Center for Health Statistics/World Health Organization (NCHS/WHO) international reference population.

According to the WHO classification:

- appropriate height for age of a child reflects linear growth and can measure long-term growth faltering or *stunting*;

- appropriate weight for height reflects proper body pro-portion or the harmony of growth. Weight-for-height is particularly sensitive to acute growth disturbances and is useful to detect the presence of *wasting*;
- weight for age represents a convenient synthesis of both linear growth and body proportion and can thus be used for the diagnosis of *underweight* children.

If a child has a low height for age, that is, below two standard deviations (-2 SD or Z-scores, where the numerical value of the Z-score specifies the distance from the mean) of the reference population, then such a child is categorized as stunted. Similarly, a low weight for age is diagnostic of an underweight child, while a low weight for height is indicative of wasting. In a popu-lation, the growth retardation prevalence for the under-five preschool child is estimated by the proportion of weight for age, height for age and weight for height below -2 SD (Z-score) which is the accepted cut-off for the diagnosis of undernutrition and hence indica-tive of an increase in risk of morbidity and mortality.

The additional advantages of the use of these anthropometric indicators of the nutritional status of infants and preschool children include the ability to display the prevalence of overweight due to overnu-trition as measured by the proportion of children with weight for height above $+2$ SD (or $+2$ Z-scores). This methodology thus allows for the display of the preva-lence of the different types of childhood malnutrition manifested as growth retardation, i.e. underweight, stunting and wasting and the degree of severity of each by the means, SD and Z-scores. It also permits strati-fication of the results of the survey according to age, gender, region, rural/urban or other sociodemo-graphic characteristics of the population.

Surveys throughout the world (Table 15.1) demon-strate the very high prevalence of stunting throughout

Table 15.1 Estimated prevalence (and numbers in millions) of under-nourished children in developing countries by region, in the year 2000

Region	Underweight % ($n \times 10^6$)	Stunted % ($n \times 10^6$)
Africa	28.5 (38.32)	35.2 (47.30)
Asia	29.0 (107.91)	34.4 (127.8)
Latin America and Caribbean	6.3 (3.40)	12.6 (6.82)
Developing countries	26.7 (149.63)	32.5 (181.92)

Adapted from ACC/SCN (2000). Reproduced with permission of the World Health Organization.

the developing world, but particularly in Asian children. Their continued stunting may reflect not only their lower nutrient intakes from local diets but also the constant impact of infection, mostly from infected water and food. The dramatic effect of ridding a child of a gastrointestinal infection is shown by the remarkable spurt in height when children with worm infection are dewormed. Thus, the stunting of children may prove to be the result of a complex interaction between the quality and quantity of the child's food intake and the burden of chronic low-grade intestinal, respiratory and other infections. The persistence of infections is in part a reflection of the immune deficit in malnutrition, and deficiencies of many vitamins (such as vitamin A) and minerals (such as zinc) are clearly associated with an excess susceptibility to infection. The infection itself, however, places increased demands on nutrient requirements and often leads to anorexia, thus mechanistically nutrition and infection are closely intertwined. Wasting and stunting are two types of nutritionally mediated growth deficits in childhood. Wasting indicated by a low weight for height can occur at any age. Stunting is seen when a child's height is low for their age and reflects poor nutrition during the early growth period, which is often the result of infectious episodes during this period. Physical stunting is associated with poor mental development and socioeconomic deprivation. Stunting is more common in southern Asia and seems to be related to the high incidence of LBW (<2500 g) in this region.

A largely neglected issue of immense societal and public health importance is the issue of brain development and learning in undernourished children in developing societies. Recent research has demonstrated that children who are stunted and living in deprived circumstances develop poorly and have major deficits in intellectual and cognitive development and social behavior. It has been shown that children's scholastic ability in their teens can be strongly influenced by interventions in the second and third years of life. Children who are involved in simple parent-assisted play with the use of simple blocks, which can be assembled in a stack or sequence, learn early to improve their mental processing in nonverbal skills. By supplementing their diet with extra food rich in nutrients, the children's mental development is again improved. The combination of extra food and mental stimulation has an effect in boosting mental development which is so remarkable that the combined effect allows children almost to catch up with the mental development of those reared in a very advantageous environment. Fur-

thermore, imposing this combination of food and environmental stimulation on children for 1 year when they are 6 months to 3 years old leads to a long-term gain in children's scholastic performance many years later.

The dependence of brain development on good nutrition has been recognized for decades, with iodine deficiency in its extreme form leading to cretinism. Even if cretinism is avoided, postnatal iodine deficiency can lead to slowing of mental processing that results in permanent impairment of mental development because of the need for adequate nutrition during early periods of development. Similarly, it has now been clearly demonstrated that anemia induced by iron deficiency can permanently handicap children at a crucial time in their scholastic development. Experimentally, however, iron is required for the synthesis of many cerebral enzymes, so a biochemical basis for selective nutritional effects on mental processing is clear. Although selective nutrient deficiencies can lead to impaired brain function, studies also show that food that stimulates longitudinal bone growth also stimulates brain development, thus implying a more generic demand for a range of nutrients provided by adequate amounts of good-quality, safe food if mental function is to improve. These studies of childhood nutrition and brain development have profound public health significance. Until now there has been a reluctance to infer that many groups in developing societies are mentally handicapped as a result of nutritional insults. However, 20–50% of the children living in developing societies are physically stunted (Table 15.1), while anemia and iodine deficiency threaten a proportion of the world's children (Table 15.2). We need to therefore recognize that the human capital of developing societies is limited by inadequate provision of food and good nutrition for the proper development, physical and mental, of its children. This then acquires huge economic and public health significance since the future adults who are slow and less able to adapt may become a societal burden rather than an asset. These examples illustrate

Table 15.2 Global prevalence (%) of iron-deficiency anemia

	0–4 years	5–14 years	Nonpregnant women	Pregnant women	Men	Elderly
Developing	42	53	43	55	35	51
Developed	17	8	11	19	5	12

From ACC/SCN (2000). Reproduced with permission of the World Health Organization.

the importance of food and nutrition in the development of human capital in developing countries.

Undernutrition among adolescents

Adolescents comprise a significant proportion of the world's population and some estimates put the numbers of youth at over 30% of the global population. The proportion of adolescents within a population group is also rising relative to other age groups and an overwhelming proportion of young adolescents live in developing countries. Increases in height as well as weight occur during adolescence. About 25% of an individual's attained height is achieved during adolescence as a result of the pubertal growth spurt, and this period marks the end of the growth in height. Variations in adolescent body size and the timing of maturational events are determined genetically in populations whose environment allows full expression of the genotype. Where this is limited by environmental constraints, including nutrition, the observed growth and maturation during adolescence reflects environmental rather than inherited potential. Growth differences among groups are related to nutritional status, socioeconomic and other factors, since growth in adolescence may be limited by prolonged undernutrition, infections and chronic disease. Stunting or short stature in adolescence is not only indicative of past undernutrition during childhood but also a cumulative indicator of nutritional status during adolescence. Stunting among adolescents reflects increased health risks, particularly among females who also tend to have a small pelvis, which is more likely to result in obstructed labor during childbirth. Undernutrition in girls during adolescence is characterized by low body weight and results in poor pregnancy outcomes, particularly an increased risk of LBW. Undernutrition may also limit school achievement and work productivity in later years.

The diagnostic criterion for defining stunting in adolescents is height for age less than the third percentile of the WHO reference data or less than -2 Z-scores. Undernutrition or thinness in adolescence is indicated by a body mass index (BMI, weight/height^2) less than the fifth percentile of the WHO reference data. A BMI for age greater than the 85th percentile in adolescence indicates a risk of overweight.

Adult undernutrition

The emphasis until recently has been on the nutrition and health of vulnerable groups in society, that is, children, pregnant and nursing mothers and possibly the elderly, because they were considered to be particularly susceptible to nutritional deficiencies and insults. It is becoming increasingly apparent that the condition of adult undernutrition has been neglected and this may have profound significance for the economic development of poor countries. A chronic state of undernutrition in the adult has its cost in terms of risk to health and impairment of function, which may include a lowered work capacity, a reduced ability to sustain economically productive work or even socially desirable physical activities, and possibly an impaired immune function with a predisposition to repeated infections and consequent absenteeism. The ability to develop effective economies, particularly in rural societies, may therefore be limited by the well-being of the adults on whom the vulnerable in society depend.

The lack of a true definition for the assessment of adult undernutrition has been addressed recently, as it has been difficult to establish satisfactory reference standards for normality and to delineate cut-offs to help to distinguish between well-nourished and under-nourished individuals in population groups. The BMI is considered to be the most suitable, objective anthropometric indicator of nutritional status of the adult. BMI was chosen since this indicator, derived from measures of weight and height of individuals of both genders, was consistently and highly correlated with body weight and was relatively independent of the stature or height of the adult. A BMI < 18.5 was considered as the cut-off for the diagnosis of chronic undernutrition in adults, along with a series of cut-offs that were provided to delineate the degrees of severity of undernutrition. BMI as the anthropometric indicator of adult undernutrition has similar advantages to weight for height in children in that it reflects the degree of severity of undernutrition and can also be used to assess overnutrition in adults by enabling the classification of underweight, normal weight, overweight and obese individuals in the same population. BMI is not only a sensitive index of adult nutritional status but also allows variations in weight in relation to socioeconomic status, dietary intakes and seasonal fluctuations in the availability of food in the community to be demonstrated. Below a BMI of 17.0 considerable impairment of physical well-being and exercise capacity is evident, with individuals becoming more lethargic and susceptible to illness.

These anthropometric measures of adult as well as childhood malnutrition now provide an opportunity for objective measures of the prevalence of undernutrition worldwide. In practice, children and adults may adapt to a shortage of food by reducing their physical activity without changing their body weight. Thus, measures of the prevalence of low weight for height provide only a minimum index of underfeeding; physical activity is fundamental to children's play and exploration and therefore to their mental development. Similarly, in adults physical activity is desirable not only for physiological well-being and for limiting the development of chronic disease, but also to allow societies to prosper through physically demanding economic activity and those developmental processes that rely on an energetic and enterprising population.

Anthropometric surveys of the nutritional status of adults with objective assessments of the numbers of undernourished adults are rare because the issue of adult undernutrition in the developing regions of the world has also largely been ignored until recently. Table 15.3 provides some data compiled since 1995 for some countries in Africa, South America and Asia based on the use of BMI.

Nutrition of the elderly

Adults aged 60 years of age and older represent the fastest growing segment of populations throughout the world. Decline in height with age is well-documented in the elderly and reduction in weight also occurs with increasing age, although the pattern of change in weight is quite different from that of height and varies with the gender of the individual. The use of anthropometry is relatively recent in the elderly and the anthropometric index of choice is BMI. Thus, height, weight and BMI are good indicators of nutritional status and the risk of morbidity and mortality in the elderly population. Measurement of height can be a problem in the elderly as a result of increasing spinal curvature with age. There are no guidelines regarding the degree of spinal curvature that would invalidate the measurement of height. Height can be estimated preferably from knee height or from arm span in the elderly. The WHO recommends knee height as being more satisfactory than arm span and the estimated height can then be used to derive the BMI. The same BMI categories as for adults apply to the elderly. Given these practical problems with obtaining accurate BMI measurements, the mid-upper arm circumference has

Table 15.3 Estimates of underweight (BMI < 18.5) and obese (BMI > 30) adult women in developing countries

	Mean age (years)	Underweight (%)	Obese (%)
Africa			
Benin (1996)	29.4	14.1	3.2
Central African Republic (1995)	28.5	15.3	2.1
Chad (1997)	28.9	19.8	2.7
Comoros (1996)	30.0	8.6	5.0
Egypt (1996)	29.5	1.8	19.4
Kenya (1998)	28.3	10.7	5.0
Madagascar (1997)	28.9	19.9	0.6
Niger (1998)	29.0	19.4	1.8
Tanzania (1996)	29.6	8.9	3.5
Uganda (1995)	28.3	9.3	2.4
Zambia (1995)	28.9	8.5	2.7
Latin America			
Bolivia (1998)	30.3	0.7	11.6
Brazil (1996)	28.9	6.6	9.9
Colombia (1995)	28.9	3.5	9.6
Dominican Republic (1996)	27.9	6.4	10.5
Guatemala (1995)	29.5	3.3	7.4
Honduras (1996)	30.7	8.6	8.3
Nicaragua (1998)	28.7	3.5	11.6
Peru (1996)	30.0	1.0	9.2
Asia			
Bangladesh (1996)	27.3	51.3	2.0
India (1999)	27.5	39.1	1.2
Nepal (1996)	28.1	27.4	0.1
Uzbekistan (1996)	26.8	11.1	3.7

BMI: body mass index.

been evaluated and appears to be a more sensitive index than BMI in the elderly.

There are few studies from the developing world that have looked at the nutritional status of elderly in their populations. Those that have looked the elderly in their midst suggest that undernutrition in the elderly is a serious problem; one study in India reported the prevalence to be as high as 35% in the elderly of both genders.

Public health initiatives that deal with the problems of undernutrition worldwide need to recognize that the basic causes of undernutrition are clearly political and socioeconomic factors. Revolutions in the twentieth century in Russia and China resulted in great improvements in food supplies for the whole population. Agricultural revolutions such as the "green revolution" have also increased food availability and helped to meet the food needs of the population. However, poverty is often the basis of a failure to obtain food even when it is available. The most important determinants of hunger in developing countries are employment, personal levels of income and the prices that individuals pay for food. Accelerated food production will alleviate hunger to the extent that the resources used in the process reduce poverty and lower food prices more than they would if used in other ways.

15.3 Hidden hunger: the global problem of micronutrient deficiency

Micronutrient deficiencies that have long been ignored have more recently moved to center stage. With the earlier preoccupation largely on increased production of food to meet the serious problem of food adequacy worldwide, the recognition of the extensive micronutrient deficiencies that existed globally and their cost to societies resulted in the usage of the term "hidden hunger" to characterize the large-scale vitamin and mineral deficiencies. From a public health perspective, the most important micronutrient deficiencies are iron, iodine and vitamin A deficiency.

Iron deficiency

Iron deficiency is probably the most common nutritional deficiency disorder in the world (see Table 15.2). The highest prevalence figures for iron deficiency are found in infants, children, teenagers and women of childbearing age. Hence, it is a major public health problem with adverse consequences, especially for women of reproductive age and for young children. The predominant cause of iron deficiency worldwide is nutritional, the diet failing to provide for the body's requirements of iron. In tropical countries, intestinal parasitosis exacerbates iron deficiency by increasing the loss of blood from the gastrointestinal tract. The increase in malaria in these countries further contributes to the anemia. A low intake of iron or its poor absorption, or both, then fails to meet the enhanced demands for iron and anemia results.

The consequences of iron deficiency are numerous as iron plays a central role in the transport of oxygen in the body and is also essential in many enzyme systems. Not only does iron deficiency affect neurotransmitter systems in the brain with changes in behavior, such as attention, memory and learning in infants and small children, but it also negatively influences the normal defence systems against infection. T-lymphocyte function, phagocytosis and the killing of bacteria by neutrophilic leukocytes are affected. In pregnant women iron deficiency contributes to maternal morbidity and mortality, and increases the risk of fetal morbidity, mortality and LBW. Long-standing iron deficiency in general terms also results in a reduction in physical work capacity and productivity of adults in both agricultural and industrial work situations. These functional impairments are economically important.

Iron-deficiency disorders encompass a range of body iron depletion states. The least severe is diminished iron stores, diagnosed by decreased serum ferritin levels, which may not be associated with adverse physiological consequences. Iron deficiency without anemia is severe enough to affect production of hemoglobin without hemoglobin levels falling below the clinical criteria indicative of anemia. This condition is characterized by decreased transferrin saturation levels and increased erythrocyte protoporphyrin. The major clinical manifestation of iron deficiency is iron-deficiency anemia (IDA). IDA seems to be a particular problem of developing countries (Table 15.2) and the dominant cause is nutritional iron deficiency. Even in industrialized, developed countries the prevalence of IDA varies between 2 and 8%. The availability of iron in the diet for absorption is affected by both the form of iron and the nature of foods concurrently ingested. Iron exists in the diet in two forms:

- heme iron is found only in animal sources, is readily available for absorption and is not influenced by other constituents of the diet
- inorganic iron is not readily available and is strongly influenced by factors present in foods ingested at the same time.

Both animal foods and ascorbic acid (vitamin C) promote the absorption of inorganic iron. Diets that are primarily cereal and legume based may contain much iron but, in the absence of cofactors such as ascorbic acid, they may provide only a low level of available iron.

Anemia affects nearly 2000 million people worldwide, while iron deficiency is estimated to affect nearly 5000 million. Overall, globally, 39% of preschool children are anemic and 52% of pregnant women are anemic; of these, more than 90% live in developing countries. Many school-aged children are also anemic, even in developed countries. IDA thus affects all age groups and has a far-reaching impact since it has profound negative effects on human health and development.

The WHO is active in developing strategies to combat iron deficiency. These include:

- iron supplementation
- iron fortification of certain foods
- dietary modification to improve the bioavailability of dietary iron by modifying the composition of meals
- parasitic disease control.

Iron and folate supplementation programs for pregnant women are currrently widely implemented in several countries; about 50 countries have a universal preventive supplementation policy during pregnancy. Iron supplementation aimed at preschool or school-aged children is being carried out in over 23 countries. Fortification of foods with iron is a preventive measure aimed at improving and sustaining adequate iron nutrition over a longer term. Many industrialized countries such as Canada, the UK and the USA have fortified foods with iron. Recently, large studies in developing countries have demonstrated the effectiveness of iron fortification of foods, provided these programs are based on careful planning and follow well-established guidelines. Improvement in the supply, consumption and the bioavailability of iron in food is an important strategy to improve the iron status of populations. The bioavailability of iron in foods is influenced by the composition of the meal and food preparation methods. The consumption of ascorbate-rich foods enhances iron absorption, whereas limiting the content of phytate, which inhibits iron absorption, will improve the bioavailability of iron from the diet. Malaria and intestinal parasites (especially hookworm) are important contributors to IDA in endemic areas. In populations where hookworm is prevalent, effective treatment of this helminthic infection has reduced IDA in school-aged children.

Iodine deficiency

The term iodine deficiency disorder (IDD) refers to a complex of effects arising from iodine deficiency. The mountainous areas of the world are likely to be iodine deficient because the rain leaches the iodine from the rocks and soils. The most severely deficient areas are the Himalayas, the Andes, the European Alps and the vast mountainous regions of China. Although iodine deficiency is likely to occur in all elevated regions subject to glaciation and higher rainfall which runs off into rivers, it also occurs in the flooded river deltas of Bangladesh, India and Burma. The Great Lake basins of North America are also iodine deficient. Excessive intakes of goitrogens in food, such as the consumption of cassava or the *brassica* group of vegetables, and in water (water-borne goitrogens in Latin America), as well as the deficiency of certain trace elements in the soil or food chain (such as selenium), may interfere with the uptake and metabolism of iodine in the body and can thus cause or amplify the effects of iodine deficiency.

IDD in humans is predominantly the result of a primary deficiency of iodine in the diet. Both water and foods are sources of iodine, with marine fish being the richest source of iodine. Milk and meat are also rich sources of iodine. Fruits, legumes and vegetables as well as freshwater fish are important additional sources. Plant foods are likely to show a reduced content of iodine if the iodine content of the soils in which they are grown is low. Goitrogens in the diet are of secondary importance as etiological factors in IDD. Recently, it has been shown that staple foods from developing countries, such as cassava, maize, sweet potatoes and lima beans, contain cyanogenic glucosides that release a goitrogen thiocyanate. Cassava is now implicated as an important contributor to iodine deficiency and results in endemic goitre and cretinism in non-mountainous Zaire and in Sarawak in Malaysia. There is also increasing evidence that selenium deficiency in the soil can result in manifestations of IDD in the presence of modest iodine deficiency, since selenium is an important trace element that is essential for thyroid metabolism. Selenium deficiency is now increasingly recognized as an etiological factor in IDD in several regions of China.

Iodine is readily absorbed from the diet and forms a very important element in the synthesis of thyroid hormones in the body. Thyroid hormones are essential for normal growth and development. Just before birth, the levels of the biologically active triiodothyronine (T_3) increase and prepare the organism for the transition from intrauterine to extrauterine life. Failure to synthesize sufficient T_3 as a result of iodine deficiency may be a factor in the stillbirths that occur as a part of the spectrum of IDD in humans. Thyroid hormone deficiency leads to severe retardation of the growth and maturation of all organs. The brain is particularly susceptible to damage during the fetal and early post-natal periods. It has been confirmed that the thyroidal control of neonatal brain development is more important than fetal brain development since early and optimal thyroid hormone treatment after birth can lead to a substantial improvement in thyroid function.

The prevalence of IDD varies globally and at present is confined to developing countries, largely because public health initiatives such as iodization of salt have been introduced in the developed, industrialized world. Iodine deficiency and goitre are still widely prevalent and are a significant public health problem in 130 countries, affecting a total of 740 million people. Despite the remarkable progress achieved in eradicating IDD there are over 16 million cretins and 49.5 million people are still affected by lesser degrees of IDD-related brain damage.

The public health initiatives for correcting iodine deficiency require the provision of adequate iodine to the individual. IDD are excellent examples of nutritional deficiency disorders of public health importance that can readily be abolished if mass community programs are undertaken. This reduction in IDD has been achieved by several methods.

Iodization of salt

Iodization of salt has been the most favored method and has greatly reduced the prevalence of IDD in Switzerland, the USA, Yugoslavia and New Zealand. Since its first successful introduction in the 1920s in Switzerland, successful programs have been reported more recently in Central and South America, Europe (Finland) and Asia (China and Taiwan). However, several developing countries have encountered problems with their salt iodization programs because it is difficult to produce and maintain enough high-quality iodized salt for large populations such as in India. The extra costs of iodized salt and problems with its availability and distribution to remote regions can also be a problem. These issues may be compounded by cultural prejudices about the use of iodized salt and the loss of iodine with cooking if salt is not added after cooking.

Iodized oil injections

Iodized oil injections have been used to prevent goitre and cretinism in New Guinea. Iodized oil is suitable for mass programs and can be carried out alongside mass immunization programs. These methods have been successful in China, Indonesia and Nepal. The major problems with iodized oil are the cost, the initial discomfort and the potential disadvantage associated with the transmission of hepatitis B and the human immunodeficiency virus (HIV) with the use of needles. The need for a primary health care team to inject the iodized oil can be a further disadvantage.

Iodized oil by mouth

Iodized oil by mouth may be an effective alternative and has been tried as a single oral dose for children in South America and Burma. Oral iodized oil has also been tried in women and primary health centers can readily administer this scheme. However, the effects of oral iodized oil seem to last for only half as long as a similar dose of injected iodized oil. They do not, however, suffer from the disadvantages of iodized oil injections, so this is a preferred method for use in remote areas.

Vitamin A deficiency

Vitamin A deficiency leads to xerophthalmia and may result in blindness in children. Xerophthalmia continues to be a major cause of childhood blindness, despite the intensive prevention programs undertaken since the 1980s. It is a widespread problem and the parts of the world most seriously affected include southern and eastern Asia, and many countries in Africa, Latin America and the Near East. Vitamin A is the parent of a class of compounds called retinoids. Provitamin A carotenoids, chiefly β-carotene, are also included in the vitamin A family. Preformed vitamin A is chiefly found in dairy products such as milk, butter, cheese and egg yolk, in some fatty fish and in the livers of farm animals and fish. Carotenes are generally abundant in yellow fruits (papayas, mangoes, apricots, peaches) and vegetables (carrots). Absorption of vitamin A is about 80% complete in the presence of an adequate fat intake, while the absorption of carotenoids is highly dependent on bile salts. Vitamin A (retinol and retinoic acid) plays a very important role in the body in cellular development and differentiation. Retinol also has a vital role in normal vision, particularly in the rods in the retina. Thus, one of the earliest manifestations of vitamin A deficiency is night blindness. Vitamin A deficiency is now known to decrease children's resistance to infections and increase mortality. Vitamin A is also involved in fetal development, cell-mediated immunity, hematopiesis, spermatogenesis, appetite and physical growth.

Vitamin A deficiency (VAD) is a major public health problem affecting preschool children and pregnant women in low-income developing countries. VAD is the leading cause of preventable severe visual impairment and blindness. Between 250 000 and 500 000 children with VAD become blind every year. In addition, VAD increases the risk of illness and the consequent morbidity and mortality. In VAD-prevalent countries pregnant women often suffer night blindness, with reported prevalences as high as 10–20%. The deficient state continues into early lactation, with the infants acquiring the increased risk of VAD owing to low vitamin A levels in breast milk. It has been estimated that VAD is a public health problem in 96 countries. Africa has the highest prevalence of clinical VAD, while the highest numbers affected are in south and southeast Asia. Among the under fives with VAD, 3 million have signs of xeropthalmia, while 140–250 million children with VAD have only subclinical manifestations and live with the increased risk of morbidity and mortality due to infectious diseases.

There is now increasing evidence that vitamin A supplements in deficient populations can reduce morbidity, mortality and blindness. Xerophthalmia has become less prevalent in recent years in hyperendemic areas such as Indonesia and India. Intervention strategies that may have contributed to this include periodic megadose vitamin A supplementation in the form of capsules or syrup, or as an injected dose. The fortification of dietary items that are universally consumed, such as sugar in Central America and monosodium glutamate in Indonesia has had a favorable impact on the vitamin A status of the whole population. The problems with food fortification are essentially logistical and technological. Food supplies from different regions of the world show limited vitamin A availability, but the problem is exacerbated by a tendency to withhold vegetables and fruits from children and from pregnant and lactating women for cultural and other reasons. In Asia, there is a particular problem because the average availability of vitamin A is less than that required and the problem is also exacerbated by the maldistribution within the population of foods rich in vitamin A. Nutrition education is the only answer when vitamin A deficiency develops despite fruit and vegetable sources of the vitamin being in plentiful supply. These foods are not incorporated into the diets of young children and mothers, because of either a lack of knowledge or cultural biases. Nutrition education together with practical advice and help with growing cheap, nutritious vegetables in home kitchen gardens may help to eradicate vitamin A deficiency.

This chapter has dealt with only some of the more important nutritionally determined deficiency disorders of public health importance. It is important to recognize that segments of populations in the world suffer from other nutritional disorders, such as those due to the deficiency of fluoride, zinc, selenium, B group vitamins and ascorbic acid. Some of these seem to occur during seasonal deficiencies in their availability, and accompany famine and conflict situations when they are seen in refugee camps. It is important to recognize that apart from these specific situations, in all regions of the world there are still some populations affected by one or more of these deficiencies, despite the significant advances that have been made in controlling nutritional deficiency disorders. In some regions of the world, largely as a result of increasing population size, the numbers of undernourished people are increasing, even though the population prevalence is declining. In many there is shift in the severity of the deficiency diseases, with decreasing numbers with severe deficiency and increasing numbers with mild to moderate deficiencies. For a majority of these countries there is still the need to pursue vigorous policies and targeted action to combat the various nutritional deficiency disorders as a part of the comprehensive health-orientated national food and nutrition policies.

15.4 Food, nutrition and the emerging burden of obesity and chronic diseases

In stark contrast to the global problem of nutritional inadequacies are diet and nutrition related non communicable diseases (NCD) such as cancer and heart disease, which have their roots partly in poor nutrition. The relationships between patterns of diet and nutrient intake and NCD are not as clear-cut as those for nutrient intake and macronutrient and micronutrient deficiency disorders and, consequently, the solutions for one may not be suitable for the other. NCD are generally multifactorial in nature, with diet just one of several elements involved.

NCD take an enormous toll in lives and health worldwide. They now account for nearly 60% of deaths globally, mostly due to heart disease, stroke, cancer, diabetes and lung diseases. The rapid rise of NCD represents one of the major health challenges to global development in the twenty-first century and threatens the economic and social development of nations as well

Table 15.4 Global distribution of deaths from three groups of causes by region

Region	Infectious causes (%)	Noncommunicable causes (%)	Injuries (%)
Established market economies	6.2	87.6	6.2
Former socialist economies	3.6	86.8	9.6
China	15.1	73.4	11.5
Latin America	32.3	57.9	9.8
Middle Eastern crescent	46.2	44.8	8.9
India	43.3	50.2	6.5
Sub-Saharan Africa	68.2	23.9	7.9
Other Asia and islands	41.8	49.6	8.6
World	33.4	58.1	8.5

Adapted from Murray and Lopez (1994). Reproduced with permission of the World Health Organization.

Box 15.1 Determinants of noncommunicable diseases in developing societies

- Demographic changes in population
- Epidemiological transition
- Urbanization and migration from rural to urban areas
- Changes in food consumption and dietary patterns
- Lifestyle changes (physical activity patterns, sociocultural changes, stress)
- Impact of birth weight and the effects of early life programing
- Infections and their associations with chronic disease risk
- Effects of malnutrition and nutrient deficiencies that increase risk
- Poverty, inequalities and social exclusion, which increase risk and reduce access
- Deleterious effects of environmental degradation and pollution
- Impact of globalization of diet and lifestyles

as the lives and health of millions of people. In 1998 alone, NCD were estimated to have contributed to 31.7 million deaths globally and 43% of the global burden of disease. Based on current trends, it is expected that by 2020, NCD will account for 73% of deaths and 60% of the disease burden.

Until recently it was believed that NCD were a minor or even nonexistent problem in the developing countries. A recent analysis of mortality trends from NCD suggests that large increases in NCD have occurred in developing countries, particularly those in rapid nutritional transition such as China and India (Table 15.4). According to these estimates at least 40% of all deaths in developing countries are attributable to NCD, while in industrialized countries NCD account for 75% of all deaths. Low- and middle-income countries suffer the greatest impact of NCD. The rapid increase in these diseases is seen disproportionately in poor and disadvantaged populations and is contributing to widening health gaps between and within countries. In 1998, of the total number of deaths attributable to NCD, 77% occurred in developing countries, and of the disease burden they represent, 85% was borne by low- and middle-income countries.

It is important to recognize that these trends are indicative of an increase in NCD in developing countries that may be partly confounded by factors such as an increase in life expectancy, a progressive reduction in deaths due to communicable diseases in adulthood, and improvements in case detection and reporting.

However, the increase in the incidence of these chronic degenerative diseases is real, and the complex range of factors (Box 15.1) that interact to determine the nature and course of this epidemic needs to be understood so that preventive strategies may be adopted to help developing societies to deal with this burgeoning problem. Developing countries, in particular those in rapid transition and economic development, will face the consequences of both nutritional deficits and excesses and will be subject to the double burden of persisting undernutrition in the midst of a growing epidemic of obesity (see Figure 15.1) and NCD. Both forms of malnutrition will contribute substantially to the increasing loss of disability-adjusted life years, continued reduction in economic growth and national productivity, and increases in health burden and the consequent costs.

Obesity deserves special mention since this nutritional condition underlies and contributes to the comorbidities of NCD. Obesity is a serious problem in the developed countries of the world and is becoming an increasing problem in developing countries as incomes rise. Some countries have increasing rates of obesity in the midst of a high incidence of childhood malnutrition and stunting. As developing countries embrace the dominant Western economic ways of development, and industrialize and urbanize, the living standards of their populations rise and are associated with dramatic changes in diet and lifestyles, leading to weight gains and obesity, which then pose a growing threat to health.

Interventions to prevent these diseases should focus on controlling the risk factors in an integrated manner and at the family and community level, since the causal risk factors are deeply entrenched in the

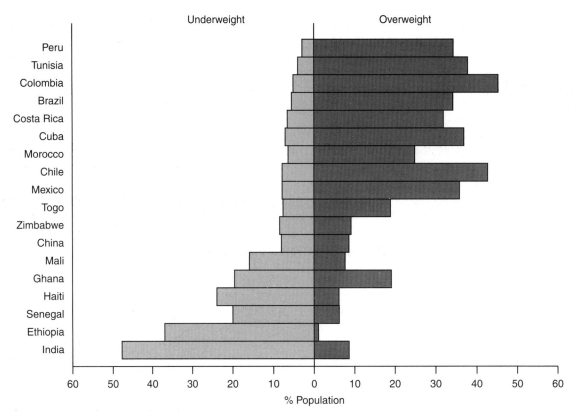

Figure 15.1 Reciprocal relationship in the prevalence of underweight [body mass index (BMI) < 18.5] and overweight (BMI > 25.0) in developing countries. The "double burden" of both forms of malnutrition among adults is illustrated.

social and cultural framework of society. Developing countries, in particular, have to recognize that the emerging epidemic of obesity and NCD is a cause for concern and that it needs to be dealt with as a national priority. They have to learn from the experience of industrialized and affluent countries to tackle this crisis, since the emerging health burden of chronic disease will affect the economically productive adult population and will consume scarce resources.

15.5 Food and nutrition and the promotion of public health

The public health approach to the prevention of nutrition and diet-related diseases requires the adoption of health-orientated nutrition and food policies for the whole population. In most developing countries, the first priority must be ensuring the production or procurement of an adequate food supply, and its equitable distribution and availability to the whole population,

along with the elimination of the various forms of nutritional deficiencies, which include protein–energy malnutrition, vitamin, mineral and trace element deficiencies. Efforts must also be made to improve the quality of the food, which includes reducing spoilage and contamination of foods as well as diversifying the availability and use of foods. In agrarian societies, consideration must be given to the short- and long-term effects of agricultural policies that affect the income and buying power of the small producers. Particular attention needs to be paid to the impact that the promotion of cash crops has on the availability and ability to procure the principal staples in the diet, as well as to the feasibility of fortification of foods to deal with localized or widespread deficiencies of iodine and iron, as a mass intervention measure.

In developed countries, the burgeoning costs of tertiary health care related to the diagnosis and management of the increasing occurrence and the associated morbidity of chronic diet-related diseases have had an impact. There is increasing recognition of the need for prevention-orientated health and nutrition policies and changes in behavior and lifestyle to reduce the occurrence of these diseases. Some developed countries have been active in the field of public education, using national dietary guidelines as a major stimulus. It is important to remember that nutrition education of the public operates in an area where advice is given on a balance of probabilities, rather than irrefutable evidence or any degree of certainty, and that consensus is based on the balance of the available evidence. The causes of these chronic diseases are complex and dietary factors are only a part of the explanation. Individuals differ in their susceptibility to the adverse health effects of specific dietary factors or deficiencies of others. Within the context of public health the focus is the health of the whole population and interventions are aimed at lowering the average level of risk to the health of the whole population.

Changes in consumer preferences have emerged, initially among the upper socioeconomic and educated masses. The media attention, along with the behavioral changes in food preferences and food choices, are in turn influencing industry in the modification of the systems for food production and processing. However, progress in changing consumer behavior and preferences is intrinsically slow and has until recently largely occurred with support for public policies in the health sector. The process of changing unsatisfactory dietary practices and lifestyles and thus promoting health is not easy to achieve both socially and politically. Despite these limitations, the occurrence of and mortality associated with some diet-related chronic diseases such as coronary heart disease have declined, reflecting possible changes in the lifestyles of the population.

The dynamic relationship between changes in a population's diet and changes in its health is reflected well in two critical situations. One is the change in disease and mortality profiles of migrant populations moving from a low-risk to a high-risk environment. An example of this is the change in disease pattern of Japanese migrants to the USA. The other more important and rapid change is seen within a country as rural to urban migration occurs, or more frequently as a developing country undergoes rapid industrialization and development, and in the process acquires a dietary change characteristic of the latter, as well as the disease, morbidity and premature mortality profile of a developed country. Several other developing countries have urban pockets of affluent diet and lifestyles and

similar disease burdens in the midst of problems typical of a poor, developing country. Such countries in transition, such as India and Brazil, bear the dual burdens of diseases of affluence and the widespread health problems of a poor country. Developing countries can benefit by learning from the experience of dietary change and adverse health effects characteristic of the developed world. In developing countries the aim should be to avoid the diseases and premature deaths related to the affluent diet and lifestyle. By recognizing this problem, governments of developing countries can gain for their people the health benefits of avoiding nutritional deficiencies without encouraging the development of diet-related NCD that invariably accompany economic and technological development.

It is thus possible for a country to achieve a reduction in infant and childhood mortality and an increase in life expectancy by pursuing health and nutrition policies that aim to provide adequate and equitable access to hygienic and nutritious food, and at the same time to minimize the occurrence of diet-related chronic diseases. This, in turn, will help to avoid the social and economic costs of morbidity and premature death in middle age, a period of highest economic activity and productivity to the nation and to society at large. If such a socially and economically desirable goal is to be achieved, then national governments in both developing and developed countries must aim towards achieving population-based dietary and lifestyle changes that promote the health of their people.

15.6 Perspectives on the future

The ultimate goal of all stakeholders in the arena of food and nutrition is to achieve a world where every individual has access to adequate quantities of good-quality and safe food, to promote optimal physical and mental development, and to sustain a healthy and productive life in communities where all forms of malnutrition are absent. Despite the recognition of the importance of this objective, food insecurity and nutritional problems exist widely throughout the world. Inadequate consumption of energy and deficient intakes of micronutrients such as iodine and vitamin A persist alongside the increasing burden of obesity and diet-related NCD. While food and nutrition are accepted as being integral to meeting the basic needs of people and as a human rights issue, they are also increasingly being recognized as an investment in human capital that raises productivity and ensures returns on investment in education and health care. Economists have estimated the costs of hunger and malnutrition by arguing that raising per capita calorie consumption above the minimum threshold increases the per capita gross domestic product (GDP) growth rate of countries, and that nutrition affects economic growth rate both directly, through its impact on labor productivity, and indirectly, through improvements in life expectancy.

The major global challenges in food and nutrition that continue to persist while others are emerging are outlined in Box 15.2.

These include, when looked at from a life-course perspective:

- the persisting huge problems of LBW
- childhood malnutrition, particularly underweight and stunting
- micronutrient deficiencies, in particular those of iron, iodine and vitamin A
- adult undernutrition, more specifically underweight among mothers which predisposes to IUGR
- diseases of urbanization and affluence: obesity and its comorbidities in NCD are emerging as important issues.

In addition to these serious problems we are faced with challenges of refugees and internally displaced peoples as a result of natural disasters, conflict and other complex emergencies. These groups are increasingly vulnerable to food and nutritional deficiencies. The changing demographic profile and the increasing numbers of elderly people in the world, even in developing societies, is another global challenge that needs to be addressed. Emerging epidemics of HIV and the acquired immunodeficiency syndrome (AIDS) contribute to food and nutritional problems in many ways, resulting in a dramatic reduction in the adult economically productive population and thus contribute to a reduction in agricultural output and increase food insecurity at the household level. Widening income disparities and inequalities in developed and developing societies are contributing to variations in health and access to health care despite sustained economic development. Environmental changes and globalization are other factors that contribute to the burgeoning challenges that outpace the achievement of the ultimate goal of food and nutrition security at the household level.

The links between malnutrition and food insecurity are well established. Food security is said to exist "when all people at all times have physical, social and economic access to sufficient (quantity), nutritious (quality) and safe food which meets their dietary needs and food preferences for an active and healthy life". Despite the remarkable achievements in increasing food production, attributable largely to the impact of the "green revolution" in several developing countries, the current level of food insecurity in the developing world is unacceptable. Over 800 million people, or one-sixth of the developing world's population (including 280 million in southern Asia, 240 million in eastern Asia and 180 million in sub-Saharan Africa), do not have access to sufficient food to lead healthy, productive lives. Food insecurity is closely associated with poverty: about 1.2 billion people in the developing world are absolutely poor, with only a dollar a day or less to meet food, shelter and other basic needs. The majority of the world's poor live in rural areas and are dependent on agriculture, either directly or indirectly, for their employment, income and food security.

The first two decades of the twenty-first century will see a further increase in the world's population (estimated to be a 24% increase), almost all of it in developing countries and much of it in urban areas. The rapid urbanization will have its effects on diet and lifestyles, and have profound effects on food preferences and food demands. Food production has hitherto kept pace with the increase in population growth, and

---

Box 15.2 Current major global challenges in food and nutrition

- Low birth weight (LBW) and intrauterine growth retardation (IUGR) (30 million LBW births; 23.8% of all births are LBW in developing countries)
- Childhood malnutrition among preschool children (149.6 million underweight; 206 million stunted)
- Iodine deficiency disorders (IDD) (Significant public health problem in 130 countries; 740 million affected)
- Vitamin A deficiency (VAD) (Between 140 and 250 million children affected)
- Iron-deficiency anemia (IDA) (2000 million have anemia; 39% of preschool children and 52% of pregnant women)
- Adult undernutrition (Undernourished mothers are at increased risk of having LBW outcomes)
- Overweight and obesity (Increasing prevalence globally; coexisting with undernutrition in developing countries)
- Increasing incidence of noncommunicable diseases (NCD) (Increasingly significant contributor to disability and premature death in developed and developing societies)

the prospects for economic growth in the developing world also appear to be favorable. The large projected increases in food needs (mainly cereal demands) will have to be met by increases in productivity. Since the opportunities for ecologically and economically sound land use are limited, much of this will have to be achieved by improving crop yields. Cereal production is projected to increase in developing countries, but will not keep pace with increased demands contributed by the strong growth in demand for meat in developing societies, which are not ecologically sustainable in the long run.

Investments in increasing food production to cope with the increasing demand as the population rises are essential to achieving food security. A wide range of policies must be in place to promote this goal, including investment in public sector research in biotechnology, developing efficient and effective markets for agricultural inputs and outputs, investment in infrastructure including transportation, water and power, and pursuing macroeconomic trade and sectoral policies that increase the food security of people on low incomes.

However, although making more food available is essential, it is not an adequate condition to ensure food security. Ensuring that people have access to food is vital. Policy initiatives that guarantee access to food and reduce malnutrition are crucial, and these include addressing issues such as women's educational attainment and status in society and increasing rural employment opportunities. Considerable progress has been made in the alleviation of poverty, malnutrition and food insecurity, but this has been slow and insufficient. This is one of the greatest challenges that we face in the new millennium.

Further reading

United Nations Administrative Committee on Coordination, Sub-Committee on Nutrition (ACC/SCN), in collaboration with the International Food Policy Research Institute (IFPRI). 4th Report of the World Nutrition Situation: Nutrition Throughout the Life Cycle, 2000.

Murray CJ, Lopez AD. Global and regional cause of death patterns. Bulletin World Health Organization 1994; 72: 447–480.

Index

Page references in **bold** refer to information in figures or boxes only, those in *italics* are to information in tables only. Abbreviations used in subheadings are: ALP = atherogenic lipoprotein phenotype; BMI = body mass index; BMR = basal metabolic rate; INFOODS = International Food Data System Project; IVNAA = *in vivo* neutron activation analysis; NCDs = noncommunicable diseases; PUFA = polyunsaturated fatty acids; RMR = resting metabolic rate; TAG = triacylglycerol.

acaeruloplasminemia 203
acceptable daily intake (ADI) 267,
    308, 309–10
acrodermatitis enteropathica 199
additives 315–16
adipose tissue 14, **15**
    determination 19, 21, 25, 28
    fatty acids 100
    lipoprotein metabolism 98
adolescent undernutrition 323
alcohol 32, 145, 146
algal toxins 312, 313, *314*
amino acid metabolism 46–7
    biology of requirements 54–9, 61
        and disease 57, 66–7
        estimation 61–3
        factors affecting 66–7
        meeting 63–6
    chemistry 49–50
    classification 50–4
    dietary sources 65–6
    digestibility 64, 65
    functions *47, 48*
    future studies 67
    metabolites from 56–7
    nonspecific nitrogen sources 52–3
    nutritional quality 64–5
    turnover 54–7
    vitamin B₆ 154, 155
amino acids 49–50, *51*
    metabolism *see above*
anemia
    iron-deficiency 195–6, 197,
        325–6
    vitamin-deficiency 159, 164, 165,
        172
animal husbandry 308, 311
animal models 123–4, 281–3

anorexia nervosa 42
anthropometric indices 22–4, 27, 28,
    29, 43, 321, 323–4
antioxidant function **209**
    bioflavonoids 175
    phytoceuticals 176
    selenium 207, 208
    vitamin A 130, 132
    vitamin C 171–2
    vitamin E 139, 140–1
appetite 32, 33
ascorbic acid *see* vitamin C
astroviruses 303
atherogenic lipoprotein phenotype
    (ALP) 97, 112, 113
atherosclerosis 93, 98, 139, 140

Bacillus cereus 297, 298, 300
bacteria, food-borne 294, 295–301
balance studies 122
Bartter's syndrome 185
basal metabolic rate (BMR) 31, 35,
    56, 244–5
Benn index 22
beriberi 145–6
bioavailability 258–9
bioelectrical impedance *15,* 25–6, 27,
    28
bioflavonoids 175
biomarkers 37–9, 123, 243–5
biotechnology 274
biotin *126,* 166–7
blindness 132, 327–8
blood clotting 141–2, 143
blood nutrient levels 33, 73–4, 123,
    173
blood pressure 190–1
body cell mass (BCM) 19

body composition 12–13
    atomic level 13, 14–15
    cellular level 14–15
    determination methods 15–29, 43
    molecular level 13–15
    tissue level 14–15
    whole body level 14–15
body fat, mass *see* fat mass
body mass index (BMI) 22, 27, 29,
    43, 321, 323–4
body water 13, 14
    determination method choice 28
    direct determination 16
    doubly indirect determination 23,
        25
    indirect determination 18, 20–1
bone 14
    calcium 178, 179, 180–2
    fluoride 216–17
    phosphorus 186, 187, 188
    vitamin D 133, 134, 137, 138
    vitamin K 142–3
botulism 296
bovine spongiform encephalopathy
    (BSE) 295, 307–8
brain
    and food intake 33
    iodine deficiency 326–7
    lipids 106, 109
    malnourished children 322
    polyunsaturates 108
    spongiform encephalopathies
        307–8
    thiamin deficiency 146
Broca index 22
burns patients 42

calciferol *see* vitamin D

calcium 178–83
  body composition 13, 178, 180
  dietary recommendations 122,
    182, *182–3*
  micronutrient interactions
    fluoride 217
    iron 183
    magnesium 183, 186
    phosphorus 183, 187, 188
    potassium 193–4
    sodium 190, 192
    vitamin D 133, 134, 136–7, 181,
      183
    zinc 183, 200
calorimetry 34–6
Campylobacter jejuni 295, 296, *298*
carbohydrate(s) *5*, 69–70
  and biotin deficiency 167
  body composition 14
  dental caries 79–80
  digestion 70–2, 74–6
  energy content 31
  energy metabolism 32, 72–3
    expenditure 35, 36, 37
    obesity 42–3
    short chain fatty acids 78, **79**
    vitamin B₁ 144–5, 146
  fatty acid synthesis 100
  fermentation 74, 76, 77–9
  food sources *71*, 77
  future studies 80
  glycemic 70, 72–4
  glycemic index 73–4, 259
  and health 71–2, 75, 79–80
  nonglycemic 74–9
  and serum TAG 112
carbon 13
carbon dioxide 34–6, 72
carbon recycling 102
carcass analysis 15–16, *27*
cardiovascular disease
  burden of 328–30
  flavonoids 175
  folate 163–4, 165
  and lipids
    ALP 97, 112, 113
    cholesterol-lowering fatty acids
      110
    chylomicron remnants 95
    dietary–serum cholesterol levels
      111
    fish oils 112
    future studies 114, 115

LDL receptor pathway 95, 96
    partially hydrogenated 107, 110
    postprandial lipemia 93, 112
    reverse cholesterol transport 96
    TAG hypothesis 98
    vitamin E 139, 140
  potassium 193
  selenium 207
caries 79–80, 216, 217
carnitine 175
cestodes 304
chemicals, safety 295, 308–16
children
  amino acid requirement 61, 62–3
  BMI 22, 321, 323
  carnitine 175
  copper 201, 203, 204
  dietary recommendations 119
  energy balance 40, 42, 45
  fluoride 216, 217
  food-borne illness 292–3, 294, 295,
    301, 311, 320, 322
  global malnutrition 5, 6, 320–4
  iodine 211, 212, 322, 326–7
  iron intake 197, 325
  obesity 45
  protein requirement 59, *60*
  protein synthesis 55–6
  selenium 206, 208
  vitamin A 132, 133, 327–8
  vitamin B₆ 154–5
  vitamin D 137
  vitamin E 140
  vitamin K 143
  zinc 199, 200
chloride 189–92
cholesterol 85, 86
  absorption 89–91, 111
  dietary sources 86, 87
  digestion 88
  heart disease 95, 96, 97, 98, 110,
    111
  hormone effects 98
  lipoproteins 91, 93, 94, 97, 98,
    109–10
    LDL receptor pathway 95–6,
      112–13
  regulation 109
  reverse transport 96
  serum, and diet 109–10, 111,
    112–13
  structural lipid pool 99
  synthesis 109

choline 121, 175
chromium 217–19
circumferences *15*, 24, 43
clinical nutrition 7, 9
Clostridium botulinum 296, *297*
Clostridium perfringens 298, 300
cobalimin *see* vitamin B₁₂
Codex Alimentarius Commission
    (CAC) 269–70, 273, 292,
    317
coenzyme Q (ubiquinone) 176
community nutrition 7, 9
computed tomography (CT) *15*,
    21–2, *27*
copper 200–5
  and fatty acids 106
  micronutrient interactions
    iron 197
    molybdenum 205, 215
    phosphorus 189
    selenium 208
    vitamin C 171
    zinc 200, 204–5
Coxsackie virus 206–7, 303
creatinine excretion *15*, 26, *27*
cretinism 211, 212, 322, 327
Creutzfeldt–Jakob disease 307, 308
Cryptosporidium parvum 295, *307*
CT scanning *15*, 21–2, *27*
cultural beliefs 7
Cyclospora cayetanensis 295, *307*

data analysis 278–80, 291
densitometry *15*, 16–17, 18, *27*, 28
dental caries 79–80, 216, 217
deprivation studies 122, 173
deuterium-labeled water 38, 244
deuterium oxide dilution *15*, 18, 28
developing countries
  food-borne illness 294, 295, 320,
    322
  malnutrition 5–6, 319–25, 332–3
  micronutrients 325–8
  NCDs 329
  obesity 329–30
  protein sources 65–6
  public health promotion 330, 331
diabetes 73–4, 176, 218
diameters, measuring *15*, 24
diet–gene interactions *see* gene–diet
    interactions
diet histories 230, 234, **236**, 239,
    241–2

dietary fats, use of term 87
  see also lipids, dietary
dietary fiber 76–7, 78
dietary reference intake (DRI) 116,
    117, **118**, 121
dietary reference standards 116–24
dietary reference value (DRV) 117,
    118
digestibility, proteins 63–4, 65
dilution techniques, body
    composition *15*, 18, *27*, 28
doubly labeled water (DLW) 37–9,
    42, 243–4
Down's syndrome 203–4
dual-energy X-ray absorptiometry
    (DXA; DEXA) *15*, **18**, 19, **20**, *27*,
    28

ecological studies 290
eicosanoids 82, 103–6
elderly people
    dietary recommendations 119–20
    energy balance 40–1
    folate 165
    food-borne illness 294, 301
    malnutrition 324–5, 332
    protein requirements 60, 66
    vitamin B_{12} 157, 158, 165
    vitamin D 137
electrical conductivity 25–6, *27*
electrolytes *15*, 25
endocrine control *see* hormones
energy metabolism
    BMR 26, 31, 35, 244–5
    carbohydrate fermentation 78,
        79
    energy balance 30–2
        future studies 45
        obesity 42–5
        special groups 40–2, 45
    energy expenditure 31–2, 34
        food intake validation 243–4
        measurement 34–6, 37–9, 243–4
        obesity 38, 43–5
        physical activity 31, 36, 37, *38*,
            39, 41, 43–4
        protein turnover 56
        RMR 31, 36–7, 39–40, 41, 42
        special groups 40–2, 45
        thermic effect of feeding 31, 35,
            37
    energy intake 31, 32–4
        measuring 38

nutrient recommendations 117,
    119
    obesity 43–4
    protein turnover 56
    underreporting 243–6
    see also food intake
energy requirements 39–40
    physical activity 39, 40, 41
    of special groups 40–2, 122–3
energy storage 31, 42–3
and health status 40–1, 42
n-6:n-3 PUFA ratio 111
obesity 38, 40, 42–5
oxidation of fatty acids 101
RMR 31, 36–7, 39–40, 41, 42
tissue fatty acid profiles 106
vitamins in
    niacin 151
    pantothenic acid 167
    ubiquinone 176
    vitamin B_1 144–5, 146
    vitamin B_2 146, 147–8, 149
energy–protein malnutrition 320
environmental contaminants 311–12
epidemiology 283, 285–91
epilepsy 165–6
Escherichia coli 294, 295, 296, *298*
Eurocode 2 food coding 252–3
exercise *see* physical activity
experimental design
    animal models 281–3
    epidemiological studies 285–8
    human studies 283–91
    in vitro studies 280–1
    and statistical analysis 275–80
extracellular fluids 14, 18, 25
extracellular solids 14

factorial dietary determination 122–3
Fanconi syndrome 188
fat-free mass (FFM) 12–13
    determination 16, **17**, 18, 19, 25,
        26, 28
    RMR 36
fat mass 13
    and BMI 22, 27
    determination method choice
        27–8, 43
    doubly indirect determination 22,
        23–4, 25–6, 28
    indirect determination 16–17, 18,
        19, 20–1, 28
    obesity 43

and RMR 36, 39
fats, dietary, use of term 87
    see also lipids, dietary
fats (nonsimple lipids) *see* lipids
fats (simple lipids) 85
    body composition 13, *14*, **15**
    classification *82*
    contamination 311
    daily intake 87
    dietary sources 86, 87, 112
    digestion 88
    n-6:n-3 PUFA ratio 111–12
    triacylglycerols *see* triacylglycerols
fatty acids 5, 82–5
    absorption 88
    and biotin 167
    body lipid pools 98–100, 101
    carbon recycling 102
    and carnitine 175
    chain elongation 103
    chain shortening 103
    classification *82*
    colonic fermentation 78–9
    desaturation 103
    diet–gene interactions 114
    dietary sources 87, 112
    digestion 88–9, 91
    effects on serum lipids 109–12
    eicosanoids 82, 103–6
    essential 107–8
    future studies 114–15
    health effects 107–9, 110, 111–12
    history of 81–2
    hydrogenation 85, 87, 103, 107,
        110
    ketogenesis 101–2
    and lipoproteins 92, 94, 98,
        109–12, 114
    metabolic effects 107–9, 112
    metabolism of long-chain
        100–7
    n-6:n-3 PUFA ratio 109, 111–12
    nutritional effects 107–9
    nutritional regulation 106–7
    oxidation 101
    peroxidation 102–3, 139, 140–1,
        171–2
    plasma 99
    postprandial lipemia 92, 98, 112
    and serum cholesterol 109–10, 111
    and vitamin E 139, 140–1
feeding, thermic effect 31, 35, 37
fiber, dietary 76–7, 78

fish, causing illness 301, 303–4, 313, *314*
fish oils 112, 311
flavonoids 175
fluoride 79–80, 215–17
folic acid 159, 160–6, 172
food additives 315–16
Food and Agriculture Organization (FAO) 6
  food balance sheets 227, 228, 247, 265
  food composition tables 249
  food policy 264, 265, 269, 271–2, 273
  food safety 292, 308, 309–10
  INFOODS 247, 251, 256, *261*
  model food law 267–8
food assistance programs 272
food balance sheets 227, 228, 247, 265
food choices 265, 270–2
food classification 247, 251–3
food composition tables 249–50
  access to 260
  analytical methods 254–5
  bioavailability 258–9
  composite dishes 258, 259, *260*
  data presentation 256
  data quality 237, 256–7
  data source information 257
  food classification 247, 251–3
  food description 251
  and food intake 237–8, 261
  food preparation effects 257–8
  food variability 253
  food–nutrient conversion 260–1
  glycemic index 259
  inclusion criteria 251, 255
  international systems 251, 252–3, 255, 256, 261
  missing values 258
  portion sizes 260
  sampling for 253, *254*
  uses 249, *250*
food disappearance data *226*, 228
food fortification 223, 270, 326, 328
food frequency questionnaires 230, 234–5, **236**, 239, 241–2, 248
food insecurity *see* food security
food intake
  factors influencing 33–4
  food composition data 237–8, 261

measurement 225–7
  adequacy assessment 246–8
  day-to-day variations 239–40
  direct *226*, 229–35, 248
  errors in 231, 235–9
  and food policy 265
  food safety assessments 248
  future studies 248
  indirect *226*, 227–9
  method selection 240–3, 248
  terminology **227**, **230**
  underreporting 240, 244–6, 265
  validation tools 243–5, 248
nutritional status assessment 225, 321, 323–4
reference standards 116–24
regulation 32–3
food labeling 268–9
food poisoning 293, 294, 296, *297–8*, 300, 312–15
food policy 263–4
  data for 264–5, 272–3
  fortification 270, 326, 328
  future 273–4
  global 273, 318–19
    future 331–3
    malnutrition 5–6, 8–9, 319–25, 332–3
    micronutrients 325–8
    NCDs 318–19, 328–30
    obesity 329–30
    public health promotion 330–1
  guiding food choice 270–2
  and production 265–6, 268, 274, 332–3
  research 272–3
  safety regulation 266–70, 316–17
  trade 269–70
food portions 238, 260
food production
  and policy 265–6, 268, 274, 332–3
  and safety 312, 315, 316–17
food quality 266–70, 316–17
food safety 10, 292–3
  assessment 247
  chemicals 295, 308–16
  food-borne illness 292–3
    bacterial 294, 295–301
    childhood malnutrition 320, 322
    chronic effects 293–4, 320
    economic consequences 295
    health consequences 294–5

natural toxins 293, 294, 296, *297–8*, 300, 312–15
parasitic 294–5, 303–7, 322, 326
pathogen numbers 295–6
plant toxins 313, 315
toxic contaminants 309, 310–12
viral 206–7, 301–3
vulnerable groups 294–5
future 317
regulation 266–70, 316–17
risk analysis 267, 316–17
food security/insecurity 5–6, 264–5, 272, 332–3
  see also global nutrition
food supply data *226*, 227–8
food technologies 274
food trade 269–70, 293
fructose
  absorption 70, 72, 75
  dental caries 79
  metabolic utilization 72, 74
  transportation 70, **71**
  in vegetable dishes *71*
functional foods 9–10, 77, 223, 270
fungal toxins 312, *313*

galactose 70, *71*, 72, 75, 79
gene–diet interactions 319
  lipids 113–14
  minerals 223–4
  research techniques 280–1
  vitamin A 130, 133
Gitelman's syndrome 185
global food trade 269–70, 293
global nutrition 318–19
  assistance programs 272
  food policy 264–5, 272
  future 331–3
  malnutrition 5–6, 8–9, 319–25, 332–3
  micronutrients 325–8
  NCDs 318–19, 328–30
  obesity 329–30
  public health promotion 330–1
gluconeogenesis 73
glucose 70
  absorption 70, 72, 75
  diabetes 73–4
  dietary management 73–4
  metabolic utilization 72, 73
  and micronutrients 167, 218
  regulation 73

transportation 70, **71**
in vegetable dishes *71*
glycemic index (GI) 73–4, 259
glycogen 42, 43, 73
goitres 211, 327

hemochromatosis 196, 218
hazard analysis critical control point
(HACCP) system 316–17
health, nutrition and 3–4
food policy 263
data for 264–5, 272–3
fortification 270, 326
future 273–4
guiding food choice 270–2
labeling 268–9
production 265–6, 268, 274
regulations 266–70, 316–17
research 272–3
malnutrition 5–6, 8–9, 319–25,
332–3
micronutrient deficiency 325–8
NCDs 318–19, 328–30
obesity 329–30
public health promotion 330–1
see also food safety
heart disease *see* cardiovascular
disease
heavy metals 208, 309, 311–12
height *see* weight/height indices
hepatitis A virus 301, 302
hormones
calcium regulation 179, 180–1
food intake 33
lipoprotein metabolism 97–8,
113
selenium 208
thyroid 208, 210–11, 212, 326–7
tissue fatty acids 106
veterinary drugs 311
vitamin B$_6$ 154, 155, 157
household food surveys *226*, 228–9
hunger 32, 33
hydrogen 13
hypomagnesemia 185
hypophosphatemia 188
hypothesis testing 277
hypothyroidism 211, 212

illness, food-borne *see* food safety,
food-borne illness
imaging techniques *15*, 21–2, *27*
immune function 132, 207

immunocompromised individuals
294, 295, 301, 332
impedance *15*, 25–6, *27*, 28
in vitro studies 280–1
in vivo neutron activation analysis
(IVNAA) 15, 16, *27*
industrial contaminants 311–12
infants *see* children
infections
carbohydrate absorption 71
food-borne 293–308, 320, 322
protein metabolism 66–7
infrared interactance *15*, 25, *27*
inositol 175–6
insulin 73, 97–8, 106, 113, 218
International Food Data System
Project (INFOODS) 247, 251,
256, *261*
intestinal flukes *305–6*
intoxications 293, 294, 296, *297–8*,
300, 312–15
intracellular water (ICW) 18, 25
iodine 208–12, 223, 322, 326–7
iron 194–7
deficiency 195–6, 197, 325–6
dietary recommendations 123,
196–7
fatty acids 107
food fortification 223, 326
micronutrient interactions
calcium 183
chromium 218
manganese 214
phosphorus 189
selenium 208
vitamin B$_2$ 149
vitamin C 171, 172, 174
zinc 197

Kashin–Beck disease 206, 212
Keshan disease 206, 207, 208
ketogenesis 101–2
kwashiorkor 320

lactation
amino acids 61
energy requirement 41, 122–3
proteins 59, *60*
vitamin A 328
vitamin B$_6$ 155
lactose 70–1, 75, 79
LanguaL 251, *252*, *261*
legislation 266, 267–8, 316, 317

lipemia 92–3, 98, 112
lipids *5*, 13, *14*, **15**, 81
absorption 89–91, 111
atherosclerosis 93, 98, 139, 140
biotin 167
and body fat 99, 101
classification 82
contamination 311
diet–gene interactions 113–14
dietary effects on serum
109–14
digestion 87–91
energy content 31
energy metabolism 32
expenditure 35, 36, 37
fatty acid oxidation 101
n-6:n-3 PUFA ratio 111
obesity 42, 43
tissue fatty acid profiles 106
enterohepatic circulation 90–1
future studies 114–15
heart disease *see* cardiovascular
disease
history 81–2
and hormones 97–8, 106
hydrogenation 85, 87, 103, 107,
110
lipid pools 98–100
lipoproteins 87, 91–8
long-chain fatty acid metabolism
100–7
membrane 98–9, 106, 109
metabolic effects 107–9
nutritional effects 107–9
nutritional regulation 106–7
peroxidation 102–3, 139, 140–1,
171–2
solubilization 88–9
sources 86–7, 112
storage 98, 99
terminology 82–6, 87
transportation 91–5
vitamin B$_2$ 148
vitamin E 139, 140–1
see also fat mass
lipoproteins 87, 91–8, 109–14, 139,
140
Listeria monocytogenes 294, 295–6,
298, 301
liver flukes *305*
lung fluke *306*

magnesium 183–6

magnetic resonance imaging *15*,
  21–2, *27*
malaria 148, 326
malnutrition **4**, 5–6, 8–9, 319–25
  assessment 225, 321, 323–4
  economic consequences 332
  food-borne illness 294, 320, 322
  vitamin A deficiency 132
maltose 70, *71*, 75, 79
manganese 205, 212–14
marasmus 320
meal-induced thermogenesis 31, 35,
  37
megaloblastic anemia 164, 165, 172
Menkes' syndrome 203
mental development 322–3
mental illness 109
menu records *226*, 230, 232
methionine load test 156
3-methylhistidine excretion 26
microbial toxins 293, 294, 296,
  297–8, 300, 312–14
micronutrients *see* minerals and
  trace elements; vitamins
milk lipids 99
minerals and trace elements 5,
  177–219
  body composition 14, 16, 18–19,
    20–1, *27*
  and fatty acids 106, 107
  future studies 219, 223–4
  global deficiency 325–7
  ultratrace elements 205, 219,
    220–3
  see also specific minerals
molecular biology techniques
  280–1
molecular nutrition 9
  see also gene–diet interactions
molybdenum 205, 214–15
motor neurone disease 203
MRI *15*, 21–2, *27*
muscle 14, 26, 43
mycotoxins 312, *313*

nematodes 304
nerve conduction, sodium 190
nerve function
  carnitine 175
  folate supplements 165
  inositol 176
  pantothenic acid 168–9
  vitamin B_1 145, 146

vitamin B_6 157
vitamin B_{12} 157, 159, 164, 165
neurology, and food intake 33
niacin (vitamin B_3) 126–7, 149–53
nitrogen
  body composition 13
  protein metabolism 46, 48–9
    amino acid classification 51,
      52–4
    amino acid structure 49–50
    biology of requirements 54–60,
      61, 63
    food intake validation 243
    and infection 66–7
    nitrogen balance 59–60, 61, 63
    protein digestibility 63–4
    sources of nonspecific 52–3
    urea cycle 57–8
nitrosamines 174
noncommunicable diseases (NCDs)
  318–19, 328–30
  see also cardiovascular disease
nonstarch polysaccharide (NSP)
  76–7, 78
Norwalk-like viruses 301, 302–3
nutraceuticals 176
nutrients 4–5
  dietary reference standards 116–24
  food composition tables 249–51
    analytical methods 254–5
    bioavailability 258–9
    composite dishes 258, 259, *260*
    data presentation 256
    data quality 256–7
    data source information 257
    food description in 251
    food preparation effects 257–8
    food variability 253
    food–nutrient conversion 260–1
    inclusion criteria 251, 255
    missing values 258
  food policy 270–2, 273
  intake adequacy assessment
    246–8
  see also carbohydrate(s); lipids;
    minerals; protein(s); vitamins
nutrition, and health *see* food safety;
  health, nutrition and
nutrition research, food policy 272–3
nutrition research methodology 275
  animal models 281–3
  epidemiology 283, 285–91
  future 291

human studies 283–91
in vitro studies 280–1
statistical analysis 275–80
nutrition science 1–11
nutritional status, assessment 225,
  321, 323–4

obesity 329–30
  definition 43
  determination 22, 27, 28, 43
  energy metabolism 38, 42–5
  etiology 43–4
observational studies 288–90
oil, iodized 327
oils (simple lipids) 85, 86, 87, 112,
  311
oral contraceptives 156–7
osteomalacia 134, 137, 138, 188
osteoporosis 137, 180, 181, 190, 216
overnutrition **4**, 6, 8, 321
oxygen 13, 34–6, 72

pantothenic acid 167–9
parasites 294–5, 303–7, 322, 326
pellagra 149–50, 152
Pendred's syndrome 211–12
pernicious anemia 159
pesticides 310–11
phospholipids *82*, 85–6, 87, 88, 175–6
phosphorus 13, 183, 184, 186–9
physical activity 31, 37, *38*
  energy requirements 39, 40, 41
  obesity 40, 43–5
  RMR 36, 39, 41
  undernutrition 324
phytoceuticals 176
picornaviruses 302, 303
plant toxins 313, 315
population growth 332–3
population reference intake (PRI)
  117, **118**, 122
portion sizes 238, 260
postprandial lipemia 92–3, 98, 112
potassium 18–19, *27*, 192–4
power calculations 277–8
pregnant women
  amino acids 61
  body fat 99–100
  dietary recommendations 122–3
  energy requirements 41
  folic acid 160, 164, 165
  food-borne illness 294–5, 301
  iodine deficiency 326–7

iron 197, 325
  malnutrition 319–20
  proteins 59, *60*
  vitamin A 133, 327–8
  vitamin B$_6$ 157
  zinc 199, 200
prostaglandins 82, 104–5
protein–energy malnutrition 320
protein(s) *5*
  body composition 14, 16, 20–1,
    54–6
  copper-containing *202*, 203, 204
  dietary sources 64–6
  energy content 31
  energy metabolism 32
    expenditure 35, 36, 37, 56
    obesity 42, 43
  functions *47*
  metabolism 46–8
    biology of requirements 54–67
    body protein mass 54
    chemistry of amino acids
      49–50
    classification of amino acids
      50–4
    digestibility 63–4, 65
    and disease 57, 66–7
    estimating requirements 59–63
    factors affecting 66–7
    food intake validation 243
    future studies 67
    and health status 66–7
    history 48–9
    meeting requirements 63–6
    niacin in 151–2
    structure of amino acids 49–50,
      51
    turnover 54–7
    vitamin B$_6$ 154, 155
  nutritional quality 63, 64–5
  selenoproteins 206
protozoa 294, 295, 307
public health nutrition 7, 9, 318–33
pyridoxine *see* vitamin B$_6$

Quetelet index 22

recall studies *226*, 230, 233–4, **236**,
  238–9
recommended dietary allowances
  (RDAs) 116–17, **118**
records, food intake 230, 232–3, **236**,
  239–40, 241–2, 248

regulations, food safety 266–70,
  316–17
research methodology *see* nutrition
  research methodology
respiratory gas analysis 34–5
resting metabolic rate (RMR) 31,
  36–7, 39–40, 41, 42
retinol *see* vitamin A
riboflavin (vitamin B$_2$) 123, *126*,
  146–9
rickets 134, 137, 138, 181, 188
risk analysis 267, 316–17
rotaviruses 303
roundworms 304

safety *see* food safety
Salmonella spp 295, 296, *299*, 300–1
salt 189, 190, 191–2, 327
satiety 32, 33
scurvy 169, 172
seafood toxins 312, 313, *314*
selenium 140–1, 205–8, 212, 326
sex hormones 98, 154, 157
shellfish 301, 313, *314*
Siri's formula 17
skeletal diameters 24
skinfold thickness *15*, 23–4, 27, 28
sodium 189–92, 193
spongiform encephalopathies 295,
  307–8
Staphylococcus aureus 296, *297*
starch *71*, 74, 75, 76, 77, 79
statistical analysis 275–80
sterols *82*, 85, 86, 111
  cholesterol *see* cholesterol
sucrose 70, 71–2, 75, 79

tapeworms 304
taurine 176
teeth 79–80, 216, 217
thermic effects 31, 35, 37
thermogenesis 31, 32, 35, 37
thiamin (vitamin B$_1$) *126*, 143–6
thyroid hormones 208, 210–11, 212,
  326–7
tissue nutrient levels 123
tocopherols *see* vitamin E
total body electrical conductivity
  (TOBEC) 26, *27*
toxic contaminants 309, 310–12
toxins 309
  food poisoning 293, 294, 296,
    297–8, 300, 312–15

Toxoplasma gondii 294, 295, *307*
trace elements *see* minerals and trace
  elements
tracer studies 61–2, 122
trauma 42, 57, 67
trematodes 303–4, *305–6*
triacylglycerols (triglycerides; TAG)
  82, 85
  absorption 89
  body composition 13, **15**
  daily intake 87
  dietary sources 86, 87
  digestion 88
  heart disease 93, 97, 98, 112,
    113
  and lipoproteins
    assembly 91
    diet–gene interactions 114
    dietary effects 112, 113, 114
    endocrine control 98, 113
    interrelationships 97
    postprandial lipemia 92–3
    TAG hypothesis 93, 98
    transport pathways 94, 95
  n-6:n-3 PUFA ratio 112
  re-esterification 91
  serum 97, 111–12, 113, 114
  storage lipid pool 99
triglycerides *see* triacylglycerols
tryptophan load test 155–6

ubiquinone 176
ultrasound 25
ultratrace elements 205, 219,
  220–3
undernutrition *4*, 5–6, 8, 319–25
United Nations (UN) organizations
  5–6
  amino acids 62, 63
  food coding 247, 251
  food policy 273
  food security 264
  proteins 60, 64–5
  see also Food and Agriculture
    Organization (FAO); World
    Health Organization (WHO)
urea cycle 57–8
urinary nitrogen 243

veterinary drugs 311
Vibrio spp 295, *299*, 301
viruses 206–7, 301–3
vision 108, 130, 132, 327–8

vitamins 5, 125–7
  ascorbic acid *see* vitamin C
  biotin *126*, 166–7
  folic acid 159, 160–6, 172
  future studies 174–6
  niacin 126–7, 149–53
  pantothenic acid 167–9
  riboflavin *see* vitamin B_2
  thiamin *see* vitamin B_1
vitamin A 123, *126*, 127–33, 327–8
vitamin B_1 *126*, 143–6
vitamin B_2 123, *126*, 146–9
vitamin B_5 *see* pantothenic acid
vitamin B_6 *126*, 149, 153–7
vitamin B_{12} *126*, 157–60, 164, 165
vitamin C 121, 122, 123, 140, 169–74, 208
vitamin D 126–7, 133, 134–8, 181, 183, 184
vitamin E 121, *126*, 138–41, 205, 208
vitamin H *see* biotin

vitamin K 123, *126*, 141–3
"vitamin Q" 176

water
  body *see* body water
  doubly labeled (DLW) 37–9, 42, 243–4
  fluoride in 79–80, 216
weighed records *226*, 230, 232–3, **236**, 242
weight/height indices *15*, 22–3, 27, 29, 43, 321, 323–4
Wernicke–Korsakoff syndrome 145, 146
Wilson's disease 203, 215
women
  lactating *see* lactation
  pregnancy *see* pregnant women
World Food Summit 6, 264
World Health Organization (WHO) 6
  adolescent undernutrition 323

BMI 22, 321, 323, 324
  childhood malnutrition 321
  food policy 269, 271–2, 273
  food safety 292–3, 308, 309–10
  iron deficiency 326
  model food law 267–8
  nutrient recommendations 117–18
World Trade Organization (WTO) 269–70, 273, 292
worm infections 303–4

X-linked hypophosphatemia 188
X-rays 19, 21
xerophthalmia 132, 327, 328

Yersinia enterocolitica 299, 301

zinc 197–200
  and fatty acids 107
  micronutrient interactions 183, 189, 200, 204–5, 208

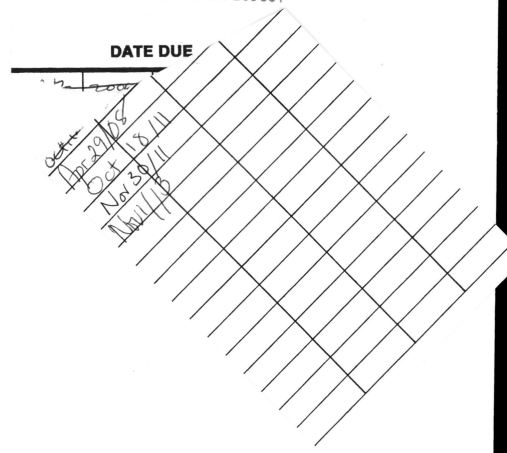